STROKE REHABILITATION

STROKE REHABILITATION

Insights from Neuroscience and Imaging

EDITED BY Leeanne M. Carey, PhD

HEAD, NEUROREHABILITATION AND RECOVERY
AND AUSTRALIAN RESEARCH COUNCIL FUTURE FELLOW
NATIONAL STROKE RESEARCH INSTITUTE
FLOREY NEUROSCIENCE INSTITUTES
MELBOURNE BRAIN CENTRE
AND
PROFESSOR
DEPARTMENT OF OCCUPATIONAL THERAPY
SCHOOL OF ALLIED HEALTH
FACULTY OF HEALTH SCIENCES
LA TROBE UNIVERSITY
MELBOURNE, AUSTRALIA

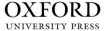

OXFORD
UNIVERSITY PRESS

OXFORD
UNIVERSITY PRESS

Oxford University Press, Inc., publishes works that further
Oxford University's objective of excellence
in research, scholarship, and education.

Oxford   New York
Auckland   Cape Town   Dar es Salaam   Hong Kong   Karachi
Kuala Lumpur   Madrid   Melbourne   Mexico City   Nairobi
New Delhi   Shanghai   Taipei   Toronto

With offices in
Argentina   Austria   Brazil   Chile   Czech Republic   France   Greece
Guatemala   Hungary   Italy   Japan   Poland   Portugal   Singapore
South Korea   Switzerland   Thailand   Turkey   Ukraine   Vietnam

Copyright © 2012 by Oxford University Press, Inc.

Published by Oxford University Press, Inc.
198 Madison Avenue, New York, New York 10016
www.oup.com

Oxford is a registered trademark of Oxford University Press

Library of Congress Cataloging-in-Publication Data
Carey, Leeanne M.
Stroke rehabilitation : insights from neuroscience and imaging / Leeanne M. Carey.
p. ; cm.
Includes bibliographical references and index.
ISBN 978-0-19-979788-2 (hardcover : alk. paper)
I. Title.
[DNLM: 1. Stroke—rehabilitation.   2. Brain—physiopathology.
3.   Neuroimaging. WL 356]
616.8′106—dc23
2011048829

1 3 5 7 9 8 6 4 2
Printed in China
on acid-free paper

I would like to dedicate this book to the many individuals who have inspired and challenged me during their journey of recovery after stroke. These individuals have the goal to 'be the best they can be'. It is a goal we collectively aspire to. This book offers hope, discovery, and translation. It is hoped that the partnership between the stroke survivor and informed therapist will ensure that this journey does not end, but rather keeps open the 'window of opportunity'.

I would like to thank all the contributors to this book. These authors come from backgrounds of basic science, neuroimaging, neuroscience, psychology, neurophysiology, clinical sciences, neurology, occupational therapy, physiotherapy, and nursing. All are dedicated to researching and translating evidence from these fields to address the challenges of stroke rehabilitation. Thank you for sharing your knowledge and insights.

I would also like to thank all the other individuals who have contributed to the book. To colleagues and friends who have assisted with proofing and editing, to Oxford University Press and their team for their ongoing support, and most importantly to the individuals who have volunteered to be research participants in the numerous studies referred to in this book.

Finally I would like to acknowledge and thank my colleagues, friends and family who have 'lived through' and supported this journey. Thank you to the many colleagues and friends across the globe who have shared their knowledge, mentored, challenged, and inspired along the way. To my parents who opened the door with their belief, to my husband who provides support, and to my children who have got their futures ahead.

PREFACE

The aim of *Stroke Rehabilitation: Insights from Neuroscience and Imaging* is to inform and challenge rehabilitation clinicians to adopt more restorative and scientific approaches to stroke rehabilitation based on current evidence from the neuroscience and neuroimaging literatures. The fields of cognitive neuroscience and neuroimaging are advancing rapidly and providing new insights into human behavior and learning. Similarly, improved knowledge of how the brain processes information after injury and recovers over time is providing new perspectives on what we aim to achieve through rehabilitation.

Historically, rehabilitation has focused on compensatory strategies rather than addressing the underlying mechanisms and brain changes associated with impairment and recovery. To improve function and adopt a more restorative approach to rehabilitation, clinicians are challenged to consider how we can "change the brain to change the behavior." It is envisaged that in the not too distant future, clinicians will have the opportunity to design treatment for an individual stroke patient based on knowledge of the individual's viable brain networks that may be accessed in therapy. This knowledge, together with a clinical appreciation of physical and cognitive capacities, mood, and patient goals, will help to bridge the current gap in achieving optimal outcomes.

Clinicians are encouraged to read the neuroscience and imaging literature so that we can better select intervention approaches that are founded on neuroscience and have relevance for therapy. Equally, we may need to make an informed decision not to continue a given intervention, even if it has been historically part of routine clinical practice. Many clinicians are excited by the potential to "change the brain" in therapy but as yet do not have the knowledge and skills to do so. The challenging, yet critical, task we must achieve is the translation of neuroscience to clinical practice. It is the intention of this book to stimulate clinicians to reflect on how we can apply this science within the context of stroke rehabilitation.

Recent discoveries in neuroscience suggest it is timely for neuroscientists and clinicians to work together to develop a framework and language to facilitate this translation. In this book our aim is to provide a framework that is meaningful and accessible to clinicians. It includes a model of rehabilitation, core concepts related to neural plasticity and imaging, and neuroscience evidence for creating the right learning environment for rehabilitation. This is followed by a series of chapters that review current neuroscience and imaging evidence in relation to common functions, and provide examples of how this evidence can be translated and operationalized within the context of rehabilitation. Finally, the book concludes with key chapters on new perspectives and directions for stroke rehabilitation research.

This book is intended for clinicians, rehabilitation specialists, and neurologists who are interested in using these new discoveries in neuroscience and imaging to achieve more optimal outcomes. Equally important, it is intended for neuroscientists, clinical researchers, and imaging specialists to help frame important clinical questions and to better understand the context in which their discoveries may be used.

Leeanne Carey.

CONTENTS

Contributors   xv

PART A
CORE CONCEPTS   1

1. INTRODUCTION   3
Leeanne M. Carey

1.1 Stroke Rehabilitation: An Ongoing Window of Opportunity   3

1.2 The Scope of the Problem: Prevalence and Impact of Stroke and Increasing Need for Stroke Rehabilitation   4

1.3 Recovery and Rehabilitation: Definitions   5

1.4 Neural Plasticity and Learning as a Basis for Stroke Rehabilitation   5

1.5 Neuroimaging and How it May Inform Stroke Rehabilitation   7

1.6 Paradigm Shift in Stroke Rehabilitation   8

2. STROKE REHABILITATION: A LEARNING PERSPECTIVE   11
*Leeanne M. Carey, Helene J. Polatajko,
Lisa Tabor Connor, and Carolyn M. Baum*

2.1 Stroke Rehabilitation: Facilitation of Adaptive Learning   11

2.2 A Common Language for Rehabilitation Science   12

2.3 Experience and Learning-Dependent Plasticity: Implications for Rehabilitation   13

2.4 Role of Brain Networks in Information Processing and Recovery   14

2.5 Skill Acquisition—A Learning Perspective   14

    2.5.1 Explicit, Task-Specific, and Goal-Driven   15

    2.5.2 Involve Active Problem Solving and Be Responsive to Environmental Demands   16

    2.5.3 Provide Opportunities for Variation and Practice   16

2.6 Application in Context of Recovery after Stroke   17

2.7 Rehabilitation Learning Model: Rehab-Learn   17

2.8 Selected Learning-Based Approaches to Rehabilitation   18

    2.8.1 Cognitive Orientation to Daily Occupational Performance (CO-OP)   19

    2.8.2 SENSe: A Perceptual Learning Approach to Rehabilitation of Body Sensations after Stroke   19

    2.8.3 Language: Constraint-Induced Aphasia Therapy   20

2.9 Measuring Response to Learning-Based Rehabilitation   20

2.10 Summary and Conclusion   21

3. NEURAL PLASTICITY AS A BASIS FOR STROKE REHABILITATION   24
*Michael Nilsson, Milos Pekny, and
Marcela Pekna*

3.1 Neural Plasticity after Brain and Spinal Cord Injury   24

    3.1.1 Experience-Dependent Plasticity of the Cerebral Cortex   24

    3.1.2 Spontaneous Recovery of Function after Stroke   24

    3.1.3 Cortical Map Rearrangements   24

    3.1.4 Contralateral Hemisphere Involvement   25

    3.1.5 Contralesional Axonal Remodeling of the Corticospinal System   25

3.2 Implications for Stroke Rehabilitation   26

3.3 Increasing Neural Plasticity through Behavioral Manipulations and Adjuvant Therapies   26

    3.3.1 Enriched Environment and Multimodal Stimulation   26

    3.3.2 Noninvasive Brain Stimulation   27

    3.3.3 Pharmacological Modulators of Neural Plasticity   28

      3.3.3.1 D-amphetamine   28

      3.3.3.2 Sigma-1 Receptor Agonists   28

      3.3.3.3 Fluoxetine   28

      3.3.3.4 Niacin   29

      3.3.3.5 Inosine   29

      3.3.3.6 Nugo-A Inhibition   29

      3.3.3.7 Reducing Tonic Inhibition   30

    3.3.4 Emerging Targets   30

      3.3.4.1 Stem Cells   30

      3.3.4.2 Targeting the Astrocytes   30

3.4 Individualized Therapy   31

4. IMAGING TECHNIQUES PROVIDE NEW INSIGHTS   35

J-Donald Tournier, Richard A. J. Masterton, and Rüdiger J. Seitz

4.1 Introduction to Neuroimaging Techniques and Their Potential to Provide New Insights   35

4.2 What Neuroimaging Can Tell Us   35

     4.2.1 Measuring Brain Perfusion   35

     4.2.2 Measuring Water Diffusion (Diffusion-Weighted Imaging)   37

     4.2.3 Measuring Regional Cerebral Metabolism   38

     4.2.4 Assessing Structural Brain Lesions   38

4.3 Measuring Brain Function with MRI   39

     4.3.1 The BOLD Image Contrast   39

     4.3.2 The BOLD Response to Neuronal Activity   40

         4.3.2.1 The Time Course of Evoked BOLD Signal Changes   40

         4.3.2.2 Neurovascular Coupling   41

     4.3.3 fMRI Experimental Design and Analysis   41

         4.3.3.1 Task-Related Activation Studies   41

         4.3.3.2 "Resting-state" Studies of Brain Function   42

     4.3.4 Applications of fMRI in Stroke Rehabilitation   43

4.4 Structural Connectivity, Including Tractography   44

     4.4.1 Modeling Diffusion in White Matter   44

         4.4.1.1 Diffusion Tensor Imaging   45

         4.4.1.2 Higher-Order Models   46

     4.4.2 Estimating Biologically Relevant Parameters   46

         4.4.2.1 Estimating Fiber Orientations   47

         4.4.2.1 Tractography   47

     4.4.3 Application to Stroke Recovery   49

5. MULTIMODAL NEUROPHYSIOLOGICAL INVESTIGATIONS   54

Cathrin M. Buetefisch and Aina Puce

5.1 Introduction   54

5.2 Magnetoencephalography (MEG) and Electroencephalography (EEG)   55

     5.2.1 Methodological Considerations   55

         5.2.1.1 Site of Recording in EEG and MEG   55

         5.2.1.2 Source Modeling of EEG and MEG Data   55

         5.2.1.3 Considerations when Studying Reorganization of the Motor System with Multimodal MEG/EEG   56

         5.2.1.4 Neurophysiological Rhythms and Potential Insights into Stroke Recovery   57

     5.2.2 Multimodal MEG/EEG Studies of Activity in Primary Sensorimotor Cortex in Stroke Recovery   58

5.3 Transcranial Magnetic Stimulation (TMS)   60

     5.3.1 Methodological Considerations   60

     5.3.2 TMS Measures of Motor Cortex   60

         5.3.2.1 Motor Threshold   60

         5.3.2.2 MEP Amplitude   60

         5.3.2.3 MEP Latency and Central Motor Conduction Time   61

         5.3.2.4 Cortical Silent Period   62

         5.3.2.5 Input–Output Curves   62

         5.3.2.6 Short Interval Cortical Inhibition (SICI)   62

         5.3.2.7 Intracortical Facilitation (ICF)   62

         5.3.2.8 Interhemispheric Inhibition (IHI)   62

     5.3.3 Repetitive Transcranial Magnetic Stimulation (rTMS)   62

     5.3.4 Multimodal TMS/Brain Imaging Studies of Stroke Recovery   64

5.4 The Future? Neurorehabilitative Studies of Stroke Recovery and the Brain–Computer Interface   66

PART B

STROKE PATHOPHYSIOLOGY AND RECOVERY   73

6. STROKE: PATHOPHYSIOLOGY, RECOVERY POTENTIAL, AND TIMELINES FOR RECOVERY AND REHABILITATION   75

Rüdiger J. Seitz and Geoffrey A. Donnan

6.1 Introduction   75

6.2 Pathophysiology   75

     6.2.1 From Cerebral Ischemia Toward Brain Infarction   75

     6.2.2 Reversal of Ischemia   76

     6.2.3 Patterns of Residual Brain Infarcts after Thrombolysis   77

     6.2.4 Functional Consequences of Brain Infarcts   78

6.3 Recovery Potential   79

     6.3.1 The Role of the Penumbra   79

     6.3.2 Perilesional Plasticity   79

     6.3.3 Infarct-Induced Disconnections   81

     6.3.4 Regenerative Therapies using Stem Cell Approaches   82

     6.3.5 Rehabilitative Effect of Physical Training   83

     6.3.6 Rehabilitative Effect of Mental Training   83

6.4 Timelines for Recovery and Rehabilitation   84

6.5 Conclusions   84

PART C

STROKE REHABILITATION: CREATING
THE RIGHT LEARNING CONDITIONS FOR
REHABILITATION   91

7. ORGANIZATION OF CARE   93

*Dominique A. Cadilhac, Tara Purvis, Julie Bernhardt,
and Nicole Korner-Bitensky*

7.1 Introduction   93

7.2 Models of Stroke Rehabilitation Services   94

    7.2.1 Inpatient Care   94

    7.2.2 Community-Based Rehabilitation as an
           Alternative to Inpatient Rehabilitation   95

    7.2.3 Current Perspectives on the Way Forward
           for Providing Stroke Rehabilitation   95

    7.2.4 Characteristics of Stroke Rehabilitation
           Services   96

7.3 Factors Affecting Access to Organized Stroke
     Rehabilitation   97

    7.3.1 Staffing Resources and the Interdisciplinary
           Approach to Rehabilitation   98

7.4 Ensuring the Quality of Care   99

    7.4.1 Monitoring and Improving the Quality
           of Care in Rehabilitation for Stroke   99

    7.4.2 What Clinical Audits Tell Us about Quality
           of Rehabilitation   100

    7.4.3 Establishing Programs to Increase the
           Uptake of Evidence into Clinical
           Practice   101

7.5 Innovations in Rehabilitation and Application
     in Clinical Practice   103

7.6 Summary of Key Messages   103

8. MOTIVATION, MOOD AND THE RIGHT
   ENVIRONMENT   106

*Thomas K. A. Linden, Leeanne M. Carey, and
Michael Nilsson*

8.1 Introduction   106

    8.1.1 Frequency and Nature of Post-Stroke
           Depression   106

    8.1.2 Impact of Post-Stroke Depression   107

    8.1.3 Etiology of Depression after Stroke   107

8.2 Is Post-Stroke Depression a Specific
     Disorder?   108

8.3 Predictors of Post-Stroke Depression   108

8.4 Functional and Structural Brain Changes with
     Depression   109

    8.4.1 Functional Brain Changes   109

    8.4.2 Morphological Brain Changes   110

    8.4.3 Depression, Cognition, and Brain
           Networks   110

8.5 Treatment of Depression in Stroke Patients   110

    8.5.1 Nonpharmacological Treatment
           Options   111

    8.5.2 Enriched Environment   111

    8.5.3 Cortical Stimulation and Depression   111

    8.5.4 Physical Activity   112

9. TRAINING PRINCIPLES TO ENHANCE
   LEARNING-BASED REHABILITATION AND
   NEUROPLASTICITY   116

*Paulette van Vliet, Thomas A. Matyas, and
Leeanne M. Carey*

9.1 Introduction   116

9.2 Task-Specific Activation of Brain Regions   116

9.3 Influence of Task Characteristics on
     Sensorimotor Performance   117

9.4 Task-Specific Nature of Motor Learning   118

9.5 Task Complexity   119

9.6 Behavioral Evidence for Task-Specific Training   119

9.7 Mental Practice of Tasks to Enhance Motor
     Learning   120

9.8 Increasing Repetitions to Enhance Motor
     Learning   121

9.9 Transfer of Training Effects   121

9.10 Implicit and Explicit Learning   123

9.11 Key Clinical Messages   124

10. ADJUNCTIVE THERAPIES   128

Charlotte J. Stagg and Heidi Johansen-Berg

10.1 Introduction and Rationale   128

    10.1.1 Insights from Animal Models   128

       10.1.1.1 The Need for Multiple
                 Sessions of Stimulation   128

       10.1.1.2 Combination with Physical
                 Therapy   129

10.2 Pharmacological Studies   129

    10.2.1 Amphetamines   129

    10.2.2 Dopaminergic Agents   130

    10.2.3 Cholinergic Agents   130

    10.2.4 Serotoninergic Agents   130

10.3 Transcranial Stimulation Techniques   131

    10.3.1 Abnormal Interhemispheric
            Balance   131

    10.3.2 Introduction to the Techniques   132

       10.3.2.1 Transcranial Magnetic
                 Stimulation (TMS)   132

       10.3.2.2 Transcranial Direct Current
                 Stimulation (tDCS)   133

       10.3.2.3 Placebo Controls   133

    10.3.3 rTMS Trials   133

       10.3.3.1 Acute Stroke   133

       10.3.3.2 Chronic Stroke   134

    10.3.4 tDCS trials   134

    10.3.5 The Necessity for Individually
            Targeted Treatments   135

    10.3.6 Safety of Transcranial Stimulation
            Approaches   135

10.4 Novel Therapeutic Approaches 135
    10.4.1 Direct Cortical Stimulation 135
    10.4.2 Robotic Therapy/Neuroprosthetics 136
    10.4.3 Stem Cell Therapy 136
    10.4.4 Growth Factors 137
10.5 Conclusions 137

PART D
REHABILITATION OF COMMON FUNCTIONS 141

11. MOVEMENT 143

Cathy Stinear and Isobel J. Hubbard

11.1 Introduction 143
11.2 Repetitive Task-Specific Training 143
    11.2.1 Description 143
    11.2.2 Behavioral Effects 143
    11.2.3 Neural Mechanisms 143
    11.2.4 Summary 145
11.3 Constraint-Induced Movement Therapy 145
    11.3.1 Description 145
    11.3.2 Behavioral Effects 145
    11.3.3 Neural Mechanisms 145
    11.3.4 Summary 147
11.4 Mental Practice 147
    11.4.1 Description 147
    11.4.2 Behavioral Effects 147
    11.4.3 Neural Mechanisms 148
    11.4.4 Summary 148
11.5 Electrostimulation and EMG Biofeedback 148
    11.5.1 Description 148
    11.5.2 Behavioral Effects 148
    11.5.3 Neural Mechanisms 149
    11.5.4 Summary 150
11.6 Robot-Assisted Training 150
    11.6.1 Description 150
    11.6.2 Behavioral Effects 150
    11.6.3 Neural Mechanisms 151
    11.6.4 Summary 151
11.7 Virtual Reality and Visuomotor Tracking Training 151
    11.7.1 Description 151
    11.7.2 Behavioral Effects 152
    11.7.3 Neural Mechanisms 152
    11.7.4 Summary 153
11.8 Other Approaches 153
11.9 Conclusions 153

12. TOUCH AND BODY SENSATIONS 157

Leeanne M. Carey

12.1 Somatosensory Function 157
12.2 Somatosensory Loss after Stroke 157
12.3 Central Processing of Somatosensory Information 158
    12.3.1 A Model of Somatosensory Processing 159
    12.3.2 Key Features of Central Processing of Somatosensory Information 160
12.4 Neural Correlates of Sensory Recovery after Stroke 161
12.5 Treatment Principles and Strategies Arising from Neuroscience 162
    12.5.1 Goal-Directed Attention and Deliberate Anticipation 163
    12.5.2 Calibration Across Modality and Within Modality 164
    12.5.3 Graded Progression Within Sensory Attributes and Across Sensory Attributes and Tasks 165
12.6 Current Approaches to Sensory Rehabilitation 165
    12.6.1 Passive Stimulation and Bombardment 166
    12.6.2 Attended Stimulation of Specific Body Sites 166
    12.6.3 Graded Sensory Exercises with Feedback 166
    12.6.4 Eclectic Approach Involving Sensorimotor Exercises 166
    12.6.5 Perceptual Learning and Neuroscience-Based Approach: Stimulus-Specific and Transfer-Enhanced Training 167
12.7 Toward a Neuroscience-Based Model of Sensory Rehabilitation 168

13. VISION 173

Amy Brodtmann

13.1 Introduction 173
13.2 Anatomy of Visual Pathways 173
    13.2.1 The Retinogeniculate Pathway 173
    13.2.2 The Geniculostriate Pathway 175
    13.2.3 Extrageniculostriate Pathways 175
13.3 Ipsilateral Representation of the Visual Hemifield 176
13.4 Striate–Extrastriate Connections—The "What" and "Where" Pathways 177
13.5 Ventral Extrastriate Cortex: Visual Object Recognition and Processing 177
13.6 Color and Movement 178
    13.6.1 Dorsal Extrastriate Cortex: Visual Motion perception 178
13.7 Visual Syndromes Caused by Stroke 178
    13.7.1 Visual Field Deficits Following Stroke 179
        13.7.1.1 Monocular Visual Deficits 179
    13.7.2 Homonymous Visual Deficits 179

13.7.2.1 Lateral Geniculate Nucleus Lesions 179

13.7.2.2 Quandrantanopic visual field defects 179

13.7.2.3 Hemianopic Visual Field Defects 179

13.7.3 Disorders of Higher Visual Cognition Commonly Caused by Stroke 180

13.8 Mechanisms of Recovery Following Stroke 180

13.8.1 Neural Plasticity Post-Stroke 180

13.8.2 Mechanisms of Recovery Following Injury to the Visual System 181

13.8.3 Cross-Modal Plasticity in The Visual System 181

13.8.3.1 The Dorsal Extrastriate Pathway—A Possible Site for Surrogacy 181

13.9 Visual Recovery Hypotheses 182

13.9.1 Experiments in Visual Recovery Following Stroke 182

13.9.1.1 PET Studies in the Visual System Following Stroke 182

13.9.1.2 MRI Studies in the Visual System Following Stroke 183

13.9.1.2.1 Insights from Blindsight 183

13.9.1.2.2 Insights from Visual Field Deficits 184

13.10 Restorative Therapies: Rehabilitating the Human Visual System 184

13.11 Summary 185

14. GOAL-DRIVEN ATTENTION AND WORKING MEMORY 190

Sheila Gillard Crewther, Nahal Goharpey, Louise C. Bannister, and Gemma Lamp

14.1 Introduction 190

14.1.1 Factors Affecting Stroke Rehabilitation 190

14.1.2 Goal-Directed Action and the Visual System 191

14.2 What is Attention? 191

14.2.1 Neuroanatomical Interaction between the Attention and Visual Systems 192

14.2.2 Attention and Multisensory Integration 194

14.3 Learning Needs Attention, Working Memory, and Motivation 195

14.3.1 Neural Plasticity: Learning in the Brain 195

14.3.2 Attention and Working Memory 195

14.3.3 Selective Attention is Also Guided by Emotive and Motivational Evaluation of the Target Stimuli 196

14.3.4 The Case of Depression 197

14.4 The Effect of Brain Lesions on Attention 197

14.5 Rehabilitation Post-Stroke 198

14.5.1 Training Attention Post-Stroke 199

14.6 Summary and Conclusion 201

15. EXECUTIVE FUNCTIONS 208

Susan M. Fitzpatrick and Carolyn M. Baum

15.1 Stroke Rehabilitation: The Role of Executive Functions 208

15.2 Overview of a Multi-Level Understanding of Executive Functions 210

15.3 Neural Substrates of Executive Functions 211

15.3.1 Neural Measures and Interventions 213

15.4 Behavioral Measures and Interventions 214

15.4.1 Measures to Identify Brain-Related Behaviors 215

15.4.2 Measures to Identify the Behavioral Consequences of Stroke 215

15.4.3 Performance-Based Tests 216

15.5 Behavioral and Performance Interventions 217

15.5.1 Interventions at the Behavioral Level 217

15.5.2 Interventions at the Performance Level 218

15.6 Conclusions 218

16. LANGUAGE 222

Lisa Tabor Connor

16.1 Neuroscience of Language: Neuropsychological and Lesion-Symptom Mapping Evidence 222

16.2 Functional Neuroimaging of Language and Recovery 223

16.2.1 White Matter Tractography 223

16.2.2 Functional Connectivity MRI 224

16.3 Current Models of Language Rehabilitation 225

16.4 Treatment Principles/Strategies Arising from Neuroscience and Cognitive Neuroscience 226

16.5 Toward a Neuroscientifically Based Model of Aphasia Rehabilitation 227

PART E

NEW PERSPECTIVES AND DIRECTIONS FOR STROKE REHABILITATION RESEARCH 231

17. TARGETING VIABLE BRAIN NETWORKS TO IMPROVE OUTCOMES AFTER STROKE 233

Cathy Stinear and Winston Byblow

17.1 Introduction 233

17.2 Measuring Connectivity to Predict Motor Outcomes 233

17.2.1 Functional Integrity of Motor Pathways 234

17.2.1.1 Crossed Corticospinal Tract 234

17.2.1.2 Uncrossed Corticospinal Tract 234

17.2.1.3 Interhemispheric Pathways 235

17.2.2 Structural Imaging of Motor Pathways 235

17.2.3 Combined Approaches 235

17.2.4 Algorithm for Predicting Upper Limb
Motor Outcomes   236

17.2.5 The Lower Limb   236

17.2.6 Conclusions   237

17.3 Priming Approaches   237

17.4 Conclusions   238

**18. DIRECTIONS FOR STROKE REHABILITATION
CLINICAL PRACTICE AND RESEARCH**   240

Leeanne M. Carey

18.1 Introduction   240

18.2 Key Findings for Stroke Rehabilitation
Clinical Practice   240

18.3 Beyond the Lesion: Impact of Focal
Lesion on Brain Networks and
Rehabilitation   242

18.4 Use of Network-Based Models of Recovery
in Stroke Rehabilitation   243

18.5 Targeting Stroke Rehabilitation to the
Individual   244

18.6 Guidelines to Facilitate the Translation of
Evidence to Clinical Practice   245

18.7 Perspectives and Directions for Stroke
Rehabilitation Research   246

18.8 Conclusions   248

Index   251

CONTRIBUTORS

LOUISE C. BANNISTER BA, BSc (Hons)
DPsych Candidate
School of Psychological Science
La Trobe University
Melbourne, Australia

CAROLYN M. BAUM, PhD, OTR/L, FAOTA
Professor
Occupational Therapy and Neurology and Elias Michael
  Director
Program in Occupational Therapy
Washington University School of Medicine
St. Louis, MO

JULIE BERNHARDT, PhD
Associate Professor, Director
AVERT Early Intervention Research Program
Australian Research Council Future Fellow
National Stroke Research Institute
Florey Neuroscience Institutes
Melbourne Brain Centre
Melbourne, Australia

AMY BRODTMANN, PhD
Co-division Head
Behavioural Neuroscience
Florey Neuroscience Institutes
University of Melbourne
Melbourne, Australia

CATHRIN M. BUETEFISCH, MD, PhD
Associate Professor
Departments of Neurology and Rehabilitation Medicine
  and Radiology
Emory University School of Medicine
Atlanta, GA

WINSTON BYBLOW, PhD
Director
Movement Neuroscience Laboratory
Department of Sport & Exercise Science
Centre for Brain Research
University of Auckland
Auckland, New Zealand

DOMINIQUE A. CADILHAC, PhD
Associate Professor and Head
Translational Public Health and Evaluation Unit
NHMRC/NHF Research Fellow
Stroke and Ageing Research Centre
Department of Medicine
Monash Medical Centre Southern Clinical School
Monash University, and
National Stroke Research Institute
Florey Neuroscience Institutes
Melbourne Brain Centre
Melbourne, Australia

LEEANNE M. CAREY, PhD
Head, Neurorehabilitation and Recovery
and Australian Research Council Future Fellow
National Stroke Research Institute
Florey Neuroscience Institutes
Melbourne Brain Centre
and
Professor
Department of Occupational Therapy
School of Allied Health
Faculty of Health Sciences
La Trobe University
Melbourne, Australia

LISA TABOR CONNOR, PhD
Assistant Professor
Program in Occupational Therapy
Departments of Radiology and Neurology
Washington University School of Medicine
St. Louis, MO

SHEILA GILLARD CREWTHER, PhD
Professor
School of Psychological Science
La Trobe University
Melbourne, Australia

GEOFFREY A. DONNAN, MD, PhD
Professor and Director
Florey Neuroscience Institutes
University of Melbourne
Melbourne Brain Centre
Melbourne, Australia

SUSAN M. FITZPATRICK, PhD
Vice-President
James S. McDonnell Foundation, and
Adjunct Associate Professor
Department of Anatomy and Neurobiology
Program in Occupational Therapy
Washington University School of Medicine
St. Louis, MO

NAHAL GORHARPEY, PhD
Assistant First Year Coordinator
School of Psychological Science
La Trobe University
Melbourne, Australia

ISOBEL J. HUBBARD, MOT
Lecturer, Academic Researcher, and PhD Candidate
School of Medicine and Public Health Faculty of Health
University of Newcastle
Newcastle, Australia

HEIDI JOHANSEN-BERG, DPhil, MSc
Wellcome Trust Senior Research Fellow
FMRIB Centre
Nuffield Department of Clinical Neurosciences
University of Oxford
John Radcliffe Hospital
Oxford, United Kingdom

NICOL KORNER-BITENSKY, PhD
Associate Professor
School of Physical and Occupational Therapy
McGill University
Montreal, Canada

GEMMA LAMP, BSc (Hons)
Research Officer
National Stroke Research Institute
Florey Neuroscience Institutes
Melbourne Brain Centre, and
Brain & Psychological Sciences Research Centre
Faculty of Life and Social Sciences
Swinburne University of Technology
Melbourne, Australia

THOMAS K. A. LINDÉN, MD, PhD
Senior Consultant/Researcher
Centre for Brain Research and Rehabilitation
Sahlgrenska Academy
Gothenburg University
Gothenburg, Sweden; and
Visiting Professor
Florey Neuroscience Institutes
Melbourne, Australia

RICHARD A. J. MASTERTON, PhD
Postdoctoral Fellow
Brain Research Institute
Florey Neuroscience Institutes
Brain Research Institute
Melbourne Brain Centre
Melbourne, Australia

THOMAS A. MATYAS, PhD
Adjunct Professor
School of Psychological Science
La Trobe University
Honorary Professorial Fellow
National Stroke Research Institute
Florey Neuroscience Institutes, and
Adjunct Associate Professor
School of Physiotherapy
University of Melbourne
Faculty of Medicine
Melbourne, Australia

MICHAEL NILSSON, MD, PhD
Professor, Director
Center for Brain Repair and Rehabilitation
Department of Clinical Neuroscience and
    Rehabilitation
Institute of Neuroscience and Physiology
Sahlgrenska Academy at the University of
    Gothenburg
Gothenburg, Sweden; and
Professor and Director
Hunter Medical Research Institute (HMRI),
Newcastle, Australia

MARCELA PEKNA, MD, PhD
Associate Professor
Center for Brain Repair and Rehabilitation
Department of Clinical Neuroscience and
    Rehabilitation
Institute of Neuroscience and Physiology
Sahlgrenska Academy at the University of Gothenburg
Gothenburg, Sweden

MILOS PEKNY, MD, PhD
Professor
Laboratory of Astrocyte Biology and
    CNS Regeneration
Center for Brain Repair and Rehabilitation
Department of Clinical Neuroscience
    and Rehabilitation
Institute of Neuroscience and Physiology
Sahlgrenska Academy at the University of Gothenburg
Gothenburg, Sweden

HELENE. J. POLATAJKO, PhD, FCAOT, FCAHS
Professor
Department of Occupational Science and Occupational
  Therapy
Graduate Department of Rehabilitation Science
Dalla Lana School of Public Health
University of Toronto Neuroscience Program (UTNP)
University of Toronto
Toronto, Canada

AINA PUCE, PhD
Eleanor Cox Riggs Professor & Director
Research Imaging Facility
Indiana University
Bloomington, IN

TARA PURVIS, BPhys (Hons), MSci
Research Officer
Translational Public Health Unit Stroke and Ageing
  Research Centre (STARC)
Department of Medicine
Monash Medical Centre Southern Clinical School
Monash University
Melbourne, Australia

RÜDIGER J. SEITZ, MD, PhD
Professor of Neurology
Department of Neurology
University Hospital Düsseldorf
Biomedical Research Centre
Heinrich-Heine-University
Düsseldorf, Germany

CHARLOTTE J. STAGG, PhD
Biomedical Research Centre Fellow
FMRIB Centre
Nuffield Department of Clinical
  Neurosciences
University of Oxford
John Radcliffe Hospital
Oxford, United Kingdom

CATHY STINEAR, PhD
Senior Lecturer
Department of Medicine
Faculty of Medical and Health
  Sciences
University of Auckland
Auckland, New Zealand

J-DONALD TOURNIER, PhD
Postdoctoral Fellow
Brain Research Institute
Florey Neuroscience Institutes
Melbourne Brain Centre
Melbourne, Australia

**PAULETTE VAN VLIET, BAppSc (Physio),
  MSc, PhD**
Professor of Stroke Rehabilitation, ARC
  Future Fellow
School of Health Sciences
Faculty of Health
University of Newcastle
Newcastle, Australia

PART A | CORE CONCEPTS

1 | INTRODUCTION

LEEANNE M. CAREY

1.1 STROKE REHABILITATION: AN ONGOING WINDOW OF OPPORTUNITY

Stroke rehabilitation has potential to directly influence positive, adaptive changes in the brain and as such provides an ongoing window of opportunity for improvement. The foundations for this change will become evident as you read through the chapters in this book. Evidence will be provided and discussed in relation to mechanisms of neural plasticity. The conditions under which these adaptive changes may be achieved will be discussed in relation to learning and the everyday functions the brain has to perform. The focus will be on new insights from neuroscience and imaging.

Neural plasticity refers to the neurobiological phenomenon that underlies the ability to adapt and learn during development, throughout the normal lifespan, and in response to injury. The question for stroke clinicians and researchers is: How can rehabilitation directly influence positive, adaptive changes in the brain in association with functional recovery after stroke?

Insights from neuroscience and neuroimaging are providing a new foundation for rehabilitation outcomes. Today, more than ever before, we need to take heed of the advice from pioneers in the field that "individuals in rehabilitation will have to revise their previous knowledge to bring it in line with the new theories, which are giving the researchers and therapists valuable insights into the recovery potentials of the central nervous system following a lesion" (Moore, 1986, p. 460).

The aim of *Stroke Rehabilitation: Insights from Neuroscience and Imaging* is to inform and challenge rehabilitation specialists to adopt more restorative and scientific approaches to stroke rehabilitation based on evidence from neuroscience. Embedded within a rehabilitation framework, this book presents the evidence from neuroscience and imaging literature that underpins an active, restorative approach to stroke rehabilitation.

In Part A (Chapters 1–5), core concepts underlying stroke rehabilitation and neural plasticity are discussed, and some of the tools that may be used to provide new insights into recovery are described. We begin by proposing a model of stroke rehabilitation that is based on a learning perspective and identifies outcomes from brain systems to performance and participation. The main structural and functional constituents of neural plasticity are then explored from macro and micro perspectives, with the applications and implications for rehabilitation highlighted. One tool that is helping to provide new insights into recovery is neuroimaging. Neuroimaging approaches, such as task-related activation, functional connectivity, and white matter tractography are introduced in the context of what they can tell us. A multimodal approach is needed to help unravel the process of recovery. Two techniques that are commonly used in stroke recovery research, magnetoencephalography (MEG) and transcranial magnetic stimulation (TMS), are presented. In Part B (Chapter 6) the pathophysiology of stroke and the timelines for recovery and rehabilitation are discussed.

In Part C (Chapters 7–10) we address issues related to creating an optimal environment and learning conditions for restorative stroke rehabilitation. Approaches to the organization and delivery of care and timing of stroke rehabilitation are discussed from both multidisciplinary and international perspectives. Next the impact of motivation and mood on rehabilitation and the importance of creating the right environment are discussed in the context of rehabilitation and neural plasticity. Common elements of training have been identified that are important across multiple functions. These include task-oriented training,

training for transfer, intensity, and repetition. These are discussed in the context of motor and perceptual learning and in relation to their foundations from the neuroscience and imaging literature. The potential for emerging adjunctive therapies to promote plasticity and enhance the response to behavioral learning–based training or more traditional therapies are then presented.

In Part D (Chapters 11–17) we critically review current approaches to rehabilitation of common functions in the context of neuroscience. Based on insights from neuroscience and imaging, we move toward describing a neuroscience-based model of rehabilitation for the functions described. These functions are: movement and action, touch and body sensations, vision, selective attention and awareness, working memory, executive functions, and language and communication. The brain uses these functions to solve the problems encountered during everyday living. As these functions will be our goal for rehabilitation, we have chosen to present them with a positive capacity rather than an impairment focus. The role of rehabilitation is to facilitate restoration of common functions in the context of achieving the goals of everyday living. Where possible the authors provide examples of how neuroscience evidence can be translated and operationalized within the context of rehabilitation.

In the final section, Part E (Chapters 18 and 19), we address the issue of how to select the most optimal approaches to rehabilitation for each individual based on viable brain networks. Key findings and their application to clinical practice are summarized. New perspectives and directions for stroke rehabilitation research are presented.

1.2 THE SCOPE OF THE PROBLEM: PREVALENCE AND IMPACT OF STROKE AND INCREASING NEED FOR STROKE REHABILITATION

Stroke is the leading cause of chronic adult disability (Paul et al., 2005; Mathers, Fat, Boerma, & World Health Organization, 2008; American Heart Association, 2010). One in six people experience a stroke at some time in their lives (www.strokefoundation.com.au/ retrieved July 2011). Every year globally, 15 million people suffer a stroke (MacKay, Mensah, Mendis, Greenlund, & World Health Organization, 2004; Australian Bureau of Statistics, 2009; American Heart Association, 2010). Worldwide there are 62 million stroke survivors (Strong, Mathers, & Bonita, 2007). Most people survive the initial insult and are left with impairment in one or more functions such as movement, sensation, language, thinking, memory, and emotion. One-third of these individuals have persisting and significant long-term disability (Barnes, Dobkin, & Bogousslavsky, 2005; Roger, 2011) and a further 20% require assistance for activities of daily living (Bonita, Solomon, & Broad, 1997). In a cohort study of 434 stroke

survivors at 6 months post-stroke, 54% reported problems with ability to perform housework, meal preparation, or shopping; 65% reported restrictions in reintegration into community activities; and 53% lacked a meaningful activity to fill the day (Mayo, Wood-Dauphinee, Cote, Durcan, & Carlton, 2002). The proportion of disabled stroke survivors is increasing (Carandang et al., 2006).

Stroke is a global healthcare problem that is common, disabling, and has an ongoing impact on quality of life (Langhorne, Bernhardt, & Kwakkel, 2011). It is the second leading cause of death and remains among the top six causes of burden of disease in the world, and top three in high-income countries, according to the burden of disease rankings of the World Health Organization (Mathers et al., 2008). It is estimated that 55%–75% of stroke survivors still have functional limitations and reduced quality of life months after the infarct (Levin, Kleim, & Wolf, 2009). These continuing disabilities significantly decrease their life satisfaction, and also the life satisfaction of their spouses (Ostwald, Godwin, & Cron, 2009). The importance of good recovery has been highlighted (Carod-Artal & Egido, 2009). Yet, even those with a mild stroke can experience significant and ongoing problems and reduced life satisfaction (Edwards, Hahn, Baum, & Dromerick, 2006). Stroke also has a major economic and societal impact (Cadilhac, Carter, Thrift, & Dewey, 2009; Heidenreich et al., 2011; see Chapter 7). Hence, the ongoing impact of stroke and disability is highlighted.

Stroke is one of the largest impairment categories for rehabilitation. For example, in Australia, stroke is the third largest impairment category, accounting for one in ten rehabilitation episodes (National Stroke Foundation, 2010b). The cost is considerable in healthcare dollars and ongoing quality of life and burden of care (Department of Health, UK, 2005). Clinical guidelines for stroke rehabilitation are available (Duncan et al., 2005; Intercollegiate Stroke Working Party, 2008; Lindsay et al., 2008; Management of Stroke Rehabilitation Working Group, 2010; National Stroke Foundation, 2010a), yet adherence is generally poor (National Stroke Foundation, 2010a). As stated in the National Stroke Audit of Rehabilitation Services (National Stroke Foundation, 2010b), too many who have suffered a stroke "… are not receiving the specialized care essential to their best possible recovery and return to meaningful daily activities." Equitable access to evidence-based care is a key recommendation. The "need for support and education for implementing evidence-based care" is highlighted.

More people need rehabilitation, yet rehabilitation outcomes are often limited, based on compensation and interventions that are not always evidence-based. A range of stroke rehabilitation services and models of organization of care have been described, and these are discussed in Chapter 7. In particular, the value of effective stroke rehabilitation in a "stroke unit" and interdisciplinary care are highlighted. The issue of timing of therapy is also important and is discussed in relation to recovery (Chapter 6), organization of care (Chapter 7), and potential for learning-based rehabilitation to influence recovery (Chapter 2). Based on the potential for neural plastic changes, current evidence suggests that the time window for learning-based approaches to restoring capacities and skills is open, providing ongoing hope for stroke survivors. For example, restoration of somatosensory and motor capacities is evident with specific, neuroscience-based training even months and years after stroke (L. M. Carey & Seitz, 2007; Richards, Stewart, Woodbury, Senesac, & Cauraugh, 2008; L. M. Carey, Macdonnell, & Matyas, 2011). Learning of compensatory strategies may also be important and can be ongoing. This time window is much longer than the "days to weeks for restoring impairments" and "days to months for task-oriented practice with adaptive learning and compensation strategies" sometimes suggested (Langhorne, Bernhardt, & Kwakkel, 2011).

1.3 RECOVERY AND REHABILITATION: DEFINITIONS

Recovery has been used to refer both to the restitution of damaged structures and behavioral functions, and as a term to describe clinical improvements regardless of how these may have occurred (Levin et al., 2009). Terms such as *recovery* and *compensation* are frequently used, yet there is debate over what they mean. Each term will have different meaning according to the level of outcome being investigated. Therefore, it is recommended that they should be interpreted and qualified relative to these levels. Consistent with the International Classification of Functioning, it is recommended that recovery versus compensation should be qualified at the health condition (neuronal), body function/structure (impairment), and activity (disability) levels (Levin et al., 2009). Other terms used include *restitution* or *restoration* (restoring the functionality of damaged neural tissue), *substitution* (reorganization of partly spared neural pathways to relearn lost functions), and *compensation* (improvement of the disparity between the impaired skills of a patient and the demands of their environment; (Finger & Stein, 1982; Kwakkel, Kollen, & Lindeman, 2004). It is recommended that recovery should be measured across a profile of outcomes from reorganization of brain networks to performance outcomes, independence in daily activities, and participation in daily activities and life roles (Chapter 2).

Rehabilitation can be defined in a number of ways. The World Health Organization defines rehabilitation of people with disabilities as "a process aimed at enabling them to reach and maintain their optimal physical, sensory, intellectual, psychological and social functional levels. Rehabilitation provides disabled people with the tools they need to attain independence and self-determination" (World Health Organization, http://www.who.int/topics/rehabilitation/en/ retrieved July 16, 2011). From a neuropsychology perspective it is suggested that "rehabilitation of sensory and cognitive function typically involves methods for retraining neural pathways or training new neural pathways to regain or improve neurocognitive functioning that has been diminished by disease or traumatic injury. (http://en.wikipedia.org/wiki/Rehabilitation_(neuropsychology); retrieved July 16, 2011). A related term, *neurorehabilitation*, is now in common use and is defined as "the clinical subspecialty that is devoted to the restoration and maximization of functions that have been lost due to impairments caused by an injury or disease to the nervous system" (Selzer, Clarke, Cohen, Duncan, & Gage, 2006a).

The National Institute of Neurological Disorders and Health describes rehabilitation post-stroke as a process that helps stroke survivors "relearn skills" that are lost when part of the brain is damaged. It also teaches survivors new ways of performing tasks to compensate for residual disabilities (http://www.ninds.nih.gov/disorders/stroke/poststrokerehab.htm; retrieved September 29, 2011). Similarly, the Stroke Rehab Definitions Conceptual Framework (GTA Rehab Network, 2009) described rehabilitation as "a progressive, dynamic, goal-oriented and often time-limited process, which enables an individual with impairment to identify and reach his/her optimal mental, physical, cognitive and/or social functional level." The overall objective is to improve function and/or prevent deterioration of function, and to bring about the highest possible level of independence—physically, psychologically, socially, and financially—within the limits of the persisting stroke impairment (National Stroke Foundation, 2005; Dewey, Sherry, & Collier, 2007; Consensus panel on the stroke rehabilitation system, 2007). Stroke rehabilitation has been defined as encompassing any aspect of stroke care (generally nonsurgical and nonpharmaceutical) that aims to reduce disability and handicap (promote activity and participation) (Langhorne & Legg, 2003). It can span from acute inpatient care to formal care in rehabilitation hospitals and outpatient services, through to rehabilitation in community settings such as home, school, or work environments (GTA Rehab Network, 2009).

1.4 NEURAL PLASTICITY AND LEARNING AS A BASIS FOR STROKE REHABILITATION

Neuroplasticity is defined, based on a recent consensus group meeting, as "... the ability of the nervous system to respond to intrinsic or extrinsic stimuli by reorganizing its structure, function and connections" (Cramer et al., 2011). Further, it "... can be described at many levels from molecular to cellular to systems to behaviour; and can occur during development, in response to the environment, in support of learning, in response to disease, or in relation to therapy." (Cramer et al., 2011) The ability of the brain to change or remodel itself based on experience forms the basis of the brain's capacity to retain memories, improve functions such as movement, and perform daily tasks (Bruel-Jungerman, Davis, & Laroche, 2007). As we learn, new knowledge and skills are acquired through instructions or experiences. To learn or memorize a fact or skill requires persistent functional changes in the brain that represent the new knowledge. The lifelong ability of the brain to change based on new experiences and learning is known as *neuroplasticity*.

It is important to appreciate that plasticity can be viewed as adaptive when associated with gain in function, or maladaptive when associated with negative consequences such as loss of function (Nudo, Eisner-Janowicz, & Stowe, 2006; Cramer et al., 2011). Examples of maladaptive plasticity include chronic pain and allodynia (hypersensitivity and altered body sensations); neuropathic pain triggered by lesions to the somatosensory nervous system (Costigan, Scholz, & Woolf, 2009); and focal hand dystonia (Classen, 2003; Schabrun, Stinear, Byblow, & Ridding, 2009). The phenomenon of learned non-use (Taub, 1980; Taub, Uswatte, Mark, & Morris, 2006) may also be considered an example of maladaptive plasticity. Clinicians are encouraged to recall this when they consider selecting compensatory therapeutic approaches; for example, when teaching the "unaffected limb" to take over lost functions.

There is growing evidence from animal and human studies for neural plastic changes associated with recovery after stroke (Nudo et al., 2006; Selzer, Clarke, Cohen, Duncan, & Gage, 2006b). Experience is an important ingredient in these neural plastic changes, as highlighted in animal studies (Nudo, Wise, SiFuentes, & Milliken, 1996). Nudo states, "post-injury behavioral experience appears to be critical to the reassembly of adaptive modules" (Nudo, 2007). The nature of the experience and whether it is focused on repeated performance versus skill acquisition appears to be important. In a series of studies by Nudo and colleagues, two behavioral tasks were used that separated the repetition of motor activity from the acquisition of motor skills. Regions of the brain associated with motor recovery were mapped. Repetitive motor activity during the easier task did not produce plastic changes in movement representations in the brain. Rather, neural plastic changes, involving selective expansions of movement representations in the brain, were only produced following skill acquisition on the difficult task. These persisted without further training for up to three months. Extensive additional training on the more difficult skill-based task produced further improvements in performance, and further changes in movement maps. Based on these experiments

the authors concluded that neural plasticity that is driven behaviorally through training is learning-dependent, not activity-dependent. The neural correlate of the acquired motor skills was the change in the functional representation of primary motor cortex (M1), and persistence of this change suggested its role in memory of motor skills (Plautz, Milliken, & Nudo, 2000).

The phenomena of "use-dependent" and "learning-dependent" plasticity have been described in the literature. Use-dependent plasticity, also known as experience-dependent or activity-dependent plasticity, refers to reorganization of motor-related cortical regions achieved as a consequence of motor practice (Nudo, Milliken, Jenkins, & Merzenich, 1996; Classen, Liepert, Wise, Hallett, & Cohen, 1998). Use-dependent plasticity may also be described in relation to other functions such as vision, and language. Learning-dependent plasticity involves the additional element of improvement of skill, often involving task-specific training (Plautz et al., 2000). Different patterns of plastic changes in the brain have been described following spontaneous learning involving frequent exposure to the stimulus alone, compared to task-specific learning of specific visual functions (Zhang & Kourtzi, 2010). The latter involves brain regions implicated in attention-gated learning and has been described as "learning-dependent" plasticity.

Both types of plasticity may be important in recovery. A key issue in rehabilitation is the extent to which use-dependent plasticity compared to learning-dependent plasticity may be impacted and accessible following brain injury. Frequent exposure to stimuli may be sufficient to effect a change in individuals without brain damage. In comparison, there is evidence from training of visual (Zihl, 1981) and somatosensory (L. M. Carey, Matyas, & Oke, 1993) discriminations that this is usually not sufficient following brain injury such as stroke. Use-dependent plasticity may be considered evidence of a more "spontaneous" form of associative learning. Learning-dependent plasticity has additional elements of being associated with "task-specific training" (Zhang & Kourtzi, 2010). Rehabilitation may be viewed as a trigger to facilitate plasticity, and a means by which neural plastic changes may be shaped to achieve meaningful outcomes for the individual. How this may be achieved is still being discovered and is the focus of this book.

Evidence is growing that specific interventions facilitate neural plasticity and improved motor recovery after stroke in humans (Hodics, Cohen, & Cramer, 2006; L. M. Carey & Seitz, 2007; Richards et al., 2008; Stinear, Barber, Coxon, Fleming, & Byblow, 2008). A number of promising interventions have been developed to facilitate neural plastic changes (L. M. Carey, 2007). Some of these approaches are supported, at least in part, by preliminary evidence of changes in the brain. For example, constraint-induced movement therapy (CIMT; Taub, Uswatte, &

Pidikiti, 1999) was developed following evidence of neural plastic changes in deafferented monkeys and has been associated with enlarged motor cortex map for the hand in humans (Wittenberg et al., 2003). Similarly, use of constraint in the training of language functions has been associated with positive outcomes and changes in brain activation (Pulvermuller & Berthier, 2008). Adjunct therapies such as neuropharmacology and brain stimulation have also been developed (Chapters 3 and 10) and are likely to be most optimal when combined with specific training.

A number of factors are likely to impact on the potential for neural plastic changes and ability to benefit from rehabilitation after stroke (Kolb, Teskey, & Gibb, 2010). These may include the nature and severity of stroke, time post-stroke, motivation, mood, levels of stress, the environment, ability to attend and learn, and viable brain networks with capacity for plasticity. Factors such as structural (Riley et al., 2011) and functional (Stinear et al., 2007) integrity of white matter tracts in motor recovery and integrity of functionally connected networks in recovery of neglect and attention functions (He et al., 2007) have shown to be more important in recovery than the localized site or volume of the infarct. This is consistent with the concept that neural plastic changes rely on the integrity of these pathways and networks during the process of recovery and rehabilitation.

1.5 NEUROIMAGING AND HOW IT MAY INFORM STROKE REHABILITATION

Experience can change both the brain's physical structure (anatomy) and functional organization (physiology) (Chapter 3). There are a number of modalities and techniques that may be used to investigate mechanisms of recovery post-stroke (Chapters 4 and 5). One modality is magnetic resonance imaging (MRI). MRI can provide information on brain structure and volume, white matter integrity, fiber tract connections, functional brain activation, and functional network connectivity, and so has potential to provide important insights into the mechanisms of recovery post-stroke. For example, functional brain imaging techniques allow us to visualize patterns of activity in the brain during motion, perception, cognition, and emotion (L. M. Carey & Seitz, 2007). Brain activation maps are created that identify regions and networks involved, how they differ following brain injury relative to healthy controls, and how they might change over time with recovery or rehabilitation. These imaging techniques will be explored in Chapter 4.

Neuroimaging methodologies, such as functional and structural MRI, can help to frame several key questions (L. M. Carey & Seitz, 2007). Examples include:

- What are the brain regions involved in task-related activation of common functions such as movement, sensation, language, and cognition?
- What are the brain regions and networks that work in synchrony during rest?
- How do these differ in people who experience impairments following stroke compared to unimpaired people?
- Do regions and networks differ according to whether the lesion is of cortical origin or involves interruption of pathways?
- How does interruption to the interconnected network help to explain the information processing deficit?
- Are there specific regions and networks correlated with severity of impairment and, if so, which regions show strong correlations with good recovery?
- Which brain networks have a role in recovery during spontaneous recovery, and are these common across different functions?
- Do patterns of activation vary over time? If so, how? And what do they tell us about the mechanism or residual capacities of the brain to adapt?
- How can we facilitate positive adaptive changes, rather than maladaptive changes?
- Can specific interventions facilitate adaptive changes in the brain, and which changes are associated with better recovery?

In addition to providing insight into neurobiological activity and mechanisms underlying recovery, information from neuroimaging studies has potential to be used as biomarkers and predictors of future outcome (Cramer et al., 2011). Imaging outcomes may also be used as a surrogate endpoint of recovery in clinical trials.

Different patterns of neural plastic change have been described following recovery in humans after stroke (L. M. Carey & Seitz, 2007; Johansen-Berg, 2007; Cramer et al., 2011). Major patterns of change observed in functional activation studies of motor recovery include:

- change in location of movement representation in cortical maps in the lesioned hemisphere, such as a shift to more posterior somatosensory regions or face region.
- activation in the region surrounding the infarct
- a shift in the balance of activity across hemispheres, involving changes in the presence and extent of activation in ipsilesional and contralesional hemispheres (Tecchio et al., 2007; Grefkes et al., 2008).

- involvement of remote locations (Seitz, Knorr, Azari, Herzog, & Freud, 1999), contralesional regions (Schaechter & Perdue, 2008), and distributed networks (Seitz et al., 1998; Sharma, Baron, & Rowe, 2009) that would not typically be required for the particular task, and

- change in strength of connections between nodes within a network (Grefkes et al., 2008; Sharma et al., 2009).

A recent investigation of the role of intrahemispheric and interhemispheric changes in recovery of motor and language functions highlighted the importance of interhemispheric changes (Carter et al., 2010). Changes in brain structure, such as an increase of cortical thickness in the vicinity of activation (Schaechter, Moore, Connell, Rosen, & Dijkhuizen, 2006), have also been described and are usually related to functional changes and improvement in function. There is also evidence of structural change associated with outcome. For example, changes in cortical thickness have been reported in areas that show increased activation and clinical improvement (Schaechter et al., 2006; Gauthier et al., 2008).

Current evidence highlights the importance of brain networks rather than localized regions in recovery after stroke. An important change of focus in understanding how the brain works is from one of localized regions to that of interrelated networks. The ability to facilitate positive adaptive changes in the recovering brain is dependent, at least in part, on residual brain networks and reestablishing a balance of activity across hemispheres during the process of recovery (Seitz, Bütefisch, Kleiser, & Hömberg, 2004; L. M. Carey & Seitz, 2007; Carter et al., 2010). Knowledge of brain networks and how they are interrupted following brain injury will help us better understand the behavioral manifestations of impairment and how neural plasticity can be manipulated in therapy.

1.6 PARADIGM SHIFT IN STROKE REHABILITATION

There is a growing realization that traditional approaches to rehabilitation that focus on compensation alone, rather than restoration, are unlikely to result in optimal recovery of function. If we are to improve outcome and adopt a more active or "restorative" approach to rehabilitation we need to understand that we need to "change the brain to change the behavior." It is important to realize however, that different kinds of therapy can promote different kinds of changes, not all of which are adaptive. For example, a person can learn non-use of the limb or develop dystonic postures following sensory loss or overuse of a body part.

Novel insights into how the brain adapts with recovery and experience, together with advances in learning theory, provide a strong foundation for the development of rehabilitation approaches that aim to restore lost capacity and improve clinical outcome (L. M. Carey, 2007). The emerging paradigm shift in rehabilitation highlights the need to identify the conditions under which adaptive changes in the brain can be facilitated, and to operationalize these into rehabilitation interventions. Some approaches have been developed based on evidence of brain recovery following brain injury in animals, and others have applied principles of learning shown to be effective in the non-damaged brain in humans. Both have shown positive outcomes. For example, CIMT was developed based on studies following brain injury in deafferented monkeys (Taub et al., 1999; Taub, Uswatte, & Elbert, 2002), and is associated with positive outcomes in clinical trials (Wolf, Winstein, Miller, & al, 2006) and neural plastic changes in humans (Wittenberg et al., 2003). Principles of motor learning, based on an extensive literature in healthy individuals, have also been used after stroke and were associated with improvement in finger movement and change from a contralesional to ipsilesional activation in primary and secondary motor areas (J. R. Carey et al., 2002). A perceptual learning approach that incorporates principles of neural plasticity (Chapter 12) has also been used to train somatosensory discriminations, with positive outcomes (L. M. Carey et al., 1993, 2011). While the processes of learning in the non-damaged and damaged brain likely share common mechanisms, there are also differences related to the brain injury and the fact that the task needs to be relearned that may require use of alternative strategies or pathways (Matthews, Johansen-Berg, & Reddy, 2004).

Patients vary in their ability to benefit from rehabilitation. Currently we do not have effective means of identifying individuals who may benefit, nor how to select the most optimal therapy for individuals. Neuroscience and neuroimaging may provide new insight not only into brain regions interrupted by the stroke, but also the viable brain networks with capacity for plasticity. Many factors influence plasticity and need to be considered in interpretation of findings, as well as in design of future studies. Our goal is to use the potential of viable brain networks to improve performance given optimized conditions for training.

REFERENCES

American Heart Association. (2010). Heart disease and stroke statistics—2010 Update. *Circulation, 121*, e46–e215.

Australian Bureau of Statistics. (2009). 3303.0—Causes of Death, Australia, 2009. Retrieved October 4, 2011, from http://abs.gov.au/AUSSTATS/abs@.nsf/mf/3303.0/.

Barnes, M., Dobkin, B., & Bogousslavsky, J. (2005). *Recovery after stroke*. New York: Cambridge University Press.

Bonita, R., Solomon, N., & Broad, J. B. (1997). Prevalence of stroke and stroke-related disability—Estimates from the Auckland stroke studies. *Stroke, 28*(10), 1898–1902.

Bruel-Jungerman, E., Davis, S., & Laroche, S. (2007). Brain plasticity mechanisms and memory: A party of four. *Neuroscientist, 13*(5), 492–505.

Cadilhac, D. A., Carter, R., Thrift, A. G., & Dewey, H. M. (2009). Estimating the long-term costs of ischemic and hemorrhagic stroke for Australia: new evidence derived from the North East Melbourne Stroke Incidence Study (NEMESIS). *Stroke, 40*(3), 915–921.

Carandang, R., Seshadri, S., Beiser, A., Kelly-Hayes, M., Kase, C. S., Kannel, W. B., et al. (2006). Trends in incidence, lifetime risk, severity, and 30-day mortality of stroke over the past 50 years. *The Journal of the American Medical Association, 296*(24), 2939–2946.

Carey, J. R., Kimberley, T. J., Lewis, S. M., Auerbach, E. J., Dorsey, L., Rundquist, P., et al. (2002). Analysis of fMRI and finger tracking training in subjects with chronic stroke. *Brain, 125*, 773–788.

Carey, L. M. (2007). Neuroplasticity and learning lead a new era in stroke rehabilitation. [editorial]. *International Journal of Therapy and Rehabilitation, 14*(6), 200–201.

Carey, L. M., Macdonnell, R., & Matyas, T. A. (2011). SENSe: Study of the Effectiveness of Neurorehabilitation on Sensation. A randomized controlled trial. *Neurorehabilitation and Neural Repair, 25*(4), 304–313.

Carey, L. M., Matyas, T. A., & Oke, L. E. (1993). Sensory loss in stroke patients: effective training of tactile and proprioceptive discrimination. *Archives of Physical Medicine and Rehabilitation, 74*(6), 602–611.

Carey, L. M., & Seitz, R. (2007). Functional neuroimaging in stroke recovery and neurorehabilitation: conceptual issues and perspectives. *International Journal of Stroke, 2*(4), 245–264.

Carod-Artal, F. J., & Egido, J. A. (2009). Quality of life after stroke: The importance of a good recovery. *Cerebrovascular Diseases, 27*, 204–214.

Carter, A. R., Astafiev, S. V., Lang, C. E., Connor, L. T., Rengachary, J., Strube, M. J., et al. (2010). Resting interhemispheric functional magnetic resonance imaging connectivity predicts performance after stroke. *Annals of Neurology, 67*(3), 365–375.

Classen, J., (2003). Focal hand dystonia—a disorder of neuroplasticity? *Brain, 126*, 2571–2572.

Classen, J., Liepert, J., Wise, S. P., Hallett, M., & Cohen, L. G. (1998). Rapid plasticity of human cortical movement representation induced by practice. *Journal of Neurophysiology, 79*(2), 1117–1123.

Consensus panel on the stroke rehabilitation system. (2007). *"Time is function." A report from the consensus panel on the stroke rehabilitation system to the Ministry of Health and Long-Term Care*. Ontario: Heart and Stroke Foundation of Ontario.

Costigan, M., Scholz, J., & Woolf, C. J. (2009). Neuropathic pain: A maladaptive response of the nervous system to damage. *Annual Review of Neuroscience, 32*, 1–32.

Cramer, S. C., Sur, M., Dobkin, B. H., O'Brien, C., Sanger, T. D., Trojanowski, J. Q., et al. (2011). Harnessing neuroplasticity for clinical applications. *Brain, 134*, 1591–1609.

Department of Health (UK). (2005). *Reducing brain damage: Faster access to better stroke care*. London: National Audit Office.

Dewey, H. M., Sherry, E. J., & Collier, J. (2007). Stroke rehabilitation 2007—what should it be? *International Journal of Stroke, 2*(3), 191–200.

Duncan, P. W., Zorowitz, R., Bates, B., Choi, J. Y., Glasberg, J. J., Graham, G. D., et al. (2005). Management of adult stroke rehabilitation care: a clinical practice guideline. *Stroke, 36*(9), E100–E143.

Edwards, D. F., Hahn, M., Baum, C., & Dromerick, A. W. (2006). The impact of mild stroke on meaningful activity and life satisfaction. *Journal of Stroke and Cerebrovascular Disease, 15*(4), 151–157.

Finger, S., & Stein, D. G. (1982). *Brain damage and recovery: Research and clinical perspectives*. New York: Academic Press.

Gauthier, L. V., Taub, E., Perkins, C., Ortmann, M., Mark, V. W., & Uswatte, G. (2008). Remodeling the brain: Plastic structural brain changes produced by different motor therapies after stroke. *Stroke, 39*, 1520–1525.

Grefkes, C., Nowak, D. A., Eickhoff, S. B., Dafotakis, M., Kust, J., Karbe, H., et al. (2008). Cortical connectivity after subcortical stroke assessed with functional magnetic resonance imaging. *Annals of Neurology, 63*(2), 236–246.

GTA Rehab Network. (2009). Stroke Rehab Definitions Network. Retrieved January 23, 2012, from http://www.gtarehabnetwork.ca/uploads/File/tools/rehab-definitions-conceptual-framework-stroke.pdf.

He, B. J., Snyder, A. Z., Vincent, J. L., Epstein, A., Shulman, G. L., & Corbetta, M. (2007). Breakdown of functional connectivity in frontoparietal networks underlies behavioral deficits in spatial neglect. *Neuron, 53*(6), 905–918.

Heidenreich, P. A., Trogdon, J. G., Khavjou, O. A., Butler, J., Dracup, K., Ezekowitz, M. D., et al. (2011). Forecasting the future of cardiovascular disease in the United States: a policy statement from the American Heart Association. *Circulation, 123*(8), 933–944.

Hodics, T., Cohen, L. G., & Cramer, S. C. (2006). Functional imaging of intervention effects in stroke motor rehabilitation. *Archives of Physical Medicine and Rehabilitation, 87*(Suppl 2), S36–S42.

Intercollegiate Stroke Working Party. (2008). *National clinical guideline for stroke* (3rd ed.). London: Royal College of Physicians.

Johansen-Berg, H. (2007). Functional imaging of stroke recovery: what we have learnt and where do we go from here? *International Journal of Stroke, 2*(1), 7–16.

Kolb, B., Teskey, G. C., & Gibb, R. (2010). Factors influencing cerebral plasticity in the normal and injured brain. *Frontiers in Human Neuroscience, 4*, Article 204.

Kwakkel, G., Kollen, B., & Lindeman, E. (2004). Understanding the pattern of functional recovery after stroke: Facts and theories. *Restorative Neurology and Neuroscience, 22*(3–5), 281–299.

Langhorne, P., Bernhardt, J., & Kwakkel, G. (2011). Stroke Care 2 Stroke rehabilitation. *Lancet, 377*(9778), 1693–1702.

Levin, M. F., Kleim, J. A., & Wolf, S. L. (2009). What do motor "recovery" and "compensation" mean in patients following stroke? *Neurorehabilitation and Neural Repair, 23*(4), 313–319.

Lindsay, P., Bayley, M., Hellings, C., Hill, M., Woodbury, E., Phillips, S., et al. (2008). Canadian best practice recommendations for stroke care (updated 2008). *Canadian Medical Association Journal, 179*(12), S1–S25.

MacKay, J., Mensah, G. A., Mendis, S., Greenlund, K., & World Health Organization. (2004). *The atlas of heart disease and stroke*. Brighton, UK: Myriad Editions Limited.

Management of Stroke Rehabilitation Working Group. (2010). *VA/DoD clinical practice guideline for the management of stroke rehabilitation*. Washington, DC: Veterans Health Administration, Department of Defense.

Mathers, C., Fat, D. M., Boerma, J. T., & World Health Organization. (2008). *Global burden of disease: 2004 update*. Geneva, Switzerland: World Health Organization.

Matthews, P. M., Johansen-Berg, H., & Reddy, H. (2004). Non-invasive mapping of brain functions and brain recovery: applying lessons from cognitive neuroscience to neurorehabilitation. *Restorative Neurology and Neuroscience, 22*, 245–260.

Mayo, N. E., Wood-Dauphinee, S., Cote, R., Durcan, L., & Carlton, J. (2002). Activity, participation, and quality of life 6 months poststroke. *Archives of Physical Medicine and Rehabilitation, 83*(8), 1035–1042.

Moore, J. C. (1986). Recovery potentials following CNS lesions: A brief historical perspective in relation to modern research data on neuroplasticity. *American Journal of Occupational Therapy, 40*, 459–463.

National Stroke Foundation. (2005). *Clinical guidelines for stroke rehabilitation and recovery*. Melbourne: National Stroke Foundation.

National Stroke Foundation. (2010a). *Clinical guidelines for stroke management 2010*. Melbourne, Australia.

National Stroke Foundation. (2010b). *National stroke audit rehabilitation services*. Melbourne, Australia.

Nudo, R. J. (2007). Postinfarct cortical plasticity and behavioral recovery. *Stroke, 38[part2]*, 840–845.

Nudo, R. J., Eisner-Janowicz, I., & Stowe, A. M. (2006). Plasticity after brain lesions. In M. E. Selzer, S. Clarke, L. G. Cohen, P. W. Duncan & F. H. Gage (Eds.), *Textbook of neural repair and rehabilitation: Vol 1. Neural repair and plasticity* (Vol. 1, pp. 228–247). Cambridge: Cambridge University Press.

Nudo, R. J., Milliken, G. W., Jenkins, W. M., & Merzenich, M. M. (1996). Use-dependent alterations of movement representations in primary motor cortex of adult squirrel monkeys. *Journal of Neuroscience, 16*, 785–807.

Nudo, R. J., Wise, B. M., SiFuentes, F., & Milliken, G. W. (1996). Neural substrates for the effects of rehabilitative training on motor recovery after ischemic infarct. *Science, 272*(5269), 1791–1794.

Ostwald, S. K., Godwin, K. M., & Cron, S. G. (2009). Predictors of life satisfaction in stroke survivors and spousal caregivers after inpatient rehabilitation. *Rehabilitation Nursing, 34*(4), 160–174.

Paul, S. L., Sturm, J. W., Dewey, H. M., Donnan, G. A., Macdonell, R. A., & Thrift, A. G. (2005). Long-term outcome in the North East Melbourne Stroke Incidence Study: predictors of quality of life at 5 years after stroke. *Stroke, 36*, 2082–2086.

Plautz, E. J., Milliken, G. W., & Nudo, R. J. (2000). Effects of repetitive motor training on movement representations in adult squirrel monkeys: role of use versus learning. *Neurobiology of Learning and Memory, 74*, 27–55.

Pulvermuller, F., & Berthier, M. L. (2008). Aphasia therapy on a neuroscience basis. *Aphasiology, 22*(6), 563–599.

Richards, L. G., Stewart, K. C., Woodbury, M. L., Senesac, C., & Cauraugh, J. H. (2008). Movement-dependent stroke recovery: a systematic review and meta-analysis of TMS and fMRI evidence. *Neuropsychologia, 46*(1), 3–11.

Riley, J. D., Le, V., Dar-Yeghianian, L., See, J., Newton, J. M., Ward, N. S., et al. (2011). Anatomy of stroke injury predicts gains from therapy. *Stroke, 42*, 421–426.

Roger, V. L., Lloyd_Jones, D. M., Adams, R. J., Berry, J. D., Brown, T. M., Carnethon, M. R., et al. (2011) Heart disease and stroke statistics- 2011 update: A report from the American Heart Association. *Circulation, 123*, e18–e209.

Schabrun, S. M., Stinear, C. M., Byblow, W. D., & Ridding, M. C. (2009). Normalizing motor cortex representations in focal hand dystonia. *Cerebral Cortex, 19*(9), 1968–1977.

Schaechter, J. D., Moore, C. I., Connell, B. D., Rosen, B. R., & Dijkhuizen, R. M. (2006). Structural and functional plasticity in the somatosensory cortex of chronic stroke patients. *Brain, 129*(10), 2722–2733.

Schaechter, J. D., & Perdue, K. L. (2008). Enhanced cortical activation in the contralesional hemisphere of chronic stroke patients in response to motor skill challenge. *Cerebral Cortex, 18*(3), 638–647.

Seitz, R. J., Bütefisch, C. M., Kleiser, R., & Hömberg, V. (2004). Reorganization of cerebral circuits in human ischemic brain disease. *Restorative Neurology and Neuroscience, 22*, 207–229.

Seitz, R. J., Hoflich, P., Binkofski, F., Tellmann, L., Herzog, H., & Freund, H.-J. (1998). Role of the premotor cortex in recovery from middle cerebral artery infarction. *Archives of Neurology, 55*(8), 1081–1088.

Seitz, R. J., Knorr, U., Azari, N. P., Herzog, H., & Freud, H.-J. (1999). Visual network activation in recovery from sensorimotor stroke. *Restorative Neurology and Neuroscience, 14*, 25–33.

Selzer, M., Clarke, S., Cohen, L., Duncan, P., & Gage, F. (2006a). Neural repair and rehabilitation: an introduction. In M. E. Selzer, S. Clarke, L. G. Cohen, P. W. Duncan & F. H. Gage (Eds.), *Textbook of neural repair and rehabilitation: Vol II Medical neurorehabilitation* (Vol. II, pp. xxvii–xxxv). Cambridge: Cambridge University Press.

Selzer, M. E., Clarke, S., Cohen, L. G., Duncan, P. W., & Gage, F. H. (2006b). *Textbook of neural repair and rehabilitation: Vol I. Neural repair and plasticity* (Vol. 1). Cambridge: Cambridge University Press.

Sharma, N., Baron, J. C., & Rowe, J. B. (2009). Motor imagery after stroke: Relating outcome to motor network connectivity. *Annals of Neurology, 66*(5), 604–616.

Stinear, C. M., Barber, P. A., Coxon, J. P., Fleming, & Byblow, W. D. (2008). Priming the motor system enhances the effects of upper limb therapy in chronic stroke. *Brain, 131*(5), 1381–1390.

Stinear, C. M., Barber, P. A., Smale, P. R., Coxon, J. P., Fleming, M. K., & Byblow, W. D. (2007). Functional potential in chronic stroke patients depends on corticospinal tract integrity. *Brain, 130*, 170–180.

Strong, K., Mathers, C., & Bonita, R. (2007). Preventing stroke: Saving lives around the world. *Lancet Neurology, 6*(2), 182–187.

Taub, E. (1980). Somatosensory deafferentation research with monkeys: implications for rehabilitation medicine. In L. P. Ince (Ed.), *Behavioral psychology in rehabilitation medicine: Clinical applications* (pp. 371–401). Baltimore: Williams & Wilkins.

Taub, E., Uswatte, G., & Elbert, T. (2002). New treatments in neurorehabilitation founded on basic research. *Nature Reviews Neuroscience, 3*(3), 228–236.

Taub, E., Uswatte, G., Mark, V. W., & Morris, D. M. (2006). The learned nonuse phenomenon: implications for rehabilitation. *Eura Medicophys, 42*(3), 241–256.

Taub, E., Uswatte, G., & Pidikiti, R. (1999). Constraint-induced movement therapy: a new family of techniques with broad application to physical rehabilitation—a clinical review. *Journal of Rehabilitation Research and Development, 36*, 237–251.

Tecchio, F., Zappasodi, F., Tombini, M., Caulo, M., Vernieri, F., & Rossini, P. M. (2007). Interhemispheric asymmetry of primary hand representation and recovery after stroke: a MEG study. *Neuroimage, 36*(4), 1057–1064.

Wittenberg, G. F., Chen, R., Ishii, K., Bushara, K. O., Eckloff, S., Croarkin, E., et al. (2003). Constraint-induced therapy in stroke: magnetic-stimulation motor maps and cerebral activation. *Neurorehabilitation and Neural Repair, 17*, 48–57.

Wolf, S., Winstein, C., Miller, J., et al. (2006). Effect of constraint induced movement therapy on upper extremity function among patients 3–9 months following stroke: The EXCITE randomized clinical trial. *Journal of the American Medical Association, 296*, 2095–2104.

Zhang, J. X., & Kourtzi, Z. (2010). Learning-dependent plasticity with and without training in the human brain. *Proceedings of the National Academy of Sciences of the United States of America, 107*(30), 13503–13508.

Zihl, J. (1981). Recovery of visual functions in patients with cerebral blindness: Effect of specific practice with saccadic localization. *Experimental Brain Research, 44*, 159–169.

2 | STROKE REHABILITATION: A LEARNING PERSPECTIVE

LEEANNE M. CAREY, HELENE J. POLATAJKO, LISA TABOR CONNOR, and CAROLYN M. BAUM

2.1 STROKE REHABILITATION: FACILITATION OF ADAPTIVE LEARNING

A learning-based approach to stroke rehabilitation is consistent with the specialty of neurorehabilitation. *Neurorehabilitation* is a term now in common use. It is defined as "the clinical subspecialty that is devoted to the restoration and maximization of functions that have been lost due to impairments caused by an injury or disease to the nervous system" (Selzer, Clarke, Cohen, Duncan, & Gage, 2006). A key element of this definition is the restoration of functions that may be affected by the impairment. In the literature, the term *recovery* has been used both to refer to the restoration of damaged systems and behavioral functions, and to describe clinical improvements regardless of how these may have occurred (Levin, Kleim, & Wolf, 2009). The focus of active learning approaches is on the restoration and maximization of damaged systems and behavioral functions. Ideally, recovery will span clinically significant and objectively measured improvements for a profile of outcomes.

Rehabilitation informed by neuroscience and learning may view outcomes related to restoration using a framework that spans interrelated levels and functions (Baum, 2011). Functions can be considered in relation to the brain, behavior, performance and participation of the individual. The restoration or maximization of these functions may span a number of levels that include: molecular/cellular mechanisms, such as synaptic plasticity; biomedical mechanisms, such as motor inhibition and functional connectivity of the brain; body function/body structure, such as touch sensation and action; functional limitations, such as grasp; activities, such as writing; and participation in tasks and roles that use these functions, such as family, work, and community life.

We propose a definition of rehabilitation that includes "facilitation of adaptive learning." This definition is founded on compelling evidence that neural changes occur in the adult human brain as a result of learning and following injury. This phenomenon, often referred to as "neural plasticity," acknowledges the capacity of the brain to learn new ways of achieving lost functions (Nudo, 2007; Kolb, Teskey, & Gibb, 2010). This differs from the previously held belief that the brain was "hard wired" and did not have capacity for repair and regeneration. Learning is a central part of the process, as discussed below. The proposed definition also recognizes that neural plastic changes facilitated by rehabilitation are required to be adaptive, given evidence of both adaptive and maladaptive plasticity.

Neural plastic changes are enhanced by experience and learning (Nudo, 2007; Kolb et al., 2010). One of the most potent modulators of cortical structure and function is behavioral experience, consistent with a learning-dependent model of plasticity. There is clear evidence from animal studies that experience and training are critical ingredients for neural plastic changes. For example, Nudo et al. (Nudo, Wise, SiFuentes, & Milliken, 1996) reported shrinkage of motor representation of the hand area of the brain in primates that did not receive rehabilitation compared to an extension of the motor representation in those who did receive task-specific motor training that was associated with functional recovery. Neural plastic changes may also involve reorganization and rerouting of intracortical pathways to completely novel territories (Nudo, 2007). Again the "post-injury behavioral experience appears to be critical to the reassembly of adaptive modules" (Nudo, 2007), highlighting the importance of skill training and learning in facilitating neural plastic changes.

In humans, evidence from functional imaging studies indicates that specific interventions can lead to changes in the brain associated with improved outcomes after stroke (Hodics, Cohen, & Cramer, 2006; L. M. Carey & Seitz, 2007; Rossini et al., 2007; Richards, Stewart, Woodbury, Senesac, & Cauraugh, 2008). Specific training paradigms have included constraint-induced movement therapy (Dong, Dobkin, Cen, Wu, & Winstein, 2006), task-oriented motor training (Nelles, Jentzen, Jueptner, Muller, & Diener, 2001; J. R. Carey et al., 2002), and constraint induced aphasia treatment (Meinzer et al., 2004; Pulvermüller, Hauk, Zohsel, Neininger, & Mohr, 2005). While the evidence is currently based on relatively small numbers, it does constitute proof of principle, demonstrating the potential for neural plastic changes associated with clinically effective interventions and recovery. Together this evidence provides new, long-term hope for stroke survivors and a foundation for more restorative approaches to rehabilitation.

Despite this potential the translation of these approaches into clinical practice has been limited and slow (Cheeran et al., 2009), and rehabilitation often involves use of compensatory strategies (Levin et al., 2009) rather than aiming for restoration of functions through learning or relearning. For example, a compensatory approach may involve teaching an individual to perform a task via use of adaptive equipment or use of the non-affected limb. While the approach may have a benefit in terms of increased independence, this approach may also have negative consequences; for example, the person may learn not to use their affected limb. This "learned non-use" may be viewed as an example of maladaptive plasticity relative to goals of restoration of function. A more active or "restorative" rehabilitation approach would involve learning or relearning to use the affected function in the context of the task for which it would normally be required. In this approach parts of the central nervous system are retrained to engage lost functions (Cheeran et al., 2009).

A model of stroke rehabilitation based on neuroscience and learning requires identification and recognition of core principles that underlie change. We propose the **Rehabilitation Learning Model** (**Rehab-Learn**) of stroke rehabilitation (described in detail below). In this model we define rehabilitation as "an active process focused on facilitation of adaptive learning." We propose that learning or relearning is central to rehabilitation. Rehabilitation happens after loss of performance capabilities, and the focus of rehabilitation, or neurorehabilitation, would most optimally be on restoring those capabilities. Much of performance is skill based; therefore, these skills need to be reacquired; relearned or learned in a new way. As clinicians we aim to facilitate change. The additional element clinicians bring to rehabilitation is the facilitated learning. The question for us as rehabilitation specialists and researchers is: How can we **build on** and **shape** the ability of the brain to adapt and learn after injury such as a stroke?

2.2 A COMMON LANGUAGE FOR REHABILITATION SCIENCE

Rehabilitation science contributes knowledge to employ rehabilitation and habilitation approaches with individuals whose lives are compromised by impairments or potentially disabling conditions. Advances in rehabilitation science are shaping new rehabilitation interventions. A multimodal approach is likely to be beneficial (Chapter 3) and addresses brain network, movement, sensation, cognition, language, and mood outcomes that impact performance in daily activities and participation. The knowledge to impact these systems will be generated by scientists who study mechanisms at different levels.

For basic and rehabilitation scientists and clinicians to be effective in achieving the goal of neuroscience-founded rehabilitation we need to take some time to define the shared values and science that we bring to the task, as well as the language we can use to best communicate these ideas. Table 2.1 is a rehabilitation language table that was constructed to help scientists see where their work fits

TABLE 2.1 The Language of Rehabilitation Science

BIOMEDICAL MOLECULAR/CELLULAR MECHANISMS	BIOMEDICAL MECHANISMS	BODY FUNCTION/ BODY STRUCTURE	FUNCTIONAL LIMITATIONS	ACTIVITY	PARTICIPATION	ENVIRONMENT
• Plasticity • Synapse • Receptor • Neurotrophic Factors • Neurotransmitters • Neuromodulators	• Attentional Control • Motor Inhibition • Anatomical Connectivity • Pattern Recognition • Cerebellar Activation • Motor Control • Metabolism • Sleep	• Executive Function • Vision/Audition • Mood • Motivational State • Motor Planning • Language • Attention • Arousal • Sleep	• Gait • Strength • Postural Control • Grasp/Pinch • Problem Solving • Range • Mobility • Endurance	• Stair Climbing • Standing • Writing • Dressing • Grooming/ Hygiene • Walking • Listening • Learning	• Education • Work • Community Life • Recreation/ Leisure • Religion/ Spirituality • Civic Life • Child Care	• Social Support • Social Capital • Assistive Technology • Workplace Accommodations • Receptivity • Access to Services

SOURCE: From Baum, 2011 with permission from Elsevier.

into rehabilitation. Some scientists work at the biomedical molecular-cellular mechanism level and others along a continuum that eventually rests at the sociocultural level of environment. In rehabilitation we are all interested in improving the human condition. In rehabilitation, that human condition is known as *participation*: participation in home, work, leisure, and community life.

The complexity of rehabilitation science is that when a person has a neurological injury there is not one single impairment or mechanism interrupted. In stroke we see people with primary language, primary sensory, primary motor, and/or primary cognitive impairments. Most patients have multiple impairments, and there are psychological factors that relate to any or all of these conditions. For these reasons we address the language of rehabilitation science. We also seek out interventions that ensure that patients and their families have the knowledge they need to manage the consequences of stroke in both the acute and chronic phases of recovery.

2.3 EXPERIENCE AND LEARNING-DEPENDENT PLASTICITY: IMPLICATIONS FOR REHABILITATION

There are a number of terms used in relation to plasticity: synaptic plasticity, experience-dependent plasticity; use-dependent plasticity; activity-dependent plasticity, and learning-dependent plasticity. Donald Hebb described a basic mechanism for synaptic plasticity, wherein an increase in synaptic efficacy arises from the presynaptic cell's repeated and persistent stimulation of the postsynaptic cell (http://en.wikipedia.org/wiki/Hebbian_theory; retrieved August 20, 2011). The theory is commonly summarized as "cells that fire together, wire together" (Doidge, 2007). It attempts to explain "associative learning," where simultaneous activation of cells leads to increases in synaptic strength between the cells. The idea is that the previous history of each synapse's activity determines its current plasticity. Such learning is known as *Hebbian learning*.

Use-dependent plasticity, also referred to as experience-dependent or activity-dependent plasticity, involves the strengthening of existing neural connections and formation of new connections. These neural plastic changes are founded on changes in long-term potentiation (LTP) and long-term depression (LTD) that underlie learning (Hess & Donoghue, 1996). The efficacy of synaptic connections is modifiable in an activity-dependent manner, resulting in long-term potentiation (LTP; Abraham, 2008). Activity-dependent plasticity (http://en.wikipedia.org/wiki/Activity-dependent_plasticity, retrieved August 23, 2011), also referred to as *metaplasticity* (Abraham, 2008), plays a large role in learning and in the ability to understand new things. It is responsible for helping to adapt an individual's brain according to the relative amount of usage

and functioning. In essence, the brain's ability to retain and develop memories based on activity-driven changes of synaptic strength allows strong learning of information. It is thought to be the growing and adapting quality of dendritic spines that provide the basis for synaptic plasticity connected to learning and memory (Sala, Cambianica, & Rossi, 2008). Direct manipulation of motor and sensory experience can modify brain plasticity and functional outcome after experimental lesions (Walker-Batson, Smith, Curtis, & Unwin, 2004).

Learning-dependent plasticity has the additional elements of being goal-driven and task-oriented. It involves active problem solving, is responsive to environmental demands, and may be necessary for functional reorganization of cortical maps. Evidence from animal studies showed that neural plastic changes in cortical maps was only present following motor skill learning of a more difficult task compared to repeated practice of a simple task (Plautz, Milliken, & Nudo, 2000). Repetitive motor activity alone did not produce functional reorganization of cortical maps; instead, researchers proposed that motor skill acquisition (motor learning) was a prerequisite factor in driving plasticity in primary motor cortex. Similarly, plasticity of primary somatosensory cortex paralleled sensorimotor skill recovery from stroke in adult monkeys (Xerri, Merzenich, Peterson, & Jenkins, 1998). Thus the behavioral experience that induces long-term plasticity in motor and sensory maps after brain injury appears to be limited to experiences that involve the development of new skills (Walker-Batson et al., 2004).

Similar associations between motor learning and neural plasticity have also been inferred in human studies (Hallett, 2001). For example, brain representations of the finger muscles used in Braille are significantly enlarged in Braille readers compared to blind, non–Braille reading controls (Chen, Cohen, & Hallett, 2002). Different patterns of plastic changes in the brain have been described under conditions of frequent exposure alone, compared to task-specific learning of specific visual functions (Zhang & Kourtzi, 2010). The latter implicates brain regions involved in attention and learning and has been described as *learning-dependent plasticity*.

In the application of this knowledge to rehabilitation, pioneers in neural plasticity through to current-day scientists and clinical researchers have all stressed the importance of training to obtain functional recovery following brain injury (Bach-y-Rita, 1980a; Moore, 1980; Finger & Stein, 1982; Nudo et al., 1996; Kolb et al., 2010). Key elements, such as forced use with guided practice of the affected limb and intensive training, have been positively correlated with return of function (Wolf et al., 2006; French et al., 2007). Task-specific training has also been shown to facilitate the development of skills such as motor control and perceptual discrimination abilities. For example, Zihl and Von Cramon (Zihl & Von Cramon, 1979;

Zihl, 1981) reported recovery of visual functions such as contrast sensitivity and visual acuity following systematic, intensive practice in localization of visual stimuli along the impaired visual field border coupled with anticipatory information on the targets to be presented. Factors such as motivation, an enriched environment, active participation, and functional demand on the system have also been advocated to facilitate recovery (Bach-y-Rita, 1980b; Kolb et al., 2010; Cramer et al., 2011).

In healthy individuals, the brain can be altered by a wide variety of experiences throughout the lifespan, including sensory and motor experiences, task learning, motivation, stress, rewards, aging, diet, hormones, drugs, neurotrophic factors, and electrical stimulation (Kolb et al., 2010). However, we cannot assume that the normal and injured brain respond in the same way to the same experience (Kolb et al., 2010). Some experiences can also produce maladaptive plastic changes in the brain. For example, recent research has implicated maladaptive plasticity as the cause of some varieties of tinnitus (Engineer et al., 2011). Noise exposure is thought to modify the frequency map in primary auditory cortex. Some success has been reported in treating tinnitus with frequency-notched musical exposure, in effect remapping the auditory frequency map by facilitating adaptive learning (Okamoto, Stracke, Stoll, & Pantev, 2010).

There is emerging evidence that the rules governing plasticity are distinctly different in different cerebral regions and are time dependent (Kolb et al., 2010). Whereas the sensory and motor regions show large long-term changes in response to complex housing, the prefrontal regions show only transient changes that disappear after a few days (Kolb, Gorny, Soderpalm, & Robinson, 2003; Comeau, McDonald, & Kolb, 2010; Kolb et al., 2010). This has important implications for designing therapies based on not only where the injury is, but also the integrity of interconnected networks and the time post-stroke. For example, prefrontal regions may be accessed early via goal-directed attention, planning, and prediction of thoughts and actions, functions known to be associated with this region, in order to facilitate access to primary regions that may have been affected by the infarct. Repeated focus may need to be given to involvement of these regions given the transient nature of the plasticity observed.

2.4 ROLE OF BRAIN NETWORKS IN INFORMATION PROCESSING AND RECOVERY

One of the foundation principles of neuroscience is that neurons do not function in isolation. They are organized into neural networks that act together (Purves et al., 2004). The neural networks of the brain process information impinging upon the organism through sensory systems such as those responsible for seeing, hearing, sensing temperature, and so forth. Neural networks are also responsible for producing responses to those inputs via a neural network to accomplish movement. Early investigations supposed that neural circuits were able to be relatively isolated; for example, that the visual system was made up of subsystems that perform specific operations. This may be true to an extent in primary sensory areas of the brain, but neuroscientists have learned that even the systems in primary sensory areas are quite complex, as pointed out famously by Felleman and VanEssen (Felleman & Van Essen, 1991) in their wiring diagram of the visual system. Despite the complexity of the system, some core organizational principles were revealed. In sensory and motor systems, the brain is organized such that relevant features of the environment or body are preserved in the neural circuitry. The primary visual cortex has a map of the visual environment with spatial information about the world being represented. Distortions in that cortical map include enlarged representations relative to expected representations from peripheral receptors (Hubel & Wiesel, 1962).

With the advent of neuroimaging, it has become easier to investigate how these well-understood, elementary sensory and motor systems are connected into broader systems that include regions not as well studied. Functional neuroimaging studies have revealed that primary sensory areas of the brain are modulated by more cognitive regions of the brain (Shulman et al., 1997; Boly et al., 2007). Larger networks in which neurons fire together in correlated patterns, uncovered through functional MRI connectivity studies, correspond to what scientists have learned through human brain lesion studies (Fox, Snyder, Vincent, & Raichle, 2007). The evolution of neuroscience to include the examination of network functions is an exciting development for neurorehabilitation, as we now have a noninvasive method for uncovering changes in the plasticity of these systems as patients recover from neurological insults (He, Shulman, Snyder, & Corbetta, 2007). Using these tools we may soon be able to investigate how specific therapies affect neural systems in individual patients.

2.5 SKILL ACQUISITION—A LEARNING PERSPECTIVE

A primary goal post-stroke is to regain the functions or skills that were lost as a result of the stroke. Present-day perspectives on the acquisition, or reacquisition, of skills is that skills, even motor-based skills, are learned; to quote Gentile, "learning processes mediate acquisition of functional skills" (Gentile, 1998, p. 7). Learning is defined "as an enduring change in behavior or in capacity to behave in a given fashion, which results from practice or other forms of experience" (Shuell, 1986). Learning is always the responsibility of the learner or, in the case of neurorehabilitation, the patient (Gentile, 1998). The role of the neurorehabilitation clinician is to promote learning.

The literature on learning is immense. It emanates from several disciplines including education, psychology, human movement science and, more laterally, rehabilitation. As well, the literature offers several perspectives on learning, including behavioral, social, cognitive, and ecological (Shumway-Cook & Woollacott, 2012). Taken together, it offers a wealth of information, albeit at times contradictory, on learning and how to promote it. The emerging literatures in neuroscience and neuroimaging point to particular elements of learning that have particular potency in optimizing adaptive neural plasticity. These, in turn, suggest differing approaches therapists can use to promote functional skill learning. Accordingly, to promote learning, intervention is recommended to be explicit, task-specific, and goal-driven; involve active problem solving; and be responsive to environmental demands; and provide opportunities for variation and practice.

There are numerous techniques available to clinicians for promoting learning; what follows are only a few, chosen for their relevance to promoting the elements of functional skill learning that, as discussed above, have been identified as germane to adaptive neural plasticity.

2.5.1 EXPLICIT, TASK-SPECIFIC, AND GOAL-DRIVEN

These three elements have been grouped as they all refer to the target of learning and are interrelated. Together they represent the starting point for skill learning. Much of the current literature suggests that intervention for individuals with functional problems that have a motor component should be task-oriented; in other words, task-specific and explicit (Shumway-Cook & Woollacott, 2012). A number of features need to be considered in this regard: which task, who chooses the task, the nature of the task, specific training techniques and, as relevant, whole or part training and in what sequence.

To promote learning, the task is recommended to have real world relevance for the client and be a task the client wants to or needs to perform. It can be beneficial for the task to be chosen by the client, or at least in collaboration with the client, as they alone know the relevance of the task for their world and the motivation for performing it. Once chosen, the task and its performance need to be considered, as the nature of the task affects performance. Consideration is given to the complexity of the task and areas of performance breakdown. To facilitate identification of performance breakdown, tools such as dynamic performance analysis (Polatajko, Mandich, & Martini, 2000) are useful. In relation to complexity, various aspects of the task are considered including body orientation, object manipulation, task structure, and the environment

(Figure 2.1). Knowledge of these can be used to provide a framework for structuring explicit task-specific learning (Shumway-Cook & Woollacott, 2012).

Once the specifics of what is to be learned are clear, a number of techniques can be used to promote explicit, skill-specific learning. These include:

Shaping, the technique of reinforcing successive approximations of the desired skill. Shaping is used when the desired skill or behavior does not yet exist, but some approximation can be performed.

Chaining, the technique of reinforcing steps that make up the desired skill in sequence. Chaining is used when a behavior or skill has multiple steps that need to be performed in succession. Chaining can be done forward (each step of the skill is taught in chronological sequence) or backward (the steps are taught in reverse sequence).

Fading, the gradual removal, over a number of learning trials, of a prompt or some other stimulus that has supported skill performance. Fading is used when learning has been supported by aids that are not part of the task itself. Fading goes hand in hand with chaining and shaping, and should accompany the use of other well-known therapeutic techniques such as handling, physical support, or hand-over-hand, each of which must be faded out if independent skill performance is to be learned.

Prompting, the act of providing a cue to help initiate the desired performance. Prompts are used to elicit the desired performance and are given in immediate proximity, temporal or geographic, to the performance, often in conjunction with shaping and chaining to enhance learning. When using prompts, care needs to be taken to use prompts that are readily available to the individual or to fade the prompt once the desired behavior or skill is established.

Modeling, the demonstration of a skill or part of a skill. Modeling is used when the desired skill does

Level of Complexity			
LOW			HIGH
Body Orientation	Stability		Transportation
Object Manipulation	Absent		Present
Task Structure	Discrete	Serial	Continuous
Environment	Stationary	in Motion	Variability

Figure 2.1 Motor Performance Complexity. From Polatajko & Mandich, 2004, with permission.

not yet exist, or when a complex skill does not yet exist in its entirety. It is effective in promoting learning if attention is drawn to salient features of the skill that are to be imitated.

Verbal guidance, the act of providing direct verbal instruction to support performance. It can be provided by the therapist, or by the client him/herself.

Direct teaching, the act of providing direct instruction on task performance. It is used when the client does not have sufficient task knowledge to perform the task. This often takes the form of specific verbal or written information.

Learning is affected by its consequences, specifically by reinforcement and feedback, which are closely associated.

Reinforcement is the provision of a reinforcer when the desired skill is performed. A reinforcer is any stimulus that follows a response and increases the likelihood of that response occurring again. Reinforcers can be extrinsic, such as praise or money, or intrinsic, such as food or the feeling of success; wherever possible, intrinsic reinforcers are recommended to be used.

Feedback is the provision of information regarding performance post hoc. Feedback is closely associated with reinforcement. The feedback can act as a verbal reinforcer, especially when it is a specific, realistic positive statement about how well the performance is doing. Feedback is essential for motor learning. There are several types of feedback that can be used to enhance the learning process.

2.5.2 INVOLVE ACTIVE PROBLEM SOLVING, AND BE RESPONSIVE TO ENVIRONMENTAL DEMANDS

Cognitive perspectives on learning point to the importance of strategies to support the learning process. Learning involves number of processes starting with the acquisition of new performance strategies that are chosen for their effectiveness from among a number of alternatives, with increasing reliance on the most effective strategies and their increasingly fast, accurate, and effortless execution (Siegler, 2004). Problem-solving strategies actively engage the client in the identification of performance strategies. Problem solving is the ability to combine previously learned knowledge in a new way to solve a new problem.

Specific techniques to support active problem solving include:

Problem-solving strategy, a cognitive tool that supports the process of problem solving. A number of

strategies have been identified to support problem solving; among them is Meichenbaum's GOAL-PLAN-DO-CHECK, which is the centerpiece of the Cognitive Orientation to daily Occupational Performance (CO-OP) approach described below (Polatajko & Mandich, 2004).

Guided discovery is the act of leading the client step by step in the discovery of strategies to solve performance problems. It is used to actively engage the client in the learning process; it supports problem solving and convergent thinking.

Problem-solving strategies, as other executive strategies, are important for generalization and transfer of learning—key issues within a learning paradigm (Shumway-Cook & Woollacott, 2012). *Generalization* refers to the degree that a specific skill, learned in a specific context, can be performed in another context. *Transfer of learning* refers to the degree to which learning one skill influences the learning of another skill. Achieving generalization and transfer is important to ensure that learning is responsive to the environment, such that the client can draw on previous experiences to perform the same or similar skills in a new context. Generalization can be improved by varying the conditions under which something is learned, making sure it is well learned, practicing the skill in a variety of contexts, progressively approximating the context for generalization, and ensuring motivation for performance is high (Shumway-Cook & Woollacott, 2012). Transfer can be promoted in much the same way as generalization.

2.5.3 PROVIDE OPPORTUNITIES FOR VARIATION AND PRACTICE

Variation and practice both support generalization and transfer, and consolidate and fine-tune learning (Shumway-Cook & Woollacott, 2012). There are several ways to arrange practice schedules (Shumway-Cook & Woollacott, 2012). Each is known to impact learning in a different way. In general, practice variability promotes learning and retention. Practice can be *random*, where conditions on each trial vary, or it can be *blocked*, where conditions remain the same across trials. With the latter, learning is quicker, but with the former retention is longer and generalization and transfer are facilitated (Shumway-Cook & Woollacott, 2012). It can be *massed*, where there are many repetitions in succession, or *distributed*, where there is rest between practices. The former is best for discrete skills, while the latter is more effective than massed practice when the physical demands are high, or when the skill is complex or motivation is low (Magill, 1998). Further practice can be *whole*, where the skill is practiced in its entirety, or *in part*, where the task is broken down and practiced in part. The former is beneficial for discrete tasks that are quick to perform, the latter for more complex, protracted tasks (Shumway-Cook & Woollacott, 2012). The latter requires that chaining techniques be used to bring the parts together.

2.6 APPLICATION IN CONTEXT OF RECOVERY AFTER STROKE

Learning is synonymous with neural plastic changes in the brain. The question for clinicians and researchers is how we can best facilitate this learning in an individual with brain injury. Rehabilitation focused on learning and relearning of skills and functions provides an ongoing window of opportunity to facilitate positive adaptive changes in the brain and recovery. It may be viewed as a trigger to facilitate plasticity. The behavioral experience and learning conditions provided in rehabilitation need to be designed to shape neural plastic changes to achieve meaningful outcomes for the individual. Common core and function-specific active learning strategies that may be used are outlined in section 2.7 below.

Adjunct therapies that may enhance training-induced cognitive and motor learning, such as brain stimulation and neuropharmacological interventions, have also been identified (Cramer et al., 2011; see also Chapters 3 and 10). As promising as these therapies may be, they are focused on modulating the brain systems underlying learning rather than producing behavioral changes themselves. These therapies may change the underlying neurotransmitter balance or cause the receptivity of the neural systems to change. Clinicians still need to provide the learning opportunities to effect the changes that will maximize recovery of functional abilities. It is critical that we do not lose sight of the learning goal and the conditions that are known to facilitate learning and neural plasticity.

While in the non–brain damaged person learning may occur spontaneously with exposure to specific stimuli, there is evidence that this may not always be the case following brain damage (L. M. Carey, Matyas, & Oke, 1993). Facilitated, active learning has been shown to achieve positive outcomes. For example, approaches that are founded on studies of learning in non–brain damaged individuals have shown improved motor performance and functional skills following stroke (J. R. Carey et al., 2002; French et al., 2007; McEwen, Polatajko, Huijbregts, & Ryan, 2009; Henshaw, Polatajko, McEwen, Ryan, & Baum, 2011). Similarly, a perceptual learning-based approach to sensory rehabilitation has shown to be effective (L. M. Carey et al., 1993; L. M. Carey, Macdonnell, & Matyas, 2011). Knowledge of optimal conditions of training and how they impact learning and neural changes in distributed networks provide the basis for a learning-based approach to rehabilitation. In the coming years, rehabilitation researchers need to further investigate and elucidate the principles for opti-

mizing relearning after stroke to enhance the delivery of effective neurorehabilitation. The extent to which we can guide patients to access residual networks in the brain with capacity for plasticity is paramount to ongoing and self-mediated recovery.

2.7 REHABILITATION LEARNING MODEL: REHAB-LEARN

We propose a model of rehabilitation that highlights the central role of learning and relearning in recovery after stroke. The **Rehab**ilitation **Learn**ing Model, **Rehab-Learn** (Figure 2.2) has a number of key elements, as described below:

The gap: The Rehab-Learn model identifies learning and relearning as a central concept to help bridge the gap between *brain function* and *function in everyday life* following stroke. *Rehabilitation* is the vehicle to facilitate adaptive neural plastic changes primarily through application of learning strategies; the focus of *Rehab-Learn*. The goal is to improve neuroperformance skills—such as movement, sensation, cognition, and language—that support performance of the everyday activities of living. This learning is achieved taking into account the *environment and context of learning* and may also be facilitated by adjunctive therapies such as *pharmacological and stimulation approaches*. The focus of the Rehab-Learn model is on rehabilitation-facilitated change rather than spontaneous recovery or healing.

Learning Strategies/Principles: Rehabilitation-facilitated learning is explicit, in comparison to more implicit learning. There are common-core and skill-specific principles

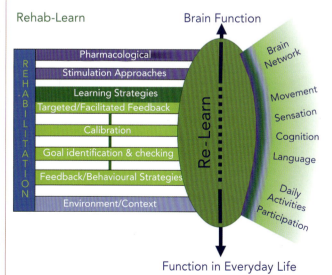

Figure 2.2 The **Rehab**ilitation **Learn**ing Model: **Rehab-Learn**

and strategies that are identified as being important in facilitation of adaptive learning. The *core active learning principles* include: Motivated, Goal Directed, Practice, Intensive, Graded, and Variation. Motivation is important in learning and in recovery after brain injury (Bachy-Rita, 1980a; Johansson, 2011; also Chapter 8) and the brain responds to meaningful goals (Nudo et al., 1996) and rewards (Pleger, Blankenburg, Ruff, Driver, & Dolan, 2008). Goal-directed learning aids the modulation of attention, which has an important role in learning and in inducing cortical plasticity (Jagadeesh, 2006; Chapter 14). The anterior cingulate cortex and orbitofrontal cortex have been proposed as key regions linking attention, emotion, and motivation (Raymond, 2009). Practice and intensity of training are important on the basis that repetition over time, with an increasing number of coincident events, serves to strengthen synaptic connections (Merzenich & Kaas, 1982; Byl & Merzenich, 2000; also Chapter 9). Graded progression facilitates differentiation, especially of complex stimuli (Goldstone, 1998). Variation of task and training conditions is important to facilitate transfer of training effects (Schmidt & Lee, 2005).

Skill-specific learning processes, such as targeted or facilitated feedback, calibration, goal identification and checking, and use of behavioral strategies are elements of the learning process that are linked to learning-based rehabilitation of specific functions. For example, *targeted or facilitated feedback* is important in a cognitive-based approach to motor learning and executive function; *calibration* within and across modalities is critical in perceptual learning of sensory functions; *goal identification and checking* is important to learning of executive functions; *feedback and behavioral strategies* are important in language training. Examples of how these specific strategies are used in training are provided below. Chapters 11 to 16 will elaborate further on these principles and review evidence of the neuroscience foundations related to treatment of these functions.

Environment/Context: The environment and situated learning are also important elements in the process. An enriched environment has been associated with better recovery after experimental stroke (Janssen et al., 2010), and it is suggested that multisensory training protocols better approximate natural settings and are more effective for learning in healthy subjects (Shams & Seitz, 2008; Johansson, 2011; Chapter 3). Neuroscience evidence supports the importance of the environment in learning, including in adulthood. For example, violinists have enlarged neural representations for their left fingers (Elbert, Pantev, Wienbruch, Rockstroh, & Taub, 1995) and London taxi drivers who learn street maps in intense detail demonstrate enlarged representations in brain regions responsible for spatial representation and navigation (Maguire et al., 2000). This type of plasticity involves environment-specific learning in complex environments. Situated learning is

learning that takes place in the same context in which it is applied (http://en.wikipedia.org/wiki/Situated_learning; retrieved 3rd October 3, 2011). Lave and Wegner (1991) argue that learning as it normally occurs is a function of the activity, context, and culture in which it occurs (i.e., it is *situated*). Observation of actions embedded in context may also impact on motor learning via the "mirror neuron" system, and has been associated with increased activation in premotor cortex using fMRI compared to observing actions without a context (Iacoboni & Dapretto, 2006). The clinician has an important role in enabling the learning environment and providing cues that may facilitate the learning to occur. The types of human cues can be verbal prompts, gestural prompts, direct verbal guidance, or physical assistance (Baum et al., 2008). Environmental cues range from the use of Post-it notes and personal data technology (e.g., PDAs), signage, objects, organized work stations. These are all tools that most people use; they become critical tools for individuals that require cues to maintain their daily routines because of brain injury.

Adjunct therapies: Pharmacological and stimulation approaches, such as transcranial magnetic stimulation (TMS) and cortical brain stimulation, have been demonstrated to have a positive effect on use dependent plasticity (Chapters 3 and 10). They may be viewed as therapies to use in conjunction with experience and learning-based behavioral interventions (Chapter 10). It is anticipated that a combination of therapies are likely to maximize outcomes and plasticity.

Outcomes: The Rehab-Learn model identifies a profile of outcomes important in measuring rehabilitation effectiveness and in understanding the link between brain function and function in everyday life. For example, it is expected that learning-dependent changes will impact brain networks. Changes in brain networks may be measured using tools such as MRI, as outlined in Chapter 4. Clinical outcomes span performance capacities such as movement, sensation, cognition, and language, through to daily life activities and participation. Cognitive capacities of importance include specific functions that may have been affected by the stroke, such as executive function and spatial attention, as well as those that are core to learning, attention, and memory. The extent to which improvements are specific to the capacity/task trained, or transfer to novel stimuli/tasks trained, is critical (see Chapter 9). The goal is improvement in performance in the activities of everyday living and return to participation in activities and life roles important to the individual.

2.8 SELECTED LEARNING-BASED APPROACHES TO REHABILITATION

A number of learning-based approaches to rehabilitation have been developed. A small selection of these are outlined below and evaluated in the context of the Rehab-Learn model. Specific learning strategies applied in these programs are highlighted.

2.8.1 COGNITIVE ORIENTATION TO DAILY OCCUPATIONAL PERFORMANCE (CO-OP)

Cognitive **O**rientation to daily **O**ccupational **P**erformance, **CO-OP** is "a client-centred, performance-based, problem solving, approach that enables skill acquisition through a process of strategy use and guided discovery" (Polatajko & Mandich, 2004, p. 2). The approach draws on cognition (*Cognitive Orientation to …*), most especially cognitive strategy use, to enhance performance in the everyday activities of living (… *daily Occupational Performance*). As the name, in brief, implies, the CO-OP approach is a collaborative one, where the client is required to actively participate in solving performance problems and work with the therapist to identify plans to meet performance goals. To quote one client, "There's a real plan here, and I am responsible for that plan" (McEwen, Polatajko, Davis, Huijbregts, & Ryan, 2010, p. 540). Consistent with client-centeredness, the performance goals addressed—that is, the skills to be acquired—are those identified as important by the client. Skill acquisition is achieved through the use of a global problem-solving strategy and a number of domain-specific strategies. The former is directly taught to the client; the therapist guides the client in the discovery and evaluation of the latter.

A task-oriented approach, CO-OP is embedded in a learning paradigm. It is derived from a combination of learning, motor learning, and cognitive-behavioral theories, and was designed to enable skill acquisition and strategy use, generalization to the real world, and transfer to new skills. A key and unique feature of CO-OP is its approach to skill acquisition. Rather than using direct skill training, CO-OP uses guided discovery, an approach whereby the clinician uses specific techniques to actively engage the client in creating his or her own strategies for problem solving. It guides the client to analyze his/her own performance and to notice problems, identify potential strategy solutions, evaluate them, and identify and test alternatives.

Originally developed for use with children with motor-based performance problems (Polatajko, Mandich, Miller, & Macnab, 2001), CO-OP has a number of features that suggest that it will be useful as a neurorehabilitation approach for individuals who have had a stroke; for example, CO-OP is goal-driven, activity-based, explicit, and involves task-specific learning, active participation, and problem solving. A number of recent studies have supported its use with this population, providing evidence of improved skill acquisition (McEwen et al., 2009; Henshaw et al., 2011) and transfer (McEwen, Polatajko, Huijbregts, & Ryan, 2010). A small pilot study has indi-

cated that it may be more effective than standard intervention (Polatajko, McEwen, Ryan, & Baum, 2012). New evidence also suggests that the approach improves self-regulation in both children (Hyland & Polatajko, 2011) and adults (Schneiderman, McEwen, Kinslikh, & Polatajko, 2008). The approach may also be used to facilitate skill acquisition in people who experience executive function problems, as described in Chapter 15. Taken together, the evidence suggests that CO-OP may be a useful approach for building on and shaping the ability of the brain to adapt and learn after injury such as a stroke, and that it may support activity and learning-dependent plasticity.

2.8.2 SENSᴇ: A PERCEPTUAL LEARNING APPROACH TO REHABILITATION OF BODY SENSATIONS AFTER STROKE

The SENSe approach to sensory rehabilitation is consistent with the Rehab-Learn model of rehabilitation. **SENSe** (**S**tudy of the **E**ffectiveness of **N**eurorehabilitation on **Se**nsation) is a rehabilitation intervention shown to be effective in improving discrimination of body sensations after stroke (L. M. Carey et al., 2011). The SENSe approach is based on perceptual learning, consistent with "learning-dependent" neural plasticity (L. M. Carey, 2006) and is designed to facilitate transfer of training effects to novel stimuli (L. M. Carey & Matyas, 2005).

Learning is central to the program and is operationalized in the procedures used in training. The program includes both the core principles of active learning as well as function-specific principles, such as calibration (L. M. Carey et al., 1993; L. M. Carey, 2006; L. M. Carey et al., 2011). Calibration is a key element of the training. It requires the individual to calibrate his or her impaired touch sensation internally by reference to a more normal touch sensation experienced through the "unaffected" hand (intramodal calibration) and via vision (cross-modal calibration). When two modalities are trained at the same time and provide feedback for each other, a higher level of performance is possible than if they remained independent (Becker, 1996). In addition, cross-modal plasticity in sensory systems may facilitate alternate and new neural connections (Sathian, 2006), and visual cortical activity is regularly associated with the neural processing of tactile inputs (Sathian, 2005). Core principles associated with learning include use of goal-directed tasks with regular opportunities for success to encourage motivation, use of attentive exploration of stimuli and anticipation trials to enhance salience of important sensory attributes and learning, and intensive training involving 3 sessions a week over 6 weeks and including a high number of repetitions (L. M. Carey, 2006; L. M. Carey et al., 2011).

The program also employs principles of learning specifically designed to facilitate transfer of training effects (L. M. Carey & Matyas, 2005). These include variation in stimuli and training conditions employed (Goldstone, 1998; Schmidt & Lee, 1999) and intermittent feedback on accuracy of response (L. M. Carey & Matyas, 2005). Progressive difficulty is defined across stimulus sets using a matrix of large, medium, and fine differences. Training includes exposure to novel stimuli with opportunity for feedback on the act of generalization (L. M. Carey & Matyas, 2005; see Chapter 12 for details).

2.8.3 LANGUAGE: CONSTRAINT-INDUCED APHASIA THERAPY

Constraint-induced learning approaches that have been successful in motor retraining have also been successfully applied to aphasia rehabilitation (Pulvermüller et al., 2001; Maher et al., 2006). Constraint treatments involve (i) constraining the patient by forcing use of the affected function, (ii) providing extensive practice, and (iii) shaping the desired performance by rewarding successive approximations to the target behavior.

In the case of constraint treatment for aphasia, Constraint-Induced Aphasia Therapy (CIAT), the constraint is accomplished by requiring verbal output rather than other typical compensatory communication strategies (e.g., gesturing, drawing, writing) that persons with aphasia learn to rely on to avoid the use of their impaired verbal abilities. In fact, barriers are erected between patient and communication partners to prevent other communication exchanges from taking place. Patient verbal output is gradually shaped during treatment to approximate grammatically correct and informationally rich sentences through extensive practice (Pulvermüller et al., 2001; Maher et al., 2006). In CIAT, this shaping effect is attained by gradually increasing the length, complexity, and overall difficulty of the utterance required of the subject (Meinzer, Elbert, Djundja, Taub, & Rockstroh, 2007). Hallmarks of this treatment are that verbal communication is required and that treatment is intense.

Recently, Connor and colleagues (Connor, Tucker, Cross, Burch, & Fucetola, 2011) have tested the extent to which training in CIAT generalizes, or transfers, to novel verbal production tasks. They focused on determining whether quantity of language (number of content units produced), quality of language (the number of content units produced per minute), or both, increased with CIAT. Although CIAT improved language output during treatment in people with chronic aphasia, gains made in treatment generalized for most participants only modestly to novel verbal production tasks that were more like everyday communication. More work needs to be done to explicitly train generalization to the types of language tasks that people need to do in daily life.

2.9 MEASURING RESPONSE TO LEARNING-BASED REHABILITATION

A learning-based approach to rehabilitation is likely to influence outcome at a number of levels. Response to therapy can be measured across different levels, for example from reorganization of brain networks to performance capacities, return to previous life activities, and optimal participation. For example, it is expected that learning-dependent changes will impact brain networks. Changes in activity across brain networks may be measured in vivo using magnetic resonance imaging (MRI) and neuroimaging paradigms, such as task-related activation of specific functions, resting state functional connectivity, probabilistic estimation of white matter fiber tracts, and cortical thickness (see Chapter 4). Multimodal modalities such as magnetoencephalography (MEG) and transcranial magnetic stimulation (TMS; see Chapter 5) can be used to gain insight into related biomedical mechanisms such as motor inhibition and attention. Investigation of these changes over time, and the relationships among them, is necessary to provide insight into changes associated with learning and rehabilitation.

Performance outcomes to be assessed include movement, sensation, cognition, and language functions. These can be assessed at the level of body function/body structure, as well as in relation to functional limitations in performance of core tasks that require these functions, such as grasp, walking, and reading. A large number of tools have been developed for use in clinical and laboratory settings. At this level it is important to determine whether improvements are specific to the skill trained, or demonstrate transfer to tasks that have not been trained. Measures of core information processing, including attention and learning, need also to be considered, particularly in the context of being able to benefit from learning-based rehabilitation (see Chapter 14). One might also ask whether there are common features of neuroperformance across functions that might be impacted by learning.

Measurement of ability to perform daily life functions can be considered core for all patients. The relationship between brain and behavior is well established; however, there is a large gap between brain and behavior and daily life measures (Baum, 2011). In order to assess the link between neuroperformance and activity outcomes it is recommended that the measure include observation and quantification of the method and quality of strategies and skill used in performing the activity, as well as the level of independence. Actual participation in personal, home, leisure, social, and work activities is also a critical outcome. Yet, it is often not adequately addressed. This outcome is important in maintaining learned skills and in quality of life. Similarly, measures of health-related quality of life are important to understand the impact of the stroke and current performance levels from the perspective of the individual.

2.10 SUMMARY AND CONCLUSION

Clinicians and researchers may benefit from using a framework to understand and apply principles of neuroscience in the context of rehabilitation. As for any translational science, neurorehabilitation requires a process for transforming basic science knowledge into clinically effective interventions, according to the rules of evidence-based practice.

Learning is synonymous with neural plasticity, and facilitated learning is synonymous with rehabilitation. In this chapter we presented a learning-based model—**Rehab-Learn**—for stroke rehabilitation that identified common-core and skill-specific behavioral strategies under which training may be facilitated. The role of adjunct therapies and environmental context that may impact on this skill-based learning was highlighted.

The model also highlighted that learning-based approaches may impact the individual across a profile of outcomes, from changes in brain systems to performance and participation. In order to facilitate communication across the continuum of outcomes, the authors identified a language of rehabilitation science that spans biomedical mechanisms to participation and environment.

Our aim is for the Rehab-Learn model to stimulate clinicians to consider new ways of thinking about stroke rehabilitation so that they incorporate an active learning approach into their rehabilitation approach, rather than relying on compensation alone. In Part D—Rehabilitation of Common Functions—the authors review current interventions and provide insights for future clinical practice of these common functions based on neuroscience. It is intended that this information will help clinicians to take active steps forward in achieving a learning-based approach to rehabilitation after stroke, founded on neuroscience.

REFERENCES

Abraham, W. C. (2008). Metaplasticity: tuning synapses and networks for plasticity. *Nature Reviews Neuroscience, 9*(5), 387–399.

Bach-y-Rita, P. (1980a). Brain plasticity as a basis for therapeutic procedures. In P. Bach-y-Rita (Ed.), *Recovery of function: theoretical considerations for brain injury rehabilitation* (pp. 225–263). Vienna: Hans Huber.

Bach-y-Rita, P. (1980b). *Recovery of function: theoretical considerations for brain injury rehabilitation*. Vienna: Hans Huber.

Baum, C. M. (2011). Fulfilling the promise: supporting participation in daily life. *Archives of Physical Medicine and Rehabilitation, 92*(2), 169–175.

Baum, C. M., Connor, L. T., Morrison, T., Hahn, M., Dromerick, A. W., & Edwards, D. F. (2008). Reliability, validity, and clinical utility of the Executive Function Performance Test: a measure of executive function in a sample of people with stroke. *American Journal of Occupational Therapy, 62*(4), 446–455.

Becker, S. (1996). Mutual information maximization: models of cortical self-organization. *Network Computation in Neural Systems, 7*, 7–31.

Boly, M., Balteau, E., Schnakers, C., Degueldre, C., Moonen, G., Luxen, A., et al. (2007). Baseline brain activity fluctuations predict somatosensory perception in humans. *Proceedings of the National Academy of Science U S A, 104*(29), 12187–12192.

Byl, N. N., & Merzenich, M. M. (2000). Principles of neuroplasticity: implications for neurorehabilitation and learning. In E. S. Gonzalez, S. Myers, J. Edelstein, J. S. Liebermann & J. A. Downey (Eds.), *Downey and Darling's physiological basis of rehabilitation medicine* (pp. 609–628). Boston: Butterworth-Heinemann.

Carey, J. R., Kimberley, T. J., Lewis, S. M., Auerbach, E. J., Dorsey, L., Rundquist, P., et al. (2002). Analysis of fMRI and finger tracking training in subjects with chronic stroke. *Brain, 125*, 773–788.

Carey, L. M. (2006). Loss of somatic sensation. In M. E. Selzer, S. Clarke, L. G. Cohen, P. W. Duncan & F. H. Gage (Eds.), *Textbook of neural repair and rehabilitation. Vol II. Medical neurorehabilitation* (Vol. II, pp. 231–247). Cambridge: Cambridge University Press.

Carey, L. M., Macdonnell, R., & Matyas, T. A. (2011). SENSe: Study of the Effectiveness of Neurorehabilitation on Sensation: a randomized controlled trial. *Neurorehabilitation and Neural Repair, 25*(4), 304–313.

Carey, L. M., & Matyas, T. A. (2005). Training of somatosensory discrimination after stroke: facilitation of stimulus generalization. *American Journal of Physical Medicine and Rehabilitation, 84*(6), 428–442.

Carey, L. M., Matyas, T. A., & Oke, L. E. (1993). Sensory loss in stroke patients: effective training of tactile and proprioceptive discrimination. *Archives of Physical Medicine and Rehabilitation, 74*(6), 602–611.

Carey, L. M., & Seitz, R. (2007). Functional neuroimaging in stroke recovery and neurorehabilitation: conceptual issues and perspectives. *International Journal of Stroke, 2*(4), 245–264.

Cheeran, B., Cohen, L., Dobkin, B., Ford, G., Greenwood, R., Howard, D., et al. (2009). The future of restorative neurosciences in stroke: driving the translational research pipeline from basic science to rehabilitation of people after stroke. *Neurorehabilitation and Neural Repair, 23*(2), 97–107.

Chen, R., Cohen, L. G., & Hallett, M. (2002). Nervous system reorganization following injury. *Neuroscience, 111*(4), 761–773.

Comeau, W. L., McDonald, R. J., & Kolb, B. E. (2010). Learning-induced alterations in prefrontal cortical dendritic morphology. *Behavioural Brain Research, 214*(1), 91–101.

Connor, L. T., Tucker, F. M., Cross, J., Burch, K., & Fucetola, R. P. (2011). *Constraint treatment for chronic aphasia: do treatment gains generalize to story retelling?* Paper presented at the Clinical Aphasiology Conference. Ft. Lauderdale, Florida.

Cramer, S. C., Sur, M., Dobkin, B. H., O'Brien, C., Sanger, T. D., Trojanowski, J. Q., et al. (2011). Harnessing neuroplasticity for clinical applications. *Brain, 134*, 1591–1609.

Doidge, N. (2007). *The brain that changes itself*. Melbourne, Australia: Scribe Publications.

Dong, Y., Dobkin, B. H., Cen, S. Y., Wu, A. D., & Winstein, C. J. (2006). Motor cortex activation during treatment may predict therapeutic gains in paretic hand function after stroke. *Stroke, 37*, 1552–1555.

Elbert, T., Pantev, C., Wienbruch, C., Rockstroh, B., & Taub, E. (1995). Increased cortical representation of the fingers of the left hand in string players. *Science, 270*(5234), 305–307.

Engineer, N. D., Riley, J. R., Seale, J. D., Vrana, W. A., Shetake, J. A., Sudanagunta, S. P., et al. (2011). Reversing pathological neural activity using targeted plasticity. *Nature, 470*(7332), 101–104.

Felleman, D. J., & Van Essen, D. C. (1991). Distributed hierarchical processing in the primate cerebral cortex. *Cerebral Cortex, 1*(1), 1–47.

Finger, S., & Stein, D. G. (1982). *Brain damage and recovery: Research and clinical perspectives*. New York: Academic Press.

Fox, M. D., Snyder, A. Z., Vincent, J. L., & Raichle, M. E. (2007). Intrinsic fluctuations within cortical systems account for intertrial variability in human behavior. *Neuron, 56*(1), 171–184.

French, B., Thomas, L. H., Leathley, M. J., Sutton, C. J., McAdam, J., Forster, A., et al. (2007). Repetitive task training for improving functional ability after stroke. *Cochrane Database of Systematic Reviews* (4), CD006073.

Gentile, A. M. (1998). Implicit and explicit processes during acquisition of functional skills. *Scandinavian Journal of Occupational Therapy, 5*, 7–16.

Goldstone, R. L. (1998). Perceptual learning. *Annual Review of Psychology, 49*, 585–612.

Hallett, M. (2001). Plasticity of the human motor cortex and recovery from stroke. *Brain Research Reviews, 36*(2–3), 169–174.

He, B. J., Shulman, G. L., Snyder, A. Z., & Corbetta, M. (2007). The role of impaired neuronal communication in neurological disorders. *Current Opinions in Neurology, 20*(6), 655–660.

Henshaw, E., Polatajko, H., McEwen, S., Ryan, J. D., & Baum, C. M. (2011). Cognitive approach to improving participation after stroke: two case studies. *American Journal of Occupational Therapy, 65*(1), 55–63.

Hess, G., & Donoghue, J. P. (1996). Long-term depression of horizontal connections in rat motor cortex. *European Journal of Neuroscience, 8*(4), 658–665.

Hodics, T., Cohen, L. G., & Cramer, S. C. (2006). Functional imaging of intervention effects in stroke motor rehabilitation. *Archives of Physical Medicine and Rehabilitation, 87*(Suppl 2), S36–S42.

Hubel, D. H., & Wiesel, T. N. (1962). Receptive fields, binocular interaction and functional architecture in cats visual cortex. *Journal of Physiology-London, 160*(1), 106–154.

Hyland, M., & Polatajko, H. (2011). Enabling children with Developmental Coordination Disorder to self-regulate through the use of Dynamic Performance Analysis: evidence from the CO-OP approach. *Human Movement Science*, doi:10.1016/j.humov.2011.09.003.

Iacoboni, M., & Dapretto, M. (2006). The mirror neuron system and the consequences of its dysfunction. *Nature Neuroscience, 7*, 942–951.

Jagadeesh, B. (2006). Attentional modulation of cortical plasticity. In M. E. Selzer, S. Clarke, L. G. Cohen, P. W. Duncan & F. H. Gage (Eds.), *Textbook of neural repair and rehabilitation: Vol 1. Neural repair and plasticity.* (Vol. 1, pp. 194–206). Cambridge: Cambridge University Press.

Janssen, H., Bernhardt, J., Collier, J. M., Sena, E. S., McElduff, P., Attia, J., et al. (2010). An enriched environment improves sensorimotor function post-ischemic stroke. *Neurorehabilitation and Neural Repair, 24*(9), 802–813.

Johansson, B. B. (2011). Current trends in stroke rehabilitation. A review with focus on brain plasticity. *Acta Neurologica Scandinavica, 123*(3), 147–159.

Kolb, B., Gorny, G., Soderpalm, A. H. V., & Robinson, T. E. (2003). Environmental complexity has different effects on the structure of neurons in the prefrontal cortex versus the parietal cortex or nucleus accumbens. *Synapse, 48*(3), 149–153.

Kolb, B., Teskey, G. C., & Gibb, R. (2010). Factors influencing cerebral plasticity in the normal and injured brain. *Frontiers in Human Neuroscience, 4*, Article 204.

Lave, J., & Wenger, E. (1991). *Situated learning: legitimate peripheral participation.* Cambridge, UK: Cambridge University Press.

Levin, M. F., Kleim, J. A., & Wolf, S. L. (2009). What do motor "recovery" and "compensation" mean in patients following stroke? *Neurorehabilitation and Neural Repair, 23*(4), 313–319.

Magill, R. A. (1998). *Motor learning: Concepts and applications* (5th ed.). Boston, MA: MacGraw Hill.

Maguire, E. A., Gadian, D. G., Johnsrude, I. S., Good, C. D., Ashburner, J., Frackowiak, R. S. J., et al. (2000). Navigation-related structural change in the hippocampi of taxi drivers. *Proceedings of the National Academy of Sciences of the United States of America, 97*(8), 4398–4403.

Maher, L. M., Kendall, D., Swearengin, J. A., Rodriguez, A., Leon, S. A., Pingel, K., et al. (2006). A pilot study of use-dependent learning in the context of constraint induced language therapy. *Journal of the International Neuropsychological Society, 12*(6), 843–852.

McEwen, S. E., Polatajko, H. J., Davis, J. A., Huijbregts, M., & Ryan, J. D. (2010). "There's a real plan here, and I am responsible for that plan": participant experiences with a novel cognitive-based treatment approach for adults living with chronic stroke. *Disability and Rehabilitation, 32*(7), 540–550.

McEwen, S. E., Polatajko, H. J., Huijbregts, M. P., & Ryan, J. D. (2009). Exploring a cognitive-based treatment approach to improve motor-based skill performance in chronic stroke: Results of three single case experiments. *Brain Injury, 23*(13–14), 1041–1053.

McEwen, S. E., Polatajko, H. J., Huijbregts, M. P. J., & Ryan, J. D. (2010). Inter-task transfer of meaningful, functional skills following a cognitive-based treatment: Results of three multiple baseline design experiments in adults with chronic stroke. *Neuropsychological Rehabilitation, 20*(4), 541–561.

Meinzer, M., Elbert, T., Djundja, D., Taub, E., & Rockstroh, B. (2007). Extending the constraint-induced movement therapy (CIMT) approach to cognitive functions: Constraint-induced aphasia therapy (CIAT) of chronic aphasia. *Neurorehabilitation, 22*(4), 311–318.

Meinzer, M., Elbert, T., Wienbruch, C., Djundja, D., Barthel, G., & Rockstroh, B. (2004). Intensive language training enhances brain plasticity in chronic aphasia. *BMC Biology, 2*(20), 1–9.

Merzenich, M. M., & Kaas, J. H. (1982). Reorganization of somatosensory cortex in mammals following peripheral nerve injury. *Trends in Neurosciences, 5*, 434–436.

Moore, J. (1980). Neuroanatomical considerations relating to recovery of function following brain injury. In P. Bach y Rita (Ed.), *Recovery of function: Theoretical considerations for brain injury rehabilitation* (pp. 3–90). Baltimore: University Park Press.

Nelles, G., Jentzen, W., Jueptner, M., Muller, S., & Diener, H. C. (2001). Arm training induced brain plasticity in stroke studied with serial positron emission tomography. *NeuroImage, 13*, 1146–1154.

Nudo, R. J. (2007). Postinfarct cortical plasticity and behavioral recovery. *Stroke, 38*[part2], 840–845.

Nudo, R. J., Wise, B. M., SiFuentes, F., & Milliken, G. W. (1996). Neural substrates for the effects of rehabilitative training on motor recovery after ischemic infarct. *Science, 272*(5269), 1791–1794.

Okamoto, H., Stracke, H., Stoll, W., & Pantev, C. (2010). Listening to tailor-made notched music reduces tinnitus loudness and tinnitus-related auditory cortex activity. *Proceedings of the National Academy of Sciences of the United States of America, 107*(3), 1207–1210.

Plautz, E. J., Milliken, G. W., & Nudo, R. J. (2000). Effects of repetitive motor training on movement representations in adult squirrel monkeys: role of use versus learning. *Neurobiology of Learning and Memory, 74*, 27–55.

Pleger, B., Blankenburg, F., Ruff, C. C., Driver, J., & Dolan, R. J. (2008). Reward facilitates tactile judgments and modulates hemodynamic responses in human primary somatosensory cortex. *Journal of Neuroscience, 28*(33), 8161–8168.

Polatajko, H. J., & Mandich, A. (2004). *Enabling occupation in children: The Cognitive Orientation to daily Occupations Performance (CO-OP) approach.* Ottawa, ON: CAOT publications ACE.

Polatajko, H. J., Mandich, A., & Martini, R. (2000). Dynamic performance analysis: A framework for understanding occupational performance. *American Journal of Occupational Therapy, 54*(1), 65–72.

Polatajko, H. J., Mandich, A. D., Miller, L., & Macnab, J. (2001). Cognitive Orientation to daily Occupational Performance: Part II—The evidence. *Physical & Occupational Therapy in Paediatrics, 20*(2/3), 83–106.

Polatajko, H. J., McEwen, S. E., Ryan, J. D., & Baum, C. M. (2012). Brief Report - Pilot randomized controlled trial investigating cognitive strategy use to improve goal performance after stroke. *American Journal of Occupational Therapy, 66*, 104–109.

Pulvermüller, F., Hauk, O., Zohsel, K., Neininger, B., & Mohr, B. (2005). Therapy-related reorganization of language in both hemispheres of patients with chronic aphasia. *NeuroImage, 28*(2), 481–489.

Pulvermüller, F., Neininger, B., Elbert, T., Mohr, B., Rockstroh, B., Koebbel, P., et al. (2001). Constraint-induced therapy of chronic aphasia after stroke. *Stroke, 32*(7), 1621–1626.

Purves, D., Augustine, G. J., Fitzpatrick, D., Hall, W. C., LaMantia, A.-S., & Williams, S. M. (2004). *Neuroscience* (3rd ed.). Sunderland, MA: Sinauer Associates, Inc.

Raymond, J. (2009). Interactions of attention, emotion and motivation. In N. Srinivasan (Ed.), Progress in Brain Research: *Attention* (Vol. 176, pp. 293–308). Amsterdam: Elsevier.

Richards, L. G., Stewart, K. C., Woodbury, M. L., Senesac, C., & Cauraugh, J. H. (2008). Movement-dependent stroke recovery: a systematic review and meta-analysis of TMS and fMRI evidence. *Neuropsychologia, 46*(1), 3–11.

Rossini, P. M., Altamura, C., Ferreri, F., Melgari, J.-M., Tecchio, F., Tombini, M., et al. (2007). Neuroimaging experimental studies on brain plasticity in recovery from stroke. *Eura Medicophys, 43*, 241–254.

Sala, C., Cambianica, I., & Rossi, F. (2008). Molecular mechanisms of dendritic spine development and maintenance. *Acta Neurobiologiae Experimentalis, 68*(2), 289–304.

Sathian, K. (2005). Visual cortical activity during tactile perception in the sighted and the visually deprived. *Developmental Psychobiology, 46*(3), 279–286.

Sathian, K. (2006). Cross-modal plasticity in sensory systems. In M. E. Selzer, S. Clarke, L. G. Cohen, P. W. Duncan & F. H. Gage (Eds.), *Textbook of neural repair and rehabilitation: Vol 1. Neural repair and plasticity.* (Vol. I, pp. 180–193). Cambridge, UK: Cambridge University Press.

Schmidt, R. A., & Lee, T. D. (1999). *Motor control and learning: a behavioral emphasis*. Illinois: Human Kinetics.

Schmidt, R. A., & Lee, T. D. (2005). *Motor control and learning: A behavioral emphasis* (4th ed.). Champaign, Ill: Human Kinetics.

Schneiderman, A., McEwen, S., Kinslikh, D., & Polatajko, H. (2008). *On route to novel strategies for adult stroke rehabilitation*. Canadian Association of Occupational Therapists Conference Whitehorse, Yukon. June 12.

Selzer, M. E., Clarke, S., Cohen, L. G., Duncan, P. W., & Gage, F. H. (2006). Neural repair and rehabilitation: an introduction. In M. E. Selzer, S. Clarke, L. G. Cohen, P. W. Duncan & F. H. Gage (Eds.), *Textbook of neural repair and rehabilitation: Vol II. Medical neurorehabilitation* (Vol. II, pp. xxvii-xxxv). Cambridge, UK: Cambridge University Press.

Shams, L., & Seitz, A. R. (2008). Benefits of multisensory learning. *TRENDS in Cognitive Sciences, 12*(11), 411–417.

Shuell, T. J. (1986). Cognitive conceptions of learning. *Review of Educational Research, 56*(4), 411–436.

Shulman, G. L., Corbetta, M., Buckner, R. L., Raichle, M. E., Fiez, J. A., Miezin, F. M., et al. (1997). Top-down modulation of early sensory cortex. *Cerebral Cortex, 7*(3), 193–206.

Shumway-Cook, A., & Woollacott, M. J. (2012). *Motor control: translating research into clinical practice*. Philadelphia: Wolters Kluwer Health/Lippincott Williams & Wilkins.

Siegler, R. S. (2004). Learning about learning. *Merrill-Palmer Quarterly, 50*(3), 353–368.

Walker-Batson, D., Smith, P., Curtis, S., & Unwin, D. H. (2004). Neuromodulation paired with learning dependent practice to enhance post stroke recovery? *Restorative Neurology and Neuroscience, 22*, 387–392.

Wolf, S., Winstein, C., Miller, J., Taub, E., Uswatte, G., Morris, D. et al. (2006). Effect of constraint induced movement therapy on upper extremity function among patients 3–9 months following stroke: The EXCITE randomized clinical trial. *Journal of the American Medical Association, 296*, 2095–2104.

Xerri, C., Merzenich, M. M., Peterson, B. E., & Jenkins, W. M. (1998). Plasticity of primary somatosensory cortex paralleling sensorimotor skill recovery from stroke in adult monkeys. *Journal of Neurophysiology, 79*, 2119–2148.

Zhang, J. X., & Kourtzi, Z. (2010). Learning-dependent plasticity with and without training in the human brain. *Proceedings of the National Academy of Sciences of the United States of America, 107*(30), 13503–13508.

Zihl, J. (1981). Recovery of visual functions in patients with cerebral blindness: Effect of specific practice with saccadic localization. *Experimental Brain Research, 44*, 159–169.

Zihl, J., & Von Cramon, D. (1979). Restitution of visual function in patients with cerebral blindness. *Journal of Neurology, Neurosurgery, and Psychiatry, 42*, 312–322.

3 | NEURAL PLASTICITY AS A BASIS FOR STROKE REHABILITATION

MICHAEL NILSSON, MILOS PEKNY, and MARCELA PEKNA

3.1 NEURAL PLASTICITY AFTER BRAIN AND SPINAL CORD INJURY

3.1.1 EXPERIENCE-DEPENDENT PLASTICITY OF THE CEREBRAL CORTEX

Cerebral cortex is an assembly of neuronal cells that are highly interconnected. The morphology as well as function of these complex and spatially distributed networks is modulated or even controlled by the glial component of the central nervous system (CNS). The ability to adapt in response to the changing environment is the most fundamental property of the nervous tissue and constitutes the basis for learning. Neural plasticity is the neurobiological basis for the ability to adapt and learn in an experience-dependent manner. At the structural level, neural plasticity could be defined in terms of dendritic and axonal arborization, spine density, synapse number and size, receptor density, and, in some brain regions, also the number of neurons. These structural constituents of neural plasticity jointly determine the complexity of neuronal networks and their activity, and contribute to recovery of function after stroke and other CNS injury (Figure 3.1).

3.1.2 SPONTANEOUS RECOVERY OF FUNCTION AFTER STROKE

Loss of function due to stroke is caused by cell death in the infarcted region, as well as cell dysfunction in the areas surrounding the infarct. In addition, the function of remote brain regions, including the contralateral areas that are connected to the area of tissue damage, is compromised due to hypometabolism, neurovascular uncoupling, and aberrant neurotransmission, jointly called *diaschisis* (Wieloch & Nikolich, 2006). Some recovery of function occurs spontaneously following stroke in humans, as well as in animal models. It is believed that this functional recovery involves three, to some extent overlapping, phases: first, reversal of diaschisis, activation of cell genesis, and repair; second, changing the properties of existing neuronal pathways; and third, neuroanatomical plasticity leading to the formation of new neuronal connections (Wieloch & Nikolich, 2006). The basic processes underlying phases two and three are also involved in normal learning, and it has indeed been recognized that functional improvement after CNS injury is a relearning process (Warraich & Kleim, 2010).

3.1.3 CORTICAL MAP REARRANGEMENTS

As stated above, the brain, and especially the cerebral cortex, has a capacity to alter the structure and function of neurons and to reorganize its neural networks in response to the changes in input and output demands. Thus, when the normal input to particular area of the primary somatosensory cortex (SI) is lost due to injury, rapid structural and functional reorganization results in this area being activated by sensory stimulation of the surrounding intact body regions. Thus, spinal cord injuries lead to both unmasking of existing latent connections as well as changes in SI anatomy due to the growth of new lateral connections (Merzenich et al., 1983; Wrigley et al., 2009; Henderson, Gustin, Macey, Wrigley, & Siddall, 2011). Similarly, the motor maps in the primary motor cortex change in response to task-specific training or after injury. Training human subjects or animals to perform a specific task leads to an increase in the area of motor cortex that controls the muscles used during the task (reviewed in Warraich & Kleim, 2010). Injury to the motor cortex leads to the recruitment of motor areas

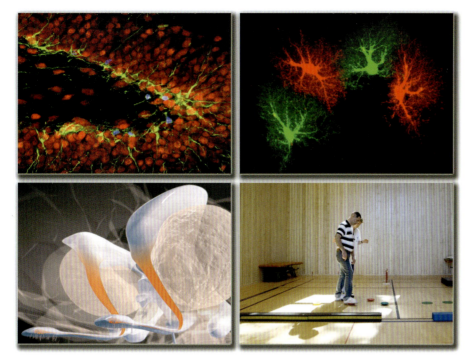

Figure 3.1 Neuroplasticity is an important basis for stroke rehabilitation. The ongoing research in this area spans from molecular and cellular studies to disease modeling in experimental animals to clinical and population-based studies. From top left clockwise: New neural cells are continuously born and cellular connections are made in the hippocampus, a part of the brain associated with learning and memory; astrocytes, cells with bush-like appearance, form a cellular network that controls many of the brain's functions; in rodent experimental models, cells can travel over relatively long distances in the brain, reaching, for example, specific parts of the brain or side of the ischemic injury; modern rehabilitation approaches are increasingly based on the newly emerging knowledge of brain plasticity and regeneration. Photos courtesy of Professor Milos Pekny, Professor Michael Nilsson, Professor Georg Kuhn, Dr. Maurice Curtis, Dr. Ulrika Wilhelmsson (all CBR, Clinical Neuroscience, Sahlgrenska Academy at the University of Gothenburg, Sweden), Professor Mark Ellisman, and Dr. Erik Bushong (both NCMIR, UCSD, San Diego, USA).

that were not making significant contribution to the lost function prior to the injury. For example, in macaque monkeys, recovery of dexterity after unilateral motor cortex lesion is mediated by the ipsilesional premotor cortex. Inactivation of this region abolishes recovered movement, whereas it does not affect the performance in uninjured monkeys (Liu & Rouiller, 1999). The notion that the activity of cortical areas recruited after injury plays a role in functional recovery in humans is supported by a study showing that in well-recovered stroke patients, the ipsilesional dorsal motor cortex shows increase in activity (Gerloff et al., 2006). Even stronger evidence stems from clinical studies showing that when the function within such a newly recruited area is disrupted using transcranial magnetic stimulation, the recovered movement of the limb affected by stroke is impaired (Feydy et al., 2002; Werhahn, Conforto, Kadom, Hallett, & Cohen, 2003; Fridman et al., 2004; Bütefisch, Kleiser, & Seitz, 2006). Functional redundancy due to substantial degree of overlap within and across brain regions can also contribute to the brain's ability to adapt to injury (Warraich & Kleim, 2010).

3.1.4 CONTRALATERAL HEMISPHERE INVOLVEMENT

The contralesional hemisphere has the capacity to contribute to movement on the ipsilateral side, but does not make any significant contribution in healthy subjects (Jankowska & Edgley, 2006). However, significant increases in contralesional motor cortex activity

can be observed in stroke patients during movement of the affected foot or arm (Chollet et al., 1991; Zemke, Heagerty, Lee, & Cramer, 2003; Enzinger et al., 2008). These and other studies have convincingly demonstrated that in the early phase of the stroke recovery process there is an increased activation of the motor areas in both hemispheres, but it is substantially more pronounced on the contralesional side. The contralesional activation is often reduced in the later stages of recovery. Although there is no general consensus concerning the role of contralesional somatosensory and motor area activation in recovery of function, it appears that the best recovery is associated with an early recruitment of the supplementary motor areas on the ipsilesional side, whereas persistent activation of the contralesional prefrontal and parietal cortex predicts a slower and less complete recovery and is also often associated with larger infarct (reviewed in Murphy & Corbett, 2009; Xerri, 2011). Notably, a recent functional magnetic resonance imaging (fMRI) study has shown that the pattern of brain activation present in the early phase after stroke could be predictive of subsequent recovery of motor functions (Marshall et al., 2009).

3.1.5 CONTRALESIONAL AXONAL REMODELING OF THE CORTICOSPINAL SYSTEM

Whereas the capacity for functional and structural rearrangements has been studied for decades and is well documented for the neural networks within the cerebral cortex, the plasticity responses induced by experimental stroke at the level of the spinal cord have been demonstrated only recently. Using a rat stroke model, Liu and coworkers showed that the spontaneous behavioral motor recovery highly correlates with the remodeling of corticospinal tract axons in the cervical spinal cord, as well as the reorganization of pyramidal neurons in the cerebral cortex of both hemispheres. Consistent with conclusions from human imaging studies, they further showed that functional recovery is highly correlated with contralesional cortical wiring only in the acute phase, with a negative correlation later on (Liu, Zhang, Li, Cui, & Chopp, 2009). Although the capacity for remodeling of the corticospinal tract axons at the spinal cord level remains to be demonstrated in stroke patients, these findings add a new dimension to the rehabilitative efforts for improved functional recovery post-stroke.

3.2 IMPLICATIONS FOR STROKE REHABILITATION

Based on the current knowledge of the mechanisms underlying neural plasticity, as well as a large number of experimental and clinical studies, several general principles appear to underpin the process of stroke rehabilitation. First, stroke rehabilitation should be provided by a multidisciplinary team. Specialized multidisciplinary stroke rehabilitation units are associated with improved functional outcomes, reduced mortality, shorter lengths of hospital stay, and reduced need for institutionalization in patients suffering from a moderate to severe stroke. Second, good rehabilitation outcome is strongly associated with high patient and family motivation and engagement. Third, rehabilitative training should target the goals that are relevant for the specific needs of each patient, and should be preferably given in the patient's own environment and context. Fourth, greater intensities of physical, occupational, and speech therapy positively influence functional recovery after stroke. The best way of providing this increased level of training seems to be a task-specific approach. In animals, functional reorganization is more pronounced when the tasks are meaningful to the subject. Repetitive activity alone is not sufficient to produce increased motor cortical representations. Instead, a component of skilled motor learning is required in addition to repetition for the activation of mechanisms underlying cortical plasticity and reorganization. Fifth, rehabilitation should begin as soon as possible after stroke. Numerous animal studies have shown that if rehabilitative intervention is delayed for several weeks after a stroke, activation of mechanisms underlying brain plasticity, brain reorganization, and recovery are severely reduced. These findings are also in line with results from clinical studies where outcomes after stroke rehabilitation were significantly improved after early mobilization and initiation of rehabilitation. Sixth, multimodal training and stimulation generate positive affect and promote recovery of function. Seventh, physical and cardiovascular fitness training should be integrated into every stroke rehabilitation program. Eighth, rehabilitation should continue after the patient has been discharged from the hospital (for a detailed review see Murie-Fernández, Irimia, Martínez-Vila, Meyer, & Teasell, 2010; Langhorne, Bernhardt, & Kwakkel, 2011).

3.3 INCREASING NEURAL PLASTICITY THROUGH BEHAVIORAL MANIPULATIONS AND ADJUVANT THERAPIES

Evidence accumulated during the past two decades together with recent advances in the field of stroke recovery clearly show that the effects of neurorehabilitation can be enhanced by behavioral manipulations and combination with adjuvant therapies that stimulate the endogenous neural plasticity. However, the dose, timing after stroke, and coupling with appropriate physical training may be critical for the outcome.

3.3.1 ENRICHED ENVIRONMENT AND MULTIMODAL STIMULATION

A large number of animal studies have demonstrated that experience in an enriched environment—that is, housing conditions that facilitate enhanced sensory, cognitive, and motor stimulation—stimulate all the structural and functional components of neural plasticity and cognitive performance in healthy animals, as well as promote recovery of sensorimotor function after experimental stroke (reviewed in Nithianantharajah & Hannan, 2006; Janssen et al., 2010). A human equivalent of environmental enrichment is multimodal stimulation and multisensory training protocols. These have been shown to be more effective for learning in healthy subjects (Ghazanfar & Schroeder, 2006; Shams & Seitz, 2008; Johansson, 2011). However, we are only beginning to understand how to translate the positive effects of enriched environment in experimental animal research to humans. The effects of multisensory stimulation most likely constitute important parts in the mechanism underlying the beneficial effects observed in several recent studies in humans that evaluated the effects of, for example, tactile massage, therapeutic gardens, music, rhythm and dancing, cardiovascular training, cognitive challenges, and so forth on functional recovery after brain injury (Johansson, 2011). Other specific examples of multisensory neurorehabilitation include mirror therapy and action observation, motor imagery and mental training, virtual reality training, and music-related therapies.

In mirror therapy, the illusion of movement in the affected limb is created by the reflection of the moving unaffected limb while the affected arm is hidden behind the mirror. The strongest evidence in support of the effectiveness of this approach has come from a study of subacute stroke patients who received a program of 30 minutes of mirror therapy per day, consisting of wrist and finger flexion and extension movements, in addition to a conventional program for 4 weeks. Compared to a control group who received a sham instead of mirror therapy, the mirror-training patients showed a more improved distal hand functioning at the end of therapy period, as well as at 5-month follow-up (Yavuzer et al., 2008). Similarly, Dohle and coworkers reported that severely hemiparetic patients who received mirror therapy regained more distal function after 6 weeks of training 30 minutes a day, 5 days a week for 6 weeks (Dohle et al., 2009). However, little is known about which patients are likely to benefit from mirror therapy and how such a therapy should preferentially be applied (Rothgangel, Braun, Beurskens, Seitz, & Wade, 2011). Action observation for 4 weeks also led to enhanced motor performance in stroke patients, and this functional improvement was still present at 8 weeks follow-up (Ertelt et al., 2007). Action observation on motor training in combination with concurrent physical training of the observed action enhanced the positive effects of task practice alone (Celnik, Webster, Glasser, & Cohen, 2008).

Mental training is based on conscious activation of brain regions and networks involved in movement preparation and execution. In a placebo-controlled trial on chronic stroke patients, therapist-guided mental practice was associated with increased dexterity and changes in patterns of cortical activation (Page, Levine, & Leonard, 2007). Since motor imagery is not dependent on the actual ability to execute movements, it can be used early in the rehabilitation process and even in severely paretic patients, although it can be difficult in patients with left parietal or left lateral prefrontal lesions (Lotze & Halsband, 2006).

Virtual reality technologies provide multimodal, interactive, and realistic 3-D environments with a high-level control of the sensory input to suit each user's needs. Despite the growing interest in this research area, the evidence of the effectiveness of virtual reality training in stroke rehabilitation thus far is very limited, with most studies underpowered and lacking controls (Carter, Connor, & Dromerick, 2010). Recently, Saposnik and coworkers reported that Wii™ gaming technology represents a safe, feasible, and potentially effective alternative to promote motor recovery. Their conclusions are based on the comparison of a Nintendo Wii gaming system with recreational therapy in groups of 9 and 8 stroke patients, respectively (Saposnik et al., 2010). A rehabilitation gaming system was found to facilitate the functional recovery of the upper extremities as compared to intense occupational therapy or nonspecific interactive games for stroke patients who received this adjuvant therapy in combination to conventional rehabilitation (da Silva Cameirão, Bermúdez, Badia, Duarte, & Verschure, 2011).

A number of studies suggest that listening to music can enhance a variety of cognitive functions, such as attention, learning, communication, and memory, both in healthy subjects and in various patient groups (Zatorre & McGill, 2005; Chen, Penhune, & Zatorre, 2008; Kim, Wigram, & Gold, 2008). Music can also affect the subject's mood and motivation, and thus could be an easy-to-conduct and inexpensive means to facilitate cognitive and emotional recovery in numerous neurological and psychiatric disorders. Indeed, a recently published study on listening to music after stroke clearly demonstrated that patients who listened to self-selected music had better cognitive recovery and mood compared with those who listened to self-selected audiobooks or those with no listening material (Särkämö et al., 2008). Further, listening to music or speech in the acute phase after ischemic stroke induced long-term plastic changes in early sensory processing that correlated with improvement in verbal memory and focused attention (Särkämö et al., 2009). Patients with chronic post-stroke visual neglect who performed tasks while listening to music of their choice showed enhanced visual awareness of contralesional targets relative to when tasks were performed either with unpreferred music or in silence. Functional MRI data showed enhanced activity in the orbitofrontal cortex and the cingulate gyrus associated with emotional responses when tasks were performed with preferred music relative to unpreferred music, suggesting that listening to preferred music induced a positive affect (Soto et al., 2009).

3.3.2 NONINVASIVE BRAIN STIMULATION

Noninvasive brain stimulation (NIBS) can be performed using repetitive transcranial magnetic stimulation (rTMS) and transcranial direct current stimulation (tDCS). These therapies have the potential to enhance neuroplasticity during stroke rehabilitation, thereby supporting recovery of motor and cognitive impairments (reviewed in Bolognini, Pascual-Leone, & Fregni, 2009; Dimyan & Cohen, 2011). The differences between tDCS and TMS are based on presumed mechanisms of action, where TMS acts both as a neurostimulator and neuromodulator, while tDCS acts as a neuromodulator. Depending on the frequency, duration of the stimulation, strength of the magnetic field, and shape of the coil, TMS can activate or suppress the activity in different cortical regions. In tDCS, weak polarizing currents are delivered to the cerebral cortex, inducing sustained changes in neural cell membrane potential and leading to either hyperpolarization or depolarization. The basic cellular mechanisms underpinning the effects of these techniques are only partially known. Based on the broad, rather nondirected interventional approach of these techniques, the prediction would be that NIBS induces a wide array of effects in the brain tissue. For example, in animal studies it has been demonstrated that the effects of TMS could be analogous to other interventions inducing long-term potentiation (LTP) or depression (LTD) in the hippocampus. Different neurotransmitters and neuromodulators, such as gamma-aminobutyric acid (GABA), glutamate, dopamine, and serotonin have been shown to be affected in defined regions of the brain after stimulation with both rTMS and tDCS. The potential of these techniques to infer plasticity changes is also supported by findings showing that NIBS can modulate gene expression. Immediate early genes like c-fos and genes coding for neurotrophic factors like BDNF are shown to be expressed in the rat brain after rTMS (reviewed in Bolognini et al., 2009; Dimyan & Cohen, 2011).

In humans, both rTMS and tDCS are shown to induce long-term effects on cortical excitability that are demonstrated to last for months after the intervention (Dimyan & Cohen, 2011), which may, in turn, lead to long-lasting behavioral modifications. These effects are believed to engage mechanisms of neural plasticity, rendering NIBS well-suited to promote recovery of cognition and motor functions, especially when it is provided together with other types of rehabilitative interventions. In promoting stroke recovery, both techniques have been tested and appear promising. Results from several studies show, for example, that active stimulation of either the affected or unaffected motor cortex in combination with physical and occupational therapy improves motor outcome after stroke (Lindenberg, Renga, Zhu, Nair, & Schlaug, 2010). For more detailed information about the effects of noninvasive brain stimulation in stroke see the more comprehensive review of NIBS provided in Chapter 10.

3.3.3 PHARMACOLOGICAL MODULATORS OF NEURAL PLASTICITY

Recently, several promising approaches that promote the recovery of function after stroke through the stimulation of neural plasticity have been identified through experimental animal research. Importantly, some of these compounds are already in clinical use for other indications or are already being tested in clinical trials.

3.3.3.1 D-AMPHETAMINE

There is large body of laboratory work showing that administration of amphetamine—a potent psychomotor stimulant that induces neuronal release of norepinephrine, dopamine, and serotonin—coupled with motor practice can enhance motor recovery in animal models of stroke or other brain injury, and these functional improvements are associated with increased axonal plasticity and the formation of new anatomical pathways (reviewed in Cheatwood, Emerick, & Kartje, 2008; Goldstein, 2009).

Several double-blind placebo-controlled clinical studies have evaluated the effects of amphetamine on poststroke motor recovery in humans (reviewed in Goldstein, 2009). A meta-analysis concluded that there is no indication for the routine use of amphetamines to improve recovery after stroke and that further research is needed considering the possible positive effect on motor recovery (Martinsson, Hardemark, & Eksborg, 2007). Given the potentially critical differences in trial designs, however, the interpretation of the results of this meta-analysis is not clear (Goldstein, 2009). As pointed out by L. B. Goldstein (2009), several principles pertinent to the trial design have been elucidated by the animal studies. First, the dose–effect relationship for amphetamine-promoted motor recovery has an inverted "U" shape. The drug is relatively ineffective at lower and higher doses. Second, the effects of certain drugs (e.g., amphetamine) on recovery are dependent on concomitant behavioral experience. Third, the timing of the drug administration/experience intervention is critical and also varies with the number and frequency of treatment sessions. Fourth, some drugs (e.g., haloperidol) impair recovery. Thus, the clinical value of D-amphetamine in combination with physical therapy remains to be determined through new clinical trials. The National Institute of Health–sponsored Amphetamine-Enhanced Stroke Recovery (AESR) trial to evaluate the impact of the timing and duration of therapy was started in 2003. Regrettably, this trial was put on hold in 2009 pending application for further funding, and the data remain unanalyzed.

3.3.3.2 SIGMA-1 RECEPTOR AGONISTS

The expression of sigma-1 receptor (Sig-1R) was found to be upregulated in brain tissue from rats that were housed in an enriched environment after focal cerebral ischemia (Ruscher et al., 2011). A more detailed analysis of the involvement of Sig-1R in recovery after stroke showed that the expression of Sig-1R is upregulated in the surviving cells, in particular astrocytes, in the peri-infarct region of animals with good recovery of neurological function (Ruscher et al., 2011). Sig-1R was found to be located in membrane rafts of astrocytes and neurons, and plays an essential role in membrane raft trafficking and neurite outgrowth. Importantly, a potent and selective Sig-1R agonist, SA45031, enhanced functional recovery in rat models of stroke when administered within 2 days after stroke induction (Ruscher et al., 2011). This promising compound is presently investigated in a stroke clinical phase II trial.

3.3.3.3 FLUOXETINE

Selective serotonin reuptake inhibitors (SSRIs) are among the most widely prescribed drugs in psychiatry. The "monoamine hypothesis" of depression, which is based on the notion that depression is caused by decreased monoamine function in the brain, originated from early clinical observations. However, even if monoamine-based agents are potent antidepressants, the cause of depression is far from being a simple deficiency of central monoamines (Krishnan & Nestler, 2008). Recent studies demonstrated that acute increases in the amount of synaptic monoamines induced by antidepressants produce secondary long-term neuroplastic changes and involve transcriptional and translational changes that mediate molecular and cellular plasticity. For example, it is shown in human postmortem tissue and in different animal models that the transcription factor cyclic-AMP-response-element-binding protein (CREB) is upregulated in the hippocampus after chronic administration of SSRIs (Pinnock, Blake, Platt, & Herbert, 2010).

Monoaminergic drugs have also been shown to modulate brain plasticity after stroke and to reduce neurological deficit and subsequent disability. Only a limited amount of animal studies exist on the effects of selective serotonin (5-HT) reuptake inhibitors (SSRIs) on the post-ischemic brain. These studies show that SSRIs are neuroprotective through their anti-inflammatory effects, and that they could improve ischemia-induced spatial cognitive deficits by promoting hippocampal neurogenesis in the rat (Homberg et al., 2011). Interestingly, SSRIs have been investigated in clinical trials and the results from those studies all demonstrate positive effects on recovery after stroke. A few small clinical studies provided initial support to the suggestion of a recovery-promoting effect of SSRIs after stroke. A larger study, Fluoxetine for motor recovery after acute ischemic stroke (FLAME), extended these promising findings, demonstrating in a larger cohort of patients (n = 118) with moderate to severe hemiplegia after ischemic stroke that early treatment with fluoxetine enhances motor recovery and reduces the number of dependent patients when linked with physical training (Chollet et al., 2011). These very interesting results call for even larger and more comprehensive trials with an extended focus on functional outcome parameters. In addition, SSRIs are not a homogeneous category of drugs and additional experimental and pharmacological studies will be needed to further deepen the understanding of their mechanism of action.

3.3.3.4 NIACIN

Niacin (nicotinic acid, vitamin B_3) is the most effective drug currently available for the treatment of dyslipidemia (Vosper, 2009). Treatment with Niaspan®, a prolonged-release formulation of niacin, starting 24 hours after focal brain ischemia improved functional outcome in rats, conceivably through a combination of its effects on angiogenesis (Chen et al., 2007), arteriogenesis (Chen et al., 2009), and increased synaptic plasticity and axon growth (Cui et al., 2010). The clinical usefulness and efficacy of niacin in treatment of stroke remain to be shown.

3.3.3.5 INOSINE

Inosine is a naturally occurring purine nucleoside. Intracerebral infusion of inosine starting immediately after unilateral stroke induction stimulated neurons on the undamaged side of the brain to extend new projections to denervated areas of the midbrain and spinal cord and improved behavioral outcome in rats (Chen, Goldberg, Kolb, Lanser, & Benowitz, 2002). Inosine alters gene expression in neurons contralateral to a stroke that is associated with an enhanced ability of these neurons to form connections on the denervated side of the spinal cord (Zai et al., 2009). Inosine combined with a Nogo receptor blocker (see below) or with environmental enrichment augmented the effects of these two treatment modalities on the restoration of skilled forelimb use after stroke (Zai et al., 2011). These intriguing results demonstrate that the combination of behavioral and pharmacological adjuvant therapies may have additive or even synergistic effect in promoting the recovery of function after stroke. A two-year-long inosine treatment was safe and well tolerated in multiple sclerosis patients (Gonsette et al., 2010). As inosine is currently in clinical trial for Parkinson's disease, it appears to be a particularly attractive candidate for increasing brain plasticity and improving outcome in stroke patients.

3.3.3.6 NOGO-A INHIBITION

Nogo-A is a myelin-associated protein that limits plasticity and recovery after CNS injury through neurite outgrowth inhibition. Anti-Nogo-A antibody treatment enhanced functional recovery and promoted reorganization of the corticospinal tract and axonal plasticity originating in the uninjured hemisphere to re-innervate deafferented areas after cortical lesions (Papadopoulos et al., 2002; Wiessner et al., 2003; Tsai et al., 2007), as well as increased dendritic arborization and spine density of pyramidal neurons in the contralesional sensorimotor cortex (Papadopoulos et al., 2006). Genetic manipulation of the Nogo-Nogo receptor system or the use of peptides that block the signaling through the Nogo receptor have similar effects on axonal plasticity and recovery of function after experimental stroke (Lee, Kim, Sivula & Strittmatter 2004). Remarkably, a recent study showed that Nogo-A immunotherapy leads also to the improvement of chronic neurological deficits and enhancement of neuronal plasticity, and that this therapy may be used to restore function even when administered intracerebroventricular (i.c.v.) for 2 weeks starting 9 weeks after stroke (Tsai, Papadopoulos, Schwab, & Kartje, 2011). An obstacle in using the anti-Nogo-A antibodies or peptide blockers could be their limited delivery into the brain parenchyma after systemic administration due to the inability to cross the blood-brain barrier (BBB). This hindrance to clinical testing of therapeutic strategies based on Nogo-Nogo receptor inhibition may have now been removed. Recently, Gou and coworkers generated a biologically active Nogo receptor blocker, NEP1-40 fusion protein, which crosses the BBB in vivo after systemic delivery (Gou, Wang, Yang, Xu, & Xiong, 2011). A phase I clinical trial applying anti-Nogo-A antibody to subjects with acute spinal cord injury has been successfully conducted, and a multicenter and a multinational phase II trial is in preparation (Zörner & Schwab, 2010).

3.3.3.7 REDUCING TONIC INHIBITION

After stroke, the peri-infarct zone shows increased neuroplasticity, which allows sensorimotor functions to remap from damaged areas (Cramer, 2008; Brown, Aminoltejari, Erb, Winship, & Murphy, 2009). However, this peri-infarct neuroplasticity, critically important for rehabilitation, is counteracted by tonic neuronal inhibition mediated by extrasynaptic $GABA_A$ receptors and is caused by an impairment in the ability of astrocytes to take up GABA (Clarkson, Huang, Macisaac, Mody, & Carmichael, 2010). L-655 708 is a cognition enhancing drug that acts as benzodiazepine inverse agonist specific for the α5 subunit of GABA receptors (Atack et al., 2006). Chronic treatment with L-655 708 starting 3 days after stroke counteracted the excessive GABA-mediated tonic inhibition and resulted in an early and sustained recovery of function in mice. In contrast, stroke volume was increased in mice treated with L-655 708 from stroke onset, showing that tonic inhibition in the acute phase is neuroprotective and the timing of drug delivery is critical for the treatment outcome (Clarkson et al., 2010). These results provide a rational basis for the development of novel pharmacological strategies to promote recovery after stroke.

3.3.4 EMERGING TARGETS

3.3.4.1 STEM CELLS

In the adult human brain, neural stem cells keep producing new neurons, astrocytes, and oligodendrocytes in two very well defined regions: the dentate gyrus of the hippocampus and the subventricular zone, albeit at a much lower rate than during earlier ontogenetic stages (Alvarez-Buylla & Lim, 2004). As demonstrated by Curtis and colleagues, a structure analogous to the rostral migratory stream in rodents connecting the subventricular zone with the olfactory bulb exists also in the human brain (Curtis et al., 2007). Having originated from dividing neural stem cells, differentiating cells migrate through the rostral migratory stream to the olfactory bulb. In the animal stroke models, some of these cells were shown to divert from the rostral migratory stream and reach the ischemic penumbra, where some of them transiently persist and others turn into both neurons and astrocytes (Arvidsson, Collin, Kirik, Kokaia, & Lindvall, 2002), with some possibly persisting for over a year after experimental stroke in mice (Osman, Porritt, Nilsson, & Kuhn 2011). To what extent this applies to the human brain, in which the migratory distances are much larger, remains to be established.

We do not know yet the functional significance of the adult mammalian neurogenesis, since no animal models exist in which neurogenesis could be specifically inhibited without simultaneous inhibitory or modulatory effects on other plasticity responses. However, it has been very well documented that enriched environment applied to adults of various vertebrate species stimulates both baseline as well as ischemia-triggered neurogenesis. Thus it is possible that the newly formed neural stem cell–derived, partially differentiated cells of neuronal or glial lineages, or newly formed neurons, astrocytes, or oligodendrocytes would positively affect brain plasticity and functional recovery after stroke. Interestingly, gap junctional coupling occurs between introduced neural stem cells and residential neuronal cells, at least in a mouse central nervous system, and this coupling was shown to be essential for the neuroprotective effect of neural stem cells on the endogenous neuronal cells (Jäderstad et al., 2010). Thus, apart from the plasticity-promoting "trophic" effects of newly born and partially differentiated neuroectodermal cells, these cells might protect the cells of the ischemic penumbra also by a direct cell–cell transfer of signaling and other molecules.

3.3.4.2 TARGETING THE ASTROCYTES

The emergence of astrocytes as a target in stroke intervention in the future is intriguing. Astrocytes were shown to control blood flow (Mulligan & MacVicar, 2004), a function highly relevant for both physiological and pathological situations such as stroke. Also, in the ischemic brain lesions, astrocytes are the major source of vascular endothelial growth factor (VEGF) and thus the main driving force behind the formation of new blood vessels. This facilitates highly coupled neurorestorative processes including synaptogenesis, which positively contributes to functional recovery (Beck & Plate, 2009). Astrocytes are considered to be of major importance in the detoxification process of different reactive oxygen species after cellular stress, which is a major component of ischemic stroke (Sims, Nilsson, & Muyderman, 2004; Hertz, 2008). Beta-lactam antibiotics were shown to be potent stimulators of the glutamate transporter GLT1 (EAAT2) in astrocytes. They had a neuroprotective effect on in vitro models of ischemic injury, and delayed progression of amyotrophic lateral sclerosis (ALS) in an animal model (Rothstein et al., 2005). Both ischemic and hemorrhagic stroke lead to massive activation of astrocytes and prominent reactive gliosis in the ischemic penumbra (Pekny & Pekna, 2004; Pekny & Nilsson, 2005; Sofroniew, 2009; Sofroniew & Vinters, 2010). We showed that attenuation of reactive gliosis in ischemic stroke by genetic ablation of GFAP and vimentin (proteins that constitute the highly dynamic astrocyte intermediate filament, or nanofilament, system) leads to increased infarction and proposed that reactive astrocytes play an important role in the protection of the ischemic penumbra (Li et al., 2008). We proposed that modulation of reactive gliosis and other aspects of astrocyte activity may provide novel therapeutic paradigms for ischemic stroke (Li et al., 2008).

Astrocytes were also shown to directly control the number and the function of neuronal synapses (Ullian, Sapperstein, Christopherson, & Barres, 2001). We demonstrated that mice deficient for GFAP and vimentin exhibit attenuated reactive gliosis and have a more pronounced loss of synapses in the hippocampus in the acute phase after partial deafferentation of the dentate gyrus of the hippocampus by entorhinal cortex lesion, but show remarkable synaptic recovery later on (Wilhelmsson et al., 2004). An interesting link exists between astrocytes, thrombospondins, and synaptic response and axonal sprouting in ischemic stroke. Thrombospondins 1 and 2 are members of a family of extracellular glycoproteins with synaptogenic properties secreted by astrocytes (Christopherson et al., 2005). Their deficiency leads to reduced synaptic density during development (Christopherson et al., 2005). Astrocyte expression of thrombospondins 1 and 2 is increased after experimental stroke (Liauw et al., 2008). Compared to wild-type (normal) mice, mice deficient in thrombospondins 1 and 2 exhibited synaptic density and axonal sprouting deficit associated with impaired motor function recovery after stroke, despite no differences in infarct volume and blood vessel density (Liauw et al., 2008).

Recent data suggest that astrocytes also play a role in the elimination of supernumerary synapses during development and possibly also in a pathological context. Immature astrocytes in the developing brain seem to be a source of a signal that triggers the expression of complement component C1q in developing neurons (Stevens et al., 2007). C1q localizes to synapses that are thus tagged for elimination through the activation of the complement cascade and deposition of C3b, an opsonin derived from the proteolytic activation of the third complement component (C3; Stevens et al., 2007). Both mice deficient in C1q and mice deficient in C3 showed significant and sustained defects in CNS synapse elimination (Stevens et al., 2007). Although the role of the astrocyte-induced mechanism of synaptic elimination and remodeling in post-stroke plasticity remains to be addressed, the complement-mediated elimination of synapses seems to be reactivated in neuropathologies such as glaucoma.

Given the immense molecular complexity of the response of reactive astrocytes to brain ischemia, it is likely that future treatment protocols will target multiple molecular pathways. It is also likely that their effects will be relatively gentle (Lipton, Gu, & Nakamura, 2007). Most probably, the future treatment and secondary prevention paradigms will be used to adjust multiple equilibriums

and will be combined with other modalities that promote regeneration, both pharmacological (Busch & Silver, 2007) and nonpharmacological, the latter including targeted rehabilitation, exercise, or multisensory stimulation (Nilsson & Pekny, 2007).

3.4 INDIVIDUALIZED THERAPY

Personalized medicine is a rapidly advancing field of health care that is directed by the unique clinical, genetic, genomic, and environmental information of each person. Because these factors are different for every person, the nature of the diseases, their onset, their course, and how they might respond to drugs and other interventions is as individual as the people who have them. Personalized medicine is defined as a way of making the treatment as individualized as the disease. It involves identifying genetic, genomic, and clinical information that allows predictions to be made about a person's susceptibility to developing disease, the course of disease, and its response to treatment. In order for personalized medicine to be used effectively by healthcare providers and their patients, these findings must be translated in precise diagnostic tests and targeted therapies. This has begun to happen in certain areas, such as testing patients genetically to determine their likelihood of having serious adverse reactions to various cancer drugs (van't Veer & Bernards, 2008).

The targeted therapies that are defined under the umbrella of personalized medicine typically include only pharmacological intervention (Clayton et al., 2006; Shastry, 2006; Clayton, Baker, Lindon, Everett, & Nicholson, 2009). However, there are other efficient therapeutic modalities, such as rehabilitation, that potentially could qualify as a part of the personalized medicine concept. For instance, modern stroke rehabilitation should comprise individually tailored programs that are based on a careful analysis of the nature of the brain damage, including its anatomical localization and functional consequences. In addition, a comprehensive review of the individual's anamnesis must be performed, including a mapping of the premorbid personality, motivational and personal drivers, individual interests and preferences, support from family and friends, professional background, social situation, mood, biological age, and so forth. Together with results from functional neuroimaging techniques, evaluation of early clinical signs of predictive value, and analysis of biomarkers linked to prediction of recovery and outcome, a platform for an individually tailored rehabilitation intervention could be shaped.

In a future perspective, genetic and genomic analyses unraveling genetic differences and polymorphisms might also be added to the review process of each individual's capacity to recover from, for example, a stroke. Indeed, there are already some clinical data on healthy individuals supporting this hypothetical view. Brain-derived growth factor (BDNF) has been proven in several studies to be critical for activity-dependent modulation of synaptic plasticity in the human motor cortex. Reduced secretion of BDNF is coupled to reduction of activity-related cortical plasticity in response to motor training, reduced capacity of short-term motor learning, and reduced cognitive performance in the elderly. It is also shown to modulate the response to rTMS, which is suggested to underpin some of the individual differences of the effect of stimulation. A common single nucleotide polymorphism (BDNF val66-met) is shown to reduce secretion of BDNF in the brain and, as a result, affected individuals experience problems as described above (reviewed in Johansson, 2011). This and presumed other genetic differences can potentially influence outcome after a stroke, and might contribute to the personal profile underlying individually tailored rehabilitation programs. Personalized medicine should, in the light of this reasoning, possibly also include individually profiled rehabilitation. Personalized medicine would then be defined in terms of how we integrate information necessary for individual patient care.

REFERENCES

Alvarez-Buylla, A., & Lim, D. A. (2004). For the long run: maintaining germinal niches in the adult brain. *Neuron, 41,* 683–686.

Arvidsson, A., Collin, T., Kirik, D., Kokaia, Z., & Lindvall, O. (2002). Neuronal replacement from endogenous precursors in the adult brain after stroke. *Nature Medicine, 8,* 963–970.

Atack, J. R., Bayley, P. J., Seabrook, G. R., Wafford, K. A., McKernan, R. M., & Dawson, G. R. (2006). L-655,708 enhances cognition in rats but is not proconvulsant at a dose selective for alpha5-containing GABAA receptors. *Neuropharmacology, 51,* 1023–1029.

Beck, H., & Plate, K. H. (2009). Angiogenesis after cerebral ischemia. *Acta Neuropathololologica, 117,* 481–496.

Bolognini, N., Pascual-Leone, A., & Fregni, F. (2009). Using non-invasive brain stimulation to augment motor training-induced plasticity. *Journal of Neuroengineering and Rehabilitation, 6,* 8.

Brown, C. E., Aminoltejari, K., Erb, H., Winship, I. R., & Murphy, T. H. (2009). In vivo voltage-sensitive dye imaging in adult mice reveals that somatosensory maps lost to stroke are replaced over weeks by new structural and functional circuits with prolonged modes of activation within both the peri-infarct zone and distant sites. *Journal of Neuroscience, 29,* 1719–1734.

Busch, S. A., & Silver, J. (2007). The role of extracellular matrix in CNS regeneration. *Current Opinions in Neurobiology, 17,* 120–127.

Bütefisch, C. M., Kleiser, R., & Seitz, R. J. (2006). Post-lesional cerebral reorganisation: evidence from functional neuroimaging and transcranial magnetic stimulation. *Journal of Physiology, 99,* 437–454.

Carter, A. R., Connor, L. T., & Dromerick, A. W. (2010). Rehabilitation after stroke: current state of the science. *Current Neurology and Neuroscience Reports, 10,* 158–166.

Celnik, P., Webster, B., Glasser, D. M., & Cohen, L. G. (2008). Effects of action observation on physical training after stroke. *Stroke, 39,* 1814–1820.

Cheatwood, J. L., Emerick, A. J., & Kartje, G. L. (2008). Neuronal plasticity and functional recovery after ischemic stroke. *Topics in Stroke Rehabilitation, 15,* 42–50.

Chen, J., Cui, X., Zacharek, A., Ding, G. L., Shehadah, A., Jiang, Q., et al. (2009). Niaspan treatment increases tumor necrosis factor-alpha-converting enzyme and promotes arteriogenesis after stroke. *Journal of Cerebral Blood Flow and Metabolism, 29,* 911–920.

Chen, J., Cui, X., Zacharek, A., Jiang, H., Roberts, C., Zhang, C., et al. (2007). Niaspan increases angiogenesis and improves functional recovery after stroke. *Annals of Neurology, 62,* 49–58.

Chen, J. L., Penhune, V. B., & Zatorre, R. J. (2008). Listening to musical rhythms recruits motor regions of the brain. *Cerebral Cortex, 18,* 2844–2854.

Chen, P., Goldberg, D. E., Kolb, B., Lanser, M., & Benowitz, L. I. (2002). Inosine induces axonal rewiring and improves behavioral outcome after stroke. *Proceedings of the National Acadamy of Science U S A, 99,* 9031–9036.

Chollet, F., DiPiero, V., Wise, R. J., Brooks, D. J., Dolan, R. J., & Frackowiak, R. S. (1991). The functional anatomy of motor recovery after stroke in humans: a study with positron emission tomography. *Annals of Neurology, 29,* 63–71.

Chollet, F., Tardy, J., Albucher, J. F., Thalamas, C., Berard, E., Lamy, C., et al. (2011). Fluoxetine for motor recovery after acute ischaemic stroke (FLAME): a randomised placebo-controlled trial. *Lancet Neurology, 10.*

Christopherson, K. S., Ullian, E. M., Stokes, C. C., Mullowney, C. E., Hell, J. W., Agah, A., et al. (2005). Thrombospondins are astrocyte-secreted proteins that promote CNS synaptogenesis. *Cell, 120,* 421–433.

Clarkson, A. N., Huang, B. S., Macisaac, S. E., Mody, I., & Carmichael, S.T. (2010). Reducing excessive GABA-mediated tonic inhibition promotes functional recovery after stroke. *Nature, 468,* 305–309.

Clayton, T. A., Baker, D., Lindon, J. C., Everett, J. R., & Nicholson, J. K. (2009). Pharmacometabonomic identification of a significant host-microbiome metabolic interaction affecting human drug metabolism. *Proceedings of the National Acadamy of Science U S A, 106,* 14728–14733.

Clayton, T. A., Lindon, J. C., Cloarec, O., Antti, H., Charuel, C., Hanton, G., et al. (2006). Pharmaco-metabonomic phenotyping and personalized drug treatment. *Nature, 440,* 1073–1077.

Cramer, S. C. (2008). Repairing the human brain after stroke: I. Mechanisms of spontaneous recovery. *Annals of Neurology, 63,* 272–287.

Cui, X., Chopp, M., Zacharek, A., Roberts, C., Buller, B., Ion, M., et al. (2010). Niacin treatment of stroke increases synaptic plasticity and axon growth in rats. *Stroke, 41,* 2044–2049.

Curtis, M. A., Kam, M., Nannmark, U., Anderson, M. F., Axell, M., Wikkelso, C., et al. (2007). Human neuroblasts migrate to the olfactory bulb via a lateral ventricular extension. *Science, 315,* 1243–1249.

da Silva Cameirão, M., Bermúdez, Badia, S., Duarte, E., & Verschure, P. F. (2011). Virtual reality based rehabilitation speeds up functional recovery of the upper extremities after stroke: A randomized controlled pilot study in the acute phase of stroke using the Rehabilitation Gaming System. *Restorative Neurology and Neuroscience, 29,* 287–298.

Dimyan, M. A., & Cohen, L. G. (2011). Neuroplasticity in the context of motor rehabilitation after stroke. *Nature Reviews Neurology, 7,* 76–85.

Dohle, C., Püllen, J., Nakaten, A., Küst, J., Rietz, C., & Karbe, H. (2009). Mirror therapy promotes recovery from severe hemiparesis: a randomized controlled trial. *Neurorehabilitation and Neural Repair, 23,* 209–217.

Enzinger, C., Johansen-Berg, H., Dawes, H., Bogdanovic, M., Collett, J., Guy, C., et al. (2008). Functional MRI correlates of lower limb function in stroke victims with gait impairment. *Stroke, 39,* 1507–1513.

Ertelt, D., Small, S., Solodkin, A., Dettmers, C., McNamara, A., Binkofski, F., et al. (2007). Action observation has a positive impact on rehabilitation of motor deficits after stroke. *NeuroImage, 36,* T164–T173.

Feydy, A., Carlier, R., Roby-Brami, A., Bussel, B., Cazalis, F., Pierot, L., et al. (2002). Longitudinal study of motor recovery after stroke: recruitment and focusing of brain activation. *Stroke, 33,* 1610–1617.

Fridman, E. A., Hanakawa, T., Chung, M., Hummel, F., Leiguarda, R. C., & Cohen, L. (2004). Reorganization of the human ipsilesional premotor cortex after stroke. *Brain, 127,* 747–758.

Gerloff, C., Bushara, K., Sailer, A., Wassermann, E. M., Chen, R., Matsuoka, T., et al. (2006). Multimodal imaging of brain reorganization in motor areas of the contralesional hemisphere of well recovered patients after capsular stroke. *Brain, 129,* 791–808.

Ghazanfar, A. A., & Schroeder, C. E. (2006). Is neocortex essentially multisensory? *Trends in Cognitive Science, 10,* 278–285.

Goldstein, L. B. (2009). Amphetamine trials and tribulations. *Stroke, 40,* S133–S135.

Gonsette, R. E., Sindic, C., D'hooghe, M. B., De Deyn, P. P., Medaer, R., Michotte, A., et al. (2010). Boosting endogenous neuroprotection in multiple sclerosis: the ASsociation of Inosine and Interferon beta in relapsing—remitting Multiple Sclerosis (ASIIMS) trial. *Multiple Sclerosis, 16,* 455–462.

Gou, X., Wang, Q., Yang, Q., Xu, L., & Xiong, L. (2011). TAT-NEP1-40 as a novel therapeutic candidate for axonal regeneration and functional recovery after stroke. *Journal of Drug Targeting, 19,* 86–95.

Henderson, L. A., Gustin, S. M., Macey, P. M., Wrigley, P. J., & Siddall, P. J. (2011). Functional reorganization of the brain in humans following spinal cord injury: evidence for underlying changes in cortical anatomy. *Journal of Neuroscience, 31,* 2630–2637.

Homberg, J. R., Olivier, J. D., Blom, T., Arentsen, T., van Brunschot, C., Schipper, P., et al. (2011). Fluoxetine exerts age-dependent effects on behavior and amygdala neuroplasticity in the rat. *Public Library of Science ONE, 6,* e16646.

Jäderstad, J., Jäderstad, L. M., Li, J., Chintawar, S., Salto, C., Pandolfo, M., et al. (2010). Communication via gap junctions underlies early functional and beneficial interactions between grafted neural stem cells and the host. *Proceedings of the National Academy of Science U S A, 107,* 5184–5189.

Jankowska, E., & Edgley, S. A. (2006). How can corticospinal tract neurons contribute to ipsilateral movements? A question with implications for recovery of motor functions. *Neuroscientist, 12,* 67–79.

Janssen, H., Bernhardt, J., Collier, J. M., Sena, E. S., McElduff, P., Attia, J., et al. (2010). An enriched environment improves sensorimotor function post-ischemic stroke. *Neurorehabilitation and Neural Repair, 24,* 802–813.

Johansson, B. B. (2011). Current trends in stroke rehabilitation. A review with focus on brain plasticity. *Acta Neurologica Scandinavia, 123,* 147–159.

Kim, J., Wigram, T., & Gold, C. (2008). The effects of improvisational music therapy on joint attention behaviors in autistic children: a randomized controlled study. *Journal of Autism and Developmental Disorders, 38,* 1758–1766.

Krishnan, V., & Nestler, E. J. (2008). The molecular neurobiology of depression. *Nature, 455,* 894–902.

Langhorne, P., Bernhardt, J., & Kwakkel, G. (2011). Stroke rehabilitation. *Lancet, 377,* 1693–1702.

Lee, J. K., Kim, J. E., Sivula, M., & Strittmatter, S. M. (2004). Nogo receptor antagonism promotes stroke recovery by enhancing axonal plasticity. *Journal of Neuroscience, 24,* 6209–6217.

Li, L., Lundkvist, A., Andersson, D., Wilhelmsson, U., Nagai, N., Pardo, A. C., et al. (2008). Protective role of reactive astrocytes in brain ischemia. *Journal of Cerebral Blood Flow and Metabolism, 28,* 468–481.

Liauw, J., Hoang, S., Choi, M., Eroglu, C., Choi, M., Sun, G. H., et al. (2008). Thrombospondins 1 and 2 are necessary for synaptic plasticity and functional recovery after stroke. *Journal of Cerebral Blood Flow and Metabolism, 28,* 1722–1732.

Lindenberg, R., Renga, V., Zhu, L. L., Nair, D., & Schlaug, G. (2010). Bihemispheric brain stimulation facilitates motor recovery in chronic stroke patients. *Neurology, 75,* 2176–2184.

Lipton, S. A., Gu, Z., & Nakamura, T. (2007). Inflammatory mediators leading to protein misfolding and uncompetitive/fast off-rate drug therapy for neurodegenerative disorders. *International Review of Neurobiology, 82,* 1–27.

Liu, Y., & Rouiller, E. M. (1999). Mechanisms of recovery of dexterity following unilateral lesion of the sensorimotor cortex in adult monkeys. *Brain Research, 128,* 149–159.

Liu, Z., Zhang, R. L., Li, Y., Cui, Y., & Chopp, M. (2009). Remodeling of the corticospinal innervation and spontaneous behavioral recovery after ischemic stroke in adult mice. *Stroke, 40,* 2546–2551.

Lotze, M., & Halsband, U. (2006). Motor imagery. *Journal of Physiology, 99,* 135–140.

Marshall, R. S., Zarahn, E., Alon, L., Minzer, B., Lazar, R. M., & Krakauer, J. W. (2009). Early imaging correlates of subsequent motor recovery after stroke. *Annals of Neurology, 65,* 596–602.

Martinsson, L., Hardemark, H. G., & Eksborg, S. (2007). Should amphetamines be given to improve recovery after stroke? *Stroke, 38,* 2400–2401.

Merzenich, M. M., Kaas, J. H., Wall, J., Nelson, R. J., Sur, M., & Felleman, D. (1983). Topographic reorganization of somatosensory cortical areas 3b and 1 in adult monkeys following restricted deafferentation. *Neuroscience, 8,* 33–55.

Mulligan, S. J., & MacVicar, B. A. (2004). Calcium transients in astrocyte endfeet cause cerebrovascular constrictions. *Nature, 431,* 195–199.

Murie-Fernández, M., Irimia, P., Martínez-Vila, E., Meyer, M., & Teasell, R. (2010). Neuro-rehabilitation after stroke. *Neurologia, 25,* 189–196.

Murphy, T. H., & Corbett, D. (2009). Plasticity during stroke recovery: from synapse to behaviour. *Nature Reviews Neuroscience, 10,* 861–872.

Nilsson, M., & Pekny, M. (2007). Enriched environment and astrocytes in central nervous system regeneration. *Journal of Rehabilitative Medicine, 39,* 345–352.

Nithianantharajah, J., & Hannan, A.J. (2006). Enriched environments, experience-dependent plasticity and disorders of the nervous system. *Nature Reviews Neuroscience, 7,* 697–709.

Osman, A. M., Porritt, M. J., Nilsson, M., & Kuhn, H. G. (2011). Long-term stimulation of neural progenitor cell migration after cortical ischemia in mice. *Stroke, 42*(12), 3559–3565.

Page, S. J., Levine, P., & Leonard, A. (2007). Mental practice in chronic stroke: results of a randomized, placebo-controlled trial. *Stroke, 38,* 1293–1297.

Papadopoulos, C. M., Tsai, S. Y., Alsbiei, T., O'Brien, T. E., Schwab, M. E., & Kartje, G. L. (2002). Functional recovery and neuroanatomical plasticity following middle cerebral artery occlusion and IN-1 antibody treatment in the adult rat. *Annals of Neurology, 51,* 433–441.

Papadopoulos, C. M., Tsai, S. Y., Cheatwood, J. L., Bollnow, M. R., Kolb, B. E., Schwab, M. E., et al. (2006). Dendritic plasticity in the adult rat following middle cerebral artery occlusion and Nogo-a neutralization. *Cerebral Cortex, 16,* 529–536.

Pekny, M., & Nilsson, M. (2005). Astrocyte activation and reactive gliosis. *Glia, 50,* 427–434.

Pekny, M., & Pekna, M. (2004). Astrocyte intermediate filaments in CNS pathologies and regeneration. *Journal of Pathology, 204,* 428–437.

Pinnock, S. B., Blake, A. M., Platt, N. J., & Herbert, J. (2010). The roles of BDNF, pCREB and Wnt3a in the latent period preceding activation of progenitor cell mitosis in the adult dentate gyrus by fluoxetine. *Public Library of Science ONE, 5,* e13652.

Rothgangel, A. S., Braun, S. M., Beurskens, A. J., Seitz, R. J., & Wade, D. T. (2011). The clinical aspects of mirror therapy in rehabilitation: a systematic review of the literature. *International Journal of Rehabilitation Research, 34,* 1–13.

Rothstein, J. D., Patel, S., Regan, M. R., Haenggeli, C., Huang, Y. H., Bergles, D. E., et al. (2005). Beta-lactam antibiotics offer neuroprotection by increasing glutamate transporter expression. *Nature, 433*, 73–77.

Ruscher, K., Shamloo, M., Rickhag, M., Ladunga, I., Soriano, L., Gisselsson, L., et al. (2011). The sigma-1 receptor enhances brain plasticity and functional recovery after experimental stroke. *Brain, 134*, 732–746.

Saposnik, G., Teasell, R., Mamdani, M., Hall, J., McIlroy, W., Cheung, D., et al. (2010). Effectiveness of virtual reality using Wii gaming technology in stroke rehabilitation: a pilot randomized clinical trial and proof of principle. *Stroke, 41*, 1477–1484.

Särkämö, T., Pihko, E., Laitinen, S., Forsblom, A., Soinila, S., Mikkonen, M., et al. (2009). Music and speech listening enhance the recovery of early sensory processing after stroke. *Journal of Cognitive Neuroscience, 22*, 2716–2727.

Särkämö, T., Tervaniemi, M., Laitinen, S., Forsblom, A., Soinila, S., Mikkonen, M., et al. (2008). Music listening enhances cognitive recovery and mood after middle cerebral artery stroke. *Brain, 131*, 866–876.

Shams, L., & Seitz, A. R. (2008). Benefits of multisensory learning. *Trends in Cognitive Science, 12*, 411–407.

Shastry, B. S. (2006). Pharmacogenetics and the concept of individualized medicine. *Pharmacogenomics, 6*, 16–21.

Sims, N.R., Nilsson, M. & Muyderman, H. (2004). Mitochondrial glutathione: a modulator of brain cell death. *Journal of Bioenergetics and Biomembranes, 36*, 329–333.

Sofroniew, M. V. (2009). Molecular dissection of reactive astrogliosis and glial scar formation. *Trends in Neuroscience, 32*, 638–647.

Sofroniew, M. V., & Vinters, H. V. (2010). Astrocytes: biology and pathology. *Acta Neuropathologica, 119*, 7–35.

Soto, D., Funes, M. J., Guzmán-García, A., Warbrick, T., Rotshtein, P., & Humphreys, G. W. (2009). Pleasant music overcomes the loss of awareness in patients with visual neglect. *Proceedings of the National Academy of Science U S A, 106*, 6011–6016.

Stevens, B., Allen, N. J., Vazquez, L. E., Howell, G. R., Christopherson, K. S., Nouri, N., et al. (2007). The classical complement cascade mediates CNS synapse elimination. *Cell, 131*, 1164–1178.

Tsai, S. Y., Markus, T. M., Andrews, E. M., Cheatwood, J. L., Emerick, A. J., Mir, A. K., et al. (2007). Intrathecal treatment with anti-Nogo-A antibody improves functional recovery in adult rats after stroke. *Experimental Brain Research, 182*, 261–266.

Tsai, S. Y., Papadopoulos, C. M., Schwab, M. E. & Kartje, G. L. (2011). Delayed anti-nogo-a therapy improves function after chronic stroke in adult rats. *Stroke, 42*, 186–190.

Ullian, E., Sapperstein, S. K., Christopherson, K. S., & Barres, B. A. (2001). Control of synapse number by glia. *Science, 291*, 657–661.

van't Veer, L. J., & Bernards, R. (2008). Enabling personalized cancer medicine through analysis of gene-expression patterns. *Nature, 452*, 564–570.

Vosper, H. (2009). Niacin: a re-emerging pharmaceutical for the treatment of dyslipidaemia. *British Journal of Pharmacology, 158*, 429–441.

Warraich, Z., & Kleim, J. A. (2010). Neural plasticity: the biological substrate for neurorehabilitation. *Physical Medicine and Rehabilitation, 2*, S208–S219.

Werhahn, K. J., Conforto, A. B., Kadom, N., Hallett, M., & Cohen, L. G. (2003). Contribution of the ipsilateral motor cortex to recovery after chronic stroke. *Annals of Neurology, 54*, 464–472.

Wieloch, T., & Nikolich, K. (2006). Mechanisms of neural plasticity following brain injury. *Current Opinions in Neurobiology, 16*, 258–264.

Wiessner, C., Bareyre, F. M., Allegrini, P. R., Mir, A. K., Frentzel, S., Zurini, M., et al. (2003). Anti-Nogo-A antibody infusion 24 hours after experimental stroke improved behavioral outcome and corticospinal plasticity in normotensive and spontaneously hypertensive rats. *Journal of Cerebral Blood Flow and Metabolism, 23*, 154–165.

Wilhelmsson, U., Li, L., Pekna, M., Berthold, C. H., Blom, S., Eliasson, C., et al. (2004). Absence of GFAP and vimentin prevents hypertrophy of astrocytic processes and improves post-traumatic regeneration. *Journal of Neuroscience, 24*, 5016–5021.

Wrigley, P. J., Press, S. R., Gustin, S. M., Macefield, V. G., Gandevia, S. C., Cousins, M. J., et al. (2009). Neuropathic pain and primary somatosensory cortex reorganization following spinal cord injury. *Pain, 141*, 52–59.

Xerri, C. (2011). Plasticity of cortical maps: Multiple triggers for adaptive reorganization following brain damage and spinal cord injury. *Neuroscientist*. doi: 10.1177/1073858410397894.

Yavuzer, G., Selles, R., Sezer, N., Sütbeyaz, S., Bussmann, J. B., Köseoğlu, F., et al. (2008). Mirror therapy improves hand function in subacute stroke: a randomized controlled trial. *Archives of Physical Medicine and Rehabilitation, 89*, 393–398.

Zai, L., Ferrari, C., Dice, C., Subbaiah, S., Havton, L. A., Coppola, G., et al. (2011). Inosine augments the effects of a Nogo receptor blocker and of environmental enrichment to restore skilled forelimb use after stroke. *Journal of Neuroscience, 31*, 5977–5988.

Zai, L., Ferrari, C., Subbaiah, S., Havton, L. A., Coppola, G., Strittmatter, S., et al. (2009). Inosine alters gene expression and axonal projections in neurons contralateral to a cortical infarct and improves skilled use of the impaired limb. *Journal of Neuroscience, 29*, 8187–8197.

Zatorre, R., & McGill, J. (2005). Music, the food of neuroscience? *Nature, 434*, 312–315.

Zemke, A. C., Heagerty, P. J., Lee, C., & Cramer, S. C. (2003). Motor cortex organization after stroke is related to side of stroke and level of recovery. *Stroke, 34*, e23–e28.

Zörner, B., & Schwab, M. E. (2010). Anti-Nogo on the go: from animal models to a clinical trial. *Annals of the New York Academy of Science, 1198*, E22–E34.

4 | IMAGING TECHNIQUES PROVIDE NEW INSIGHTS

J-DONALD TOURNIER, RICHARD A. J. MASTERTON, and RÜDIGER J. SEITZ

4.1 INTRODUCTION TO NEUROIMAGING TECHNIQUES AND THEIR POTENTIAL TO PROVIDE NEW INSIGHTS

Before the advent of neuroimaging, understanding of the brain was based either on the study of its disorders, or of its anatomy. The pioneering findings of Broca (1824–1880) and Wernicke (1848–1905) were all made possible by correlating lesion location in the brains of patients with their affected function, while those of Brodmann (1868–1918) and Dejerine (1849–1917) were made possible with the advent of postmortem histological and gross dissection techniques. These approaches undeniably led to tremendous advances in neuroscience and now form the foundation of our current understanding of the brain. However, there are many questions about the brain and its disorders that could not be answered with these approaches.

Modern neuroimaging techniques allow the brain to be studied in vivo, and the many techniques now available can provide information about a range of different aspects of brain anatomy and function. It is now possible for example to identify areas of the brain involved in the performance of a particular task, or to relate the size of particular brain structures to the severity of clinical symptoms in a completely noninvasive manner. These techniques have, therefore, allowed tremendous advances to be made over the last two decades in many areas of neuroscience and neurology and will undoubtedly continue to do so.

4.2 WHAT NEUROIMAGING CAN TELL US

4.2.1 MEASURING BRAIN PERFUSION

Perfusion refers to the amount of blood delivered to the tissue (via the capillary bed) per unit time, and is typically measured in milliliters of blood per minute per 100 grams of tissue. It reflects the supply of oxygen and nutrients provided to the tissue, as well as the removal of waste products. Perfusion imaging provides information on the momentary hemodynamic state of the brain tissue, which is of great clinical importance, as a blood vessel obstruction immediately impairs tissue perfusion (Warach, Gaa, Siewert, Wielopolski, & Edelman, 1995; Sorensen et al., 1996). Therefore, perfusion imaging may yield information about pathologically hypoperfused regions even before the onset of genuine structural brain tissue damage. A regional cerebral blood flow of 15–20 ml per 100g of tissue is the critical viability limit derived from animal experiments (Hossmann, 1994; Sorensen et al., 1996) and from blood flow measurements in patients using positron emission tomography (Herholz et al., 1987). Interestingly, the cerebral arteries typically reopen after thromboembolic occlusion, which results in a normalization of the perfusion data usually within 24 hours (Wittsack et al., 2002).

Measurements of cerebral blood flow or brain perfusion in man started in the 1960s using intra-arterial tracer injections in the carotid artery (Lassen & Ingvar, 1972). These studies provided lateral views of the tracer distribution in the brain. Since the advent of positron emission tomography (PET), the tracer distribution following intravenous bolus injections could be visualized in axial images with constant intensity and resolution throughout the entire brain (Phelps, Mazziotta, & Schelbert, 1985). Moreover, biological variables like the regional cerebral blood flow (rCBF) could be determined pixel-by-pixel in these tomographic images based on biomathematical modeling. The quantitative measurements of rCBF rely on rapid recording of the dynamics of tracer accumulation in the brain and on simultaneous measurements of the tracer distribution in the arterial blood following intravenous tracer administration (Figure 4.1). With appropriate modeling, and taking into account the arterial input curve, the radioactive decay of the tracer, and the dispersion of the tracer bolus in the brain, it is possible to determine the rCBF pixel-by-pixel throughout the brain. The rCBF is in the range of 45 to 70 ml/100g/min in cerebral grey matter structures and about 15 to 25 ml/100g/min in cerebral white matter. A closely related biological variable is the regional cerebral blood volume (rCBV), which can also be determined with PET. Essentially, this is the ratio of the integrated tracer concentration in the brain to that measured in the arterial blood.

Perfusion computed tomography (CT) techniques are based on similar biomathematical modeling. The CT measurements image the distribution of contrast-enhancing agents in the brain using external radiation provided by the CT scanner. Whole-brain perfusion-CT is useful to evaluate the entire brain perfusion, but can only provide information related to rCBV and therefore cannot differentiate reversible from nonreversible ischemic brain damage (Hunter et al., 1998; Lev et al., 2001). Dynamic perfusion-CT involves the dynamic acquisition of sequential CT slices during the intravenous administration of contrast (Wintermark, Reichhart, et al., 2002). This technique assesses quantitatively both rCBF and rCBV and can delineate the penumbra tissue. However, the volume of brain tissue that is imaged with perfusion-CT is limited by the current CT scanners, although new techniques have been developed to increase the amount of scanned tissue (Roberts et al., 2001). Using rapidly scanning spiral CT, rCBF and rCBV can now also be determined with computed tomography using iodinated contrast media. Rapid CT scanning does, however, expose the patient to a considerable amount of radiation, inherent in CT scanning. The penumbra tissue, defined by dynamic perfusion-CT, has been demonstrated to be accurate in comparison with acute and delayed diffusion/perfusion-weighted MRI (Wintermark, Reichhart, et al., 2002a; Wintermark, Reichhart, et al., 2002b). Pregnancy, renal failure, and allergy to contrast material are relative contraindications to performing a brain CT.

Magnetic resonance imaging (MRI) is an entirely noninvasive tomographic scanning method that relies on the magnetic properties of hydrogen nuclei. With this technique one can determine brain perfusion after an intravenous bolus injection, similarly to PET. Bolus contrast perfusion-weighted MRI requires the intravenous application of some 15 ml of a gadolinium contrast agent and provides information about the momentary state of brain tissue perfusion. The tracer concentration in the brain can be used to estimate rCBF and rCBV in a pixel-by-pixel fashion, along with the so-called mean transit time (MTT, Figure. 4.2). Calculation of rCBF in a pixel-by-pixel approach taking into account also the dispersion of the tracer bolus in the brain has been implemented in MRI measurements (Calamante &

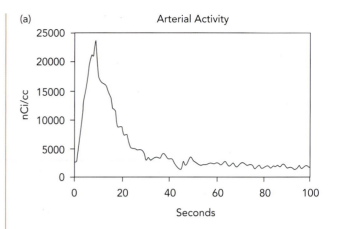

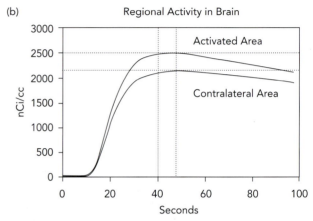

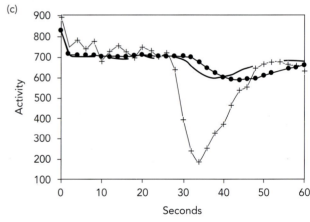

Figure 4.1 Activity data obtained with positron emission tomography needed for quantitation of rCBF (a, b). Abnormal activity changes in an acute infarct (solid line), in chronic cerebral hypoperfusion due to a carotid artery occlusion (dotted line), and in a normal brain (crossed line) as determined with MRI (c); from Surikova et al., (2006).

Connelly, 2009). Unfortunately, however, head movements of the patients, who are typically severely ill in acute stroke, preclude the routine application of this method in a clinical setting. Rather, in clinical routine the bolus concentration data are converted into relative rCBF and relative rCBV, which represent qualitative representations easy to use to identify abnormalities like an acute stroke. Furthermore, measurements of the delay of the bolus are also routinely used in clinical settings, since they are easy to calculate and

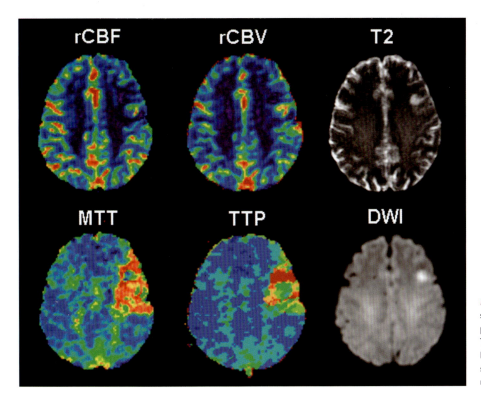

Figure 4.2 Multimodal MRI in acute stroke. Note the large area of impaired perfusion as evident from the MTT and TTP maps as compared with the small DWI lesion. The area of abnormal perfusion is less evident in the rCBF and rCBV maps.

easy to read (Figure 4.2). The most widely used measure of brain perfusion is the *time-to-peak*—the time taken for the intravenously-administered gadolinium bolus to reach peak concentration within each voxel in the tissue. This model-independent measure allows the assessment of the severity of ischemia in comparison to the non-affected hemisphere in an objective manner (Wittsack et al., 2002). In brain infarcts the accumulation of the tracer bolus is delayed as compared to healthy brain tissue (Figure 4.1). The larger the delay, the more likely the brain tissue will be damaged by ischemia. In fact, a delay of 4 seconds relative to the non-affected hemisphere will result in a functional impairment, while a delay of 6 s relative to the non-affected hemisphere shows the brain tissue that will be damaged (Neumann-Haefelin et al., 1999). More recently, so-called T_{max} images have been proposed that also reflect primarily the delay in perfusion; these are computed by deconvolution of the arterial concentration time course from the cerebral concentration time course, to give the so-called *residue function*, the maximum of which occurs at T_{max} (Calamante et al., 2010). Again, a delay greater than approximately 4–6 seconds indicates tissue at risk of infarction (Olivot et al., 2009).

Both CT and MRI have options to also image the cerebral arteries and veins. This provides important information in addition to the functional tomographic images, since it also allows investigations of the intracranial and extracranial vasculature. Both methods are therefore of key importance in acute stroke imaging. Interestingly, in MRI, time-of-flight angiography can be performed, which does not require the application of a contrast medium but uses the blood as an endogenous tracer. It does, however,

suffer from the limitation that with a severe stenosis, the severe slowing of the blood stream typically results in a loss of signal. Consequently, a subtotal stenosis may be mistaken as a complete vessel occlusion. If so, contrast-enhanced angiography is still mandatory.

4.2.2 MEASURING WATER DIFFUSION (DIFFUSION-WEIGHTED IMAGING)

Diffusion-weighted MR imaging (DWI) in addition to imaging of tissue perfusion has become an integral part of diagnostic procedures in the clinical evaluation of acute stroke, as these new MR techniques allow the delineation of the actual ischemic lesion with high sensitivity (Rordorf et al., 1998). The DWI technique provides quantitative maps of water diffusion (Figure 4.2). The quantification results in images of the apparent diffusion coefficient (ADC). In ischemic brain tissue, the movements of proton spins are restricted due to cytotoxic edema. This leads to an ADC decrease and a DWI signal intensity increase in areas of acute ischemic injury. It has been shown that ADC values below $5 \times 10^{-4} \text{mm}^2/\text{s}$ indicate a severe cytotoxic edema in brain tissue which will be irreversibly damaged by ischemia (Seitz et al., 2005).

The amount of change of the ADC depends on the temporal course of the ischemia, the development of the edema, and the resulting increase in cell volume (Moseley, Kucharczyk, et al., 1990; Baird & Warach, 1998; Tong et al., 1998). Additionally, DWI lesions are inhomogeneous and differ from normal tissue in various ways due to different temporal rates of lesion evolution toward infarction (Nagesh et al., 1998). The area with abnormal DWI is typically smaller than the area with reduced tissue perfusion (Baird et al., 1997; Schwamm et al., 1998; Tong et al., 1998). This has led to the suggestion that the region of mismatch between acute perfusion and DWI may represent pathologically underperfused tissue where structural damage has not yet taken place. The perfusion–diffusion mismatch area is considered the target for thrombolysis therapy in stroke. This area is considered the MR equivalent of the so-called *penumbra*, the area of misery perfusion. However, measurements with PET and MRI in acute stroke patients have shown that there are subtle differences between these two measures and, specifically, that the perfusion–diffusion mismatch area is not identical to the penumbra (Sobesky et al., 2005).

The DWI lesions grow within the first 24 hours and shrink thereafter, due to reparative and atrophic processes of the brain. Thus, in the early hours after stroke there is often a perfusion–diffusion mismatch such that the area of abnormal perfusion is larger than the area with abnormal ADC values. Due to the further expansion of the ADC lesion and the regression of the impaired perfusion, the lesions in perfusion imaging and DWI typically match after 8 to 10 hours (Wittsack et al., 2002). Also, the ADC values typically undergo a dynamic evolution after stroke, showing a decrease in the first day and a conversion to positive values after approximately one week (Lövblad et al., 1997; Beaulieu et al., 1999;). Rarely, head movements of the patients, who are typically severely ill, limit the use of DWI in the acute clinical setting.

4.2.3 MEASURING REGIONAL CEREBRAL METABOLISM

Measures of the rCBF and rCBV, along with a separate scan of $^{15}O_2$-accumulation in the brain, allows the determination of the regional cerebral metabolism of oxygen ($rCMRO_2$). Also, the regional cerebral metabolism of glucose can be assessed using glucose labeled with a positron-emitting isotope. During normal physiological conditions, the brain's exclusive source of energy for any sort of function is glucose (a simple, natural sugar). In fact, just to maintain the lowest level of functioning the brain needs a minimum of 120g glucose per day. PET-rCMRglc measures the rate at which different regions in the brain use—or metabolize—glucose. Most widely used has been ^{18}F fluorodeoxyglucose, which is transported into neurons and glial cells in the brain but cannot be metabolized further (Reivich et al., 1985). In the 1980s it was shown that in acute stroke the rCBF is severely depressed, while the oxygen extraction rate may be enhanced resulting in a normal $rCMRO_2$ (Baron et al., 1981; Lenzi, Frackowiak, & Jones, 1982). This area of enhanced oxygen extraction was called *area of misery perfusion* or *penumbra* and considered as target for recanalization procedures (Heiss, Grond,

Thiel, von Stockhausen, et al., 1998). Finally, it should be mentioned that PET can also be used to study neurotransmitter and neuroreceptors. In the context of this discussion it is important that binding of the GABA-receptor ligand flumazenil can be assessed. After dedicated biomedical modeling, this approach was used to demonstrate the loss of gamma-aminobutyric acid (GABAergic) interneurons in ischemic stroke (Heiss, Grond, Thiel, Ghaemi, et al., 1998).

4.2.4 ASSESSING STRUCTURAL BRAIN LESIONS

Study of localization of human brain function has a long tradition. Until the advent of CT, this could only be done retrospectively by correlating neurological deficits with brain lesions at autopsy. CT provided for the first time a means of making in vivo correlations of brain lesions with clinical deficits, allowing for prospective analyses. However, anatomical contrast and resolution are compromised in CT due to the strong attenuation caused by the skull, and the fact that only a few Hounsfield units differentiate tissue compartments within the brain. Thus, small brain lesions, particularly in white matter structures and the brain stem, are usually elusive in CT scans. The lesion-based approach for studying the brain was dramatically improved by MRI, which is far more sensitive and less prone to the confounding effects of partial-volume averaging than CT. Accordingly, MRI has become the method of choice for correlation studies between lesions and deficits, with T2-weighted images being particularly sensitive to brain lesions. It should be noted that structural brain lesions are not fixed in terms of volume, but rather are modulated in size such that they first increase due to local postlesional vasogenic edema and subsequently decrease due to brain atrophy and tissue shrinkage (Beaulieu et al., 1999; Ritzl et al., 2004).

Brain lesions usually do not follow functional divisions of the brain or cerebral cortex, but develop within the pathogenetic framework of the underlying disease. For example, brain infarctions have an individual configuration following the territories of the cerebral arteries or their branches (Bogousslavsky, Regli, & Assal, 1986; Ringelstein et al., 1992). Thus, superimposition of brain lesions of different subjects introduces noise into the group data. Nevertheless, a common area of lesion overlap is expected to demonstrate a brain area critical for a certain function.

A further limitation is that not all syndromes can be mapped in this way. For example, *motor aphasia* was not a sufficiently precise description of the deficit to pinpoint the representative speech areas in the brain (Poeck, De Bleser, & von Keyserlingk, 1984; Alexander, Naeser, & Palumbo, 1990). One explanation for this failure could be the distributed localization of brain function involving networks of different brain structures—a concept pioneered by Mesulam (1981; 1990). Accordingly, damage to any critical node within such a network interferes with the function of the network. However, there are a large number of different nodes within such a network, subserving different subfunctions and allowing for partial rewiring after damage to one or a few of these nodes. Nevertheless, well-defined neurophysiological or neuropsychological deficits can be mapped to critical nodes. Examples are the clinically similar but clearly differentiable syndromes of mirror agnosia, mirror ataxia, and visuomotor ataxia (Rondot, de Recondo, & Dumas, 1977; Binkofski et al., 1998; Binkofski, Buccino, Dohle, Seitz, & Freund, 1999). Thus, slightly different lesion locations are characterized by slightly different patterns of neurophysiological or neuropsychological deficits, which can be mapped to non-overlapping brain lesions even within the same lobe. Lesion mapping can also be done more precisely using digital atlases of brain anatomy in order to superimpose the lesions on the anatomical template (Hömke et al., 2009). This allows the identification of anatomical structures damaged by a brain lesion. It should be noted, however, that this approach requires the digital adaptation of the atlas structures to the individual configuration of the brain investigated.

More recently, Karnath and collaborators (2011) advocated the need to do lesion mapping using a statistical imaging approach. In fact, the authors compared stroke patients with spatial neglect with stroke patients with similar infarct location who do not present with neglect. By group comparisons they were able to show the areas specifically damaged in patients with neglect, both in the acute and chronic stage of the disease. Interestingly, they found considerable differences in lesion location between acute and chronic spatial neglect. They highlighted, in addition to damage of grey matter structures, the damage of white matter fiber tracts. These results raise interesting questions about the pathophysiology of spatial neglect. Similarly, severe hemiparetic stroke involves more paraventricular white matter than less severely affected patients (Seitz, Sondermann, Wittsack, & Siebler, 2009).

Other approaches have recently been proposed to identify more subtle regional changes in the amount of grey or white matter. These include the use of voxel-based morphometry (VBM) to identify regions of the brain where the density of grey or white matter differs between two groups of subjects (Ashburner & Friston, 2000), and methods to estimate the thickness of the cortex and compare these values between groups (Fischl & Dale, 2000). Both of these methods are fully automated, and require high-resolution anatomical 3D T1-weighted MR images with good grey/white matter contrast. To date, these methods have not been widely used in stroke imaging, mainly for two reasons. First, these methods are designed to pick up subtle changes in otherwise healthy-looking brains. The presence of gross lesions complicates the analysis, first because it makes it difficult to accurately segment the image into grey matter, white matter, and CSF compartments (Mehta, Grabowski, Trivedi, & Damasio, 2003), and second because it makes it difficult to establish the spatial mapping (i.e., normalization) between images from different subjects with lesions in different locations (Brett, Leff, Rorden, & Ashburner, 2001). The second reason is due to the heterogeneity of lesion locations and associated deficits. These methods are designed to identify particular regions that are consistently involved across subjects. It therefore follows that they cannot be meaningfully applied to study heterogeneous populations. Nonetheless, the methods may potentially be used to identify more subtle changes secondary to the primary insult, and hence identify regions consistently associated with particular deficits.

4.3 MEASURING BRAIN FUNCTION WITH MRI

An understanding of the functional organization of the brain, particularly the mapping of specific functional roles to specific regions, is important in the design of treatment for many neurological and mental diseases. The field of functional brain mapping has been greatly advanced in the last two decades by the development of functional MRI (fMRI) (Ogawa, Lee, Nayak, & Glynn, 1990), a neuroimaging technique that provides high-resolution images of the brain containing information about local blood flow and metabolism. Functional MRI enables noninvasive monitoring of ongoing brain activity, and can therefore be used in both patients and normal healthy subjects to identify regions that activate in response to experimentally controlled stimulation or cognitive task performance.

4.3.1 THE BOLD IMAGE CONTRAST

Functional MRI makes use of the magnetic properties of hemoglobin contained in red blood cells (Pauling & Coryell, 1936; Thulborn, Waterton, Matthews, & Radda, 1982; Ogawa et al., 1990). Within an externally applied magnetic field there is a magnetization difference between oxygenated and deoxygenated hemoglobin, and this difference can be used to detect changes in the relative concentration of these two different states of hemoglobin within the blood. Functional MRI images are said, therefore, to have blood oxygenation level dependent (BOLD) image contrast (Ogawa et al., 1990). The vast bulk of signal in MRI images comes from hydrogen nuclei (protons) contained in water molecules, and the BOLD contrast relies upon the effect of deoxyhemoglobin upon water molecules within and surrounding blood vessels in the brain. The paramagnetic deoxyhemoglobin changes the magnetic field surrounding red blood cells, which leads to a de-phasing of the proton's spins in water within and around these red blood cells, and a resulting loss of the MRI signal (Thulborn et al., 1982). This effect is greatest within the blood vessels, but also extends into the extravascular tissue (Ogawa et al., 1990), which provides sensitivity to detect the effect of deoxyhemoglobin even when the blood vessels themselves may be a relatively small percentage of the total voxel volume.

The concentration of deoxyhemoglobin in the capillaries and veins varies over time, due to changes in the local metabolic demands of the tissues. Functional MRI experiments use rapid sequential acquisition of BOLD contrast images in order to monitor these activity-dependent changes. The raw signal intensity measured by the BOLD contrast, however, does not provide a directly quantitative measure of blood oxygenation (Ogawa, Menon, Kim, & Ugurbil, 1998), as many other unrelated instrumental and physiological factors also contribute to the measured signal. Monitoring BOLD signal changes with sequential fMRI acquisition, therefore, provides a time course of relative changes in blood oxygenation rather than absolute quantitative values.

Current MRI scanners enable multi-slice BOLD-weighted images with full-brain coverage to be acquired at a spatial resolution of approximately 3x3x3 mm^3 in 3 seconds or less, or at even higher resolutions if the temporal resolution is sacrificed. Irrespective of voxel size, however, the maximum effective resolution obtainable with standard fMRI imaging—i.e., how closely the detected BOLD signal changes spatially co-localize to the underlying neuronal activity—is on the order of a few millimeters (Kâmil Ugurbil, Toth, & Kim, 2003; Kim et al., 2004). This is a consequence of the BOLD contrast being an indirect measure of brain activation that does not have an exact one-to-one spatial correspondence with the underlying active neuronal population. In particular, BOLD signal changes arise from venules and veins as well as from capillaries, so the detected BOLD signal changes can be displaced from the actual site of neuronal activity. The proximity of larger vessels, therefore, must always be considered when inferring spatial localization of neuronal activity from associated BOLD signal changes.

4.3.2 THE BOLD RESPONSE TO NEURONAL ACTIVITY

4.3.2.1 THE TIME COURSE OF EVOKED BOLD SIGNAL CHANGES

The BOLD signal change observed after sensory stimulation or task performance follows a stereotypical time course. The dominant feature is an increase in signal intensity that is delayed and dispersed in time, with a peak after approximately 5 seconds and return to baseline approximately 10 seconds after the task or stimuli (Ogawa et al., 1992). Other notable features are a prolonged signal undershoot after the initial peak, the *post-stimulus undershoot* (Krüger, Kleinschmidt, & Frahm, 1996), and an occasionally observed brief initial signal decrease, the *initial dip* (Menon et al., 1995). The prominent positive peak in the BOLD signal reflects a localized increase in blood flow that delivers oxygen exceeding the increased requirements of the activated region (P.T. Fox, Raichle, Mintun, & Dence, 1988) and results in a local decrease in the concentration of deoxyhemoglobin.

The amplitude and duration of evoked BOLD signal changes are dependent upon the generating stimulus. The BOLD signal time course closely matches the stimulus presentation time course, except with an apparent temporal shift and blurring introduced by the delay and dispersion of the BOLD signal changes (Bandettini, Jesmanowicz, Wong, & Hyde, 1993; Friston, 1994). Furthermore, increasing the intensity of the stimulus—for example, the contrast of a visual stimulation—results in a larger amplitude BOLD signal change (Boynton, Engel, Glover, & Heeger, 1996). This relationship between stimuli and BOLD signal change is approximately linear—in other words, the expected BOLD signal time course evoked by two sequential stimuli is equivalent to the addition of two copies of the expected BOLD signal time course evoked by a single stimulus (Dale & Buckner, 1997; Friston, Fletcher, et al., 1998)—and can be modeled in terms of a hemodynamic response function (HRF). The HRF has a stereotypical shape throughout the brain, and commonly used models of the HRF are based upon the average response evoked in primary sensory cortex after brief sensory stimulation (Boynton et al., 1996; Friston, Josephs, Rees, & Turner, 1998; Glover, 1999).

The peak BOLD signal increase that is evoked by a task or stimulus is in the range of a few percentage points above the baseline signal intensity (Gati, Menon, Ugurbil, & Rutt, 1997). Although this is much larger than the instrumental noise in MRI scanners, there are other sources of nonstimulus-related signal changes in BOLD-weighted images that contribute considerable noise to an fMRI experiment, such as head motion, cardiac pulsation, respiration, and spontaneous fluctuations in ongoing neuronal activity (Bandettini et al., 1993; Biswal, Yetkin, Haughton, & Hyde, 1995; Friston, Williams, Howard, Frackowiak, & Turner, 1996). The effects of such noise can be somewhat mitigated by approaches such as spatial realignment of the images to compensate for subject movement between each acquisition (Friston et al., 1995) and filtering the BOLD signal time course to remove effects due to motion, cardiac pulsation, and respiration (Friston et al., 1996; Glover, 1999). Such post-acquisition corrections cannot remove all the noise, however, and fMRI experiments generally require several minutes of scanning in order to present sufficient numbers of trials to reliably detect the BOLD signal changes associated with a given stimulus.

4.3.2.2 NEUROVASCULAR COUPLING

Functional MRI provides only an indirect measure of neuronal activity. The BOLD signal depends upon the local concentration of deoxyhemoglobin in each imaging voxel, which changes in association with cerebral blood flow (CBF), cerebral blood volume (CBV), and the cerebral metabolic rate of oxygen ($CMRO_2$; Buxton, Uluda, Dubowitz, & Liu, 2004). Although each of these physiological parameters is coupled to changes in neuronal activity, there is a complex interrelationship and a variety of different mechanisms at work. A critical requirement for the interpretation of fMRI results, therefore, is an understanding of the coupling between neuronal activity and the vascular and metabolic changes that underlie the BOLD signal.

Empirically, simultaneous recording of fMRI and intracranial EEG in monkeys have shown that the synaptic inputs rather than spiking outputs of a cortical region provide the strongest correlate of the BOLD signal changes (Logothetis, Pauls, Augath, Trinath, & Oeltermann, 2001; Goense & Logothetis, 2008). However, the underlying mechanism that links synaptic activity with these changes is complex. Synaptic activity is thought to account for most of the energy usage associated with neuronal signaling, with the majority expended in reestablishing the resting membrane potential of the postsynaptic neuron (Attwell & Iadecola, 2002). The local blood flow is also increased in the region of increased synaptic activity, although this blood flow response is not directly initiated by a deficit in glucose or oxygen per se, and does not even show an exact one-to-one relationship between energy supply and demand (Attwell & Iadecola, 2002), which suggests that increased blood flow most likely serves further roles beyond the delivery of energy substrates to the parenchymal tissue. A number of different vasoactive mediators that act upon vascular tone are thought to play a role in the blood flow response, including vasoactive neurotransmitters and ions as well as metabolic by-products and vasoactive substances triggered by neurotransmitters, and it is likely that different mechanisms operate in different parts of the brain (Lauritzen & Gold, 2003). One possible pathway is mediated by the uptake of glutamate into astrocytes, which causes an increase in intracellular Ca^{2+} within the astrocyte that triggers the release of vasoactive molecules through the astrocytic endfeet (Haydon & Carmignoto, 2006). The many potential mechanisms mediating the neurovascular coupling are still not fully understood, however, and for a more detailed discussion the reader is directed to Attwell and Iadecola, 2002; Lauritzen and Gold, 2003; Haydon and Carmignoto, 2006; and Shmuel, 2010.

4.3.3 FMRI EXPERIMENTAL DESIGN AND ANALYSIS

Functional MRI provides a powerful tool for noninvasively measuring brain function, but requires careful experimental design and analysis in order to provide useful and meaningful information from the inherently non-quantitative and noisy BOLD signal. Two broad classes of fMRI experiment are commonly used: task-related studies of evoked brain activity, and resting-state studies of spontaneous brain activity.

4.3.3.1 TASK-RELATED ACTIVATION STUDIES

Functional MRI activation studies use a structured presentation of sensory stimulation and/or task performance to provide a modulation of brain activity that allows for the isolation and localization of brain regions activated during the performance of a specific function. The most appropriate experimental design is dependent upon the particular effect of interest, but all experiments require two or more different conditions to be compared in order to infer activation based upon the relative measure of brain activity provided by the BOLD signal. For some applications, such as mapping sensory responses, it may be sufficient to compare the BOLD signal measured during stimulation or task performance with a baseline "rest" period measured without stimulation. Many cognitive experiments, however, require more sophisticated designs in order to isolate the specific cognitive process of interest.

The most simple fMRI experimental design is the block-design paradigm, which uses a series of interleaved "blocks" that alternate between two or more different conditions requiring continuous performance of a given task or stimulation. Typical experimental durations range from 2 to 10 minutes, during which many cycles of each block are performed. One of the block conditions may simply be passive rest, but often all blocks will involve some form of active task performance. Block-design experiments may also be constructed using a parametric approach by altering the "level" of the task within different blocks; for example, the intensity of stimulation or difficulty of cognitive task. Analysis of a block-design experiment to identify differences in activation between the two conditions simply requires subtraction of the average BOLD signal measured during each of the different blocks. The identified activation may be interpreted as isolating just the cognitive process that is different between the two experimental conditions, although this assumes that combining two or more cognitive processes simply leads to an addition of brain activations without any interaction between the components of the compound task. To explicitly test this assumption and identify any interactions between the different conditions, a factorial study design should be used where possible (Amaro & Barker, 2006).

An alternative approach to grouping conditions into blocks of continuous performance is to instead use an event-related design, where stimuli are presented as individual trials or events. As with the block-design approach, experiments may compare a single event type against a baseline of passive rest, or instead, multiple event types may be used. By measuring the time course of BOLD signal changes evoked by many repetitions of an event, the response to an individual trial can be estimated, which can be compared between different event types for features such as amplitude or latency (Friston, Fletcher, et al., 1998). Importantly, as a consequence of the linear nature of the BOLD response, the spacing between events may be much closer than the expected duration of BOLD signal changes to each individual event; linear analysis methods using models of the hemodynamic response function and least-squares estimation can be used to separate the overlapping responses to these closely spaced events (Friston, Fletcher, et al., 1998). However, the assumption of linearity is not appropriate for very short interstimulus intervals (Friston, Josephs, et al., 1998). In this case, the spacing between trials should typically be no shorter than 4 seconds if accurate estimation of the single-trial response shape is important (Glover, 1999). If only the location of event-related activation is important, however, then event separations as short as a second may be used (Friston, Zarahn, Josephs, Henson, & Dale, 1999). Event-related designs enable studying processes that cannot be easily blocked into epochs of continuous performance, such as an oddball-detection paradigm where the subject must identify rare target stimuli intermixed among more common stimuli (McCarthy, Luby, Gore, & Goldman-Rakic, 1997), or incorrect responses in a difficult cognitive paradigm (Kiehl, Liddle, & Hopfinger, 2000). Variable timing between the presentations of stimuli can also be used to help maintain attention across the experiment by making it more difficult for a subject to predict or anticipate events (D'Esposito, Zarahn, & Aguirre, 1999). An example of regions of activation during a verbal fluency task is provided in Figure 4.3.

In addition to identifying regions of activation, task-related fMRI experiments may also reveal regions of BOLD signal decrease associated with the task. In experiments contrasting two different active conditions, the interpretation of these decreases is generally straightforward—a region of BOLD signal decrease observed in one condition most likely reflects a region that selectively activates during the other condition. Including an explicit baseline rest condition in the experiment can confirm this. BOLD signal decreases observed in a comparison to baseline rest condition, however, may reflect a number of different underlying sources. One interpretation is that task performance has "interrupted" activity within a brain region that is tonically active at rest; this is the explanation given for task-related BOLD signal decreases commonly observed in the "default-mode" regions of the brain (Raichle et al., 2001). Alternatively, BOLD signal decreases may reflect a reduction in local synaptic activity below the baseline level, due to task-related reduced input from the neurons that project to that region (Lauritzen & Gold, 2003; Shmuel, Augath, Oeltermann, & Logothetis,

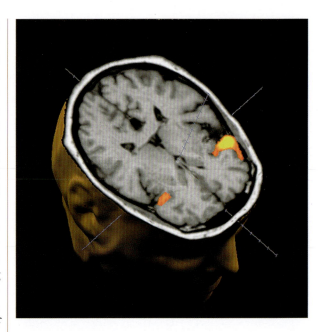

Figure 4.3 Bilateral activation areas related to a verbal fluency task in a patient who had recovered from severe motor aphasia due to an embolic infarction in the left inferior frontal gyrus.

2006). A purely vascular "stealing" effect can also lead to BOLD signal decreases in areas immediately adjacent to an activated region (Harel, Lee, Nagaoka, Kim, & Kim, 2002). A final possibility is that BOLD signal decreases may reflect local neuronal inhibition within the region (Czisch et al., 2004; Stefanovic, Warnking, & Pike, 2004), although different experiments have observed a diversity of hemodynamic responses associated with neural inhibition (Logothetis, 2008), so neuronal inhibition should not in general be assumed to result in BOLD signal decreases.

4.3.3.2 "RESTING-STATE" STUDIES OF BRAIN FUNCTION

In a resting state without overt task performance, it has been shown that spontaneous, intrinsic activity of the brain shows correlation within systemwide networks (Biswal et al., 1995; Lowe, Mock, & Sorenson, 1998)—a phenomenon referred to as *resting-state functional connectivity* (RSFC). Functional MRI can assess RSFC throughout the brain, by measuring the correlation between spontaneous fluctuations in BOLD signal measured in different brain regions. The simultaneous measurement of fMRI and intracranial electroencephalography (EEG) in monkeys has demonstrated that correlated spontaneous BOLD fluctuations are associated with a corresponding synchronization of slow fluctuations in underlying neuronal networks (Shmuel & Leopold, 2008). These synchronized fluctuations are observed under deep anesthesia (Vincent et al., 2007) and superimposed upon, rather than interrupted by, task performance (M. D. Fox, Snyder, Zacks, & Raichle, 2006). This suggests that they are not due to unconstrained, consciously directed cognitive activity, but rather are a more fundamental property of neuronal networks. Experiments using voltage-sensitive dye imaging of feline visual cortex have shown that such activity represents a set of dynamically switching cortical states that might form an internal context that reflects and/or influences memory, perception, and behavior (Kenet, Bibitchkov, Tsodyks, Grinvald, & Arieli, 2003). Spontaneous fluctuations in human primary motor cortex have also been shown to account for observed trial-to-trial variability in motor performance (M. D. Fox, Snyder, Vincent, & Raichle, 2007).

Functional MRI experiments for estimating RSFC networks acquire BOLD-weighted images while the subject is performing no explicit task. Typically from 5 to 10 minutes of scanning is acquired. These data may be analyzed using a seeded approach, where an a priori seed region of interest is chosen and a spatial map generated showing regions with significant correlation to the seed (M. D. Fox et al., 2005). Alternatively, blind-source separation techniques, such as independent components analysis, may be used in order to automatically estimate different networks based upon the observed correlated fluctuations (Beckmann & Smith, 2004). Because RSFC analyses are based upon correlation, care must be taken to filter the fMRI data to remove physiological noise arising from respiration, motion, and cardiac rate that can also lead to correlations in the BOLD signal (M. D. Fox et al., 2005).

The networks of correlated spontaneous brain activity identified by RSFC analysis correspond with many well-known functional subsystems of the brain, so this technique can provide an alternative approach to standard task-related fMRI activation experiments for functional brain mapping. For example, the BOLD signal measured in the left and right primary motor cortex shows a strong correlation at rest without explicit performance of a motor task (Biswal et al., 1995), and similar patterns of bilateral RSFC are also seen in other areas of primary cortex (Lowe et al., 1998; Cordes et al., 2000). RSFC is also observed in higher-level cognitive networks, such as between brain regions related to language processing (Hampson, Peterson, Skudlarski, Gatenby, & Gore, 2002) and "default-mode" regions that are associated with tasks such as episodic memory retrieval (Greicius, Krasnow, Reiss, & Menon, 2003). In addition to the spatial mapping of functional networks, RSFC is also thought to provide a marker of the integrity and efficiency of these networks, as RSFC has been shown to be significantly correlated with disease state (Greicius, Srivastava, Reiss, & Menon, 2004; Cherkassky, Kana, Keller, & Just, 2006; Waites, Briellmann, Saling, Abbott, & Jackson, 2006) and task performance (Hampson, Driesen, Skudlarski, Gore, & Constable, 2006).

RSFC fMRI experiments can offer a number of advantages over task-related activation experiments. They can be applied to subjects that may not be able to cooperate with the task performance in an fMRI activation experiment due to cognitive or other impairment. These experiments are also more efficient than activation studies, because a single fMRI session can be used to identify many different RSFC networks (De Luca, Beckmann, De Stefano, Matthews, & Smith, 2006), whereas activation studies require a different experiment for each network. However, whereas activation studies enable the assignment of specific functional roles to identified regional activations based upon the cognitive content of the activation task, RSFC experiments provide no context for interpretation of the identified resting-state networks.

4.3.4 APPLICATIONS OF FMRI IN STROKE REHABILITATION

Functional MRI provides the ability to monitor and assess changes in brain function as a result of stroke. Patients can be studied longitudinally to measure dynamic changes in activation patterns, which can help better understand the recovery process and allow for the assessment of the effect of either drugs or physical therapy (Calautti & Baron, 2003). An example is provided in Figure 4.3. Functional connectivity analysis can be used to assess the integrity of functional networks after stroke, and relate this to functional deficits: for example, a correlation between functional connectivity disruption in attentional networks and the severity of spatial neglect has been shown (He et al., 2007).

A certain amount of caution must be exercised when applying fMRI techniques to the study of a clinical population. Because the BOLD signal represents combined contributions from CBF, CBV and $CMRO_2$, any decoupling of these parameters can change the relationship between neuronal activity and BOLD signal change. For example, if there is no blood flow response associated with a region of excitatory synaptic activity, then the rise in $CMRO_2$ will cause a BOLD signal decrease. In diseases where the coupling between neural activity and blood flow is disturbed, therefore, BOLD signal changes should be interpreted with caution (Lauritzen & Gold, 2003). For example, it appears that the neurovascular coupling may be transiently disturbed during the early chronic phase of ischemic stroke recovery, leading to an absence of detectable BOLD signal changes in activated cortex (Ferdinand Binkofski & Seitz, 2004; Figure 4.4). The percentage increase of evoked BOLD signal changes also depends upon the baseline CBF level; this means that factors that could alter the baseline CBF of a patient group relative to a healthy population, such as anxiety or vasoactive medications, could also result in significant group differences in the BOLD response,

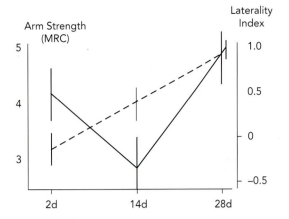

Figure 4.4 Changes in BOLD activation measured in the perilesional sensorimotor cortex related to exploratory finger movements of the affected hand after hemiparetic stroke (n = 8 patients). The solid line shows the Laterality Index (LI) calculated from BOLD signal measured in bilateral regions of interest in the sensorimotor cortex: 1 = lateralized to side of lesion; 0 = bilateral; –1 = contralateral to lesion. At the early time point, BOLD activation was bilateral, but with an emphasis in the perilesional area. After 14 days, BOLD activation was reduced in the perilesional area, leading to a more contralateral LI. After 28 days the ipsilateral BOLD activation was present again, as indicated by an LI of close to 1. Note the steady increase of grip force (dotted line) in these patients. Data from Binkofski & Seitz (2004), published in Carey & Seitz (2007).

even if the underlying neural response is the same in the two groups (Buxton et al., 2004).

4.4 STRUCTURAL CONNECTIVITY, INCLUDING TRACTOGRAPHY

An important aspect of brain function is its connectivity through its white matter tracts, which connect distant regions of the cortex to each other and the rest of the body. In recent years, the introduction of diffusion tensor imaging (DTI; Basser, 1994) has led to renewed interest in understanding the brain at this level. This is due primarily to the fact that diffusion-weighted imaging (on which DTI is based) is the only method that can provide this type of information in vivo and noninvasively, making it possible for the first time to study white matter and its disorders in patients and normal subjects.

Fundamentally, diffusion-weighted imaging (DWI) can be used to infer structural connectivity based on its sensitivity to the cellular microstructure at the micron level. In white matter, the arrangement of axonal fibers into coherent bundles leads to a pronounced orientation dependence of the diffusion-weighted (DW) signal, from which the orientation of the white matter fibers can be inferred at each point in the image (Figure 4.5). From these orientation estimates, so-called fiber-tracking or tractography algorithms can be used to delineate white matter pathways by simply following ("tracking") the direction of the fibers through the image (Figure 4.6).

4.4.1 MODELING DIFFUSION IN WHITE MATTER

Diffusion-weighted imaging (DWI) is sensitive to the diffusion of water molecules—the random walk behavior of water molecules due to their own thermal energy. This is the same process that causes a drop of ink placed in water to "spread out" from its initial position. In living tissue, it turns out that the length scales to which DWI is sensitive on a clinical system are of the order of microns—similar to that of many cellular structures. Since these structures can restrict or "hinder" the random motion of water molecules, this implies that DWI is sensitive to the microstructure of the tissue at that scale. In white matter in particular, the dense, regular arrangement of co-aligned axonal fibers leads to a pronounced difference in the distance traveled by water molecules along the axis of the fibers compared to that traveled across the fibers, since axonal membranes and myelin sheaths all constitute strong barriers to free

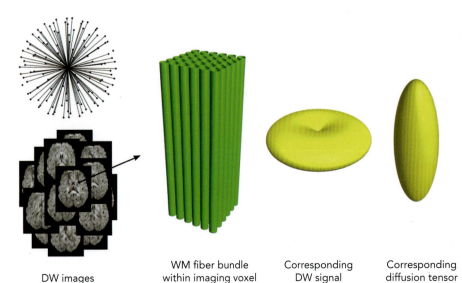

DW images

WM fiber bundle within imaging voxel

Corresponding DW signal

Corresponding diffusion tensor

Figure 4.5 From diffusion-weighted imaging to diffusion tensor. From left to right: a number of DW images are acquired, each sensitized along a different DW direction; the fiber arrangement within a particular WM voxel, with the fibers tightly packed into a single bundle; the DW signal that would be measured for that WM voxel, showing strong attenuations for DW directions aligned with the fiber direction; the diffusion tensor ellipsoid computed from the DW signal, showing preferential diffusion along the direction of the fibers. DW = diffusion weighted; WM = White Matter.

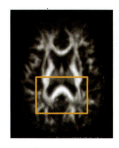

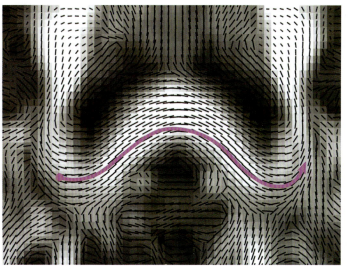

Figure 4.6 An illustration of the concept of fiber-tracking. Left: an axial fractional anisotropy image through the brain, showing the region displayed on the right. Right: the supposed direction of the WM fibers is shown as a black line within each imaging voxel. The process of fiber-tracking involves selecting a "seed point" from which to initiate the algorithm (pink dot), and following the estimated direction of the WM fibers through the image, as shown by the pink line.

motion. This translates to a strong orientation dependence of the diffusion-weighted (DW) signal, from which the orientation of the white matter fibers can be inferred within each imaging voxel (volume element). From these orientation estimates, so-called *fiber-tracking* or *tractography* algorithms can be used to delineate white matter pathways by simply following ("tracking") the direction of the fibers through the image.

MRI images are made sensitive to diffusion by introducing a pair of diffusion-weighting gradient pulses, whose purpose is essentially to respectively "label" and "unlabel" water molecules according to their position along the direction of the DW gradient. A spread of the water molecules along this DW direction between the two DW gradient pulses will cause a mismatch between the "label" and "unlabel" operations, which is detected as a drop in the corresponding DW signal. Hence, the DWI signal is reduced in regions where the diffusion is high (large displacements) along the direction of the DW gradient.

To infer the orientation of the white matter fibers, the orientation dependence of the DWI signal needs to be adequately characterized. To achieve this in practice, a number of DW images are acquired, each sensitized to a different DW orientation. These measurements can then be combined into an appropriate model, from which the orientation of the white matter fibers (among other parameters) can be estimated.

4.4.1.1 DIFFUSION TENSOR IMAGING

The model most commonly used for the purpose of characterizing the DW signal is the diffusion tensor model, leading to the well-known diffusion tensor imaging (DTI) approach. This model has been widely adopted due to its simplicity and intuitive interpretation. However, there are limitations as discussed below. The simplest way to visualize the diffusion tensor is as its characteristic ellipsoid, which represents the mean displacement of water

molecules as a function of orientation. In brain white matter, the diffusion ellipsoid is typically elongated (prolate or cigar-shaped) along the axis of the fibers, corresponding to a larger degree of diffusion along this direction rather than across it (Basser & Pierpaoli, 1996; Lin, Tseng, Cheng, & Chen, 2001).

The diffusion tensor model is fully characterized using only six independent parameters, implying that a minimum of six imaging volumes, each with a different DW direction, need to be sampled (in addition to at least one volume with no diffusion-weighting, the $b = 0$ image). In practice, a larger number of DW directions (e.g., 30) are typically acquired to improve the stability of the results (Jones, 2004). This leads to acquisition times for full brain coverage at resolutions of $2 \times 2 \times 2$ mm^3 (or greater) of approximately 5 minutes on the current generation of MRI scanners.

However, it is becoming increasingly apparent that the diffusion tensor model is simply inadequate to characterize much of the white matter (A. L. Alexander, Hasan, Lazar, Tsuruda, & Parker, 2001; Frank, 2001; D. C. Alexander, Barker, & Arridge, 2002; Behrens, Berg, Jbabdi, Rushworth, & Woolrich, 2007; Jeurissen, Leemans, Tournier, Jones, & Sijbers, 2010). This is due to the simplistic assumption that each voxel contains a single, coherently oriented bundle of fibers—this assumption is inherently made if the principal axis of the diffusion tensor is used as the fiber orientation estimate. Given that the spatial resolution of DWI (~2mm) is comparable to the width of typical WM tracts, it is likely that a significant number of voxels will contain contributions from more than a single fiber bundle—a situation often referred to as "crossing fibers." While it has long been known that DTI is unsuitable for modeling such voxels, it is only recently that the extent of the problem is truly becoming apparent: a recent study estimates that as much as 90% of brain WM voxels contain crossing fibers (Jeurissen et al., 2010), a much larger proportion than previously assumed. These findings suggest that alternative descriptions of diffusion in white matter are urgently required to replace the diffusion tensor model.

4.4.1.2 HIGHER-ORDER MODELS

For this reason, a number of alternative models have been proposed in recent years. These are commonly referred to as higher-order models, and are often based on the acquisition of so-called *high angular resolution DW imaging* (HARDI) data. This HARDI acquisition scheme is similar to that used for DTI, but with a much larger number of unique, non-collinear DW directions (e.g., 45 to 100), leading to increased scan times (e.g., ~10 minutes for 60 DW directions). These additional directions are required to fully characterize all the orientational features of the DW signal, in order to correctly extract the fiber orientations. These methods are now beginning to be used for clinical and neuroscientific investigations, with promising results. For a more in-depth review of these methods, we refer to existing literature (D. C. Alexander & Seunarine, 2010; Seunarine & Alexander, 2009; Tournier, 2010; Tournier, Mori, & Leemans, 2011).

4.4.2 ESTIMATING BIOLOGICALLY RELEVANT PARAMETERS

In practice, one of the greatest uses of DWI is to provide scalar metrics that reflect various aspects of the diffusion properties within each voxel. Of these, the most widely used is mean diffusivity (MD), also referred to as the average apparent diffusion coefficient (ADC), or the trace of the diffusion tensor. This metric corresponds to the volume of the diffusion tensor, and reflects the overall amount of diffusion, irrespective of orientation. It is widely used for two reasons. First, it is much simpler to measure in practice than any other DWI metric (only four imaging volumes need to be acquired—one $b = 0$ and three orthogonal DW directions). Second, it is exquisitely sensitive to ischemia: the MD has been shown to drop markedly minutes after the onset of ischemia, 6 hours earlier than other conventional imaging approaches (Moseley, Cohen, et al., 1990; Thomas, Lythgoe, Pell, Calamante, & Ordidge, 2000). This has led to its widespread use as a way of identifying acute stroke patients most likely to benefit from early reperfusion interventions (Warach et al., 1995; Lövblad et al., 1997; Baird & Warach, 1998).

In recent years, measures of the anisotropy of the diffusion tensor have become increasingly popular, based on the widely held belief that they can be used a surrogate markers of white matter "integrity." There are several such indices, with the most commonly used in the literature being the fractional anisotropy (FA; Basser & Pierpaoli, 1996). In essence, these measures quantify the degree to which the diffusion deviates from the isotropic, directionally unbiased case represented by a spherical diffusion ellipsoid, as would be expected, for example, in free water. In general, they range from a value of zero for perfect isotropic diffusion, to a value of one for the most anisotropic case, with diffusion occurring along a single direction only. These measures have rapidly been adopted as markers of so-called white matter "integrity" based on the observation that anisotropy is near-zero in CSF and grey matter regions, and relatively high in white matter regions (Basser & Pierpaoli, 1996), along with findings by a number of studies demonstrating an impact of various white matter pathologies on anisotropy measures (e.g., demyelination [Christian Beaulieu, 2002] or Wallerian degeneration [Pierpaoli et al., 2001]).

More recently, measures of radial and axial diffusivities (sometimes referred to as *perpendicular* and *parallel* diffusivities, respectively) have also been used in the literature. These correspond to the apparent diffusion coefficient measured respectively across and along the corresponding fiber bundle, and can be obtained relatively easily from the diffusion tensor. The advantage of these measures over anisotropy metrics is that radial and axial diffusivities have been shown to be affected differently with different types of pathology (Song et al., 2003, 2002), and hence may be capable of providing more specific information than anisotropy alone.

However, it is important to stress that these metrics all need to be used and interpreted with a great deal of caution. The original observations relating anisotropy and radial/axial diffusivities to pathology were all performed in highly controlled experiments, where the underlying fiber geometry was known to consist of a single bundle of coherently oriented axons. As mentioned above, these conditions are unlikely to be met in practice, given the abundance of crossing fiber voxels in the human white matter (Behrens et al., 2007; Jeurissen et al., 2010). In such voxels, estimates of anisotropy are severely affected and no longer reflect the intrinsic anisotropy of any of the fiber bundles present (A. L. Alexander et al., 2001). In fact, in certain cases the anisotropy has been shown to increase, contrary to the assumed biological effect (Pierpaoli et al., 2001; Tuch et al., 2005; Douaud et al., 2010). The effect on radial/axial diffusivities is greater still, since these rely on an accurate estimate of the orientation of the fiber bundle; in a crossing fiber voxel, it can readily be appreciated that such an orientation is ambiguous at best, with obvious implications for the reliability of these metrics (Wheeler-Kingshott & Cercignani, 2009). Hence, while these metrics are indeed very sensitive to changes in the diffusion of water within the tissue, their specificity in terms of biological interpretation is highly ambiguous, since changes can often be explained by crossing fiber effects. The simplistic interpretation of anisotropy or radial/axial diffusivities as surrogate markers of white matter "integrity" is, therefore, fundamentally flawed.

A number of alternative methods have been proposed based on higher-order models. These include diffusion kurtosis imaging (Jensen, Helpern, Ramani, Lu, & Kaczynski, 2005; Lu, Jensen, Ramani, & Helpern, 2006; Fieremans, Jensen, & Helpern, 2011), and q-space based approaches (e.g., Cohen & Assaf, 2002; Assaf et al., 2005). While these may eventually provide more specific biological information than DTI-derived metrics, current methods suffer from similar limitations in that they are still only valid in single-fiber regions. Furthermore, they typically require different acquisition strategies (a larger number of DW directions, at multiple b-values), leading to longer scan times that may in some cases not be clinically practical.

4.4.2.1 ESTIMATING FIBER ORIENTATIONS

As mentioned earlier, a prerequisite to tractography is the estimation of the orientation of the fibers within each imaging voxel from the DW data. The model most commonly used for this purpose is the diffusion tensor model, as used in DTI. In simple single-fiber configurations, it has been shown that the principal direction of diffusion (PDD), as given by the primary eigenvector of the diffusion tensor, provides an accurate estimate of the orientation of the fibers (Lin et al., 2001). Unfortunately, it is also well known that this simple relationship breaks down in crossing fiber regions (A. L. Alexander et al., 2001; Frank, 2001; D. C. Alexander et al., 2002; Tuch et al., 2002; Jansons & Alexander, 2003; Tournier, Calamante, Gadian, & Connelly, 2004; Tuch, 2004; D. C Alexander, 2005; Van Wedeen, Hagmann, Tseng, Reese, & Weisskoff, 2005; Behrens et al., 2007; Tournier et al., 2011). This will lead to errors in the fiber orientation estimates, with potentially serious consequences for the subsequent fiber-tracking results, with the algorithm identifying connec-

tions that do not exist in reality (Pierpaoli et al., 2001; Jeurissen, Leemans, Jones, Tournier, & Sijbers, 2011) or failing to identify connections that do exist (Kinoshita et al., 2005; Behrens et al., 2007; Jeurissen et al., 2011). As discussed above, recent evidence suggests that the prevalence of crossing fibers is much greater than previously thought (Behrens et al., 2007; Jeurissen et al., 2010), which implies that the diffusion tensor model should not be considered sufficiently reliable for use in tractography.

A number of higher-order models have been proposed to address these limitations (see Seunarine & Alexander, 2009; D. C. Alexander & Seunarine, 2010; Tournier, 2010; Tournier et al., 2011 for comprehensive reviews). These algorithms typically produce their output in one of two formats: an estimate of the number of fiber populations present and their orientation and partial volume; or a more general distribution of fiber orientations (the fiber orientation distribution, FOD, also referred to as the fiber orientation density function, fODF), as illustrated in Figure 4.7. In both cases, this information can be used for tractography and has been shown to lead to vastly improved results (Behrens et al., 2007; Van Wedeen et al., 2008; Descoteaux, Deriche, Knösche, & Anwander, 2009; Jeurissen et al., 2011).

4.4.2.2 TRACTOGRAPHY

Based on the estimated fiber orientations, the path of white matter tracts can be estimated by "fiber-tracking" or tractography algorithms. The simplest and most widely used of these algorithms is the so-called "streamlines" approach: starting from a user-specified "seed point" in the image, small steps are taken along the direction of the estimated fiber orientations until some "termination criteria" are met and the algorithm stops (as illustrated in Figure 4.6). Ideally, the sequence of points visited provides

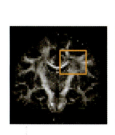 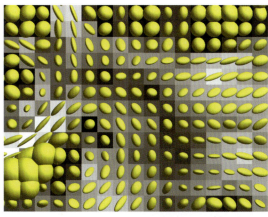 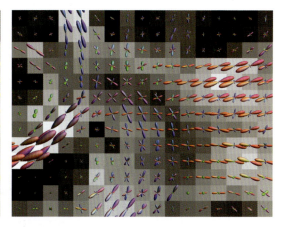

Figure 4.7 The fundamental limitation of the diffusion tensor model is its inability to adequately model the presence of crossing fibers, as demonstrated here. Left: a coronal fractional anisotropy map, showing the region of interest in the centrum semiovale. Middle: the diffusion tensor ellipsoid estimated within each voxel of the ROI. Right: the fiber orientation distributions estimated using constrained spherical deconvolution (Tournier, Calamante, & Connelly, 2007) from the same data, showing the presence of multiple fiber orientations, corresponding to the commissural fibers of the corpus callosum (left–right, red lobes), the corona radiata (inferior–superior, blue lobes), and the superior longitudinal fasciculus (anterior–posterior, green lobes).

a delineation of the supposed path of the white matter tract passing through the seed point. Termination criteria are used to ensure the algorithm does not propagate into biologically implausible regions; for example, through grey matter or CSF regions. This is typically achieved based on a simple anisotropy threshold, since anisotropy is low in these regions.

A wide range of algorithms have been proposed based on the streamlines approach. The simplest and most widely used is the well-known fiber assignment by continuous tracking (FACT) algorithm (Mori, Crain, Chacko, & van Zijl, 1999), which simply uses fiber orientation estimates obtained from the diffusion tensor's PDD. This algorithm forms part of the "deterministic" class of fiber tracking algorithms, since the path of the track produced is fully determined once the seed point has been selected—in other words, running the algorithm again from the same seed point will produce the same track.

In contrast, a number of "probabilistic" algorithms have been proposed to take the effects of noise into account (Koch, Norris, & Hund-Georgiadis, 2002; Parker, Wheeler-Kingshott, & Barker, 2002; Behrens et al., 2003; Jones, 2003; Tournier, Calamante, Gadian, & Connelly, 2003; Jones & Pierpaoli, 2005; Lazar & Alexander, 2005; Parker & Alexander, 2005; Jeurissen et al., 2011). DWI is an inherently noisy technique, since the contrast mechanism is based on signal attenuation. There will, therefore, inevitably be some uncertainty surrounding the estimated fiber orientations. Deterministic streamlines algorithms do not take this into account, and simply follow the direction as estimated from the data. While this approach provides appealing "clean" results, in reality there is a range of paths that the track could have followed, given the uncertainty inherent in the measurements. By only displaying the single most likely path, deterministic approaches give no indication as to the degree of confidence that can be placed in the results. This is a potentially serious limitation, since a small difference in the estimated fiber orientation at one point can cause the algorithm to veer into adjacent structures and follow a different tract altogether. Clearly, some indication of the range of likely paths is needed.

Probabilistic approaches were introduced to address this limitation. Most of these algorithms are based on an extension of the simple deterministic streamlines approach, but in this case the fiber orientations used by the algorithm are chosen by random sampling from the fiber orientation distribution (FOD). In simple terms, the direction of each step is now slightly perturbed about the "actual" estimated orientation, by a random amount determined by the quality of the data (i.e., signal-to-noise ratio, number of DW directions, etc.). The track generated in this way will differ from the equivalent deterministic track, yet will still be plausible based on the data available. By generating a large number of such tracks from the same seed point, an estimate of the distribution of likely paths can be obtained, with the density of tracks going through a given region reflecting in some way the probability of such a connection existing. It is also possible to seed throughout the white matter to generate whole-brain tractography results, as shown in Figure 4.8.

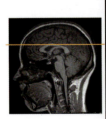
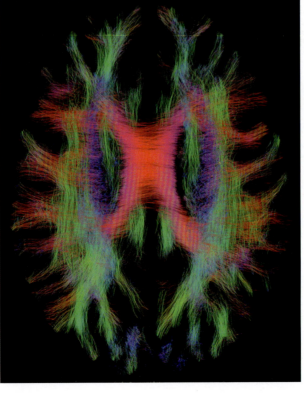

Figure 4.8 Non-DTI whole-brain tractography results obtained from a healthy volunteer. Left: a sagittal slice through a structural image showing the plane of the image displayed on the right. Right: a 2mm-thick axial section through 100,000 tracks generated by seeding randomly throughout the brain. Each track is color-coded according to its local direction (red: left–right; green: anterior–posterior; blue: inferior–superior). These results were generated using a probabilistic streamlines algorithm (Tournier, Calamante, Gadian, & Connelly, 2005) combined with fiber orientation estimates computed using constrained spherical deconvolution (Tournier et al., 2007). Note that these results were not produced using DTI, since the diffusion tensor model was not used to infer the fiber orientations—note the extensive regions of crossing fibers throughout the centrum semiovale. DWI data acquired at *b* = 3000 s/mm² along 150 DW directions, with a 2.3mm isotropic voxel size. DTI = Diffusion Tensor Imaging; DWI = Diffusion Weighted Imaging.

Note that probabilistic approaches do not bypass the limitations of the model used to estimate the fiber orientations: while the diffusion tensor model can be used with a probabilistic fiber-tracking algorithm, the results will still be biased due to systematic errors in the fiber orientations in crossing fiber regions. Probabilistic results therefore only provide an estimate of the range of likely connections that would be produced by that particular algorithm—the probabilistic aspects refer to the reproducibility of the algorithm rather than its biological accuracy (Jones, 2010).

Furthermore, while it is tempting to interpret the probability values produced by these algorithms as measures of connectivity, it is important to bear in mind that they only reflect the reproducibility of the algorithm, and have little if any relationship with the actual biological connectivity. These issues of interpretation are very well articulated in Jones, 2010.

4.4.3 APPLICATION TO STROKE RECOVERY

As already mentioned, the mean diffusivity is widely used in the clinic to identify an acute ischemic infarct before the onset of changes on conventional imaging. However, the potential of diffusion-weighted imaging as a tool to investigate white matter is even more promising. Changes can be observed in white matter tracts damaged by a stroke in regions remote from the lesion, due to Wallerian degeneration (Pierpaoli et al., 2001). Other potential applications include the correlation of infarct location with the particular pathway involved (Newton et al., 2006; Dawes et al., 2008), an approach that may lead to more refined prognostic indicators of potential for recovery and response to treatment. Even more promising is the potential of DWI to study the reorganization of the brain following pathology (Bridge, Thomas, Jbabdi, & Cowey, 2008) or intervention (Draganski et al., 2004).

REFERENCES

Alexander, A. L., Hasan, K. M., Lazar, M., Tsuruda, J. S., & Parker, D. L. (2001). Analysis of partial volume effects in diffusion-tensor MRI. *Magnetic Resonance in Medicine, 45*(5), 770–780.

Alexander, D. C., Barker, G. J., & Arridge, S. R. (2002). Detection and modeling of non-Gaussian apparent diffusion coefficient profiles in human brain data. *Magnetic Resonance in Medicine, 48*(2), 331–340.

Alexander, D. C. (2005). Multiple-fiber reconstruction algorithms for diffusion MRI. *Annals of the New York Academy of Sciences, 1064,* 113–133.

Alexander, D. C., & Seunarine, K. K. (2010). Mathematics of Crossing Fibers. In D.K. Jones (Ed.), *Diffusion MRI: Theory, Methods, and Applications.* Oxford University Press, USA.

Alexander, M. P., Naeser, M. A., & Palumbo, C. (1990). Broca's area aphasias: aphasia after lesions including the frontal operculum. *Neurology, 40*(2), 353–362.

Amaro, E., & Barker, G. J. (2006). Study design in fMRI: basic principles. *Brain Cognition, 60*(3), 220–232.

Ashburner, J., & Friston, K. J. (2000). Voxel-based morphometry—the methods. *NeuroImage, 11*(6 Pt 1), 805–821.

Assaf, Y., Chapman, J., Ben-Bashat, D., Hendler, T., Segev, Y., Korczyn, A. D., Graif, M., et al. (2005). White matter changes in multiple sclerosis: correlation of q-space diffusion MRI and 1H MRS. *Magnetic Resonance Imaging, 23*(6), 703–710.

Attwell, D., & Iadecola, C. (2002). The neural basis of functional brain imaging signals. *Trends in neurosciences, 25*(12), 621–625.

Baird, A. E., Benfield, A., Schlaug, G., Siewert, B., Lövblad, K. O., Edelman, R. R., & Warach, S. (1997). Enlargement of human cerebral ischemic lesion volumes measured by diffusion-weighted magnetic resonance imaging. *Annals of Neurology, 41*(5), 581–589.

Baird, A. E., & Warach, S. (1998). Magnetic resonance imaging of acute stroke. *Journal of Cerebral Blood Flow and Metabolism, 18*(6), 583–609.

Bandettini, P. A., Jesmanowicz, A., Wong, E. C., & Hyde, J. S. (1993). Processing strategies for time-course data sets in functional MRI of the human brain. *Magnetic Resonance in Medicine, 30*(2), 161–173.

Baron, J. C., Bousser, M. G., Rey, A., Guillard, A., Comar, D., & Castaigne, P. (1981). Reversal of focal "misery-perfusion syndrome" by extra-intracranial arterial bypass in hemodynamic cerebral ischemia. A case study with 15O positron emission tomography. *Stroke; a Journal of Cerebral Circulation, 12*(4), 454–459.

Basser, P. J. (1994). MR diffusion tensor spectroscopy and imaging. *Biophysical Journal, 66*(1), 259–267.

Basser, P. J., & Pierpaoli, C. (1996). Microstructural and physiological features of tissues elucidated by quantitative-diffusion-tensor MRI. *Journal of Magnetic Resonance, Series B, 111*(3), 209–219.

Beaulieu, C., de Crespigny, A., Tong, D. C., Moseley, M. E., Albers, G. W., & Marks, M. P. (1999). Longitudinal magnetic resonance imaging study of perfusion and diffusion in stroke: evolution of lesion volume and correlation with clinical outcome. *Annals of Neurology, 46*(4), 568–578.

Beaulieu, C. (2002). The basis of anisotropic water diffusion in the nervous system—a technical review. *NMR in Biomedicine, 15*(7–8), 435–455.

Beckmann, C. F., & Smith, S. M. (2004). Probabilistic independent component analysis for functional magnetic resonance imaging. *IEEE Transactions on Medical Imaging, 23*(2), 137–152.

Behrens, T. E. J., Woolrich, M. W., Jenkinson, M., Johansen-Berg, H., Nunes, R. G., Clare, S., Matthews, P. M., et al. (2003). Characterization and propagation of uncertainty in diffusion-weighted MR imaging. *Magnetic Resonance in Medicine, 50*(5), 1077–1088.

Behrens, T. E. J., Berg, H. J., Jbabdi, S., Rushworth, M. F. S., & Woolrich, M. W. (2007). Probabilistic diffusion tractography with multiple fiber orientations: What can we gain? *NeuroImage, 34*(1), 144–155.

Binkofski, F., Buccino, G., Dohle, C., Seitz, R. J., & Freund, H. J. (1999). Mirror agnosia and mirror ataxia constitute different parietal lobe disorders. *Annals of Neurology, 46*(1), 51–61.

Binkofski, F., Dohle, C., Posse, S., Stephan, K. M., Hefter, H., Seitz, R. J., & Freund, H. J. (1998). Human anterior intraparietal area subserves prehension: a combined lesion and functional MRI activation study. *Neurology, 50*(5), 1253–1259.

Binkofski, F., & Seitz, R. J. (2004). Modulation of the BOLD-response in early recovery from sensorimotor stroke. *Neurology, 63*(7), 1223–1229.

Biswal, B., Yetkin, F. Z., Haughton, V. M., & Hyde, J. S. (1995). Functional connectivity in the motor cortex of resting human brain using echo-planar MRI. *Magnetic Resonance in Medicine, 34*(4), 537–541.

Bogousslavsky, J., Regli, F., & Assal, G. (1986). The syndrome of unilateral tuberothalamic artery territory infarction. *Stroke, 17*(3), 434–441.

Boynton, G. M., Engel, S. A., Glover, G. H., & Heeger, D. J. (1996). Linear systems analysis of functional magnetic resonance imaging in human V1. *The Journal of neuroscience, 16*(13), 4207–4221.

Brett, M., Leff, A. P., Rorden, C., & Ashburner, J. (2001). Spatial normalization of brain images with focal lesions using cost function masking. *NeuroImage, 14*(2), 486–500.

Bridge, H., Thomas, O., Jbabdi, S., & Cowey, A. (2008). Changes in connectivity after visual cortical brain damage underlie altered visual function. *Brain, 131*(Pt 6), 1433–1444.

Buxton, R. B., Uluda, K., Dubowitz, D. J., & Liu, T. T. (2004). Modeling the hemodynamic response to brain activation. *NeuroImage, 23 Supplement 1*, S220–S233.

Calamante, F., & Connelly, A. (2009). Perfusion precision in bolus-tracking MRI: estimation using the wild-bootstrap method. *Magnetic Resonance in Medicine., 61*(3), 696–704.

Calamante, F., Christensen, S., Desmond, P. M., Ostergaard, L., Davis, S. M., & Connelly, A. (2010). The physiological significance of the time-to-maximum (Tmax) parameter in perfusion MRI. *Stroke, 41*(6), 1169–1174.

Calautti, C., & Baron, J.-C. (2003). Functional neuroimaging studies of motor recovery after stroke in adults: a review. *Stroke, 34*(6), 1553–1566.

Carey, L. M. & Seitz, R. J. (2007). Functional neuroimaging in stroke recovery and neurorehabilitation: conceptual issues and perspectives. *International Journal of Stroke* **2**(4): 245–264.

Cherkassky, V. L., Kana, R. K., Keller, T. A., & Just, M. A. (2006). Functional connectivity in a baseline resting-state network in autism. *Neuroreport, 17*(16), 1687–1690.

Cohen, Y., & Assaf, Y. (2002). High b-value q-space analyzed diffusion-weighted MRS and MRI in neuronal tissues—a technical review. *NMR in Biomedicine, 15*(7–8), 516–542.

Cordes, D., Haughton, V. M., Arfanakis, K., Wendt, G. J., Turski, P. A., Moritz, C. H., Quigley, M. A., et al. (2000). Mapping functionally related regions of brain with functional connectivity MR imaging. *American Journal of Neuroradiology, 21*(9), 1636–1644.

Czisch, M., Wehrle, R., Kaufmann, C., Wetter, T. C., Holsboer, F., Pollmacher, T., & Auer, D. P. (2004). Functional MRI during sleep: BOLD signal decreases and their electrophysiological correlates. *The European Journal of Neuroscience, 20*(2), 566–574.

D'Esposito, M., Zarahn, E., & Aguirre, G. K. (1999). Event-related functional MRI: implications for cognitive psychology. *Psychological Bulletin, 125*(1), 155–164.

Dale, A., & Buckner, R. (1997). Selective averaging of rapidly presented individual trials using fMRI. *Human Brain Mapping, 5*(5), 329–340.

Dawes, H., Enzinger, C., Johansen-Berg, H., Bogdanovic, M., Guy, C., Collett, J., Izadi, H., et al. (2008). Walking performance and its recovery in chronic stroke in relation to extent of lesion overlap with the descending motor tract. *Experimental Brain Research, 186*(2), 325–333.

Descoteaux, M., Deriche, R., Knösche, T. R., & Anwander, A. (2009). Deterministic and probabilistic tractography based on complex fibre orientation distributions. *IEEE Transactions on Medical Imaging, 28*(2), 269–286.

Douaud, G., Jbabdi, S., Behrens, T. E. J., Menke, R. A., Gass, A., Monsch, A. U., Rao, A., et al. (2011). DTI measures in crossing-fibre areas: increased diffusion anisotropy reveals early white matter alteration in MCI and mild Alzheimer's disease. *NeuroImage, 55*(3), 880–890.

Draganski, B., Gaser, C., Busch, V., Schuierer, G., Bogdahn, U., & May, A. (2004). Neuroplasticity: changes in grey matter induced by training. *Nature, 427*(6972), 311–312.

Fieremans, E., Jensen, J. H., & Helpern, J. A. (2011). White matter characterization with diffusional kurtosis imaging. *NeuroImage, 58*(1), 177–188.

Fischl, B., & Dale, A. M. (2000). Measuring the thickness of the human cerebral cortex from magnetic resonance images. *Proceedings of the National Academy of Sciences of the United States of America, 97*(20), 11050–11055.

Fox, M. D., Snyder, A. Z., Vincent, J. L., Corbetta, M., Van Essen, D. C., & Raichle, M. E. (2005). The human brain is intrinsically organized into dynamic, anticorrelated functional networks. *Proceedings of the National Academy of Sciences of the United States of America, 102*(27), 9673–9678.

Fox, M. D, Snyder, A. Z., Vincent, J. L., & Raichle, M. E. (2007). Intrinsic fluctuations within cortical systems account for intertrial variability in human behavior. *Neuron, 56*(1), 171–184.

Fox, M. D, Snyder, A. Z., Zacks, J. M., & Raichle, M. E. (2006). Coherent spontaneous activity accounts for trial-to-trial variability in human evoked brain responses. *Nature Neuroscience, 9*(1), 23–25.

Fox, P. T., Raichle, M. E., Mintun, M. A., & Dence, C. (1988). Nonoxidative glucose consumption during focal physiologic neural activity. *Science, 241*(4864), 462–464.

Frank, L. R. (2001). Anisotropy in high angular resolution diffusion-weighted MRI. *Magnetic Resonance in Medicine, 45*(6), 935–939.

Friston, K. J. (1994). Functional and effective connectivity in neuroimaging: a synthesis. *Human Brain Mapping, 2*(1–2), 56–78.

Friston, K. J., Ashburner, J., Frith, C. D., Poline, J. B., Heather, J. D., & Frackowiak, R. S. J. (1995). Spatial registration and normalization of images. *Human Brain Mapping, 3*(3), 165–189.

Friston, K. J., Fletcher, P., Josephs, O., Holmes, A., Rugg, M. D., & Turner, R. (1998). Event-related fMRI: characterizing differential responses. *NeuroImage, 7*(1), 30–40.

Friston, K. J., Josephs, O., Rees, G., & Turner, R. (1998). Nonlinear event-related responses in fMRI. *Magnetic resonance in medicine, 39*(1), 41–52.

Friston, K. J., Williams, S., Howard, R., Frackowiak, R. S., & Turner, R. (1996). Movement-related effects in fMRI time-series. *Magnetic Resonance in Medicine, 35*(3), 346–355.

Friston, K. J., Zarahn, E., Josephs, O., Henson, R. N., & Dale, A. M. (1999). Stochastic designs in event-related fMRI. *NeuroImage, 10*(5), 607–619.

Gati, J. S., Menon, R. S., Ugurbil, K., & Rutt, B. K. (1997). Experimental determination of the BOLD field strength dependence in vessels and tissue. *Magnetic Resonance in Medicine, 38*(2), 296–302.

Glover, G. H. (1999). Deconvolution of impulse response in event-related BOLD fMRI. *NeuroImage, 9*(4), 416–429.

Goense, J. B. M., & Logothetis, N.K. (2008). Neurophysiology of the BOLD fMRI signal in awake monkeys. *Current Biology, 18*(9), 631–640.

Greicius, M. D., Krasnow, B., Reiss, A. L., & Menon, V. (2003). Functional connectivity in the resting brain: a network analysis of the default mode hypothesis. *Proceedings of the National Academy of Sciences of the United States of America, 100*(1), 253–258.

Greicius, M. D., Srivastava, G., Reiss, A. L., & Menon, V. (2004). Default-mode network activity distinguishes Alzheimer's disease from healthy aging: evidence from functional MRI. *Proceedings of the National Academy of Sciences of the United States of America, 101*(13), 4637–4642.

Hampson, M., Driesen, N. R., Skudlarski, P., Gore, J. C., & Constable, R. T. (2006). Brain connectivity related to working memory performance. *Journal of Neuroscience, 26*(51), 13338–13343.

Hampson, M., Peterson, B. S., Skudlarski, P., Gatenby, J. C., & Gore, J. C. (2002). Detection of functional connectivity using temporal correlations in MR images. *Human Brain Mapping, 15*(4), 247–262.

Harel, N., Lee, S.-P., Nagaoka, T., Kim, D.-S., & Kim, S.-G. (2002). Origin of negative blood oxygenation level-dependent fMRI signals. *Journal of Cerebral Blood Flow and Metabolism, 22*(8), 908–917.

Haydon, P. G., & Carmignoto, G. (2006). Astrocyte control of synaptic transmission and neurovascular coupling. *Physiology Reviews, 86*(3), 1009–1031.

He, B. J., Snyder, A. Z., Vincent, J. L., Epstein, A., Shulman, G. L., & Corbetta, M. (2007). Breakdown of functional connectivity in frontoparietal networks underlies behavioral deficits in spatial neglect. *Neuron, 53*(6), 905–918.

Heiss, W. D., Grond, M., Thiel, A., Ghaemi, M., Sobesky, J., Rudolf, J., Bauer, B., et al. (1998). Permanent cortical damage detected by flumazenil positron emission tomography in acute stroke. *Stroke,* *29*(2), 454–461.

Heiss, W. D., Grond, M., Thiel, A., von Stockhausen, H.M., Rudolf, J., Ghaemi, M., Löttgen, J., et al. (1998). Tissue at risk of infarction rescued by early reperfusion: a positron emission tomography study in systemic recombinant tissue plasminogen activator thrombolysis of acute stroke. *Journal of Cerebral Blood Flow and Metabolism,* *18*(12), 1298–1307.

Herholz, K., Buskies, W., Rist, M., Pawlik, G., Hollmann, W., & Heiss, W. D. (1987). Regional cerebral blood flow in man at rest and during exercise. *Journal of Neurology,* *234*(1), 9–13.

Hömke, L., Amunts, K., Bönig, L., Fretz, C., Binkofski, F., Zilles, K., & Weder, B. (2009). Analysis of lesions in patients with unilateral tactile agnosia using cytoarchitectonic probabilistic maps. *Human Brain Mapping,* *30*(5), 1444–1456.

Hossmann, K. A. (1994). Viability thresholds and the penumbra of focal ischemia. *Annals of Neurology,* *36*(4), 557–565.

Hunter, G. J., Hamberg, L. M., Ponzo, J. A., Huang-Hellinger, F. R., Morris, P. P., Rabinov, J., Farkas, J., et al. (1998). Assessment of cerebral perfusion and arterial anatomy in hyperacute stroke with three-dimensional functional CT: early clinical results. *American Journal of Neuroradiology,* *19*(1), 29–37.

Jansons, K. M., & Alexander, D. C. (2003). Persistent angular structure: new insights from diffusion magnetic resonance imaging data. *Inverse Problems,* *19*(5), 1031–1046.

Jensen, J. H., Helpern, J. A., Ramani, A., Lu, H., & Kaczynski, K. (2005). Diffusional kurtosis imaging: the quantification of non-gaussian water diffusion by means of magnetic resonance imaging. *Magnetic Resonance in Medicine,* *53*(6), 1432–1440.

Jeurissen, B., Leemans, A., Jones, D. K., Tournier, J.-D., & Sijbers, J. (2011). Probabilistic fiber tracking using the residual bootstrap with constrained spherical deconvolution. *Human Brain Mapping,* *32*(3), 461–479.

Jeurissen, B., Leemans, A., Tournier, J.-D., Jones, D. K., & Sijbers, J. (2010). Estimating the number of fiber orientations in diffusion MRI voxels: A constrained spherical deconvolution study. *Proceedings of the International Society for Magnetic Resonance in Medicine* (Vol. 18, p. 573). Presented at the International Society for Magnetic Resonance in Medicine, Stockholm, Sweden.

Jones, D. K. (2003). Determining and visualizing uncertainty in estimates of fiber orientation from diffusion tensor MRI. *Magnetic Resonance in Medicine,* *49*(1), 7–12.

Jones, D. K. (2004). The effect of gradient sampling schemes on measures derived from diffusion tensor MRI: a Monte Carlo study. *Magnetic Resonance in Medicine,* *51*(4), 807–815.

Jones, D. K. (2010). Challenges and limitations of quantifying brain connectivity in vivo with diffusion MRI. *Imaging in Medicine,* *2,* 341–355.

Jones, D. K., & Pierpaoli, C. (2005). Confidence mapping in diffusion tensor magnetic resonance imaging tractography using a bootstrap approach. *Magnetic Resonance in Medicine,* *53*(5), 1143–1149.

Karnath, H.-O., Rennig, J., Johannsen, L., & Rorden, C. (2011). The anatomy underlying acute versus chronic spatial neglect: a longitudinal study. *Brain: A Journal of Neurology,* *134*(Pt 3), 903–912.

Kenet, T., Bibitchkov, D., Tsodyks, M., Grinvald, A., & Arieli, A. (2003). Spontaneously emerging cortical representations of visual attributes. *Nature,* *425*(6961), 954–956.

Kiehl, K. A., Liddle, P. F., & Hopfinger, J. B. (2000). Error processing and the rostral anterior cingulate: an event-related fMRI study. *Psychophysiology,* *37*(2), 216–223.

Kim, D., Ronen, I., Olman, C., Kim, S., Ugurbil, K., & Toth, L. (2004). Spatial relationship between neuronal activity and BOLD functional MRI. *NeuroImage,* *21*(3), 876–885.

Kinoshita, M., Yamada, K., Hashimoto, N., Kato, A., Izumoto, S., Baba, T., Maruno, M., et al. (2005). Fiber-tracking does not accurately estimate size of fiber bundle in pathological condition: initial neurosurgical experience using neuronavigation and subcortical white matter stimulation. *NeuroImage,* *25*(2), 424–429.

Koch, M. A., Norris, D. G., & Hund-Georgiadis, M. (2002). An investigation of functional and anatomical connectivity using magnetic resonance imaging. *NeuroImage,* *16*(1), 241–250.

Krüger, G., Kleinschmidt, A., & Frahm, J. (1996). Dynamic MRI sensitized to cerebral blood oxygenation and flow during sustained activation of human visual cortex. *Magnetic Resonance in Medicine,* *35*(6), 797–800.

Lassen, N. A., & Ingvar, D. H. (1972). Radioisotopic assessment of regional cerebral blood flow. *Progress in Nuclear Medicine,* *1,* 376–409.

Lauritzen, M., & Gold, L. (2003). Brain function and neurophysiological correlates of signals used in functional neuroimaging. *The Journal of Neuroscience,* *23*(10), 3972–3980.

Lazar, M., & Alexander, A. L. (2005). Bootstrap white matter tractography (BOOT-TRAC). *NeuroImage,* *24*(2), 524–532.

Lenzi, G. L., Frackowiak, R. S., & Jones, T. (1982). Cerebral oxygen metabolism and blood flow in human cerebral ischemic infarction. *Journal of Cerebral Blood Flow and Metabolism,* *2*(3), 321–335.

Lev, M. H., Segal, A. Z., Farkas, J., Hossain, S. T., Putman, C., Hunter, G.J., Budzik, R., et al. (2001). Utility of perfusion-weighted CT imaging in acute middle cerebral artery stroke treated with intra-arterial thrombolysis: prediction of final infarct volume and clinical outcome. *Stroke,* *32*(9), 2021–2028.

Lin, C. P., Tseng, W. Y., Cheng, H. C., & Chen, J. H. (2001). Validation of diffusion tensor magnetic resonance axonal fiber imaging with registered manganese-enhanced optic tracts. *NeuroImage,* *14*(5), 1035–1047.

Logothetis, N. K., Pauls, J., Augath, M., Trinath, T., & Oeltermann, A. (2001). Neurophysiological investigation of the basis of the fMRI signal. *Nature,* *412*(6843), 150–157.

Logothetis, N. K. (2008). What we can do and what we cannot do with fMRI. *Nature,* *453*(7197), 869–878.

Lövblad, K. O., Baird, A. E., Schlaug, G., Benfield, A., Siewert, B., Voetsch, B., Connor, A., et al. (1997). Ischemic lesion volumes in acute stroke by diffusion-weighted magnetic resonance imaging correlate with clinical outcome. *Annals of Neurology,* *42*(2), 164–170.

Lowe, M. J., Mock, B. J., & Sorenson, J. A. (1998). Functional connectivity in single and multislice echoplanar imaging using resting-state fluctuations. *NeuroImage,* *7*(2), 119–132.

Lu, H., Jensen, J. H., Ramani, A., & Helpern, J. A. (2006). Three-dimensional characterization of non-gaussian water diffusion in humans using diffusion kurtosis imaging. *NMR in Biomedicine,* *19*(2), 236–247.

De Luca, M., Beckmann, C. F., De Stefano, N., Matthews, P. M., & Smith, S. M. (2006). fMRI resting state networks define distinct modes of long-distance interactions in the human brain. *NeuroImage,* *29*(4), 1359–1367.

McCarthy, G., Luby, M., Gore, J., & Goldman-Rakic, P. (1997). Infrequent events transiently activate human prefrontal and parietal cortex as measured by functional MRI. *Journal of Neurophysiology,* *77*(3), 1630–1634.

Mehta, S., Grabowski, T. J., Trivedi, Y., & Damasio, H. (2003). Evaluation of voxel-based morphometry for focal lesion detection in individuals. *NeuroImage,* *20*(3), 1438–1454.

Menon, R. S., Ogawa, S., Hu, X., Strupp, J. P., Anderson, P., & Ugurbil, K. (1995). BOLD based functional MRI at 4 tesla includes a capillary bed contribution: echo-planar imaging correlates with previous optical imaging using intrinsic signals. *Magnetic Resonance in Medicine,* *33*(3), 453–459.

Mesulam, M. M. (1981). A cortical network for directed attention and unilateral neglect. *Annals of Neurology,* *10*(4), 309–325.

Mesulam, M. M. (1990). Large-scale neurocognitive networks and distributed processing for attention, language, and memory. *Annals of Neurology,* *28*(5), 597–613.

Mori, S., Crain, B., Chacko, V., & van Zijl, P. (1999). Three-dimensional tracking of axonal projections in the brain by magnetic resonance imaging. *Annals of Neurology,* *45*(2), 269, 265.

Moseley, M. E., Cohen, Y., Mintorovitch, J., Chileuitt, L., Shimizu, H., Kucharczyk, J., Wendland, M. F., et al. (1990). Early detection of regional cerebral ischemia in cats: comparison of diffusion- and T2-weighted MRI and spectroscopy. *Magnetic Resonance in Medicine, 14*(2), 330–346.

Moseley, M. E., Kucharczyk, J., Mintorovitch, J., Cohen, Y., Kurhanewicz, J., Derugin, N., Asgari, H., et al. (1990). Diffusion-weighted MR imaging of acute stroke: correlation with T2-weighted and magnetic susceptibility-enhanced MR imaging in cats. *American Journal of Neuroradiology, 11*(3), 423–429.

Nagesh, V., Welch, K. M., Windham, J. P., Patel, S., Levine, S. R., Hearshen, D., Peck, D., et al. (1998). Time course of ADCw changes in ischemic stroke: beyond the human eye! *Stroke, 29*(9), 1778–1782.

Neumann-Haefelin, T., Wittsack, H. J., Wenserski, F., Siebler, M., Seitz, R. J., Mödder, U., & Freund, H. J. (1999). Diffusion- and perfusion-weighted MRI. The DWI/PWI mismatch region in acute stroke. *Stroke, 30*(8), 1591–1597.

Newton, J. M., Ward, N. S., Parker, G. J. M., Deichmann, R., Alexander, D. C., Friston, K. J., & Frackowiak, R. S. J. (2006). Non-invasive mapping of corticofugal fibres from multiple motor areas—relevance to stroke recovery. *Brain, 129*(7), 1844–1858.

Ogawa, S., Lee, T. M., Nayak, A. S., & Glynn, P. (1990). Oxygenation-sensitive contrast in magnetic resonance image of rodent brain at high magnetic fields. *Magnetic Resonance in Medicine, 14*(1), 68–78.

Ogawa, S., Menon, R. S., Kim, S. G., & Ugurbil, K. (1998). On the characteristics of functional magnetic resonance imaging of the brain. *Annual review of biophysics and biomolecular structure, 27,* 447–474.

Ogawa, S., Tank, D. W., Menon, R., Ellermann, J. M., Kim, S. G., Merkle, H., & Ugurbil, K. (1992). Intrinsic signal changes accompanying sensory stimulation: functional brain mapping with magnetic resonance imaging. *Proceedings of the National Academy of Sciences of the United States of America, 89*(13), 5951–5955.

Olivot, J.-M., Mlynash, M., Thijs, V. N., Kemp, S., Lansberg, M. G., Wechsler, L., Bammer, R., et al. (2009). Optimal Tmax threshold for predicting penumbral tissue in acute stroke. *Stroke, 40*(2), 469–475.

Parker, G. J. M., Wheeler-Kingshott, C. A. M., & Barker, G. J. (2002). Estimating distributed anatomical connectivity using fast marching methods and diffusion tensor imaging. *IEEE Transactions on Medical Imaging, 21*(5), 505–512.

Parker, G., & Alexander, D. (2005). Probabilistic anatomical connectivity derived from the microscopic persistent angular structure of cerebral tissue. *Philosophical Transactions of the Royal Society B: Biological Sciences, 360*(1457), 902, 893.

Pauling, L., & Coryell, C. D. (1936). The magnetic properties and structure of hemoglobin, oxyhemoglobin and carbonmonoxyhemoglobin. *Proceedings of the National Academy of Sciences of the United States of America, 22*(4), 210–216.

Phelps, M. E., Mazziotta, J., & Schelbert, H. R. (Eds.). (1985). *Positron emission tomography and autoradiography: Principles and applications for the brain and heart.* New York: Raven Press.

Pierpaoli, C., Barnett, A., Pajevic, S., Chen, R., Penix, L., Virta, A., & Basser, P. (2001). Water diffusion changes in Wallerian degeneration and their dependence on white matter architecture. *NeuroImage, 13*(6), 1174–1185.

Poeck, K., De Bleser, R., & von Keyserlingk, D. G. (1984). Neurolinguistic status and localization of lesion in aphasic patients with exclusively consonant-vowel recurring utterances. *Brain, 107 (Pt 1)*, 199–217.

Raichle, M. E., MacLeod, A. M., Snyder, A. Z., Powers, W. J., Gusnard, D. A., & Shulman, G. L. (2001). A default mode of brain function. *Proceedings of the National Academy of Sciences of the United States of America, 98*(2), 676–682.

Reivich, M., Alavi, A., Wolf, A., Fowler, J., Russell, J., Arnett, C., MacGregor, R. R., et al. (1985). Glucose metabolic rate kinetic model parameter determination in humans: the lumped constants and rate constants for [18F]fluorodeoxyglucose and [11C] deoxyglucose. *Journal of Cerebral Blood Flow and Metabolism, 5*(2), 179–192.

Ringelstein, E. B., Biniek, R., Weiller, C., Ammeling, B., Nolte, P. N., & Thron, A. (1992). Type and extent of hemispheric brain infarctions and clinical outcome in early and delayed middle cerebral artery recanalization. *Neurology, 42*(2), 289–298.

Ritzl, A., Meisel, S., Wittsack, H.-J., Fink, G. R., Siebler, M., Mödder, U., & Seitz, R. J. (2004). Development of brain infarct volume as assessed by magnetic resonance imaging (MRI): follow-up of diffusion-weighted MRI lesions. *Journal of Magnetic Resonance Imaging, 20*(2), 201–207.

Roberts, H. C., Roberts, T. P., Smith, W. S., Lee, T. J., Fischbein, N. J., & Dillon, W. P. (2001). Multisection dynamic CT perfusion for acute cerebral ischemia: the "toggling-table" technique. *American Journal of Neuroradiology, 22*(6), 1077–1080.

Rondot, P., de Recondo, J., & Dumas, J. L. (1977). Visuomotor ataxia. *Brain, 100*(2), 355–376.

Rordorf, G., Koroshetz, W. J., Copen, W. A., Cramer, S. C., Schaefer, P. W., Budzik, R. F., Jr, Schwamm, L. H., et al. (1998). Regional ischemia and ischemic injury in patients with acute middle cerebral artery stroke as defined by early diffusion-weighted and perfusion-weighted MRI. *Stroke, 29*(5), 939–943.

Schwamm, L. H., Koroshetz, W. J., Sorensen, A. G., Wang, B., Copen, W. A., Budzik, R., Rordorf, G., et al. (1998). Time course of lesion development in patients with acute stroke: serial diffusion- and hemodynamic-weighted magnetic resonance imaging. *Stroke, 29*(11), 2268–2276.

Seitz, R. J., Meisel, S., Weller, P., Junghans, U., Wittsack, H.-J., & Siebler, M. (2005). Initial ischemic event: perfusion-weighted MR imaging and apparent diffusion coefficient for stroke evolution. *Radiology, 237*(3), 1020–1028.

Seitz, R. J., Sondermann, V., Wittsack, H.-J., & Siebler, M. (2009). Lesion patterns in successful and failed thrombolysis in middle cerebral artery stroke. *Neuroradiology, 51*(12), 865–871.

Seunarine, K. K., & Alexander, D. C. (2009). Multiple fibres: beyond the diffusion tensor. In H. Johansen-Berg & T. E. J. Behrens (Eds.), *Diffusion MRI: from quantitative measurement to in-vivo neuroanatomy* (pp. 56–74). San Diego, California, USA: Elsevier.

Shmuel, A. (2010). Locally measured neuronal correlates of functional MRI Signals. In C. Mulert & L. Lemieux (Eds.), *EEG—fMRI* (pp. 63–82). Springer Berlin Heidelberg. Retrieved from http://dx.doi.org/10.1007/978-3-540-87919-0_4.

Shmuel, A., Augath, M., Oeltermann, A., & Logothetis, N. K. (2006). Negative functional MRI response correlates with decreases in neuronal activity in monkey visual area V1. *Nature Neuroscience, 9*(4), 569–577.

Shmuel, A., & Leopold, D. A. (2008). Neuronal correlates of spontaneous fluctuations in fMRI signals in monkey visual cortex: Implications for functional connectivity at rest. *Human Brain Mapping, 29*(7), 751–761.

Sobesky, J., Zaro Weber, O., Lehnhardt, F.-G., Hesselmann, V., Neveling, M., Jacobs, A., & Heiss, W.-D. (2005). Does the mismatch match the penumbra? Magnetic resonance imaging and positron emission tomography in early ischemic stroke. *Stroke, 36*(5), 980–985.

Song, S.-K., Sun, S.-W., Ju, W.-K., Lin, S.-J., Cross, A. H., & Neufeld, A. H. (2003). Diffusion tensor imaging detects and differentiates axon and myelin degeneration in mouse optic nerve after retinal ischemia. *NeuroImage, 20*(3), 1714–1722.

Song, S.-K., Sun, S.-W., Ramsbottom, M. J., Chang, C., Russell, J., & Cross, A. H. (2002). Dysmyelination revealed through MRI as increased radial (but unchanged axial) diffusion of water. *NeuroImage, 17*(3), 1429–1436.

Sorensen, A. G., Buonanno, F. S., Gonzalez, R. G., Schwamm, L. H., Lev, M. H., Huang-Hellinger, F. R., Reese, T. G., et al. (1996). Hyperacute stroke: evaluation with combined multisection diffusion-weighted and hemodynamically weighted echo-planar MR imaging. *Radiology, 199*(2), 391–401.

Stefanovic, B., Warnking, J. M., & Pike, G. B. (2004). Hemodynamic and metabolic responses to neuronal inhibition. *NeuroImage, 22*(2), 771–778.

Surikova, I., Meisel, S., Siebler, M., Wittsack, H.-J., & Seitz, R. J. (2006). Significance of the perfusion-diffusion mismatch in chronic cerebral ischemia. *Journal of Magnetic Resonance Imaging, 24*(4), 771–778.

Thomas, D. L., Lythgoe, M. F., Pell, G. S., Calamante, F., & Ordidge, R. J. (2000). The measurement of diffusion and perfusion in biological systems using magnetic resonance imaging. *Physics in Medicine and Biology, 45*(8), R97–R138.

Thulborn, K. R., Waterton, J. C., Matthews, P. M., & Radda, G. K. (1982). Oxygenation dependence of the transverse relaxation time of water protons in whole blood at high field. *Biochimica et Biophysica Acta, 714*(2), 265–270.

Tong, D. C., Yenari, M. A., Albers, G. W., O'Brien, M., Marks, M. P., & Moseley, M. E. (1998). Correlation of perfusion- and diffusion-weighted MRI with NIHSS score in acute (<6.5 hour) ischemic stroke. *Neurology, 50*(4), 864–870.

Tournier, J. D. (2010). The Biophysics of Crossing Fibres. In D. K. Jones (Ed.), *Diffusion MRI: Theory, Methods, and Applications* (pp. 465–482). Oxford University Press, USA.

Tournier, J. D., Calamante, F., & Connelly, A. (2007). Robust determination of the fiber orientation distribution in diffusion MRI: Non-negativity constrained super-resolved spherical deconvolution. *NeuroImage, 35*(4), 1459–1472.

Tournier, J. D., Calamante, F., Gadian, D. G., & Connelly, A. (2003). Diffusion-weighted magnetic resonance imaging fiber tracking using a front evolution algorithm. *NeuroImage, 20*(1), 276–288.

Tournier, J. D., Calamante, F., Gadian, D. G., & Connelly, A. (2004). Direct estimation of the fiber orientation density function from diffusion-weighted MRI data using spherical deconvolution. *NeuroImage, 23*(3), 1176–1185.

Tournier, J. D., Mori, S., & Leemans, A. (2011). Diffusion tensor imaging and beyond. *Magnetic Resonance in Medicine, 65*(6), 1532–1556.

Tournier, J. D., Calamante, F., Gadian, D. G., & Connelly, A. (2005). Probabilistic fibre tracking through regions containing crossing fibres. *Proceedings of the International Society for Magnetic Resonance in Medicine* (Vol. 13, p. 1343). Presented at the International Society for Magnetic Resonance in Medicine, Miami Beach, Florida, USA.

Tuch, D. S. (2004). Q-ball imaging. *Magnetic Resonance in Medicine, 52*(6), 1358–1372.

Tuch, D. S., Reese, T. G., Wiegell, M. R., Makris, N., Belliveau, J. W., & Wedeen, V. J. (2002). High angular resolution diffusion imaging reveals intravoxel white matter fiber heterogeneity. *Magnetic Resonance in Medicine, 48*(4), 577–582.

Tuch, D. S., Salat, D. H., Wisco, J. J., Zaleta, A. K., Hevelone, N. D., & Rosas, H. D. (2005). Choice reaction time performance correlates with diffusion anisotropy in white matter pathways supporting visuospatial attention. *Proceedings of the National Academy of Sciences of the United States of America, 102*(34), 12212–12217.

Ugurbil, K., Toth, L., & Kim, D.-S. (2003). How accurate is magnetic resonance imaging of brain function? *Trends in Neurosciences, 26*(2), 108–114.

Vincent, J. L., Patel, G. H., Fox, M. D., Snyder, A. Z., Baker, J. T., Essen, D. C. V., Zempel, J. M., et al. (2007). Intrinsic functional architecture in the anesthetized monkey brain. *Nature, 447*(7140), 83–86.

Waites, A. B., Briellmann, R. S., Saling, M. M., Abbott, D. F., & Jackson, G. D. (2006). Functional connectivity networks are disrupted in left temporal lobe epilepsy. *Annals of Neurology, 59*(2), 335–343.

Warach, S., Gaa, J., Siewert, B., Wielopolski, P., & Edelman, R. R. (1995). Acute human stroke studied by whole brain echo planar diffusion-weighted magnetic resonance imaging. *Annals of Neurology, 37*(2), 231–241.

Wedeen, V. J., Wang, R. P., Schmahmann, J. D., Benner, T., Tseng, W. Y. I., Dai, G., Pandya, D. N., et al. (2008). Diffusion spectrum magnetic resonance imaging (DSI) tractography of crossing fibers. *NeuroImage, 41*(4), 1267–1277.

Wedeen, V. J., Hagmann, P., Tseng, W.-Y. I., Reese, T. G., & Weisskoff, R. M. (2005). Mapping complex tissue architecture with diffusion spectrum magnetic resonance imaging. *Magnetic Resonance in Medicine, 54*(6), 1377–1386.

Wheeler-Kingshott, C. A. M., & Cercignani, M. (2009). About "axial" and "radial" diffusivities. *Magnetic Resonance in Medicine, 61*(5), 1255–1260.

Wintermark, M., Reichhart, M., Cuisenaire, O., Maeder, P., Thiran, J.-P., Schnyder, P., Bogousslavsky, J., et al. (2002a). Comparison of admission perfusion computed tomography and qualitative diffusion- and perfusion-weighted magnetic resonance imaging in acute stroke patients. *Stroke, 33*(8), 2025–2031.

Wintermark, M., Reichhart, M., Thiran, J.-P., Maeder, P., Chalaron, M., Schnyder, P., Bogousslavsky, J., et al. (2002b). Prognostic accuracy of cerebral blood flow measurement by perfusion computed tomography, at the time of emergency room admission, in acute stroke patients. *Annals of Neurology, 51*(4), 417–432.

Wittsack, H.-J., Ritzl, A., Fink, G. R., Wenserski, F., Siebler, M., Seitz, R. J., Mödder, U., et al. (2002). MR imaging in acute stroke: diffusion-weighted and perfusion imaging parameters for predicting infarct size. *Radiology, 222*(2), 397–403.

5 | MULTIMODAL NEUROPHYSIOLOGICAL INVESTIGATIONS

CATHRIN M. BUETEFISCH and AINA PUCE

5.1   INTRODUCTION

Noninvasive neuroimaging and electrophysiological techniques allow us to study the organization and reorganization in the intact and diseased human brain. Recently, investigators started to combine multiple techniques to answer specific aspects of their research questions in more detail, thereby taking advantage of the strengths of each technique (Dale & Halgren, 2001; Shibasaki, 2008; Friston, 2009). In this chapter we review noninvasive neurophysiological methods, such as magnetoencephalography (MEG), electroencephalography (EEG), and transcranial magnetic stimulation (TMS). We then illustrate how MEG/EEG and TMS can add valuable complementary information when applied in combination with neuroimaging methods, such as functional magnetic resonance imaging (fMRI).

Functional magnetic resonance imaging (fMRI) has been able to noninvasively identify brain areas involved in motor learning (Karni et al., 1995) and recovery in human brain disorders, including stroke (Pineiro, Pendlebury, Johansen-Berg, & Matthews, 2001; Johansen-Berg et al., 2002; Ward, Brown, Thompson, & Frackowiak, 2003; Butefisch et al., 2005; see Chapter 4 for detailed discussion of this technique). Briefly, fMRI exploits the coupling between neuronal activity, blood flow, and oxygen consumption in the brain (Logothetis, Pauls, Augath, Trinath, & Oeltermann, 2001; Friston, 2009; Glover, 2011). It uses the relative changes in the ferromagnetic characteristics of oxygenated and deoxygenated blood to measure blood oxygen level (BOLD) in focal brain regions (Ogawa, Lee, Kay, & Tank, 1990; Kwong et al., 1992). As such, fMRI is an *indirect* measure of neuronal activity. A task-related increase in neuronal activity of different brain areas is thereby signaled by an increase in BOLD signal (oxygenated blood flowing in to replace deoxygenated blood) to the focal brain region. Yet, although BOLD fMRI identifies areas of increased neural activity, their specific contribution to the task under investigation is not defined. While fMRI is known for its excellent spatial resolution and the ability to localize activation within the human brain, it has relatively poor temporal resolution—typically, the hemodynamic or blood flow response peaks 4–8 seconds following the delivery of a sensory stimulus or the execution of a motor act (Glover, 2011). Therefore, if the aim is to characterize the *sequence* of task-related activation of brain areas, fMRI may not be the technique of choice (see Chapter 4 for details). Noninvasive methods that assess neural activity directly, such as MEG, EEG (see section 5.2), or transcranial magnetic stimulation (TMS; see section 5.3) have excellent temporal resolution; however, their spatial resolution is relatively poor with respect to methods such as fMRI. Hence, multimodal investigations using multiple methods can exploit the various strengths of these techniques and generate high-resolution, spatially and temporally rich datasets that can allow the characteristics of perception, cognition, and action to be studied (Dale & Halgren, 2001; Friston, 2009). Moreover, TMS can be used to perturb focal neural regions, allowing their potential functional role in an activation task to be explored in detail (Johansen-Berg et al., 2002; Paus, 2005), and this approach has been particularly successful for studying the motor system (Stoeckel, Seitz, & Buetefisch, 2009; Chouinard & Paus, 2010; Buetefisch, Hines, Shuster, Pergami, & Mathes, 2011).

5.2 MAGNETOENCEPHALOGRAPHY (MEG) AND ELECTROENCEPHALOGRAPHY (EEG)

5.2.1 METHODOLOGICAL CONSIDERATIONS

5.2.1.1 SITE OF RECORDING IN EEG AND MEG

One of the main strengths of measuring neurophysiological activity from the human brain lies in the fine-grained temporal information (millisecond accuracy) that is obtained (Aine, 1995; George et al., 1995; Aminoff, 1996; Liu, Belliveau, & Dale, 1998; Rossini & Pauri, 2000). This allows the temporal dynamics of perception, cognition, and motor output associated with any activation task to be studied as the time progresses in the experimental trial.

Neurophysiological studies in human subjects are typically performed in a noninvasive manner, and the investigator can record electrical activity at the scalp (via EEG) or magnetic fields that are emitted from the head (via MEG). Both methods require specialized instrumentation to record the tiny physiological signals that are emitted from the human brain, either spontaneously or in response to a particular stimulus or task (Dawson & Walter, 1945; Cohen, 1972; Fagaly, 1990; Dunseath & Kelly, 1995). EEG is the more established noninvasive method, and was first described by Dr. Hans Berger (1929). It has always had an important role to play in clinical studies (Bickford & Baldes, 1947; Niedermeyer, 1954, 1960) as well as research studies (Dawson, 1947; Ciganek, 1961; Sutton, Braren, Zubin, & John, 1965; Lopes da Silva & van Leeuwen, 1969) mainly due to its relatively lower cost and accessibility when compared to MEG.

Magnetoencephalography is a more recently developed technique relative to EEG, which was first described in the 1970s (Cohen, 1972). MEG developed as a research technique and remained so for many years, due to not only the specialized superconducting sensors that were required to measure the infinitesimally small magnetic fields that emanate from the head (Cohen, 1972; Fagaly, 1990), but also due to the more complex data analysis procedures that are typically used for MEG recordings (George et al., 1995; Jousmaki, 2000; Michel et al., 2004). MEG has a potential advantage relative to EEG in that magnetic fields pass through the skull unimpeded (Cuffin & Cohen, 1979; Michel et al., 2004), while electrical fields in EEG recordings are subject to low-pass filtering and spatial smearing due to the insulative properties of the skull and scalp. MEG is typically sensitive to tangential neural sources in the head (e.g., pyramidal neurons in cortical sulci), whereas EEG favors activity from radial sources (e.g., pyramidal neurons in cortical gyri; Cohen & Cuffin, 1983; Aine, 1995; Lopes da Silva, 1996; Srinivasan, Winter, & Nunez, 2006; Srinivasan, Winter, Ding, & Nunez, 2007). Therefore, both methods may offer complementary neurophysiological

data. In specific settings, concurrent recordings of MEG and EEG could provide a more complete picture of the neurophysiological profile of activity, particularly when using source modeling procedures (Baumgartner et al., 1991; Mosher, Spencer, Leahy, & Lewis, 1993; Babiloni et al., 2001; Huang et al., 2007).

5.2.1.2 SOURCE MODELING OF EEG AND MEG DATA

There is another methodological distinction between MEG and EEG which is important to consider. Traditionally, MEG studies have required some sort of modeling procedure to understand the output from the sensors that measure MEG activity, so that source modeling has typically accompanied the MEG data analysis procedures (Michel et al., 2004). EEG data have not been routinely analyzed using these methods; however, source modeling procedures can also be performed on EEG data. Source modeling of EEG or MEG data can yield accurate and reliable information, particularly with respect to activity in primary sensory or motor cortices (Elberling, Bak, Kofoed, Lebech, & Saermark, 1982; Okada, Tanenbaum, Williamson, & Kaufman, 1984; Hari & Kaukoranta, 1985; Eggermont & Ponton, 2002). Neurophysiological activity in sensory cortices has typically short latencies, well-formed components, and is focal in its distribution (Allison et al., 1989; Allison, McCarthy, Wood, Williamson, & Spencer, 1989). These qualities make it easier to source model this type of activity; hence, the development and testing of new source modeling methods typically uses these sensory systems for initial testing (see Michel, 2004).

At the heart of any source modeling procedure lies the specification of a head model. The earliest models consisted of multiple concentric spherical shells (Scherg & von Cramon, 1985; Roth, Saypol, Hallett, & Cohen, 1991) which simulated the various tissues types in the head, whereas more recent head models take a more realistic approach based on high-resolution structural MRI scans (Gevins, Brickett, Costales, Le, & Reutter, 1990; Michel et al., 2004; Hallez et al., 2007). Spherical head models were very popular in studies where activity in the sensorimotor system was being studied, as they were reasonably straightforward to calculate and computationally were relatively non-intensive (see review by Michel et al., 2004). While is it acknowledged that the human head/brain does not resemble a sphere, when one considers the nature of the curvature of the dorsal surface of the head/brain this has been accepted as being a reasonable approximation.

Irrespective of which head model is selected, each tissue type in the model is assigned different values of conductivity, based on empirical measures derived from invasive physiological studies in humans and animals (e.g., Roth et al., 1991; Schmid, Neubauer, & Mazal, 2003). A so-called forward model is first constructed, which takes into account physical characteristics such as sensor recording locations in 3-D space relative to brain structures, and tissue composition within the head and associated differences in conductivity. The activity profile on the scalp generated by putative neural structures in the brain can then be predicted and calculated. The forward model is then used to calculate a set of neural sources that can account for the topographic voltage or current patterns observed across the set of neurophysiological sensors in the real dataset (solving the so-called *inverse problem*). Unfortunately, the solution that is generated by solving the inverse problem is not unique (Cohen & Cuffin, 1987; Lopes da Silva, Wieringa, & Peters, 1991) because there are potentially multiple source distributions that can account for any observed topographic pattern in EEG or MEG sensors. The selection of the optimal solution crucially depends on its likelihood and its physiological plausibility (Michel et al., 2004). The characteristics of the head model may vary, but recent studies typically use a high-resolution structural MRI of individual subject brains for specifying a so-called "realistic head model."

MEG is by necessity a multimodal investigation, as MEG data analysis requires MRI data to specify the underlying active sources in the neural process being studied. However, the accuracy of the source modeling procedures relies on the ability to accurately co-register the MEG dataset with a high-resolution anatomical MRI dataset. This entails identifying a set of landmarks on the head that can be identified in both MRI and neurophysiological datasets for co-registration. These typically include the nasion (at the bridge of the nose) and the preauricular points next to the right and left ears, and will require the use of fiducial markers in the MRI (typically Vitamin E capsules can serve this purpose, as they have high signal contrast relative to the scalp and underlying tissue). The anatomical landmarks in the MRI data and MEG/EEG data are then aligned into a common head space which is unique (native) to each subject.

In order to make this type of alignment between the two datasets possible, the initial neurophysiological data acquisition phase must include an accurate 3-dimensional spatial sampling of the scalp regions that are being covered by the sensors. In the case of MEG, the sensor array does not contact the subject's scalp and the head can essentially move freely. Typically, a set of multiple tracking radio frequency (RF) receiver coils are attached to the subject's head/face, enabling the position of the head to be mapped relative to the fixed sensor array and an RF transmitter. This is typically part of the MEG system. Using software correction, activity sampled at each MEG sensor can then be reliably estimated (Hämäläinen & Hari, 2002).

In the case of EEG data, a commonly used electrode localization method (e.g. Polhemus, Colchester, VT, USA) is available: The subject is positioned near an RF transmitter and an RF receiver, which is typically shaped like a pen or stylus (Koessler, Maillard, Benhadid, Vignal, Braun,

& Vespignani, 2007; Engels, De Tiege, Op de Beeck, & Warzée, 2010). As each electrode is touched with the stylus, the RF signal at that position in space is recorded, so that a 3-dimensional spatial map of electrode positions can be generated. The fiducial landmark locations are also identified during this procedure and are part of the spatial map. Similar to the MEG sensor localization method, the subject also wears additional receiver coils that allow the correction of errors in electrode position that might occur from changes in head position. An alternative approach to EEG electrode localization involves capturing a photographic image of the subject with EEG sensors and fiducial markers using a multi-camera system (Russell, Jeffrey Eriksen, Poolman, Luu, & Tucker, 2005; Koessler et al., 2007). User-assisted software will then generate the 3-dimensional spatial map of electrode locations and fiducial markers that can be co-registered to a structural MRI of the head, if source modeling is being performed using a realistic head model.

5.2.1.3 CONSIDERATIONS WHEN STUDYING REORGANIZATION OF THE MOTOR SYSTEM WITH MULTIMODAL MEG/EEG

While it is clear that the location of primary sensorimotor cortex can be mapped reliably with MEG or EEG (see section 5.2.1), it is important to consider the remarkable ability of the cortex to reorganize based on sensory and motor experience or injury such as stroke (Rossini et al., 2007; Jancke, 2009). There are many studies that have reported experience-based differences in brain networks responsible for carrying out motor actions related to sport, dancing, musical, or other motor-based activities, which show clear differences between experts and novices, or as a function of an intensive training experience (Draganski et al., 2004; Jancke, 2009; Herdener et al., 2010; Wei & Luo, 2010; Petrini et al., 2011).

Taken together, these studies highlight a number of important issues to consider when studying plasticity of the motor system in humans, irrespective of intact or diseased brain. We outline these important considerations below:

i. Different baseline abilities in motor skills will exist in individuals *prior to* training and need to be considered as a potential source of variance when examining effects of sensorimotor training. Individual differences in training improvements that occur during the motor skill manipulation may in turn be correlated with differences in brain regional grey and matter characteristics (Tomassini et al., 2011).

ii. Differences in the baseline physical fitness, particularly in the elderly, may also be important for baseline (premorbid) brain health (van Praag, 2009;

Jak, 2011), and the ability to which the brain recovers may well depend on some of these factors.

iii. Changes in cortical excitability, functional connectivity, grey matter, and white matter structure can occur as a part of a short training session (Karni et al., 1995; Sanes & Donoghue, 2000; Taubert et al., 2010) or following an intensive motor training experience (Sanes & Donoghue, 2000; Taubert, Lohmann, Margulies, Villringer, & Ragert, 2011). Similarly, the lack of use of a limb (e.g., as when it has been in a plaster cast for a few weeks) can produce a striking shrinkage in the cortical motor maps (Karni et al., 1995; Liepert, Tegenthoff, & Malin, 1995; Lissek et al., 2009) or altered cortical excitability (Granert et al., 2011).

iv. Attributes such as handedness may be associated with differences in neuroanatomy (Kloppel, Mangin, Vongerichten, Frackowiak, & Siebner, 2010) and may well influence training capacity.

v. Sensorimotor cortex should be considered as an important part of an action-generation brain network, where the input of other brain structures is important in modulating the local activity within sensorimotor cortex. In this same vein, input carried by cross-callosal fibers from homologous sensorimotor cortex in the contralateral hemisphere is an important component of this brain network.

If one considers sensorimotor cortex to be part of a brain network for action execution, then other potential options for neurorehabilititative training become available. Given that activity from other parts of the brain network can act on sensorimotor cortex during action execution, it might be possible to exploit this functional connectivity in designing personalized programs to aid stroke recovery (Tomassini et al., 2011).

5.2.1.4 NEUROPHYSIOLOGICAL RHYTHMS AND POTENTIAL INSIGHTS INTO STROKE RECOVERY

Multimodal neurophysiological investigations using MEG and EEG in healthy subjects have demonstrated complex changes in oscillatory rhythmic components in the neurophysiological signal during the execution of a sensorimotor task (reviewed by (Hummel & Gerloff, 2006). The mu rhythms, which consist of a comb-like periodic pattern made up of 10 Hz and 20 Hz components, are thought to emanate from neuronal tissue in primary motor and somatosensory cortices and are best seen in MEG-based neurophysiological recordings (reviewed by Forss & Silen, 2001; Hari, 2006). These rhythms are suppressed preceding, during, and immediately after a planned or executed motor movement, and can be seen to rebound following

the movement. Strikingly, this rhythm also exhibits suppression and rebound-like behavior when the individual observes someone else carrying out the same action (Forss & Silen, 2001; Hari, 2006). Therefore, the presence of this finding could be exploited as a potential indicator of the potential health of post-stroke sensorimotor cortex and may aid in predicting potential for recovery.

Other EEG changes in the beta (13–30 Hz) and alpha (7–13 Hz) frequency ranges have also been demonstrated during the execution of skilled motor movements. Some investigators have quantified task-related changes in terms of whether these cortical rhythms are suppressed (event-related desynchronization, ERD) or whether they are augmented (event-related synchronization, ERS) and have quantified the change in the amount of signal power in each frequency range (reviewed by Forss & Silen, 2001; Hummel & Gerloff, 2006). ERS and ERD have been interpreted by some investigators to reflect cortical activation and deactivation, respectively (Neuper, Wortz, & Pfurtscheller, 2006), a view not shared by others (Hari, 2006). Induced beta rebound (ERS) has been documented following the execution of voluntary motor movements and following somatosensory stimulation of peripheral nerves (Neuper et al., 2006).

With respect to studying stroke patients, so-called *single trial analyses* of MEG/EEG data may give some further insight regarding the degree of neurological impairment from the frequency content of *induced* neurophysiological rhythms. This is a method which is being increasingly used in conjunction with the more usual *evoked* rhythms, which typically lend themselves to visualization using conventional averaging (David, Kilner, & Friston, 2006). These types of analyses have potential for studying sensorimotor actions as different oscillatory rhythms. Coherences across different brain regions can, in principle, be tracked (de Lange, Jensen, Bauer, & Toni, 2008). Single-digit hand stimulation can even show induced gamma range rhythms whose locations are spatially separable across digits (Schweitzer et al., 2001). Some preliminary work looking at these types of induced rhythms in a single case study involving a hemianopic patient with blindsight indicates that gamma rhythms correlate with visual awareness, whereas other characteristic occipital rhythms, such as alpha activity, do not show this relationship (Schurger, Cowey, & Tallon-Baudry, 2006).

A measure of synchronization or regional coupling across cortex in MEG or EEG data can be given by a coherence measure. Coherence typically varies from 0 to 1, with 1 describing perfect correspondence between the two signals (but with allowable phase delays between the two waveforms; Gross et al., 2001; Hummel & Gerloff, 2006). Phase differences between the two waveforms can also be calculated, although there is some debate about which waveform is the "cart" and which is the "horse"; only an "apparent" phase delay could be calculated, as one could not know with certainty which noninvasive neurophysiological signal really led the other. More recently developed wavelet-based coherence calculations may circumvent this problem (Lachaux et al., 2002).

An important question in stroke recovery is to what extent other structures in the sensorimotor network influence or accelerate stroke recovery via these modulating oscillatory neurophysiological rhythms. Additionally, the question can also be applied to contributions from homologous structures in the contralateral hemisphere. Measures such as MEG/EEG coherence are one way with which to estimate this type of interaction. Serrien and coworkers (2004) examined EEG coherence in different frequency bands when stroke patients performed a unimanual gripping task. For those patients who had not yet recovered, a significant contribution of task-relevant beta activity was seen in the contralesional hemisphere when the affected limb performed the task (Serrien, Strens, Cassidy, Thompson, & Brown, 2004). In contrast, this type of coherence relationship was not observed when the patients performed the task with their unaffected limb. Importantly, this same pattern of activity was also observed in patients who had shown excellent recovery from their stroke. The investigators suggested that these oscillatory rhythms that occur between sensorimotor cortices in an impaired stroke patient might have an important functional role in the recovery process (Serrien et al., 2004). Further studies are needed to more fully characterize this phenomenon so that it could be exploited in individualized neurorehabilitative strategies.

Interestingly, the induction of artificial cortical neurophysiological rhythms via TMS—so-called *theta burst TMS stimulation*, where high frequency bursts of 50 Hz TMS are applied at 5 Hz (at the 4–7 Hz frequency of the EEG theta band)—can also influence brain responses. Theta burst TMS stimulation (40-second period) applied over primary motor cortex (M1) of healthy subjects can significantly *augment* somatosensory/motor evoked potential components for over 50 minutes (Ishikawa et al., 2007). This facilitatory effect appears specific to M1stimulation. When applied 2 cm posterior to the putative location of M1, *suppression* of the somatosensory/motor evoked potential components occurred. The use of TMS in conjunction with EEG-based or MEG-based neurophysiological investigations, as well as behavioral assessment, is necessary to be able to generate a more complete picture of the status of sensorimotor cortex, especially in post-stroke recovery.

The important take-home message from this cursory discussion on the effect of experience-dependent changes on the brain's rhythms is that not only can local cortical rhythms be altered, but also rhythms from remote but functionally connected brain regions can potentially have a profound modulatory impact on a brain region. Additionally, it is clear the mere *intention* to act can also influence these rhythms.

The planning and successful execution of a complex motor act associated with intention will necessarily involve the coordinated and sequenced activity of a complex brain network. This allows for multiple potential brain pathways that could potentially be accessed to structure an individualized neurorehabilitation program. This approach may be more effective than current conventional therapeutic strategies. Mechanisms underlying brain plasticity as they apply to stroke are moving beyond the realm of research into practice (Johansson, 2011). However, multimodal investigations are crucial for an improved understanding of mechanisms underlying motor recovery after stroke and for prediction of stroke recovery. This is a necessary step toward the development of patient-tailored effective rehabilitation therapies.

5.2.2 MULTIMODAL MEG/EEG STUDIES OF ACTIVITY IN PRIMARY SENSORIMOTOR CORTEX IN STROKE RECOVERY

There is now a fairly substantial fMRI literature that has documented variable degrees of post-stroke reorganization following sensorimotor stroke, including recruitment of contralesional motor areas and additional regions in the ipsilesional hemisphere (e.g., Calautti & Baron, 2003; Butefisch et al., 2005; Carey, Abbott, Egan, Bernhardt, & Donnan, 2005; Carey et al., 2002, 2006, 2011), as discussed in detail in this book. However, fMRI, while invaluable for documenting these changes, nevertheless can be problematic in the presence of edema or hemorrhage, as neurovascular coupling mechanisms may be disrupted and produce little fMRI activation, or activation data that cannot easily be interpreted (Rossini et al., 2004; Zaca, Hua, & Pillai, 2011). It has been shown that in cases where sensorimotor fMRI activation is *absent* in the chronic phase following stroke, a reliable MEG response can still be elicited (Rossini et al., 2004). In this study, identical stimulus paradigms consisting of supramotor threshold electrical stimulation of the median nerve was utilized in both MEG and fMRI studies. Additionally, the magnitude and characteristics of the persisting MEG response appeared to be influenced by the presence of compounds in the bloodstream that signal oxidative stress (Rossini et al., 2004). We discuss this important point again later in this chapter when comparing fMRI and TMS data that were collected in the same subjects.

A second limitation for the performance of fMRI studies in the acute phase post-stroke relates to the medical instability of the patient, which may pose a contraindication for performing an MRI (Hand et al., 2005). These limitations of fMRI preclude acute post-stroke research studies of neuroplasticity, which could potentially be conducted using EEG/MEG instead. For patients who cannot easily be moved in their acute hospital setting, EEG may well be the assessment method of choice, as the equipment can be brought directly to the patient's bedside.

A number of multimodal studies involving noninvasive neurophysiological assessments have studied stroke patients in the chronic recovery period following stroke. For example, Altamura and colleagues (2007) performed an MEG-fMRI investigation of 10 patients with sensorimotor impairment of the upper limb due to either cortical or subcortical stroke (Altamura et al., 2007). Their activation paradigm consisted of electrical stimulation of the median nerve of the hand. MEG data consisted of averaged magnetic field, whose strength and likely source location were assessed using an equivalent current dipole (ECD) model. Specifically, the M20 MEG response was studied. The M20 is thought to be generated by the primary somatosensory cortex and occurs nominally at 20 ms after the delivery of the electrical stimulus to the median nerve. fMRI activation to the electrical stimulus was demonstrated relative to a rest condition in a block design.

The difference in the relative loci of MEG ECDs and fMRI activation, in terms of mean Euclidian distance, was calculated for stimulation of each hand. Interestingly, in these 10 chronic stroke survivors, no ipsilateral sensorimotor activation was observed in either the MEG or fMRI data. Functional MRI activation at 1.5 Tesla was not seen in the ipsilesional hemisphere in 4 patients, despite clearly present M20 responses (an inclusion criterion in the study was that patients should exhibit at least discernable MEG responses bilaterally). Ipsilesional M20 ECD strength was, however, significantly diminished in 3 patients, and in one individual it was significantly greater relative to the corresponding contralesional response.

There was no significant correlation between fMRI and MEG abnormalities. Mean Euclidian distances between ECD locations and the centroids of fMRI activation were around 10 mm. Interestingly, interhemispheric asymmetries were observed in M20 ECD location. ECD source activity was located outside the usual postrolandic regions in the ipsilesional hemisphere, as well as extending posteriorly beyond perirolandic regions in some patients (Altamura et al., 2007). The posterior shift of active cortex to sensorimotor stimulation has also been demonstrated in a multimodal investigation of a single case using MEG, fMRI, and TMS, in a pioneering study by investigators from this research team (Rossini et al., 1998).

Recovery from stroke does not have to be associated with activation shifts to other parts of sensorimotor cortex. MEG data in response to median nerve stimulation in patients with ischemic strokes in acute and later stages of recovery can also show changes in focal neural sources in primary somatosensory and motor cortices whose strengths increase as recovery progresses (Huang et al., 2004).

The use of an ECD model in MEG or EEG precludes an assessment of the *extent* of active cortex. It would be instructive to study individuals with both high-resolution fMRI/MRI and MEG/EEG, using parallel distributed source modeling with a realistic model of the individual's head, to assess the nature of this aberrant activation more closely. (Gross et al., 2001; Schweitzer et al., 2001;Lachaux et al., 2002; Serrien et al., 2004; David et al., 2006; Hummel & Gerloff, 2006; Schurger et al., 2006; de Lange et al., 2008).

One of the major strengths of multimodal investigations involving MEG/EEGs of stroke patients lies in the additional interpretive power that the combination of multiple datasets can provide (Dale & Halgren, 2001). A good case in point is the study by Gerloff and colleagues (2006). They studied a fairly homogeneous group of 11 right-handed chronic stroke patients with lacunes in the posterior limb of the left internal capsule and compared their multimodal data with a group of age-matched controls. Enhanced blood flow in both ipsilesional and contralesional lateral premotor cortices was noted in PET scans. EEG coherence across sites in the ipsilesional hemisphere was significantly reduced relative to the contralesional hemisphere—which the authors suggested reflected a shift in functional connectivity to the contralesional hemisphere. In the lesioned hemisphere, corticospinal transmission was observed. Consistent with results of previous TMS studies in well-recovered patients, TMS applied to contralesional M1 did not elicit reliable ipsilateral MEPs. This complex pattern of multimodal results was interpreted as being consistent with the idea that increased contralesional activity likely influences recovery via higher-order motor mechanisms, although recovery requires the use of both ipsilesional and contralesional resources (Gerloff et al., 2006).

Two methodological points regarding future multimodal MEG/EEG studies need to be made. First, data analyses using frequency decomposition or coherence measures on single trial data can be applied to continuous EEG/MEG data if higher than normal sampling rates and wider filter bands are used. This lends itself well to use with current experimental task designs. Second, an important consideration for performing MEG/EEG studies aiming to study neuroplastic mechanisms would also require continuous EMG monitoring of the limb contralateral to that being stimulated in a sensorimotor activation task. It has not been standard practice in MEG/EEG studies to monitor EMG of the muscle(s) being stimulated in these hand activation paradigms, or to monitor for mirror movements in the contralateral unstimulated limb (but see Serrien et al., 2004). It is well known that facilitation of motor evoked potentials in TMS studies can occur in response to not only contraction of the hand contralateral to the cortex being stimulated, but also potentially to mirror movements of the ipsilateral hand to stimulation (Duque et al., 2005; Garry, Loftus, & Summers, 2005). If a bilateral fMRI activation pattern is observed to sensorimotor stimulation post-stroke, then monitoring of bilateral EMG can rule out the presence of mirror movements and confirm that the bilateral activation pattern reflects motor performance that is truly unilateral (Butefisch et al., 2005). If this is not the case, and given that it is known that oscillatory rhythms in MEG/EEG studies can be bilateral and can impact remote regions of the brain (see earlier discussion), the monitoring of EMG to eliminate potential confounding effects of mirror movements would appear to be an important consideration for the interpretation of bilateral oscillatory MEG/EEG phenomena, as well as fMRI activation.

5.3 TRANSCRANIAL MAGNETIC STIMULATION (TMS)

5.3.1 METHODOLOGICAL CONSIDERATIONS

TMS allows noninvasive stimulation of the cortex through the closed skull. In principle, TMS involves a large capacitor that discharges its charge through a coil. The current in the coil creates a magnetic field around the coil that passes through the skin and bone and induces a transient current that activates the cerebral cortex under the stimulating coil (Hallett, 2007). Since the magnetic field strength falls off rapidly with the distance from the coil (Hess, Mills, & Murray, 1987), TMS as commonly applied does not directly stimulate deep structures of the brain (thalamus, basal ganglia). In addition, the greater resistance of white matter results in further reduction of the current.

Therefore, the current induced in the subcortical structures is usually small. In primary motor cortex, the transient current activates the pyramidal tract neurons through horizontal connections trans-synaptically (indirect (I) waves; Day, Thompson, Dick, Nakashima, & Marsden, 1987). This is in contrast to transcranial electrical stimulation (TES) of the brain, where the pyramidal tract neurones are predominantly stimulated directly at their axon hillock (direct (D) waves; Amassian, Quirk, & Stewart, 1990; Rothwell, 1991). Both TES and TMS result in a synchronized discharge of pyramidal tract neurons. The number and excitability of activated neurons is reflected in a potential that is recorded with surface electrodes mounted over the target muscle (motor evoked potential: MEP, Figure 5.1). The latency of TMS-evoked MEPs are longer when compared to TES-evoked MEPs due to the site of their activation.

A point should be made about the popularity and propagation of TMS methods relative to TES. TES is associated with high-voltage electrical transcranial stimulation, which typically involves a noxious stimulus and considerable physical discomfort. The first-ever study of TES was performed in anaesthetized human and monkey subjects (Gualtierotti & Paterson, 1954). Subsequent work performed years later in awake human subjects also alludes to the painful nature of the delivered stimulus, whereby the stimulation was performed only on the laboratory investigators themselves (Merton & Morton, 1980). Early TMS studies using circular coils delivered less focal stimulation, which was also associated with quite marked stimulation of the ipsilateral scalp and potentially facial and ocular musculature. Modern coils (e.g., figure-8 designs) reduce these peripheral stimulation effects and improve focality of cortical stimulation (Hallett, 2000).

5.3.2 TMS MEASURES OF MOTOR CORTEX

5.3.2.1 MOTOR THRESHOLD

The smallest stimulation intensity required to elicit an MEP (minimum of 50 μV amplitude) in 5 out of 10 trials is defined as the resting motor threshold (RMT) (Rossini et al., 1994). The MT is obtained at the so-called *hot spot*, the location of the scalp that produces the largest MEP response with the smallest intensity of stimulation. The MT is lower during voluntary contraction (active motor threshold: AMT) because resting spinal and cortical motor neurons require more excitation to reach the discharging threshold than during contraction. The AMT is usually determined during a slight voluntary tonic contraction (at 10%–20% of maximum). In this setting, the minimum MEP amplitude is usually about 100–200 μV in amplitude. Since MT is increased by drugs that block voltage-gated sodium channels (Ziemann, Lonnecker, Steinhoff, & Paulus, 1996b), it is thought that MT reflects neural membrane excitability, which is mainly dependent on ion channel conductivity. In subacute stroke patients, MT of ipsilesional M1 is usually abnormally increased (Boroojerdi, Diefenbach, & Ferbert, 1996; Liepert, Storch, Fritsch, & Weiller, 2000; Manganotti et al., 2002), while MT of contralesional M1 is normal (Boroojerdi et al., 1996; Liepert, Hamzei, & Weiller, 2000; Manganotti et al., 2002; Butefisch, Netz, Wessling, Seitz, & Homberg, 2003).

5.3.2.2 MEP AMPLITUDE

MEP amplitudes depend on the excitability of corticospinal neurons in M1, as well as spinal motor neurons. As defined in the previous section, MEP amplitude is measured at the hot spot at intensities above the MT. Typically 5 to 10 evoked responses are obtained and an average MEP amplitude is calculated. With increasing stimulation intensity and proximity of the stimulation site to the true hot spot, the reliability of the obtained MEP amplitude measurement increases (Brasil-Neto et al., 1992). Measurement of MEP amplitude is commonly used to determine alteration in motor cortex excitability (Buetefisch & Cohen, 2008). However, any changes in MEP amplitudes could be caused by alterations in excitability at either cortical or spinal level, or a combination of both.

In order to localize the site of excitability changes within the corticospinal system, additional measurements are needed. Direct recording of the TMS-evoked descending volleys with epidural electrodes is an invasive approach that can be used only in limited situations (Di Lazzaro et al., 1999). Another approach involves the comparison of MEP amplitudes elicited by TMS to those elicited by TES. As mentioned earlier, TMS activates pyramidal tract neurons, predominantly trans-synaptically (Day et al., 1987), while TES stimulates pyramidal tract neurons predominantly at their axon hillock (Amassian et al., 1990; Rothwell, 1991). If training-induced MEP changes occur at a cortical site, one would expect to observe them with TMS but not with TES. On the other hand, changes at a spinal level would elicit comparable modifications in MEP amplitudes to both TMS and TES.

TMS of the brainstem is a means to differentiate between changes at the cortical and spinal levels. MEP evoked by brainstem TMS should be relatively unaffected by changes in cortical excitability. Changes in MEP after TMS in association with unaffected spinal excitability would also support a cortical site for changes in MEP amplitude. In most TMS studies, spinal excitability is estimated by measuring changes in F-waves (Mercuri et al., 1996) or the H-reflexes (Fuhr, Agostino, & Hallett, 1991). For the F-waves, the alpha motor fiber is the afferent as well as the efferent pathway. For the H-reflex, the Ia fiber is the afferent pathway and the alpha motor fiber the efferent pathway. Therefore, both studies probe excitability of the spinal alpha motoneurons.

5.3.2.3 MEP LATENCY AND CENTRAL MOTOR CONDUCTION TIME

MEP latency is defined as the time interval between the application of the stimulus and the onset of the MEP response. The latency depends on central motor conduction

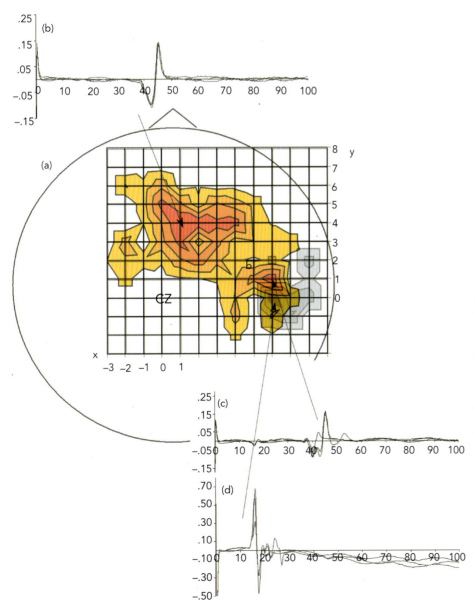

Figure 5.1 TMS of M1 reveals two motor maps of abductor hallucis (AH) in a subject with congenital upper extremity malfunction (single subject data). Average of 5 motor evoked potentials (MEPs) of the right AH muscle (orange, a and c) and right hand muscle (grey, d) are shown. Coordinates refer to positions (in cm) of the center of the coil on the mediolateral axis (left to right) and fronto-occipital axis (top to bottom) with CZ (i.e., vertex) at the origin. MEP data were normalized to the maximum mean amplitude of each map. Positions with a mean amplitude of >20%, >40%, >60% and >80% are indicated by the increasing shading with the darkest shade being the largest amplitude. The similarity of MEP latency for the two hot spots of the AH (b and c) indicate that both areas have likely monosynaptic connection to the spinal alpha motor neurons (modified from Stoeckel et al., 2009).

time (i.e., the time that elapses between the discharges of the pyramidal tract neurons and the arrival of the volley at the spinal motor neurons) and peripheral conduction time (time from the discharge of spinal motor neurons to the target muscle where the compound muscle action potential is measured). Prolongation of the MEP latency can therefore reflect processes involving central and peripheral nervous systems. In addition, as mentioned above, the MEP latency can depend on TMS coil position and intensity of the applied stimulus. Latency measures can also differentiate between types of corticospinal connections. Monosynaptic or oligosynaptic connections have a shorter latency when compared to polysynaptic projections because each synapse will delay the conduction by about 2 ms (Figure 5.1).

5.3.2.4 CORTICAL SILENT PERIOD
In the silent period paradigm, a suprathreshold TMS pulse (i.e., above MT) is applied to the contralateral M1 during tonic muscle activation of the targeted muscle. This results in the disruption of M1 activity that is reflected in EMG silence following the MEP lasting 40–300 ms. The length of this silent period depends on the target muscle, the stimulus intensity, and intake of central nervous system (CNS) active drugs. It partly reflects intracortical inhibitory activity and is probably GABA$_B$ mediated (Inghilleri, Berardelli, Cruccu, & Manfredi, 1993; Roick, von Giesen, & Benecke, 1993).

5.3.2.5 INPUT–OUTPUT CURVES
As described above, measurement of MEP amplitude is used to determine motor cortex excitability. By stimulating the hot spot at increasing intensities, an increase in the MEP amplitude is observed (also referred to as a *stimulus response curve*). Compared to the measure of MEP amplitudes at a single intensity, the input–output curve is more comprehensive, as it includes the assessment of neurons that are intrinsically less excitable or more distant from the hot spot (Ridding & Rothwell, 1997). The steepness of the recruitment curves are likely related to the strength of corticospinal projections, and are generally steeper in muscles with low MT, such as intrinsic hand muscles (Chen et al., 1998). The steepness of the input–output curve and maximum MEP amplitudes may be decreased in some patients post-stroke, but may remain similar to healthy age matched controls in other stroke patients (see section 5.3.3 for more detailed discussion (Butefisch, Wessling, Netz, Seitz, & Homberg, 2008)).

5.3.2.6 SHORT INTERVAL CORTICAL INHIBITION (SICI)
In the paired pulse paradigm, two pulses are delivered through the same coil with a short temporal relationship. A suprathreshold test stimulus (TS) is preceded by a subthreshold conditioning stimulus (CS) at different interstimulus intervals (ISI; Kujirai et al., 1993). With short interstimulus intervals (2–4 ms), test MEP responses are inhibited (conditioned MEP). This effect is mediated by GABA$_A$ receptors (Ziemann, Lonnecker, Steinhoff, & Paulus, 1996a) and arises in close proximity to the stimulated area (Di Lazzaro et al., 1998). Since the threshold for inhibitory interneurons is lower than that for excitatory interneurons, (Schafer, Biesecker, Schulze-Bonhage, & Ferbert, 1997; Chen et al., 1998; Butefisch et al., 2003) varying the intensity of the CS allows the separation of the effects mediated by these respective networks in more detail (Schafer et al., 1997; Chen et al., 1998; Fisher, Nakamura, Bestmann, Rothwell, & Bostock, 2002; Butefisch et al., 2003; Figure 5.2).

5.3.2.7 INTRACORTICAL FACILITATION (ICF)
To evaluate intracortical facilitation (ICF), a suprathreshold test stimulus (TS) is preceded by a subthreshold conditioning stimulus (CS) at different interstimulus intervals (ISI; Kujirai et al., 1993). With an ISI of 8–30 ms, the test responses are facilitated (Kujirai et al., 1993). The neuronal populations mediating ICF are less well understood but they are distinct from those mediating short interval cortical inhibition (SICI) and appear to be located in cortex (Ziemann et al., 1996a; Di Lazzaro et al., 2006).

5.3.2.8 INTERHEMISPHERIC INHIBITION (IHI)
IHI can be demonstrated by applying a conditioning stimulus (CS) to the motor cortex, which inhibits the size of the motor evoked potential (MEP) produced by the test stimulus (TS) applied to the homotopic area of the opposite motor cortex (Ferbert et al., 1992). The intensity of the CS is usually adjusted to produce a MEP of about 1.5 mV, and the interstimulus interval is typically 10 ms (Ferbert et al., 1992). Usually, the paired pulses are intermixed with single TS and single CS pulses applied at random. The amount of IHI from one motor cortex on the other motor cortex is expressed as percentage of the mean MEP amplitude of the single TS pulses (Ferbert et al., 1992), as shown in Figure 5.3.

5.3.3 REPETITIVE TRANSCRANIAL MAGNETIC STIMULATION (rTMS)
In general, rTMS applied to intact primary motor cortex (M1) at high frequency produces an excitatory effect (Pascual-Leone et al., 1994; Di Lazzaro et al., 2002; Daskalakis et al., 2006; Fitzgerald et al., 2006) and an inhibitory effect when applied at low frequency (Chen et al., 1997; Daskalakis et al., 2006; Fitzgerald et al., 2006). Low-frequency rTMS (1 Hz or less) at intensities at about MT, applied to primary motor cortex, can be used safely (Wassermann, Wedegaertner, Ziemann, George, & Chen, 1998; Chen et al., 2008) to decrease excitability in the stimulated M1 (Chen et al., 1997; Maeda, Keenan,

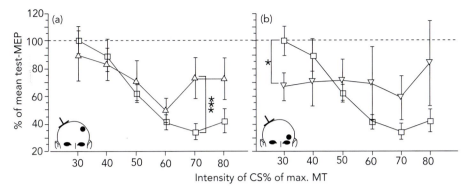

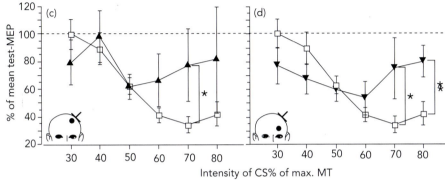

Figure 5.2 Effect of different CS intensities on the inhibitory effect on conditioned MEP amplitude in patients post-stroke (n = 23) and an age-matched healthy control population (n = 20). Upper panel: Control (square) and contralesional M1 of patients with cortical (open triangle, a) and subcortical location of infarction (open inverted triangle, b). Lower panel: Control (squares) and ipsilesional M1 of patients with cortical (black triangle, c) and subcortical location of infarction (black inverted triangle, d). Mean ± SE. * p < 0.05, ** p < 0.02, *** p < 0.01. Inserts illustrate the location of the lesion (black dot) and the site of TMS (inverted T). CS = intensity of conditioning stimulus, MT = motor threshold. (modified from Buetefisch et al., 2008).

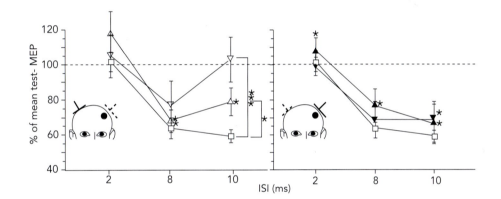

Figure 5.3 IHI in intact brain of healthy controls (n=20) and lesioned brain of patients after stroke (n = 23). EMG was recorded from the first dorsal interosseous muscle (FDI) contralateral to the conditioned M1 (inverted dotted T indicates the site of the conditioning pulse). Left panel: IHI of the ipsilesional M1 on the contralesional M1 was impaired when compared to M1 of healthy subjects. Although IHI was significant at 8 and 10 ms with cortical infarction (open triangle) it was still smaller at ISI of 10 ms when compared to M1 of healthy subjects. For subcortical infarction, IHI was impaired and significantly smaller when compared to M1 of healthy subjects at ISI of 10 ms (open inverted triangle). Right panel: IHI of the contralesional M1 on the ipsilesional M1 was intact for subcortical infarction (black inverted triangle) and cortical infarction (black triangle). The conditioned MEP amplitude is expressed as percentage of the mean test-MEP. Mean ± SE * p < 0.05, ** p < 0.02, *** p < 0.0002.

Tormos, Topka, & Pascual-Leone, 2000; Di Lazzaro et al., 2008; Sommer, Lang, Tergau, & Paulus, 2002; Bagnato et al., 2005; Fitzgerald, Fountain, & Daskalakis, 2006) , which in specific settings can produce measurable behavioral effects. In this regard, rTMS when applied to the brain area of interest is a means to probe its contribution to the studied activation task.

Low frequency rTMS of one M1 can also lead to effects remote from the stimulated cortex. For example, subthreshold 1 Hz rTMS applied to one M1 suppressed intracortical inhibition and enhanced intracortical facilitation in the opposite, nonstimulated M1 (Kobayashi,

Hutchinson, Theoret, Schlaug, & Pascual-Leone, 2004). Further, changes in metabolic rate in the (nonstimulated) contralateral motor cortex have been reported, as have increases in EEG coherence between the motor cortices, or between stimulated cortex and more anterior motor areas (Strens et al., 2002). These corticocortical and interhemispheric effects may lead to discernable changes in behavior. For example, improved motor performance in the hand *ipsilateral* to stimulated M1 has been reported by some investigators (Kobayashi, Hutchinson, Schlaug, & Pascual-Leone, 2003; Dafotakis, Grefkes, Wang, Fink, & Nowak, 2008); however, this was dependent on the specific motor

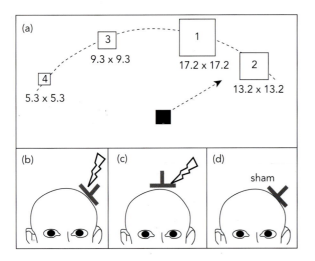

Figure 5.4 Repetitive TMS is used to probe the role of ipsilateral M1 in a motor task. **(a).** Prior to and following the stimulation, subjects had to manipulate a joystick in a pointing task with either the left or right hand. Subjects were asked to move a cursor as quickly as possible to the center of targets of different sizes upon their appearance on the screen. Targets were presented at four evenly spaced locations on the upper half field of a PC monitor (**b, c, d**). The effect of 1 Hz rTMS at 90% resting MT to iM1 (**b**) and vertex (**c**) was tested. In an additional control condition, sham rTMS was applied to iM1 (**d**). (Modified from Buetefisch et al., 2011).

demand in a more recent study (Figure 5.4; Buetefisch et al., 2011).

5.3.4 MULTIMODAL TMS/BRAIN IMAGING STUDIES OF STROKE RECOVERY

Here, we illustrate the multimodal TMS/brain imaging approach in selected studies of motor recovery post-stroke. In one of the first ever multimodal longitudinal studies, brain imaging using positron emission tomography (PET) and TMS were used to identify brain areas associated with good recovery (Binkofski et al., 1996). TMS was used to probe the integrity of the corticospinal tract while PET was used to identify paretic hand movement–related brain areas. Derived from the results of this study, the integrity of the pyramidal motor output system appeared to be one of the most important factors influencing motor recovery (Binkofski et al., 1996). As discussed above, TMS provides a means to measure the functional efficacy of the corticospinal output system early after the infarction, because the size of the MEP depends on the excitability and number of cortical, subcortical, and spinal neurons and on the integrity of the entire corticopyramidal tract.

Within the first 72 hours after stroke, an absent MEP was related to poor functional recovery (Binkofski et al., 1996; Nardone & Tezzon, 2002). This correlation was found to still hold when MEPs were measured 1 to 2 months after brain infarction, irrespective of cortical or subcortical location. Subsequent work was done using

TMS and fMRI. As pointed out at the beginning of the chapter, fMRI exploits the coupling between neuronal activity, blood flow and oxygen consumption in the brain (Logothetis et al., 2001; Friston, 2009; Glover, 2011). It uses the relative changes in the ferromagnetic characteristics of oxygenated and deoxygenated blood to measure blood oxygen level (BOLD) in focal brain regions (Ogawa et al., 1990; Kwong et al., 1992). As such, fMRI is an indirect measure of neuronal activity. Hence, a task-related increase in neuronal activity of different brain areas is signaled by an increase in BOLD signal (oxygenated blood flowing in to replace deoxygenated blood) to the focal brain region. In a serial fMRI/TMS study, eight patients with sensorimotor stroke were studied at 1 week, 2–4 weeks, and 1 month after their stroke (Binkofski & Seitz, 2004). A tactile exploration task involving finger movement was used (for fMRI) and MEPs to motor cortex stimulation were studied. MEPs were preserved at all test stages of the study while motor function was seen to improve. In comparison, fMRI activation was not observed in the expected regions in the subacute (1 week) phase of the study, but only emerged in the early chronic phase (2–4 weeks) of the study. Considering the fact that selective finger function was required for the tactile exploration task and the selective finger function depends on the integrity of primary motor cortex and its projections to spinal motoneurons (measured with TMS), the dissociation between the presence of MEPs and absent fMRI activation in M1 was interpreted as a transient neurophysiological-hemodynamic decoupling in the subacute phase of the study (Binkofski & Seitz, 2004).

A similar uncoupling of neuronal activity from fMRI activation was found in a combined MEG/fMRI study of stroke patients (Rossini et al., 2004). An electrical median nerve stimulation always produced both a stimulus-locked electromagnetic brain activity (MEG) and identifiable BOLD activation (fMRI) in healthy subjects, but frequently failed to produce a fMRI BOLD activation in stroke patients. To date, very little work has been performed to investigate this really important issue.

In a systematic review of the predictive value of the presence of MEPs obtained within the first week after infarction, sensitivity and specificity of this test was consistently high for patients with either subcortical or cortical location of their infarction. Odds ratios varied between 5.49 and 13.50 for functional recovery in the presence of an MEP (Hendricks, Zwarts, Plat, & van Limbeek, 2002). Furthermore, upon recovery, good functional outcome was associated with an increase of the initially reduced MEP amplitudes (Binkofski et al., 1996). However, there are patients with severe motor deficits in whom increased cortical inhibitory activity may cause the motor deficit, despite the presence of normal MEPs (Classen et al., 1997). Similarly, there are a few patients with excellent recovery of motor function despite an absent MEP or late

MEP reappearance (Traversa, Cicinelli, Bassi, Rossini, & Bernardi, 1997; Butefisch et al., 2003).

In imaging studies of stroke patients, the activation of contralesional motor areas has been consistently reported (Calautti & Baron, 2003). Cross-sectional functional imaging studies of stroke patients moving the affected hand revealed a shift from an initially abnormal bilateral activation of motor areas in the subacute stroke patients (Chollet et al., 1991; Weiller, Chollet, Friston, Wise, & Frackowiak, 1992; Cramer et al., 1997; Cao, D'Olhaberriague, Vikingstad, Levine, & Welch, 1998; Small, Hlustik, Noll, Genovese, & Solodkin, 2002; Ward et al., 2003; Butefisch et al., 2005) toward a more normal unilateral activation pattern of ipsilesional motor areas in chronic stroke patients (Ward et al., 2003). Importantly, this activation shift to the ipsilesional hemisphere was associated with good recovery, whereas persistence of the bilateral activation pattern was associated with poor outcome (Ward et al., 2003). On the basis of these studies, it was concluded that greater involvement of the contralesional M1 predicted poor motor outcome (Calautti & Baron, 2003; Ward et al., 2003). However, more recently, Lotze et al. (2006) used a combined approach of fMRI and rTMS to explore the behavioral contribution of motor areas in contralesional hemisphere that were identified as being active during a motor task. Using fMRI, task-related activation of premotor cortex, the superior parietal lobe, and M1 of the contralesional M1 was identified. TMS when applied over these motor areas resulted in significant interference with the recovered performance in patients, indicating a supportive role for these motor areas.

In another fMRI-TMS study of well-recovered stroke patients, paretic hand movement–related fMRI responses in both, ipsilesional- and contralesional primary sensorimotor cortex were demonstrated (Butefisch et al., 2005; Lotze et al., 2006; Nair et al., 2007). Since patients had excellent motor recovery, this increased recruitment suggests an adaptive response to the infarct. This fMRI-derived evidence is further supported by findings obtained with TMS in these patients. First, TMS of the motor cortex in the ipsilesional, but not the contralesional, hemisphere induced MEPs in the recovered hand. This indicates that the corticospinal projections from the motor cortex of the ipsilesional hemisphere were still intact. Second, using paired-pulse TMS, an increase in M1 excitability of contralesional hemisphere was demonstrated (Nair et al., 2007). This result is consistent with data from animal stroke models where the regulation of excitatory and inhibitory neurotransmitter systems may play an early role in the reorganization process in contralesional M1 (Witte, 1998; Nudo, 1999). Further, IHI was greater from contralesional motor cortex on the motor cortex of the ipsilesional hemisphere. As a comparison to IHI in healthy control subjects was not performed in this study, it is not clear whether this asymmetry in interhemispheric inhibition is due to abnormally decreased IHI from ipsilesional on contralesioned motor cortex (Butefisch et al., 2008), or abnormally increased IHI from contralesional on ipsilesional M1, as reported for the active IHI but not resting IHI in another study (Murase, Duque, Mazzocchio, & Cohen, 2004).

Gerloff et al. (2006) combined ^{15}O-PET brain imaging, EEG, and TMS to evaluate motor recovery in chronic subcortical stroke patients. Affected hand movement–related activation of brain areas was identified using ^{15}O-PET and EEG spectral analysis. Corticocortical connectivity was assessed with EEG coherence analysis (corticocortical coherence) and corticospinal connectivity with TMS. Similar to the study of chronic subcortical stroke patients, motor areas in the contralesional hemisphere were more active when compared to healthy controls. EEG coherence analysis indicated that after stroke, corticocortical connections were reduced in the ipsilesional hemisphere but were relatively increased in the contralesional hemisphere, suggesting a shift of functional connectivity towards the contralesional hemisphere. Similar to previous studies of chronic well-recovered patients, TMS of the motor cortex in the ipsilesional but not contralesional hemisphere induced MEPs in the recovered hand.

Few investigators attempt to study the effect of TMS on brain function during fMRI, due to the technical challenges imposed by the hostile and interactive magnetic environment of the MRI scanner and the TMS stimulator. In the study by Bestmann and colleagues, the role of the contralesional dorsal premotor cortex (cPMd) in motor performance of the affected hand of chronic stroke patients was explored (Bestmann et al., 2010). The cPMd was previously identified as having a role in supporting recovered motor function in the affected hand in earlier studies using TMS (see above, Johansen-Berg et al., 2002). The advantage of studying the effect of TMS applied to cPMd on a paretic hand motor task–related fMRI signal is that the brain areas involved in supporting this effect may be identified. In an initial experiment using TMS over cPMd and ipsilesional M1, a less inhibitory/more facilitatory effect of cPMd on ipsilesional M1 was demonstrated in patients with greater clinical impairment. This corresponded to their findings in the fMRI-TMS experiments, where TMS of the cPMd exerted a stronger facilitatory influence on an abnormally posteriorly shifted peak of paretic hand motor task–related fMRI signal in ipsilesional sensorimotor cortex of the more impaired patients. This may represent a mechanism by which cPMd supports recovered function after stroke.

When studying the effect of a rehabilitative treatment on cerebral reorganization in stroke patients with TMS, changes in (i) the MEP amplitude, (ii) the stimulus response curve, and (iii) the number of cortical sites from where a MEP is elicited (cortical map) are used to measure treatment-related changes in the excitability of the motor output zone. In these TMS studies a rehabilitative training-related increase was demonstrated in the number of cortical sites from where MEPs of the paretic hand could be elicited. This indicates that the cortical representation of the target muscle (muscle map) was enlarged compared to the pre-training mapping (Traversa et al., 1997; Liepert et al., 1998; Wittenberg et al., 2003). The shift of the muscle map (Liepert et al., 1998; Wittenberg et al., 2003), or the increased number of abnormal location of cortical stimulation sites (Traversa et al., 1997), indicates that the cortical motor output zone may have expanded into the adjacent spared cortex, involving cortical areas previously not dedicated to this muscle, similar to the findings in monkeys (Nudo, Wise, SiFuentes, & Milliken, 1996). In the study by Wittenberg et al. intervention-related changes on brain function were also evaluated with positron emission tomography (PET). Following the intervention, paretic hand movement–related cerebral activation decreased significantly. In the context of improved behavior and greater excitability, decreased cerebral activation during a motor task may reflect improved ability of upper motor neurons to produce movements (Wittenberg et al., 2003).

5.4 THE FUTURE? NEUROREHABILITATIVE STUDIES OF STROKE RECOVERY AND THE BRAIN–COMPUTER INTERFACE

Much of this current volume is based on neuroscience underlying plastic changes that occur in the brain as it recovers from stroke. While there is cause for much optimism regarding the ability of the brain to reorganize following traumatic, ischemic, or vascular injury, there will be limitations for its full recovery. In situations where patients are faced with a poor motor recovery from their brain injury, one exciting future direction for neurorehabilitation involves the use of external robotic prosthetic devices. These are controlled by neurophysiological activity of the patient's brain, or the so-called "brain-machine" (Joseph, 1985) or brain–computer (Wolpaw, McFarland, Neat, & Forneris, 1991) interface. Of the multiple approaches that allow the human brain to potentially control an external device, and thereby be suitable as a robotic assistant for an individual with a paralyzed limb, the most promising appear to be those which use neurophysiological signals, such as noninvasive EEG or invasive chronically implanted electrodes, which can record field potentials over strategically selected cortical regions (Friehs, Zerris, Ojakangas, Fellows, & Donoghue, 2004; Birbaumer & Cohen, 2007).

The human sensorimotor system is an ideal candidate for these devices to control hand or arm movements, as the active neural sources have been well known and precisely mapped for many years (Huttunen, Kaukoranta, & Hari, 1987; Wood et al., 1988; Allison, Wood, McCarthy,

& Spencer, 1991; Baumgartner, Barth, Levesque, & Sutherling, 1991; Puce, 1995; Vanni, Rockstroh, & Hari, 1996). Approaches using noninvasive EEG measures in conjunction with additional EMG-based feedback to the robotic device are already being explored in selected patients recovering from stroke (Yao, Sheaff, & Dewald, 2008). The use of cortical (including TMS-based) stimulation to aid stroke recovery is already being used in human subjects (see section 5.3.3). What is exciting is that studies in animal models suggest that targeted brain–machine interface approaches, using local cortical stimulation and exploiting Hebbian-based mechanisms (see discussion in section 5.3.3) in conjunction with a neuroprosthesis, might also be a potential neurorehabilitative strategy (Rebesco & Miller, 2011). Chronically implanted electrodes which record electrocorticographic (ECoG) signals and support vector machine analysis routines, which separate oscillatory neurophysiological signals into frequency bands (e.g., gamma, beta) that are modulated differentially by prosthetic arm movements, have enabled a prosthetic hand to be controlled in real time (Yanagisawa et al., 2011). A similar approach using spectral analysis of ECoG signals in a primate brain, with additional inputs from an accelerometer on the prosthetic device itself, has added an additional level of sophistication and control to the system (Rouse et al., 2011) and offers a way forward for the future refinement of personalized neuroprosthetic devices for patients recovering from stroke.

For a neuroprosthetic therapeutic approach to be feasible, practice and training is an important element. The use of neurofeedback in practice sessions allows baseline performance to be characterized and recovery to be charted from improvements in performance (Prasad, Herman, Coyle, McDonough, & Crosbie, 2010). Current neurorehabilitative approaches using brain–computer interfaces can be divided into two main approaches: (i) restorative; namely, those which aim to facilitate normalization of the brain's neurophysiological rhythms to aid motor recovery; and (ii) assistive, or those which provide electrical stimulation to peripheral muscles of the paralyzed limb to control a neuroprosthesis (Soekadar, Birbaumer, & Cohen, 2011). This latter category would, in principle, include electrical stimulation from a peripheral stimulator or from the brain itself via ECoG or EEG signals.

Most recently, brain–computer interface control signals using near-infra red spectroscopy (NIRS, or noninvasively measured local blood flow changes), fMRI, or MEG have also demonstrated real-time capability (Sudre et al., 2011). However, current NIRS, fMRI, and MEG technologies impose a limitation on patient mobility, unlike EEG systems which can be made portable and allow the individual to move through the environment wirelessly (Gramann, Gwin, Bigdely-Shamlo, Ferris, & Makeig, 2010; Gwin, Gramann, Makeig, & Ferris, 2011). Therefore, future work in the field of neurorehabilitation is likely to use electrophysiologically based control signals as measures of recovery and as control signals for neuroprostheses.

It is clear that neurophysiological methods such as EEG and MEG, as well as TMS, will play an important role in the future. They will have a clear role for evaluating the patient's potential for recovery, as well as potentially providing control signals or pulses that can monitor or control neuroprostheses or enhance the effect of motor training in the appropriate patient population. Both human and animal studies suggest that these approaches might be feasible. The ultimate success of these treatment approaches hinges on an accurate assessment of the functional state of the patient's brain post-stroke.

REFERENCES

Aine, C. J. (1995). A conceptual overview and critique of functional neuroimaging techniques in humans: I. MRI/FMRI and PET. *Critical Reviews in Neurobiology, 9*(2–3), 229–309.

Allison, T., McCarthy, G., Wood, C. C., Darcey, T. M., Spencer, D. D., & Williamson, P. D. (1989). Human cortical potentials evoked by stimulation of the median nerve. I. Cytoarchitectonic areas generating short-latency activity. *Journal of Neurophysiology, 62*(3), 694–710.

Allison, T., McCarthy, G., Wood, C. C., Williamson, P. D., & Spencer, D. D. (1989). Human cortical potentials evoked by stimulation of the median nerve. II. Cytoarchitectonic areas generating long-latency activity. *Journal of Neurophysiology, 62*(3), 711–722.

Allison, T., Wood, C. C., McCarthy, G., & Spencer, D. D. (1991). Cortical somatosensory evoked potentials. II. Effects of excision of somatosensory or motor cortex in humans and monkeys. *Journal of Neurophysiology, 66*(1), 64–82.

Altamura, C., Torquati, K., Zappasodi, F., Ferretti, A., Pizzella, V., Tibuzzi, F., et al. (2007). fMRI-vs-MEG evaluation of post-stroke interhemispheric asymmetries in primary sensorimotor hand areas. *Experimental Neurology, 204*(2), 631–639.

Amassian, V. E., Quirk, G. J., & Stewart, M. (1990). A comparison of corticospinal activation by magnetic coil and electrical stimulation of monkey motor cortex. *Electroencephalography and Clinical Neurophysiology, 77*(5), 390–401.

Aminoff, M. J. (1996). Clinical neurophysiology of cortical sensorimotor function: yesterday, today, and tomorrow. *Journal of Clinical Neurophysiology, 13*(3), 219–226.

Babiloni, F., Carducci, F., Cincotti, F., Del Gratta, C., Pizzella, V., Romani, G. L., et al. (2001). Linear inverse source estimate of combined EEG and MEG data related to voluntary movements. *Human Brain Mapping, 14*(4), 197–209.

Bagnato, S., Curra, A., Modugno, N., Gilio, F., Quartarone, A., Rizzo, V., et al. (2005). One-hertz subthreshold rTMS increases the threshold for evoking inhibition in the human motor cortex. *Experimental Brain Research, 160*(3), 368–374.

Baumgartner, C., Barth, D. S., Levesque, M. F., & Sutherling, W. W. (1991). Functional anatomy of human hand sensorimotor cortex from spatiotemporal analysis of electrocorticography. *Electroencephalography and Clinical Neurophysiology, 78*(1), 56–65.

Baumgartner, C., Doppelbauer, A., Sutherling, W. W., Zeitlhofer, J., Lindinger, G., Lind, C., et al. (1991). Human somatosensory cortical finger representation as studied by combined neuromagnetic and neuroelectric measurements. *Neuroscience Letters, 134*(1), 103–108.

Berger, H. (1929). Über das Elektroenkephalogramm des Menschen. *Archiv für Psychiatrie und Nervenkrankheiten, 87*, 527–570.

Bestmann, S., Swayne, O., Blankenburg, F., Ruff, C. C., Teo, J., Weiskopf, N., et al. (2010). The role of contralesional dorsal premotor cortex after stroke as studied with concurrent TMS-fMRI. *Journal of Neuroscience, 30*(36), 11926–11937.

Bickford, R. G., & Baldes, E. J. (1947). The electroencephalogram in tumors of the posterior fossa. *Proceedings of the Annual Meeting of the Center for Social and Clinical Research U S, 20*, 87.

Binkofski, F., & Seitz, R. J. (2004). Modulation of the BOLD-response in early recovery from sensorimotor stroke. *Neurology, 63*(7), 1223–1229.

Binkofski, F., Seitz, R. J., Arnold, S., Classen, J., Benecke, R., & Freund, H. J. (1996). Thalamic metbolism and corticospinal tract integrity determine motor recovery in stroke. *Annals of Neurology, 39*(4), 460–470.

Birbaumer, N., & Cohen, L. G. (2007). Brain-computer interfaces: communication and restoration of movement in paralysis. *Journal of Physiology, 579*(Pt 3), 621–636.

Boroojerdi, B., Diefenbach, K., & Ferbert, A. (1996). Transcallosal inhibition in cortical and subcortical cerebral vascular lesions. *Journal of Neurological Science, 144*(1–2), 160–170.

Brasil-Neto, J. P., Cohen, L. G., Panizza, M., Nilsson, J., Roth, B. J., & Hallett, M. (1992). Optimal focal transcranial magnetic activation of the human motor cortex: effects of coil orientation, shape of the induced current pulse, and stimulus intensity. *Journal of Clinical Neurophysiology, 9*(1), 132–136.

Buetefisch, C., & Cohen, L. (2008). Practice-induced changes in TMS measures. In E. Wassermann, C. Epstein, U. Ziemann, S. Lisanby, T. Paus & V. Walsh (Eds.), *Handbook of transcranial stimulation* (pp. 219–234). Oxford: Oxford University Press.

Buetefisch, C. M., Hines, B., Shuster, L., Pergami, P., & Mathes, A. (2011). Motor demand dependent improvement in accuracy following low-frequency transcranial magnetic stimulation of left motor cortex. *Journal of Neurophysiology, 106*(4), 1614–1621.

Butefisch, C. M., Kleiser, R., Korber, B., Muller, K., Wittsack, H. J., Homberg, V., et al. (2005). Recruitment of contralesional motor cortex in stroke patients with recovery of hand function. *Neurology, 64*(6), 1067–1069.

Butefisch, C. M., Netz, J., Wessling, M., Seitz, R. J., & Homberg, V. (2003). Remote changes in cortical excitability after stroke. *Brain, 126*(Pt 2), 470–481.

Butefisch, C. M., Wessling, M., Netz, J., Seitz, R. J., & Homberg, V. (2008). Relationship between interhemispheric inhibition and motor cortex excitability in subacute stroke patients. *Neurorehabilitation and Neural Repair, 22*(1), 4–21.

Calautti, C., & Baron, J. C. (2003). Functional neuroimaging studies of motor recovery after stroke in adults: a review. *Stroke, 34*(6), 1553–1566.

Cao, Y., D'Olhaberriague, L., Vikingstad, E. M., Levine, S. R., & Welch, K. M. (1998). Pilot study of functional MRI to assess cerebral activation of motor function after poststroke hemiparesis. *Stroke, 29*(1), 112–122.

Carey, L. M., Abbott, D. F., Egan, G. F., Bernhardt, J., & Donnan, G. A. (2005). Motor impairment and recovery in the upper limb after stroke: behavioral and neuroanatomical correlates. *Stroke, 36*(3), 625–629.

Carey, L. M., Abbott, D. F., Egan, G. F., O'Keefe, G. J., Jackson, G. D., Bernhardt, J., et al. (2006). Evolution of brain activation with good and poor motor recovery after stroke. *Neurorehabilitation and Neural Repair, 20*(1), 24–41.

Carey, L. M., Abbott, D. F., Harvey, M. R., Puce, A., Seitz, R. J., & Donnan, G. A. (2011). Relationship between touch impairment and brain activation after lesions of subcortical and cortical somatosensory regions. *Neurorehabilitation and Neural Repair, 25*(5), 443–457.

Carey, L. M., Abbott, D. F., Puce, A., Jackson, G. D., Syngeniotis, A., & Donnan, G. A. (2002). Reemergence of activation with poststroke somatosensory recovery: a serial fMRI case study. *Neurology, 59*(5), 749–752.

Chen, R., Classen, J., Gerloff, C., Celnik, P., Wassermann, E. M., Hallett, M., et al. (1997). Depression of motor cortex excitability by low-frequency transcranial magnetic stimulation. *Neurology, 48*(5), 1398–1403.

Chen, R., Cros, D., Curra, A., Di Lazzaro, V., Lefaucheur, J. P., Magistris, M. R., et al. (2008). The clinical diagnostic utility of transcranial magnetic stimulation: report of an IFCN committee. *Clinical Neurophysiology, 119*(3), 504–532.

Chen, R., Tam, A., Butefisch, C., Corwell, B., Ziemann, U., Rothwell, J. C., et al. (1998). Intracortical inhibition and facilitation in different representations of the human motor cortex. *Journal of Neurophysiology, 80*(6), 2870–2881.

Chollet, F., DiPiero, V., Wise, R. J., Brooks, D. J., Dolan, R. J., & Frackowiak, R. S. (1991). The functional anatomy of motor recovery after stroke in humans: a study with positron emission tomography. *Annals of Neurology, 29*(1), 63–71.

Chouinard, P. A., & Paus, T. (2010). What have we learned from "perturbing" the human cortical motor system with transcranial magnetic stimulation? *Frontiers in Human Neuroscience, 4*, 173.

Ciganek, L. (1961). The EEG response (evoked potential) to light stimulus in man. *Electroencephalogry and Clinical Neurophysiology, 13*, 165–172.

Classen, J., Schnitzler, A., Binkofski, F., Werhahn, K. J., Kim, Y. S., Kessler, K. R., et al. (1997). The motor syndrome associated with exaggerated inhibition within the primary motor cortex of patients with hemiparetic. *Brain, 120 (Pt 4)*, 605–619.

Cohen, D. (1972). Magnetoencephalography: detection of the brain's electrical activity with a superconducting magnetometer. *Science, 175*(22), 664–666.

Cohen, D., & Cuffin, B. N. (1983). Demonstration of useful differences between magnetoencephalogram and electroencephalogram. *Electroencephalography and Clinical Neurophysiology, 56*(1), 38–51.

Cohen, D., & Cuffin, B. N. (1987). A method for combining MEG and EEG to determine the sources. *Physics in Medicine and Biology, 32*(1), 85–89.

Cramer, S. C., Nelles, G., Benson, R. R., Kaplan, J. D., Parker, R. A., Kwong, K. K., et al. (1997). A functional MRI study of subjects recovered from hemiparetic stroke. *Stroke, 28*(12), 2518–2527.

Cuffin, B. N., & Cohen, D. (1979). Comparison of the magnetoencephalogram and electroencephalogram. *Electroencephalography and Clinical Neurophysiology, 47*(2), 132–146.

Dafotakis, M., Grefkes, C., Wang, L., Fink, G. R., & Nowak, D. A. (2008). The effects of 1 Hz rTMS over the hand area of M1 on movement kinematics of the ipsilateral hand. *Journal of Neural Transmission, 115*(9), 1269–1274.

Dale, A. M., & Halgren, E. (2001). Spatiotemporal mapping of brain activity by integration of multiple imaging modalities. *Current Opinions in Neurobiology, 11*(2), 202–208.

Daskalakis, Z. J., Moller, B., Christensen, B. K., Fitzgerald, P. B., Gunraj, C., & Chen, R. (2006). The effects of repetitive transcranial magnetic stimulation on cortical inhibition in healthy human subjects. *Exp Brain Res, 174*(3), 403–412.

David, O., Kilner, J. M., & Friston, K. J. (2006). Mechanisms of evoked and induced responses in MEG/EEG. *NeuroImage, 31*(4), 1580–1591.

Dawson, G. D. (1947). Cerebral Responses to Electrical Stimulation of Peripheral Nerve in Man. *Journal of Neurology, Neurosurgery and Psychiatry, 10*(3), 134–140.

Dawson, G. D., & Walter, W. G. (1945). Recommendations for the design and performance of electroencephalographic apparatus. *Journal of Neurology, Neurosurgery and Psychiatry, 8*, 61–64.

Day, B. L., Thompson, P. D., Dick, J. P., Nakashima, K., & Marsden, C. D. (1987). Different sites of action of electrical and magnetic stimulation of the human brain. *Neuroscience Letters, 75*(1), 101–106.

de Lange, F. P., Jensen, O., Bauer, M., & Toni, I. (2008). Interactions between posterior gamma and frontal alpha/beta oscillations during imagined actions. *Frontiers in Human Neuroscience, 2*, 7.

Di Lazzaro, V., Oliviero, A., Profice, P., Insola, A., Mazzone, P., Tonali, P., et al. (1999). Direct demonstration of interhemispheric inhibition of the human motor cortex produced by transcranial magnetic stimulation. *Experimental Brain Research, 124*(4), 520–524.

Di Lazzaro, V., Pilato, F., Dileone, M., Profice, P., Oliviero, A., Mazzone, P., et al. (2008). Low-frequency repetitive transcranial magnetic stimulation suppresses specific excitatory circuits in the human motor cortex. *Journal of Physiology, 586*(Pt 18), 4481–4487.

Di Lazzaro, V., Pilato, F., Oliviero, A., Dileone, M., Saturno, E., Mazzone, P., et al. (2006). Origin of facilitation of motor-evoked potentials after paired magnetic stimulation: direct recording of epidural activity in conscious humans. *Journal of Neurophysiology, 96*(4), 1765–1771.

Di Lazzaro, V., Restuccia, D., Oliviero, A., Profice, P., Ferrara, L., Insola, A., et al. (1998). Magnetic transcranial stimulation at intensities below active motor threshold activates intracortical inhibitory circuits. *Experimental Brain Research, 119*(2), 265–268.

Di Lazzaro, V., Oliviero, A., Berardelli, A., Mazzone, P., Insola, A., Pilato, F., et al. (2002). Direct demonstration of the effects of repetitive transcranial magnetic stimulation on the excitability of the human motor cortex. *Exp Brain Res, 144*(4), 549–553.

Draganski, B., Gaser, C., Busch, V., Schuierer, G., Bogdahn, U., & May, A. (2004). Neuroplasticity: changes in grey matter induced by training. *Nature, 427*(6972), 311–312.

Dunseath, W. J., & Kelly, E. F. (1995). Multichannel PC-based data-acquisition system for high-resolution EEG. *IEEE Transactions in Biomedical Engineering, 42*(12), 1212–1217.

Duque, J., Mazzocchio, R., Dambrosia, J., Murase, N., Olivier, E., & Cohen, L. G. (2005). Kinematically specific interhemispheric inhibition operating in the process of generation of a voluntary movement. *Cerebral Cortex, 15*(5), 588–593.

Eggermont, J. J., & Ponton, C. W. (2002). The neurophysiology of auditory perception: from single units to evoked potentials. *Audiology and Neurotology, 7*(2), 71–99.

Elberling, C., Bak, C., Kofoed, B., Lebech, J., & Saermark, K. (1982). Auditory magnetic fields from the human cerebral cortex: location and strength of an equivalent current dipole. *Acta Neurologica Scandinavia, 65*(6), 553–569.

Engels, L., De Tiege, X., Op de Beeck, M., & Warzée, N. (2010). Factors influencing the spatial precision of electromagnetic tracking systems used for MEG/EEG source imaging. *Clinical Neurophysiology, 40*(1), 19–25.

Fagaly, R. L. (1990). Neuromagnetic instrumentation. *Advances in Neurology, 54*, 11–32.

Ferbert, A., Priori, A., Rothwell, J. C., Day, B. L., Colebatch, J. G., & Marsden, C. D. (1992). Interhemispheric inhibition of the human motor cortex. *Journal of Physiology, 453*, 525–546.

Fisher, R. J., Nakamura, Y., Bestmann, S., Rothwell, J. C., & Bostock, H. (2002). Two phases of intracortical inhibition revealed by transcranial magnetic threshold tracking. *Experimental Brain Research, 143*(2), 240–248.

Fitzgerald, P. B., Fountain, S., & Daskalakis, Z. J. (2006). A comprehensive review of the effects of rTMS on motor cortical excitability and inhibition. *Clinical Neurophysiology, 117*(12), 2584–2596.

Forss, N., & Silen, T. (2001). Temporal organization of cerebral events: neuromagnetic studies of the sensorimotor system. *Reviews in Neurology (Paris), 157*(8–9 Pt 1), 816–821.

Friehs, G. M., Zerris, V. A., Ojakangas, C. L., Fellows, M. R., & Donoghue, J. P. (2004). Brain-machine and brain-computer interfaces. *Stroke, 35*(11 Suppl 1), 2702–2705.

Friston, K. J. (2009). Modalities, modes, and models in functional neuroimaging. *Science, 326*(5951), 399–403.

Fuhr, P., Agostino, R., & Hallett, M. (1991). Spinal motor neuron excitability during the silent period after cortical stimulation. *Electroencephalography and Clinical Neurophysiology, 81*(4), 257–262.

Garry, M. I., Loftus, A., & Summers, J. J. (2005). Mirror, mirror on the wall: viewing a mirror reflection of unilateral hand movements facilitates ipsilateral M1 excitability. *Experimental Brain Research, 163*(1), 118–122.

George, J. S., Aine, C. J., Mosher, J. C., Schmidt, D. M., Ranken, D. M., Schlitt, H. A., et al. (1995). Mapping function in the human brain with magnetoencephalography, anatomical magnetic resonance imaging, and functional magnetic resonance imaging. *Journal of Clinical Neurophysiology, 12*(5), 406–431.

Gerloff, C., Bushara, K., Sailer, A., Wassermann, E. M., Chen, R., Matsuoka, T., et al. (2006). Multimodal imaging of brain reorganization in motor areas of the contralesional hemisphere of well recovered patients after capsular stroke. *Brain, 129*(Pt 3), 791–808.

Gevins, A., Brickett, P., Costales, B., Le, J., & Reutter, B. (1990). Beyond topographic mapping: towards functional-anatomical imaging with 124-channel EEGs and 3-D MRIs. *Brain Topography, 3*(1), 53–64.

Glover, G. H. (2011). Overview of functional magnetic resonance imaging. *Neurosurgery Clinics of North America, 22*(2), 133–139.

Gramann, K., Gwin, J. T., Bigdely-Shamlo, N., Ferris, D. P., & Makeig, S. (2010). Visual evoked responses during standing and walking. *Frontiers in Human Neuroscience, 4*, 202.

Granert, O., Peller, M., Gaser, C., Groppa, S., Hallett, M., Knutzen, A., et al. (2011). Manual activity shapes structure and function in contralateral human motor hand area. *NeuroImage, 54*(1), 32–41.

Gross, J., Kujala, J., Hamalainen, M., Timmermann, L., Schnitzler, A., & Salmelin, R. (2001). Dynamic imaging of coherent sources: Studying neural interactions in the human brain. *Proceedings of the National Academy of Science U S A, 98*(2), 694–699.

Gualtierotti, T., & Paterson, A. S. (1954). Electrical stimulation of the unexposed cerebral cortex. *Journal of Physiology, 125*(2), 278–291.

Gwin, J. T., Gramann, K., Makeig, S., & Ferris, D. P. (2011). Electrocortical activity is coupled to gait cycle phase during treadmill walking. *NeuroImage, 54*(2), 1289–1296.

Hallett, M. (2000). Transcranial magnetic stimulation and the human brain. *Nature, 406*(6792), 147–150.

Hallett, M. (2007). Transcranial magnetic stimulation: a primer. *Neuron, 55*(2), 187–199.

Hallez, H., Vanrumste, B., Grech, R., Muscat, J., De Clercq, W., Vergult, A., et al. (2007). Review on solving the forward problem in EEG source analysis. *Journal of Neuroengineering and Rehabilitation, 4*, 46.

Hämäläinen, M., & Hari, R. (Eds.). (2002). *Magnetoencephalographic characterization of dynamic brain activation: Basic principles and methods of data collection and source analysis.* (2nd ed.). San Diego: Academic Press.

Hand, P. J., Wardlaw, J. M., Rowat, A. M., Haisma, J. A., Lindley, R. I., & Dennis, M. S. (2005). Magnetic resonance brain imaging in patients with acute stroke: feasibility and patient related difficulties. *Journal of Neurology, Neurosurgery and Psychiatry, 76*(11), 1525–1527.

Hari, R. (2006). Action-perception connection and the cortical mu rhythm. *Progress in Brain Research, 159*, 253–260.

Hari, R., & Kaukoranta, E. (1985). Neuromagnetic studies of somatosensory system: principles and examples. *Progress in Neurobiology, 24*(3), 233–256.

Hendricks, H. T., Zwarts, M. J., Plat, E. F., & van Limbeek, J. (2002). Systematic review for the early prediction of motor and functional outcome after stroke by using motor-evoked potentials. *Archives of Physical Medicine and Rehabilitation, 83*(9), 1303–1308.

Herdener, M., Esposito, F., di Salle, F., Boller, C., Hilti, C. C., Habermeyer, B., et al. (2010). Musical training induces functional plasticity in human hippocampus. *Journal of Neuroscience, 30*(4), 1377–1384.

Hess, C. W., Mills, K. R., & Murray, N. M. (1987). Responses in small hand muscles from magnetic stimulation of the human brain. *Journal of Physiology, 388*, 397–419.

Huang, M., Davis, L. E., Aine, C., Weisend, M., Harrington, D., Christner, R., et al. (2004). MEG response to median nerve stimu-lation correlates with recovery of sensory and motor function after stroke. *Clinical Neurophysiology, 115*(4), 820–833.

Huang, M. X., Song, T., Hagler, D. J., Jr., Podgorny, I., Jousmaki, V., Cui, L., et al. (2007). A novel integrated MEG and EEG analysis method for dipolar sources. *NeuroImage, 37*(3), 731–748.

Hummel, F. C., & Gerloff, C. (2006). Interregional long-range and short-range synchrony: a basis for complex sensorimotor processing. *Progress in Brain Research, 159*, 223–236.

Huttunen, J., Kaukoranta, E., & Hari, R. (1987). Cerebral magnetic responses to stimulation of tibial and sural nerves. *Journal of Neurologucal Science, 79*(1–2), 43–54.

Inghilleri, M., Berardelli, A., Cruccu, G., & Manfredi, M. (1993). Silent period evoked by transcranial stimulation of the human cortex and cervicomedullary junction. *Journal of Physiology, 466*, 521–534.

Ishikawa, S., Matsunaga, K., Nakanishi, R., Kawahira, K., Murayama, N., Tsuji, S., et al. (2007). Effect of theta burst stimulation over the human sensorimotor cortex on motor and somatosensory evoked potentials. *Clinical Neurophysiology, 118*(5), 1033–1043.

Jak, A. J. (2011). The impact of physical and mental activity on cognitive aging. *Current Topics in Behavioral Neuroscience.* (Online Aug 5)

Jancke, L. (2009). The plastic human brain. *Restorative Neurology and Neuroscience, 27*(5), 521–538.

Johansen-Berg, H., Rushworth, M. F., Bogdanovic, M. D., Kischka, U., Wimalaratna, S., & Matthews, P. M. (2002). The role of ipsilateral premotor cortex in hand movement after stroke. *Proceedings of the National Academy of Science U S A, 99*(22), 14518–14523.

Johansson, B. B. (2011). Current trends in stroke rehabilitation. A review with focus on brain plasticity. *Acta Neurologica Scandinavia, 123*(3), 147–159.

Joseph, A. B. (1985). Design considerations for the brain-machine interface. *Medical Hypotheses, 17*(3), 191–195.

Jousmaki, V. (2000). Tracking functions of cortical networks on a millisecond timescale. *Neural Networks, 13*(8–9), 883–889.

Karni, A., Meyer, G., Jezzard, P., Adams, M. M., Turner, R., & Ungerleider, L. G. (1995). Functional MRI evidence for adult motor cortex plasticity during motor skill learning. *Nature, 377*(6545), 155–158.

Kloppel, S., Mangin, J. F., Vongerichten, A., Frackowiak, R. S., & Siebner, H. R. (2010). Nurture versus nature: long-term impact of forced right-handedness on structure of pericentral cortex and basal ganglia. *Journal of Neuroscience, 30*(9), 3271–3275.

Kobayashi, M., Hutchinson, S., Schlaug, G., & Pascual-Leone, A. (2003). Ipsilateral motor cortex activation on functional magnetic resonance imaging during unilateral hand movements is related to interhemispheric interactions. *NeuroImage, 20*(4), 2259–2270.

Kobayashi, M., Hutchinson, S., Theoret, H., Schlaug, G., & Pascual-Leone, A. (2004). Repetitive TMS of the motor cortex improves ipsilateral sequential simple finger movements. *Neurology, 62*(1), 91–98.

Koessler, L., Maillard, L., Benhadid, A., Vignal, J. P., Braun, M., Vespignani, H. (2007) Spatial localization of EEG electrodes. *Clinical Neurophysiology 37*(2), 97–102.

Kujirai, T., Caramia, M. D., Rothwell, J. C., Day, B. L., Thompson, P. D., Ferbert, A., et al. (1993). Corticocortical inhibition in human motor cortex. *Journal of Physiology, 471*, 501–519.

Kwong, K. K., Belliveau, J. W., Chesler, D. A., Goldberg, I. E., Weisskoff, R. M., Poncelet, B. P., et al. (1992). Dynamic magnetic resonance imaging of human brain activity during primary sensory stimulation. *Proceedings of the National Academy of Science U S A, 89*(12), 5675–5679.

Lachaux, J. P., Lutz, A., Rudrauf, D., Cosmelli, D., Le Van Quyen, M., Martinerie, J., et al. (2002). Estimating the time-course of coherence between single-trial brain signals: an introduction to wavelet coherence. *Clinical Neurophysiology, 32*(3), 157–174.

Liepert, J., Hamzei, F., & Weiller, C. (2000). Motor cortex disinhibition of the unaffected hemisphere after acute stroke. *Muscle Nerve, 23*(11), 1761–1763.

Liepert, J., Miltner, W. H., Bauder, H., Sommer, M., Dettmers, C., Taub, E., et al. (1998). Motor cortex plasticity during constraint-induced movement therapy in stroke patients. *Neuroscience Letters, 250*(1), 5–8.

Liepert, J., Storch, P., Fritsch, A., & Weiller, C. (2000). Motor cortex disinhibition in acute stroke. *Clinical Neurophysiology, 111*(4), 671–676.

Liepert, J., Tegenthoff, M., & Malin, J. P. (1995). Changes of cortical motor area size during immobilization. *Electroencephalography and Clinical Neurophysiology, 97*(6), 382–386.

Lissek, S., Wilimzig, C., Stude, P., Pleger, B., Kalisch, T., Maier, C., et al. (2009). Immobilization impairs tactile perception and shrinks somatosensory cortical maps. *Current Biology, 19*(10), 837–842.

Liu, A. K., Belliveau, J. W., & Dale, A. M. (1998). Spatiotemporal imaging of human brain activity using functional MRI constrained magnetoencephalography data: Monte Carlo simulations. *Proceedings of the National Academy of Science U S A, 95*(15), 8945–8950.

Logothetis, N. K., Pauls, J., Augath, M., Trinath, T., & Oeltermann, A. (2001). Neurophysiological investigation of the basis of the fMRI signal. *Nature, 412*(6843), 150–157.

Lopes da Silva, F., & van Leeuwen, W. S. (1969). Electrophysiological correlates of behaviour. *Psychiatria, Neurologia, Neurochirurgia, 72*(3), 285–311.

Lopes da Silva, F. H. (1996). Biophysical issues at the frontiers of the interpretation of EEG/MEG signals. *Electroencephalography and Clinical Neurophysiology Suppl, 45*, 1–7.

Lopes da Silva, F. H., Wieringa, H. J., & Peters, M. J. (1991). Source localization of EEG versus MEG: empirical comparison using visually evoked responses and theoretical considerations. *Brain Topography, 4*(2), 133–142.

Lotze, M., Markert, J., Sauseng, P., Hoppe, J., Plewnia, C., & Gerloff, C. (2006). The role of multiple contralesional motor areas for complex hand movements after internal capsular lesion. *Journal of Neuroscience, 26*(22), 6096–6102.

Maeda, F., Keenan, J. P., Tormos, J. M., Topka, H., & Pascual-Leone, A. (2000). Modulation of corticospinal excitability by repetitive transcranial magnetic stimulation. *Clinical Neurophysiology, 111*(5), 800–805.

Manganotti, P., Patuzzo, S., Cortese, F., Palermo, A., Smania, N., & Fiaschi, A. (2002). Motor disinhibition in affected and unaffected hemisphere in the early period of recovery after stroke. *Clinical Neurophysiology, 113*(6), 936–943.

Mercuri, B., Wassermann, E. M., Manganotti, P., Ikoma, K., Samii, A., & Hallett, M. (1996). Cortical modulation of spinal excitability: an F-wave study. *Electroencephalography and Clinical Neurophysiology, 101*(1), 16–24.

Merton, P. A., & Morton, H. B. (1980). Stimulation of the cerebral cortex in the intact human subject. *Nature, 285*(5762), 227.

Michel, C. M., Murray, M. M., Lantz, G., Gonzalez, S., Spinelli, L., & Grave de Peralta, R. (2004). EEG source imaging. *Clinical Neurophysiology, 115*(10), 2195–2222.

Mosher, J. C., Spencer, M. E., Leahy, R. M., & Lewis, P. S. (1993). Error bounds for EEG and MEG dipole source localization. *Electroencephalography and Clinical Neurophysiology, 86*(5), 303–321.

Murase, N., Duque, J., Mazzocchio, R., & Cohen, L. G. (2004). Influence of interhemispheric interactions on motor function in chronic stroke. *Annals of Neurology, 55*(3), 400–409.

Nair, D. G., Hutchinson, S., Fregni, F., Alexander, M., Pascual-Leone, A., & Schlaug, G. (2007). Imaging correlates of motor recovery from cerebral infarction and their physiological significance in well-recovered patients. *NeuroImage, 34*(1), 253–263.

Nardone, R., & Tezzon, F. (2002). Inhibitory and excitatory circuits of cerebral cortex after ischaemic stroke: prognostic value of the transcranial magnetic stimulation. *Electromyography and Clinical Neurophysiology, 42*(3), 131–136.

Neuper, C., Wortz, M., & Pfurtscheller, G. (2006). ERD/ERS patterns reflecting sensorimotor activation and deactivation. *Progress in Brain Research, 159*, 211–222.

Niedermeyer, E. (1954). Psychomotor seizure with generalized synchronous spike and wave discharge; report of a case. *Electroencephalography and Clinical Neurophysiology, 6*(3), 495–496.

Niedermeyer, E. (1960). On a neurological-psychiatric-brain electrical syndrome on the basis of probable chronic insufficiency of the basilar artery. *Wien Klin Wochenschr, 72*, 10–13.

Nudo, J. R. (1999). Recovery after damage to motor cortical areas. *Current Opinions in Neurobiology, 9*, 740–747.

Nudo, J. R., Wise, B. M., SiFuentes, F. S., & Milliken, G. W. (1996). Neural substrates for the effects of rehabilitative training on motor recovery after ischemic infarct. *Science, 272*, 1791–1794.

Ogawa, S., Lee, T. M., Kay, A. R., & Tank, D. W. (1990). Brain magnetic resonance imaging with contrast dependent on blood oxygenation. *Proceedings of the National Academy of Science U S A, 87*(24), 9868–9872.

Okada, Y. C., Tanenbaum, R., Williamson, S. J., & Kaufman, L. (1984). Somatotopic organization of the human somatosensory cortex revealed by neuromagnetic measurements. *Experimental Brain Research, 56*(2), 197–205.

Pascual-Leone, A., Valls-Sole, J., Wassermann, E. M., & Hallett, M. (1994). Responses to rapid-rate transcranial magnetic stimulation of the human motor cortex. *Brain, 117* (Pt 4), 847–858.

Paus, T. (2005). Inferring causality in brain images: a perturbation approach. *Philosophical Transactions of the Royal Society London B: Biological Science, 360*(1457), 1109–1114.

Petrini, K., Pollick, F. E., Dahl, S., McAleer, P., McKay, L., Rocchesso, D., et al. (2011). Action expertise reduces brain activity for audiovisual matching actions: an fMRI study with expert drummers. *NeuroImage, 56*(3), 1480–1492.

Pineiro, R., Pendlebury, S., Johansen-Berg, H., & Matthews, P. M. (2001). Functional MRI detects posterior shifts in primary sensorimotor cortex activation after stroke: evidence of local adaptive reorganization? *Stroke, 32*(5), 1134–1139.

Prasad, G., Herman, P., Coyle, D., McDonough, S., & Crosbie, J. (2010). Applying a brain-computer interface to support motor imagery practice in people with stroke for upper limb recovery: a feasibility study. *Journal of Neuroengineering and Rehabilitation, 7*, 60.

Puce, A. (1995). Comparative assessment of sensorimotor function using functional magnetic resonance imaging and electrophysiological methods. *Journal of Clinical Neurophysiology, 12*(5), 450–459.

Rebesco, J. M., & Miller, L. E. (2011). Enhanced detection threshold for in vivo cortical stimulation produced by Hebbian conditioning. *Journal of Neural Engineering, 8*(1), 016011.

Ridding, M. C., & Rothwell, J. C. (1997). Stimulus/response curves as a method of measuring motor cortical excitability in man. *Electroencephalography and Clinical Neurophysiology, 105*(5), 340–344.

Roick, H., von Giesen, H. J., & Benecke, R. (1993). On the origin of the postexcitatory inhibition seen after transcranial magnetic brain stimulation in awake human subjects. *Experimental Brain Research, 94*(3), 489–498.

Rossini, P. M., Altamura, C., Ferreri, F., Melgari, J. M., Tecchio, F., Tombini, M., et al. (2007). Neuroimaging experimental studies on brain plasticity in recovery from stroke. *Eura Medicophys, 43*(2), 241–254.

Rossini, P. M., Altamura, C., Ferretti, A., Vernieri, F., Zappasodi, F., Caulo, M., et al. (2004). Does cerebrovascular disease affect the coupling between neuronal activity and local haemodynamics? *Brain, 127*(Pt 1), 99–110.

Rossini, P. M., Barker, A. T., Berardelli, A., Caramia, M. D., Caruso, G., Cracco, R. Q., et al. (1994). Non-invasive electrical and magnetic stimulation of the brain, spinal cord and roots: basic principles and procedures for routine clinical application. Report of an IFCN committee. *Electroencephalography and Clinical Neurophysiology, 91*(2), 79–92.

Rossini, P. M., Caltagirone, C., Castriota-Scanderbeg, A., Cicinelli, P., Del Gratta, C., Demartin, M., et al. (1998). Hand motor cortical area reorganization in stroke: a study with fMRI, MEG and TCS maps. *Neuroreport, 9*(9), 2141–2146.

Rossini, P. M., & Pauri, F. (2000). Neuromagnetic integrated methods tracking human brain mechanisms of sensorimotor areas "plastic" reorganisation. *Brain Research: Brain Research Reviews, 33*(2–3), 131–154.

Roth, B. J., Saypol, J. M., Hallett, M., & Cohen, L. G. (1991). A theoretical calculation of the electric field induced in the cortex during magnetic stimulation. *Electroencephalography and Clinical Neurophysiology, 81*(1), 47–56.

Rothwell, J. C. (1991). Physiological studies of electric and magnetic stimulation of the human brain. *Electroencephalography and Clinical Neurophysiology Suppl, 43*, 29–35.

Rouse, A. G., Stanslaski, S. R., Cong, P., Jensen, R. M., Afshar, P., Ullestad, D., et al. (2011). A chronic generalized bi-directional brain-machine interface. *Journal of Neural Engineering, 8*(3), 036018.

Russell, G. S., Jeffrey Eriksen, K., Poolman, P., Luu, P., & Tucker, D. M. (2005). Geodesic photogrammetry for localizing sensor positions in dense-array EEG. *Clinical Neurophysiology, 116*(5), 1130–1140.

Sanes, J. N., & Donoghue, J. P. (2000). Plasticity and primary motor cortex. *Annual Reviews of Neuroscience, 23*, 393–415.

Schafer, M., Biesecker, J. C., Schulze-Bonhage, A., & Ferbert, A. (1997). Transcranial magnetic double stimulation: influence of the intensity of the conditioning stimulus. *Electroencephalography and Clinical Neurophysiology, 105*(6), 462–469.

Scherg, M., & von Cramon, D. (1985). A new interpretation of the generators of BAEP waves I-V: results of a spatio-temporal dipole model. *Electroencephalography Clinical Neurophysiology, 62*(4), 290–299.

Schmid, G., Neubauer, G., & Mazal, P. R. (2003). Dielectric properties of human brain tissue measured less than 10 h postmortem at frequencies from 800 to 2450 MHz. *Bioelectromagnetics, 24*(6), 423–430.

Schurger, A., Cowey, A., & Tallon-Baudry, C. (2006). Induced gamma-band oscillations correlate with awareness in hemianopic patient GY. *Neuropsychologia, 44*(10), 1796–1803.

Schweitzer, G., Edlinger, G., Krausz, G., Neuper, C., Bammer, R., Stollberger, R., et al. (2001). Source localization of induced cortical oscillations during tactile finger stimulation. *Biomedical Technology (Berl), 46*(1–2), 24–28.

Serrien, D. J., Strens, L. H., Cassidy, M. J., Thompson, A. J., & Brown, P. (2004). Functional significance of the ipsilateral hemisphere during movement of the affected hand after stroke. *Experimental Neurology, 190*(2), 425–432.

Shibasaki, H. (2008). Human brain mapping: hemodynamic response and electrophysiology. *Clinical Neurophysiology, 119*(4), 731–743.

Small, S. L., Hlustik, P., Noll, D. C., Genovese, C., & Solodkin, A. (2002). Cerebellar hemispheric activation ipsilateral to the paretic hand correlates with functional recovery after stroke. *Brain, 125*(Pt 7), 1544–1557.

Soekadar, S. R., Birbaumer, N., & Cohen, L. G. (2011). Brain-computer-interfaces in the rehabilitation of stroke and neurotrauma. In: Kenji Kansaku (Ed.), *Systems-Neuroscience and Rehabilitation*, Springer Tokyo, (pp. 3–19).

Sommer, M., Lang, N., Tergau, F., & Paulus, W. (2002). Neuronal tissue polarization induced by repetitive transcranial magnetic stimulation? *Neuroreport, 13*(6), 809–811.

Srinivasan, R., Winter, W. R., Ding, J., & Nunez, P. L. (2007). EEG and MEG coherence: measures of functional connectivity at distinct spatial scales of neocortical dynamics. *Journal of Neuroscience Methods, 166*(1), 41–52.

Srinivasan, R., Winter, W. R., & Nunez, P. L. (2006). Source analysis of EEG oscillations using high-resolution EEG and MEG. *Progress in Brain Research, 159*, 29–42.

Stoeckel, M. C., Seitz, R. J., & Buetefisch, C. M. (2009). Congenitally altered motor experience alters somatotopic organization of human

primary motor cortex. *Proceedsing of the National Academy of Science U S A. 106* (7) 2395–2400.

Strens, L. H., Oliviero, A., Bloem, B. R., Gerschlager, W., Rothwell, J. C., & Brown, P. (2002). The effects of subthreshold 1 Hz repetitive TMS on cortico-cortical and interhemispheric coherence. *Clinical Neurophysiology, 113*(8), 1279–1285.

Sudre, G., Parkkonen, L., Bock, E., Baillet, S., Wang, W., & Weber, D. J. (2011). rtMEG: A Real-Time Software Interface for Magnetoencephalography. *Computational Intelligence and Neuroscience, 2011*, 327953.

Sutton, S., Braren, M., Zubin, J., & John, E. R. (1965). Evoked-potential correlates of stimulus uncertainty. *Science, 150*(700), 1187–1188.

Taubert, M., Draganski, B., Anwander, A., Muller, K., Horstmann, A., Villringer, A., et al. (2010). Dynamic properties of human brain structure: learning-related changes in cortical areas and associated fiber connections. *Journal of Neuroscience, 30*(35), 11670–11677.

Taubert, M., Lohmann, G., Margulies, D. S., Villringer, A., & Ragert, P. (2011). Long-term effects of motor training on resting-state networks and underlying brain structure. *NeuroImage, 57*(4), 1492–1498.

Tomassini, V., Jbabdi, S., Kincses, Z. T., Bosnell, R., Douaud, G., Pozzilli, C., et al. (2011). Structural and functional bases for individual differences in motor learning. *Human Brain Mapping, 32*(3), 494–508.

Traversa, R., Cicinelli, P., Bassi, A., Rossini, P. M., & Bernardi, G. (1997). Mapping of motor cortical reorganization after stroke. A brain stimulation study with focal magnetic pulses. *Stroke, 28*(1), 110–117.

van Praag, H. (2009). Exercise and the brain: something to chew on. *Trends in Neuroscience, 32*(5), 283–290.

Vanni, S., Rockstroh, B., & Hari, R. (1996). Cortical sources of human short-latency somatosensory evoked fields to median and ulnar nerve stimuli. *Brain Research, 737*(1–2), 25–33.

Ward, N. S., Brown, M. M., Thompson, A. J., & Frackowiak, R. S. (2003). Neural correlates of motor recovery after stroke: a longitudinal fMRI study. *Brain, 126*(Pt 11), 2476–2496.

Wassermann, E. M., Wedegaertner, F. R., Ziemann, U., George, M. S., & Chen, R. (1998). Crossed reduction of human motor cortex excitability by 1-Hz transcranial magnetic stimulation. *Neuroscience Letters, 250*(3), 141–144.

Wei, G., & Luo, J. (2010). Sport expert's motor imagery: functional imaging of professional motor skills and simple motor skills. *Brain Research, 1341*, 52–62.

Weiller, C., Chollet, F., Friston, K. J., Wise, R. J., & Frackowiak, R. S. (1992). Functional reorganization of the brain in recovery from striatocapsular infarction in man. *Annals of Neurology, 31*(5), 463–472.

Witte, O. W. (1998). Lesion-induced plasticity as a potential mechanism for recovery and rehabilitative training. *Current Opinions in Neurology, 11*(6), 655–662.

Wittenberg, G. F., Chen, R., Ishii, K., Bushara, K. O., Eckloff, S., Croarkin, E., et al. (2003). Constraint-induced therapy in stroke: magnetic-stimulation motor maps and cerebral activation. *Neurorehabilitation and Neural Repair, 17*(1), 48–57.

Wolpaw, J. R., McFarland, D. J., Neat, G. W., & Forneris, C. A. (1991). An EEG-based brain-computer interface for cursor control. *Electroencephalography and Clinical Neurophysiology, 78*(3), 252–259.

Wood, C. C., Spencer, D. D., Allison, T., McCarthy, G., Williamson, P. D., & Goff, W. R. (1988). Localization of human sensorimotor cortex during surgery by cortical surface recording of somatosensory evoked potentials. *Journal of Neurosurgery, 68*(1), 99–111.

Yanagisawa, T., Hirata, M., Saitoh, Y., Goto, T., Kishima, H., Fukuma, R., et al. (2011). Real-time control of a prosthetic hand using human electrocorticography signals. *Journal of Neurosurgery, 114*(6), 1715–1722.

Yao, J., Sheaff, C., & Dewald, J. P. (2008). Usage of the ACT Robot in a brain machine interface for hand opening and closing in stroke survivors. *IEEE International Conference on Rehabilitation Robotics, 2007*, 938–942.

Zaca, D., Hua, J., & Pillai, J. J. (2011). Cerebrovascular reactivity mapping for brain tumor presurgical planning. *World Journal of Clinical Oncolology, 2*(7), 289–298.

Ziemann, U., Lonnecker, S., Steinhoff, B. J., & Paulus, W. (1996a). The effect of lorazepam on the motor cortical excitability in man. *Experimental Brain Research, 109*(1), 127–135.

Ziemann, U., Lonnecker, S., Steinhoff, B. J., & Paulus, W. (1996b). Effects of antiepileptic drugs on motor cortex excitability in humans: a transcranial magnetic stimulation study. *Annals of Neurology, 40*(3), 367–378.

PART B | STROKE PATHOPHYSIOLOGY AND RECOVERY

6 | STROKE: PATHOPHYSIOLOGY, RECOVERY POTENTIAL, AND TIMELINES FOR RECOVERY AND REHABILITATION

RÜDIGER J. SEITZ and GEOFFREY A. DONNAN

6.1 INTRODUCTION

Stroke is one of the leading causes of persistent disability in Western countries (Bejot et al., 2007). It induces acute deficits of motion, sensation, cognition and emotion. In the majority of patients stroke results from an interruption of cerebral blood supply and subsequent ischemic brain damage, while more than 25% of patients suffer from intracranial hemorrhage (Intiso et al., 2003; Shiber et al., 2010). The neurological deficits after stroke may regress spontaneously after the insult depending on the severity of the initial event, the pathophysiology of stroke, and the recovery potential.

Recovery from stroke is a multifaceted process depending on different mechanisms that become operational at different phases after the acute insult ranging from hours to many months (Carey & Seitz, 2007). Importantly, acute stroke treatment such as thrombolysis has opened new avenues to substantially reverse the neurological deficits after stroke (Hacke et al., 2004, 2008; Donnan et al., 2009). In addition, recent developments in neurorehabilitation have improved the fate of stroke patients, as training approaches can be tailored depending on the time point after stroke and the residual capacities of the patients. These approaches include very early mobilization, anti-gravity support for walking, basic arm training, and arm ability training (Cumming et al., 2011; Hesse, 2008; Platz et al., 2009).

Neuroimaging and neurophysiological methods have offered means to investigate the severity of the initial event, the pathophysiology of stroke, and the recovery potential of stroke patients (Wittenberg et al., 2003; Cramer, 2008a,b). In particular, these noninvasive neuroscientific measures can be repeated at different time points that allow one to assess the times for recovery and rehabilitation.

Studies of this sort supplement clinical observations and have opened new insights into the neuroscientific basis of human stroke and stroke rehabilitation. We review here recent publications addressing the pathophysiology, recovery potential, and the timelines for recovery and rehabilitation after ischemic stroke.

6.2 PATHOPHYSIOLOGY

6.2.1 FROM CEREBRAL ISCHEMIA TOWARD BRAIN INFARCTION

Ischemic stroke results from an acute interruption of cerebral blood supply leading to disturbances of neural function and, in the most severe cases, structural brain damage caused by infarction. Typically, stroke symptoms start abruptly at the time of cerebral arterial occlusion and interruption of brain perfusion. The depression of cerebral circulation induces immediate suppression of cerebral electrical activity and peri-infarct depolarization with repeated episodes of metabolic stress (Heiss et al., 1992; Hossmann, 1994). In the acute stage of stroke, the area of impaired perfusion typically exceeds the area with a complete cessation of perfusion. In the area of impaired or misery perfusion the extraction of oxygen from blood into brain tissue is enhanced. This defines the so-called *penumbra*, which has been demonstrated in stroke patients using positron emission tomography (Heiss et al., 2004; Moustafa & Baron, 2008). Since the advent of MRI it was shown that the area of impaired perfusion typically exceeds the area of reduced water diffusion, which signifies the extent of virtually irreversible ischemic brain damage (Neumann-Haefelin et al., 1999; Rother et al., 2002; Olivot et al. 2008a). In fact, the perfusion–diffusion mismatch area has been assumed to be indicative of the penumbra. There is a good correspondence of area with enhanced oxygen extraction and the perfusion–diffusion mismatch area in acute stroke, although there is no quantitative relation between these two concepts (Sobesky, 2004, 2005).

Notably, the area of reduced diffusion undergoes a dramatic evolution within the first 24 hours after onset of brain ischemia (Beaulieu et al., 1999; Rohl et al., 2001; Wittsack et al., 2002). If an arterial occlusion persists, growth of the infarct lesion occurs up to 24 hours post-occlusion (Lee et al., 2000; Li et al., 2000). As has been shown in animal experiments, ischemic neuronal and tissue necrosis occur in proportion to the extent of the reduction of regional cerebral blood flow (rCBF; Hossmann, 1994). Thus, critical determinants of acute stroke are the occlusion of a cerebral artery, the induced local depression of rCBF, and its subsequent electrical, metabolic, and ionic changes (Dirnagl et al., 1999). Imaging and neurophysiological studies in humans have shown that, similarly to animal experiments, spreading depression occurs in severe ischemic stroke entertaining progressive infarct expansion (Dohmen et al., 2008; Dreier et al., 2009).

Beyond the acute time window of about 24 hours, secondary changes evolve, including an early phase with vasogenic edema and a later phase with inflammatory infiltration (Saleh et al. 2004). Lymphocytes and macrophages have been shown by MRI to accumulate in a perivascular distribution in infarcted brain tissue approximately 6 days after a cerebral infarction. Macrophages were labelled by uptake of iron after intravenous injection (Schroeter et al., 2004). A similar approach employed tracers against the peripheral gamma-aminobutyric acid (GABA)receptor, which is located on macrophages using positron emission tomography for imaging the distribution of inflammatory infiltrates (Price et al., 2006). Recently, it was observed that the areas with inflammatory infiltration are heterogeneously distributed within the infarct area (Saleh et al., 2007). It was speculated that due to their immunological competence these cells augment the infarct lesion. This raises the interesting hypothesis that immunosuppression may affect lesion growth in stroke (McCombe & Read, 2008).

6.2.2 REVERSAL OF ISCHEMIA

A major step in acute stroke treatment has been the advent of thrombolysis. It is targeted toward the rescue of brain tissue by early recanalization of the occluded cerebral artery. It has been shown to be effective up to 4.5 hours, with maximal efficacy within the first 90 minutes after symptom onset (Hacke et al., 2004, 2008; Merino et al., 2008). The beneficial role of early recanalization was shown by functional imaging (Heiss et al., 1998; Kidwell et al., 2002) and monitoring with transcranial Doppler

sonography (Alexandrov et al., 2000, 2001). By such studies it became evident that brain tissue at risk of ischemic damage can be salvaged by tissue reperfusion owing to arterial recanalization. In contrast, edema formation in the subacute stage of stroke can hardly be limited pharmacologically. Thus, to rescue patients from malignant brain swelling after stroke, craniectomy has been advocated as an effective therapy (Schwab et al., 1998). But this is a lifesaving action rather than treatment reducing the neurological deficit, particularly in patients older than 60 years (Arac et al., 2009). Likewise, use of immunosuppressive agents targeting the inflammatory reaction after stroke has resulted in conflicting effects (McCombe & Read, 2008).

Perfusion and diffusion imaging studies performed in the hyperacute phase of stroke before treatment onset and at follow-up have revealed that the severity and the spatial extent of the ischemic brain damage predict the volume of the subsequent infarct lesions (Figure 6.1). The most important determinants of the extent of a brain infarct are the underlying causes of the ischemic insult, the severity and duration of ischemia, the dimension and composition of the causal arterial emboli, the anatomy and the vascular changes of the cerebral arteries, and the presence of diabetic hyperglycemia (Rohl et al., 2001; Parsons et al., 2002; Almekhlafi et al., 2008).

Brain infarcts may result from cardiac or artery-to-artery-embolism, or from small penetrating vessel disease such as hyalinosis or microatheroma (Thrift et al., 2001; Dewey et al., 2003). Typically, infarcts in the territory of the posterior cerebral artery are embolic in origin and comprise the entire supply area of the affected artery (Finelli, 2008). In contrast, infarcts in the anterior cerebral artery are usually of atherosclerotic origin and more variable in lesion pattern and neurological deficit (Kang & Kim, 2008). The situation is more complicated in the middle cerebral artery (MCA) territory, given the wide arborization of the artery, the large territory supplied by the artery, and the net-like anastomoses of the downstream arterial branches with the leptomeningeal arteries.

There is accumulating evidence that in addition to the acute artery occlusion underlying stroke, there is also the impact of collaterals contributing to the initial ischemic event. The poorer the collaterals are, and the more severe arterosclerotic changes are present in the intracranial arteries, the more severe is the initial ischemic event (Seitz et al., 2005; Bang et al., 2008; Liebeskind et al., 2011). Thus, an arterial obstruction in the MCA may have different consequences for the neurological deficit and infarct manifestation depending on the site of the occlusion (Bang et al., 2005). In addition, the success of the recanalizing acute stroke therapy is of fundamental importance for the topography and volume of the resulting ischemic infarct lesion (von Kummer et al., 1994; Delgado-Mederos et al., 2007).

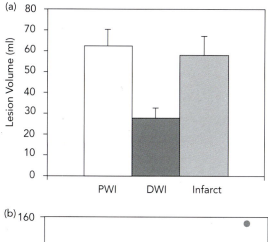

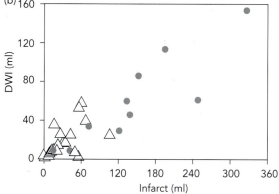

Figure 6.1 Lesion evolution after stroke. **(a)** Mean volumes of reduced perfusion (white column) and diffusion (grey column) before thrombolysis and the infarct lesions 24 hours after thrombolysis (black column). **(b)** High correlation of diffusion lesions before and 24 hours after thrombolysis in patients with recanalization (triangles) and lacking recanalization (black dots). From Seitz et al. (2011).

6.2.3 PATTERNS OF RESIDUAL BRAIN INFARCTS AFTER THROMBOLYSIS

Owing to the pathophysiology and therapeutic modification of cerebral ischemia, we have proposed recently a refined classification of ischemic brain infarcts that takes into account the affected cerebral artery and the effects of acute stroke treatment (Seitz & Donnan, 2010). We labeled circumscribed territorial infarcts as Type I strokes (Table 6.1). Depending on the size of the emboli, either a distal or a more proximal arterial branch becomes occluded, giving rise to either small infarcts entirely limited to the cerebral cortex or larger infarcts involving the cerebral cortex and the underlying white matter (Wang et al., 2006). Typically, these territorial infarcts do not destroy the entire cortical representation area, nor the complete descending motor cortical output tract or afferent sensory input tract (Binkofski et al., 1996; Crafton et al., 2003; Rey et al., 2007). This leaves sufficient adjacent cerebral tissue for perilesional reorganization to occur, as will be discussed below.

Type II strokes affect large parts of or the entire striatocapsular region (Donnan et al., 1991; Seitz & Donnan,

2010). They result from an embolic occlusion of the MCA stem (Table 6.1). If reperfusion is achieved early, only the deep perforating arteries and the arteries that supply the insular cortex remain critically affected by ischemia, thus causing infarcts limited to the lentiform nucleus and insula (Seitz et al., 2009). Notably, in these infarcts the initial ischemic event is aggravated when a compensatory redistribution of arterial blood along collaterals is impaired by arterial changes, such as vessel stenosis or occlusion in multiple cerebral arteries (Seitz et al., 2005, Bang et al., 2008). It was shown that in the more severely affected patients the hemispheric white matter is significantly damaged, resulting also in corticocortical and cortico-subcortical disconnections which contribute to the occurrence of hemispatial neglect and conduction aphasia (Saur et al., 2006; Stoeckel et al., 2007; Karnath et al., 2009).

Small-sized lacunar infarcts resulting from an occlusion of the small penetrating cerebral arteries, or even arterioles, typically occur in the anterior choroidal artery, the deep perforating lenticular MCA branches, the thalamic branches of the posterior cerebral artery, or in brainstem structures and the pons (Fisher, 1982; Boiten & Lodder, 1991). Typically, these Type III strokes proceed to full-blown infarcts (though of small spatial dimension) which, due to their strategic location in cerebral white matter, may result in well-defined lacunar deficit syndromes (Table 6.1). These include pure motor or pure sensory stroke, which may have a very limited capacity for recovery, as predicted by a loss of motor evoked potentials and asymmetry of water diffusivity on MR imaging (Binkofski et al., 1996; Stinear et al., 2007; Lindenberg et al., 2010a). The crucial role of the white matter for functional outcome can be illustrated by the observation that small cortical infarcts, for example in the precentral gyrus, typically allow for profound recovery from stroke, whereas infarcts of similar volume in the periventricular white matter or the internal capsule may induce a severe and persistent hemiparesis (Kretschmann, 1988; Wenzelburger et al., 2005). Recently, white matter damage in stroke was found in a large genome-wide association study to be related to a mutation in chromosome 17 (Fornage et al., 2011).

Patients with long-standing cerebrovascular disease and chronic occlusion of extracranial cerebral arteries, as well as younger patients who suffer from dissection of extracranial arteries, constitute Type IV strokes (Table 6.1). These patients may become symptomatic with minor neurological deficits such as transient ischemic attacks due to small arterio-embolic or hemodynamically induced watershed infarcts, particularly in cerebral white matter (Surikova et al., 2006; Blondin et al., 2009). In these patients, blood flow depression induces a reactive vasodilatation of the intracranial blood vessels, resulting in a severe delay in cerebral brain perfusion in the presence of a normal cerebral blood volume (Kurada & Houkin, 2008).

TABLE 6.1 Cerebral Stroke Subtypes

TYPE	INFARCT LOCATION	SIZE	PATHOGENESIS	EFFECT OF THROMBOLYSIS
I	**territorial**		**occlusion of cerebral artery branch**	
I.1	cortical	small	distal branch	early
I.2	cortico-subcortical	medium	proximal branch	none or delayed
II	**striatocapsular**		**occlusion of MCA stem**	
II.1	+/– insula	medium	infarct core	early
II.2	+ periventricular white matter	large	complete infarct	none or delayed
III			**lacunar hyalinosis of arterioles**	none or delayed
III.1	fiber tracts			
III.2	internal capsule (anterior choroidal artery)			
III.3	basal ganglia, lateral thalamus			
III.4	medial and anterior thalamus (perforating branches of posterior cerebral artery)			
IV			**chronic hemodynamic deficit + downstream emboli**	
IV.1	cortico-subcortical	medium	extracranial artery disease +/–	none or delayed
			intracranial large artery disease +/–	
			accompanied by reactive vasodilation	
IV.2	arterial border zone	medium	(arterial dissection, arteriosclerosis)	

SOURCE: Adapted from Seitz and Donnan (2010).

6.2.4 FUNCTIONAL CONSEQUENCES OF BRAIN INFARCTS

The functional deficit in an individual patient is determined by the location and the volume of the cerebral infarct. For example, small brain lesions may specifically erase a well-defined function which, conversely, engages this very same area when probed in healthy subjects. This was shown for simple sensorimotor functions as well as cognitive and emotional functions (Binkofski et al., 1998; Kim, 2001; Binkofski & Seitz, 2004; Schäfer et al., 2007; Barton et al., 2008; Hömke et al., 2009). In contrast, larger brain lesions or small subcortical white matter lesions may affect multiple brain systems, which results in complex neurological syndromes such as apraxia, neglect, or Gerstman's syndrome (Karnath et al., 2004; Pazzaglia et al., 2008; Rusconi et al., 2009). Moreover, measures of fiber tract damage or cortical activations have been found to explain the degree of recovery (Binkofski et al., 1996; Hamzei et al., 2008; Kim et al., 2008; Schiemanck et al., 2008; Schaechter et al., 2009). Similar observations have also been made for language functions, the somatosensory system, and the visual system (Vitali et al., 2007; Connell et al., 2008; Poggel et al., 2008; Brodtmann et al., 2009).

Beyond structural changes, there are also functional changes in the brain following stroke. Most importantly, the intracortical excitability was increased in motor cortex of both hemispheres regardless of subcortical or cortical location of infarction (Liepert et al., 2000; Bütefisch et al., 2003; Hummel et al., 2009). These changes can be assessed with transcranial magnetic stimulation (TMS) using different single and paired-pulse stimulation techniques (Bütefisch et al., 2008). These changes are thought to provide a physiological basis for the abnormal muscle activity in the hemiparetic patients. For example, a prolonged suppression of muscle activity after a TMS stimulus correlated with the severity of hemiparesis (Classen et al., 1997). Conversely, ipsilesional MEPs were more easily elicited from proximal muscles in stroke patients than in healthy subjects (Lewis et al., 2007; Misawa et al., 2008; Schwerin et al., 2008). The enhanced cortical excitability probably corresponded to the changed pattern of the GABA receptor in the perilesional vicinity after experimental ischemia (Redecker et al., 2000). Heiss and collaborators (2004) were able to show in the human that the expression of the GABA-Benzodiazepin receptor is downregulated in ischemic brain tissue, suggesting extensive neuronal damage. Similarly, the binding of flumazenil, a $GABA_A$ receptor antagonist, as measured with positron emission tomography was found to be reduced in this area in proportion to the initial hypoperfusion as assessed with perfusion CT (Guadagno et al., 2008).

In addition, there is evidence that interhemispheric connectivity is altered after stroke (Figure 6.2). In fact, the

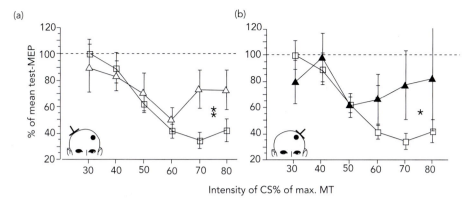

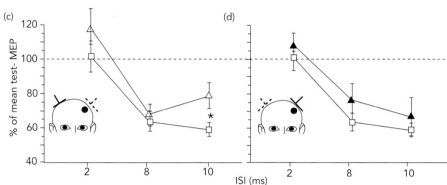

Figure 6.2 Bihemispheric excitability changes in cortical infarcts. Reduced short interval cortical inhibition (SICI) in the affected (**a**) and contralesional (**b**) hemisphere in patients with cortical infarcts (triangle) as compared with controls (squares). (**c**) Reduced interhemispheric inhibition from the affected to the contralesional hemisphere in patients with cortical infarcts. (**d**) Intact interhemispheric inhibition of the contralesional to the affected hemisphere. MEP = Motor evoked potential; MT = motor threshold; CS = conditioning stimulus. Adapted from Bütefisch et al. (2008).

interhemispheric inhibition from M1 of the lesioned on the nonlesioned hemisphere has been shown to be decreased, while it was normal from M1 of the nonlesioned to the lesioned hemisphere (Bütefisch et al., 2008). Notably, two other measures of cortical excitability, namely the motor threshold of the target muscles and the intracortical facilitation, were not affected.

6.3 RECOVERY POTENTIAL

6.3.1 THE ROLE OF THE PENUMBRA

The perfusion–diffusion mismatch, as assessed with the widely available MRI, has been the target for acute stroke treatment approaches in large clinical trials (Rother et al., 2002). In the Diffusion and Perfusion Imaging Evaluation For Understanding Stroke Evolution (DEFUSE) trial, it was found that a good clinical outcome after thrombolysis performed 3 to 6 hours after stroke onset was associated with less infarct growth in such patients with a perfusion–diffusion mismatch (Albers et al., 2006; Olivot et al., 2008b). Likewise, an acute perfusion–diffusion mismatch > 20% in left Brodmann area 37 was strongly associated with acute improvement of naming on day 3 to 5, independently of volume or percentage of total perfusion–diffusion mismatch, or abnormalities of diffusion or perfusion (Hillis et al., 2008).

In the Echoplanar Imaging Thrombolytic Evaluation Trial (EPITHET) recanalization was strongly correlated with reperfusion as assessed with MRI on day 3

to 5 (Davis et al., 2008). These data correspond to the observation that early recanalization was predictive of good outcome and reduced infarct growth as compared to failed recanalization (Neumann-Haefelin et al., 2004; Seitz et al., 2009). In contrast, reversal of the area with abnormal water diffusion in diffusion-weighted imaging was uncommon (Seitz et al., 2005; Chemmanam et al., 2010). Apparently, the residual flow associated with an intracranial occlusion before systemic thrombolysis predicts the likelihood of complete recanalization and long-term neurological outcome. However, even if there is no flow detected in transcranial Doppler, the opportunity to achieve recanalization exists (Saqqur et al., 2009). Here, good arterial collaterals have been shown to be important for stroke evolution (Surikova et al., 2006; Liebeskind et al., 2011). These data suggest that recovery from stroke commences early after the ischemic event related to rapid arterial recanalization and cerebral tissue reperfusion, since reperfusion determines the extent of salvage of brain tissue threatened by ischemia and limits the expansion of the ischemic brain lesion.

6.3.2 PERILESIONAL PLASTICITY

An important factor contributing to functional recovery is the perilesional tissue. The perilesional tissue is supposed to be structurally intact but functionally altered due to transient ischemia and subsequent reperfusion. Both factors evoke a large number of biochemical, metabolic, and immunological processes that evolve sequentially (Taoufik

& Probert, 2008). Animal experiments have shown that there is synaptic plasticity related to spontaneous recovery when animals are kept in an enriched environment or subjected to dedicated training (Nudo et al., 1996; Biernaskie & Corbett, 2001). These plastic changes have been shown to result in structural changes, such as growing of axons and formation of new synapses. These changes occur in the perilesional vicinity and in remote locations in functionally related areas in the affected and contralesional "nonaffected" hemisphere (Frost et al., 2003; Dancause et al., 2005). On the molecular level, there are changes in the expression of genes, neurotransmitters such as glutamate and GABA, as well as of neurotrophic mediators implicated as molecular substrates mediating perilesional reorganization (Witte et al., 2000; Carmichael et al., 2005; Centonze et al., 2007).

In the first 4 weeks, there is a perilesional activation which seems to be localized nearby in those portions of the motor cortical area that are not affected (Figure 6.3). After a follow-up of some 2 years it has been possible to show that cortical activation related to finger movements has moved to a more dorsal location (Hamzei et al., 2003; Jaillard et al., 2005). Recently, it has been shown by TMS that the sites of activation actually move into the region of maximal cortical disinhibition (Liepert et al., 2006).

Using paired-pulse TMS it was found that within the first 7 days after a brain infarct there is an enhanced cortical excitability in the cortex adjacent to the brain lesion, but also in the contralateral hemisphere (Cincenelli et al., 2003; Bütefisch et al., 2008; Manganotti et al., 2008). Notably, the enhanced perilesional excitability was secondary to the infarct lesion and not due to an abnormality of interhemispheric inhibition (Figure 6.2). Rather, it was transmitted to the intact motor cortex in the contralesional hemisphere. The enhanced excitability was found to be decreased in the contralesional hemisphere in the patients who showed a good recovery within the 90 days, while it persisted in those patients with poor recovery (Bütefisch et al., 2003). In keeping with these observations, functional MRI performed approximately 2 days after stroke revealed an area in the ipsilesional postcentral gyrus and posterior cingulate gyrus that correlated with motor recovery approximately 3 months after stroke (Marshall et al., 2009). Furthermore, restoration of hand function 3 months after stroke was associated with highly lateralized activation of the affected sensorimotor cortex which developed over time (Askam et al., 2009).

Noninvasive electrical anodal stimulation of the affected motor cortex was found to augment motor skill acquisition (Reis et al., 2009). The effect of 5 days anodal stimulation of the injured motor cortex improved consolidation but not long-term retention of a motor task (Reis et al., 2009). Conversely, application of 1-Hz repetitive TMS (rTMS) of 10 minutes' duration to the contralesional motor cortex which downregulates the contralesional motor cortex improved the

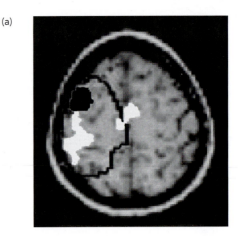

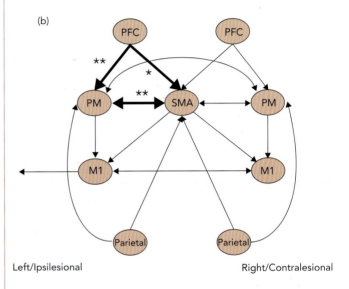

Left/Ipsilesional   Right/Contralesional

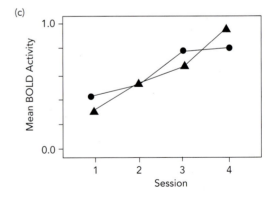

Figure 6.3 Activation in perilesional vicinity after MCA-stroke. Area of hypoperfusion (black line), lesion area (black area). Activation area in sensorimotor cortex is related to sequential finger movements of the affected hand; additional activation of the supplementary motor area is noted (from Kleiser et al., 2005). (b) Enhanced connectivity of prefrontal cortex to motor cortical areas in the affected hemisphere in the presence of a decreased connectivity between premotor cortex and supplementary motor area (from Sharma et al., 2009, with permission). (c) Increase of activity related to combined botulinum toxin treatment for spasticity and cycling arm training in the perilesional sensorimotor cortex in 8 chronic stroke patients (from Diserens et al., 2010).

kinematics of finger and grasp movements in the affected hand (Nowak et al., 2008). This resulted in overactivity in the contralesional motor and premotor cortical areas. While there was no correlation to the behavioral improvement for motor cortex activation, overactivity in contralesional premotor cortex and ipsilesional medial frontal cortex predicted improvement in movement kinematics. One may wonder if long-term retention of the induced effects can be achieved by longer-lasting stimulation or by the combination of voluntary action and direct brain stimulation.

The combination of electrical stimulation of finger extensor muscles and tracking training over 2 to 3 weeks did not result in an improvement of dexterity of the affected hand as assessed with the Jebson test greater than each intervention alone (Bhatt et al., 2007). Subjects with an intact motor cortex showed a greater improvement than those who had direct involvement of the motor cortex. However, only in the combination group did functional improvement correlate with a change of the laterality index in sensorimotor cortex and premotor cortex activation, indicating greater ipsilesional control. There was a negative correlation with the fMRI signal intensity change in the ipsilesional sensorimotor cortex and the supplementary motor area (Bhatt et al., 2007). Similarly, in chronic stroke-induced aphasia, repetitive TMS over the left inferior frontal gyrus resulted in an increase of reaction time or error rate in a semantic task, suggesting restoration of a perilesional tissue in the left hemisphere (Winhuisen et al., 2007; Marangolo et al., 2009). Accordingly, fMRI activation most likely reflects adaptation of the injured brain to the functional deficit related to spontaneous reorganization in the perilesional tissue.

6.3.3 INFARCT-INDUCED DISCONNECTIONS

The importance of corticospinal fibers for recovery of motor function after stroke has been demonstrated with different imaging modalities as well as electrophysiological measures (Fries et al., 1991; Binkofski et al., 1996; Stinear et al., 2007; Schaechter et al., 2008). Most often in human stroke it is damaged in the posterior limb of the internal capsule (Figure 6.4). Based on animal studies, it has been suggested that so-called alternate motor fibers can compensate for motor impairment after severe damage to the corticospinal tract (Lang & Schieber, 2004). In monkeys and cats, the corticoreticulospinal and corticorubrospinal tracts may mediate motor functions in case of corticospinal tract lesions (Canedo, 1997), whereas these tracts have been described as functionally redundant in healthy animals (Kennedy, 1990). Notably, estimates of the integrity of the corticospinal tract as derived from diffusion tensor imaging (DTI) correlate with gross atrophy of the cerebral peduncles (Schaechter et al., 2008, Lindenberg et al., 2010a). Also, the integrity of the corticospinal tract determines the movement-related motor cortex activation (Stinear

et al., 2007, Hamzei et al., 2008). In chronic patients without motor evoked potentials there was no recovery if the fractional anisotropy of the posterior part of the internal capsule, as assessed by diffusion tensor imaging, was asymmetric across the hemispheres (Stinear et al., 2007). In these patients bilateral fMRI activations were observed in relation to finger movements, while in the patients with a lower asymmetry there was an activation lateralized to the affected hemisphere.

There are not only changes in the efferent motor fiber tracts but also in the corticocortical and probably also cortico-subcortical fiber tract systems during recovery. In fact, motor cortical connectivity was shown by diffusion tensor imaging to be enhanced after stroke (Pannek et al., 2009). Additionally, orientation uncertainty and greater white matter complexity correlated with functional outcome (Lang et al., 2009; Pannek et al., 2009). Notably, there was correlation with lesion volume suggesting that the repair processes were possibly triggered by functional demands. In addition, it was recently found that the pyramidal tract splits up in the pons, forming a ventral and also a dorsal tract (Lindenberg et al., 2010a). Both tracts are severely affected in patients with poor recovery, while continuity of the projections in the dorsal portion was characterized by good recovery (Figure 6.4). However, the level of motor skill recovery achieved in the chronic stage after stroke was related also to the microstructural status of the corticospinal tract in the contralesional hemisphere. Patients with poorer motor skill had reduced fractional anisotropy in both corticospinal tracts, while patients with better motor skill had elevated fractional anisotropy in both corticospinal tracts (Schaechter et al., 2009). In chronic stroke patients, DTI-derived measures of transcallosal motor fibers as well as ipsilesional corticospinal tracts, pyramidal tract, and alternate fiber tract, could be used to explain the therapeutic response to rehabilitation. The more the diffusivity profiles resembled those observed in healthy subjects, the greater a patient's potential for functional recovery (Zhang et al., 2008; Lindenberg et al., 2011). While these findings need to be substantiated by further investigations, they accord with the evidence from functional imaging suggesting that the concerted action of both cerebral hemispheres is required for recovery.

It is now well established that in neurological patients with a focal brain lesion there are large-scale changes that affect the contralesional cerebral cortex and subcortical structures in a highly structured pattern, which most likely reflects functional intracerebral connectivity. These changes are related to the volume of the infarct lesion but regress over time. Thus, patients who recover from an infarct lesion have a progressively normal activation pattern (Marshall et al., 2000; Nhan et al., 2004; Askam et al., 2009). Nevertheless, even patients with an excellent recovery may show a bilateral activation pattern (Foltys et al., 2003; Bütefisch et al., 2005). This abnormal activity

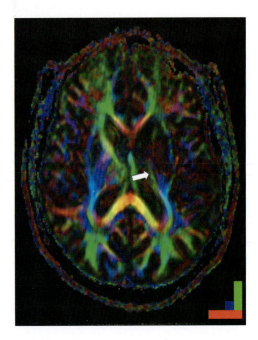

Motor Recovery
Damage of Pyramidal Tract

	Ventral	Dorsal
Good	–	–
Moderate	+	–
Poor	+	+

Figure 6.4 White matter damage after stroke in a patient with persistent hemiplegia. Note the complete destruction of the posterior limb of the internal capsule (arrow). Color bar: green fronto-occipital diffusion, red right-left diffusion, blue dorso-ventral diffusion. Motor recovery in relation to damage of the ventral and posterior portion of the pyramidal tract (right). From Lindenberg et al. (2010a) with permission.

involved premotor cortical areas and was largely reminiscent of relearning, as they represent activation patterns similar to procedural relearning and are essentially transient in nature (Bütefisch et al., 2005; Saur et al., 2006; Marshall et al., 2009). Notably, tiny activation areas in contralesional motor cortex were related to mirror movements that frequently occur initially after stroke (Nelles et al., 1998).

Apart from local activations, network types of neuroimaging data analysis can reveal abnormalities in the intrahemispheric and interhemispheric coupling between cortical areas. For example, there is a pathological interhemispheric interaction between the ipsilesional and contralesional motor cortex, as well as between the ipsilesional supplementary motor area (SMA) and contralesional motor cortex in patients with a single infarct lesion (Seitz et al., 1999; Grefkes et al., 2008). In unilateral movements of the affected hand, there was an inhibitory influence from the contralesional to the ipsilesional motor cortex which correlated with the degree of motor impairment (Grefkes et al., 2008). In bimanual movements, the interaction of the ipsilesional SMA and the contralesional motor cortex was reduced, and this correlated with impaired bimanual performance. This can be related to the observation that there was less activation in contralesional motor cortex when the motor task did not require working memory demands, and no change when the task required online visual feedback monitoring (Kimberley et al., 2008). Also, the premotor cortex was bilaterally less active when there was no working memory demand but increased activity upon online visual feedback monitoring, although there was no difference in overt performance. Motor network connectivity strength was shown to correlate with motor outcome after stroke (Sharma et al., 2009). Notably, connectivity strength of the prefrontal cortex to the premotor cortex was enhanced in relation to motor imagery, highlighting the role of the prefrontal cortex for higher-order planning of movement (Figure 6.3).

6.3.4 REGENERATIVE THERAPIES USING STEM CELL APPROACHES

Since brain infarcts result in damage of both grey and white matter, tissue repair resulting in replacement of the ischemic tissue debris by functional brain tissue for each of these compartments would be optimal. It is possible that this replacement may come from endogenous sources: experimental work in laboratory animals suggests that stem cells in the subventricular germinal zone, as well as neural progenitor cells, proliferate in response to focal ischemia (Kokaia et al., 2006; Ohab et al., 2006). They seem to be regulated by a number of different factors such as neurotrophic substances and inflammatory mediators (Schäbitz et al., 2007; Pluchino et al., 2008). However, it seems that neurons have only a limited capacity for regeneration and axons usually do not extend for long distances within the brain. The progress of their growth appears to become arrested at sites of scars within central nervous tissue lesions (Hermanns et al., 2001).

In spite of this, there is also good evidence from animal experiments that nerve fibers of intact nerve cells in the perilesional cortex may grow across considerable distances and form new synapses at their destination, in proportion to dedicated rehabilitative training (Nudo et al., 1996; Biernaskie & Corbett, 2001; Frost et al., 2003; Dancause et al., 2005). Tissue formation of stem cells transplanted into the human brain, however, faces a number of challenges that need to be targeted (Dihné et al., 2011). These include questions of which cells in addition to neurons are to be transplanted, how they are integrated into anatomical structures, whether endogenous neurogenesis can be enhanced, and how vascular regeneration can be initiated. Not least, survival of transplanted cells calls upon immunomodulation and neuroprotection.

6.3.5 REHABILITATIVE EFFECT OF PHYSICAL TRAINING

There are numerous reports about rehabilitative approaches to improve the neurological deficit following stroke (Carey & Seitz, 2007; Cramer, 2008b). Notably, the intensity of the training rather than the type of training appears to determine long-term improvement of motor function (Kwakkel et al., 1999; Boake et al., 2008). Treadmill training was found to improve walking velocity, which correlated with brain activity in the posterior cerebellum related to movement of the paretic limb (Luft et al., 2008). Passive training of wrist movements was reported to be clinically effective and associated with change in cortical activation (Lindberg et al., 2007). Even successful hand shaping and grasping of objects did not occur when there was not sufficient volitional control of finger and thumb extensions (Lang et al., 2009). These therapeutic approaches result in a widespread recruitment of motor representations in the affected hemisphere during the learning period as observed with fMRI and TMS (Wittenberg et al., 2003; Boake et al., 2008).

Repetitive training of the affected arm resulted in an increase of activation in the sensorimotor cortex related to hand movements, which initially persisted for weeks after training completion and then decreased in magnitude in relation to the functional gain (Dong et al., 2007; Mintzopoulos et al., 2008). Further, a 3-week training in chronic stroke patients using robot-assisted training resulted in gains of hand motor function, which was associated to a greater fMRI signal in sensorimotor cortex related to performance of the movements trained using the robot (Takahashi et al., 2008). This increase was task-specific, since it did not occur in relation to a nontrained supination/pronation movement with the affected hand and movements of the nontrained hand.

Not only training of the affected limb but also training targeting the non-affected limb has been proposed to be effective. For example, use of bilateral synergies has been reported to improve the motor capacity of the paretic arm (Mudie & Matyas, 2001). It was described that active-passive bilateral arm therapy can produce sustained improvements in upper limb motor function in chronic stroke patients. This was paralleled by an enhanced ipsilesional motor cortex excitability and an increased transcallosal inhibition from ipsilesional to contralesional motor cortex (Perez & Cohen, 2008).

Conversely, the concept of "learned non-use" was implemented in new approaches of rehabilitative strategies in chronic patients with brain infarction (Wolf et al., 1989; Taub et al., 1994). This concept imposed constraints on the unaffected limb by keeping it in a cast, forcing the subject to use the residual functions of the affected arm for daily purposes. This so called "constraint-induced" therapy has been shown to be successful even when applied in the chronic state to moderately affected patients (Liepert et al., 1998; Sawaki et al., 2008). This beneficial effect of constraint-induced movement therapy is likely to be composed of focusing the patient's attention to the affected side and imposing repetitive training results in improved motor function and enhanced activation in the partially damaged sensorimotor cortex (Hamzei et al., 2008; Sawaki et al., 2008), as well as in other grey matter areas including the hippocampus (Gauthier et al., 2008). Given the human postlesional changes of cortical excitability, it may be intriguing to rebalance the interhemispheric rivalry by direct cortical stimulation or peripheral stimulation (Muehlbacher et al., 2002; Floel et al., 2004; Fregni et al., 2005; Hummel et al., 2005). An even greater effect was observed when bihemispheric direct cortical stimulation activated the affected motor cortex and inhibited the contralesional motor cortex (Lindenberg et al., 2010b).

6.3.6 REHABILITATIVE EFFECT OF MENTAL TRAINING

Mental training was reported to result in better functionality of the upper extremity and in greater gains of activities of daily living than standard physiotherapy (Müller et al., 2007; Page et al., 2009). More specifically, daily treatment that involved observing actions combined with physical training for 4 weeks resulted in a significant increase in motor functions, which lasted for at least 8 weeks after training (Ertelt et al., 2007). This was associated with a significant overactivation, as compared to the control group, in the bilateral ventral premotor cortex, bilateral superior temporal gyrus, the SMA and the contralateral supramarginal gyrus related to an object manipulation task. Similarly, functional MRI revealed that motor imagery activated a widespread network of cerebral areas in motor, premotor, and parietal cortex in both cerebral hemispheres (Page et al., 2009; Sharma et al., 2009). With respect to the concept of the so-called *mirror neurons* that become active not only in relation to motor activity but also in response to observation and imagery of the same type of movements, it has been assumed that the inferior frontal cortex may play a critical role in motor recovery.

It should be mentioned, however, that the capacity to perform motor imagery can be weakened by limb loss or disuse, while the temporal characteristics of motor imagery may not be affected (Malouin et al., 2009). This is of importance, since first-person imagery of hand movements strongly activates the left inferior parietal lobe (parietal operculum and secondary somatosensory cortex) in healthy volunteers, particularly with postures compatible with a previously seen right hand movement (Lang et al., 2009). Notably, the secondary somatosensory cortex is particularly activated in successful recovery from hemiparesis (Askam et al., 2009; Thiel et al., 2007) and treatment of spasticity (Diserens et al., 2010).

6.4 TIMELINES FOR RECOVERY AND REHABILITATION

The neurological deficits can regress substantially in the early period after ischemic stroke following acute stroke treatment, but arterial recanalization and effective reperfusion need to occur fast after the insult. The processes of cerebral organization are slow and may need many months to complete. The early recovery in patients with small cortical lesions steadily evolves over weeks and levels out over the subsequent months (Duncan et al., 2000; Kwakkel et al., 2003; Jaillard et al., 2005). In the acute phase of stroke it is difficult to predict the degree of ultimate recovery, since there is a large heterogeneity of recovery over the first 3 months after stroke (Glymour et al., 2007; Cramer, 2008a). Prediction becomes progressively better the more specific and differentiated the physiological assessment measures are, and the longer the time since stroke (Connell et al., 2008; Beebe et al., 2009; Krebs et al., 2009). For example, the neurological state by day 4 predicts the long-term neurological outcome (Kwakkel et al., 2003; Sprigg et al., 2007). Notably, patients older than 65 years benefit as much as younger patients from intensive rehabilitation (Baztán et al., 2009; Krebs et al., 2009), while younger patients typically improve more on mobility, balance, walking, and grip strength (Gosselin et al., 2008).

It is important to consider that in addition to the effect of ischemia, there are also general medical considerations that impact on stroke recovery. For example, an inflammatory disease precipitating the ischemic stroke may adversely affect the patient's condition, causing an enhanced sleep demand and minor recovery (Seitz et al., 2011).

The recovery of activities of daily living usually develop within 26 weeks after the stroke insult and are often accompanied by compensatory hand use (Schepers et al., 2008; Welmer et al., 2008). In controlled trials early after stroke, mirror therapy was found to improve the neurological status immediately after the intervention and at long-term follow-up (Yavuzer et al., 2008; Dohle et al., 2009).

Most functional imaging studies of cerebral changes related to recovery of motor function, speech, and attention have been performed in the chronic stage many weeks after the ischemic stroke. Since there is a variable amount of spontaneous recovery in the acute and subacute stage after stroke (Duncan et al., 2000; Kwakkel et al., 2003), the majority of studies has been focused on the chronic stages in order to investigate the specific effect of rehabilitative training. Similarly, noninvasive cortical stimulation with anodal transcranial direct current stimulation (tDCS) and repetitive transcranial magnetic stimulation (rTMS) in patients with chronic stroke provide proof-of-principle evidence for modulation of functional representations in the human brain (see also Chapters 5 and 10). Both methods applied to the affected hemisphere, preferably in association with motor training, were observed to improve motor performance (Hummel et al., 2005; Nair et al., 2007; Talelli et al., 2007; Khedr et al., 2009). Along the same line, combining peripheral nerve stimulation to the affected hand with anodal direct current stimulation of the affected motor cortex in chronic stroke facilitates motor performance beyond levels reached with either intervention alone (Celnik et al., 2009). In patients without complete recovery after stroke, Galvanic stimulation of the median nerve resulted in a displacement of the evoked cortical response in the affected hemisphere as compared with the non-affected hemisphere, in proportion to clinical recovery (Tecchio et al., 2007).

An important and largely neglected aspect of hemiparesis, however, is the presence of spasticity that typically builds up progressively after stroke, counteracting voluntary movement. Botulinum toxin is an effective drug to alleviate spasticity and to release the affected limbs for active or passive movements in chronic stroke patients (Francis et al., 2004). When botulinum toxin was combined with repetitive bilateral arm cycling training in chronic stroke patients, spasticity could be reduced. This was also reflected by a profound change of the cerebral activation pattern (Figure 6.3). Residual sensorimotor function was a prerequisite, since patients with residual motor activity benefitted more from this treatment regime than patients with complete absence of spontaneous movement activity on the affected side (Diserens et al., 2010).

6.5 CONCLUSIONS

After stroke the human brain has the capability to regain functions which have been impaired by structural damage in cerebral grey and white matter. The greatest effect for recovery is brought about by early recanalization therapy using thrombolysis. This is followed by a slowly evolving recovery of function lasting for many months and years. It is paralleled by normalization of functional representations involving neural networks in both cerebral hemispheres. These changes can be enhanced by dedicated rehabilitation and experimental modulation of functional representations in the human brain, as evident from clinical, fMRI, and neurophysiological studies.

REFERENCES

Albers, G. W., Thijs, V. N., Wechsler, L., Kemp, S., Schlaug, G., Skalabrin, E., et al. (2006). Magnetic resonance imaging profiles predict clinical response to early reperfusion: the diffusion and perfusion imaging evaluation for understanding stroke evolution (DEFUSE) study. *Annals of Neurology, 60*, 508–517.

Almekhlafi, M. A., Hu, W. Y., Hill, M. D., & Auer. R. N. (2008). Calcification and endothelialization of thrombi in acute stroke. *Annals of Neurology, 64*, 344–352.

Alexandrov, A. V., Burgin, W. S., Demchuk, A. M., El Mitwalli, A., & Grotta. J. C. (2001). Speed of intracranial clot lysis with intravenous tissue plasminogen activator therapy: sonographic classification and short-term improvement. *Circulation, 103*, 2897–2902.

Alexandrov, A. V., Demchuk, A. M., Felberg, R. A., Christou, I., Barber, P. A., Burgin, W. S., et al. (2000). High rate of complete recanalization and dramatic clinical recovery during tPA infusion when continuously monitored with 2-MHz transcranial doppler monitoring. *Stroke, 31*, 610–614.

Pluchino, S., Muzio, L., Imitola, J., Deleidi, M., Alfaro-Cervello, C., Salani, G., et al. (2008). Persistent inflammation alters the function of the endogenous brain stem cell compartment. *Brain, 131*, 2564–2578.

Arac, A., Blanchard, V., Lee, M., & Steinberg, G. K. (2009). Assessment of outcome following decompressive craniectomy for malignant middle cerebral artery infarction in patients older than 60 years of age. *Neurosurgery Focus, 26*(6), E3.

Askam, T., Indredavik, B., Vangberg, T., & Haberg, A. (2009). Motor network changes associated with successful motor skill relearning after acute ischemic stroke: a longitudinal functional magnetic resonance imaging study. *Neurorehabilitation and Neural Repair, 23*, 295–304.

Bang, O. Y., Lee, P. H., Heo, K. G., Joo, U. S., Yoon, S. R., & Kim, S. Y. (2005). Stroke specific DWI lesion patterns predict prognosis after acute ischaemic stroke within the MCA territory. *Journal of Neurology, Neurosurgery and Psychiatry, 76*, 1222–1228.

Bang, O. Y., Saver, J. L., Buck, B. H., Alger, J. R., Starkman, S., Ovbiagele, B., et al. (2008). Impact of collateral flow on tissue fate in acute ischaemic stroke. *Journal of Neurology, Neurosurgery and Psychiatry, 79*, 625–629.

Barton, J. J. (2008). Structure and function in acquired prosopagnosia: lessons from a series of 10 patients with brain damage. *Journal of Neuropsychology, 2*, 197–225.

Baztán, J. J., Gálvez, C. P., & Soccoro, A. (2009). Reocvery of functional impairment after acute illness and mortality: one-year follow-up study. *Gerontology, 55*, 269–274.

Beaulieu, C., de Crespigny, A., Tong, D. C., Moseley, M. E., Albers, G. W., & Marks, M. P. (1999). Longitudinal magnetic resonance imaging study of perfusion and diffusion in stroke: evolution of lesion volume and correlation with clinical outcome. *Annals of Neurology, 46*, 568–578.

Beebe, J. A., & Lang, C. E. (2009). Active range of motion predicts upper extremity function 3 months after stroke. *Stroke, 40*, 1772–1792.

Bejot, Y., Benatru, I., Rouaud, O., Fromont, A., Besancenot, J. P., Moreau, T., et al. (2007). Epidemiology of stroke in Europe: geographic and environmental differences. *Journal of Neurological Science, 262*, 85–88.

Bhatt, E., Nagpal, A., Greer, K. H., Grunewald, T. K., Steele, J. L., Wiemiller, J. W., et al. (2007). Effect of finger tracking combined with electrical stimulation on brain reorganization and hand function in subjects with stroke. *Experimental Brain Research, 182*, 435–447.

Biernaskie, J., & Corbett D. (2001). Enriched rehabilitative training promotes improved forelimb motor function and enhanced dendritic growth after focal ischemic injury. *Journal of Neuroscience, 21*, 5272–5280.

Binkofski, F., Dohle, C., Posse, S., Stephan, K M., Hefter, H., Seitz, R. J. et al. (1998). Human anterior intraparietal area subserves prehension. A combined lesion and functional MRI activation study. *Neurology, 50*, 1253–1259.

Binkofski, F., Seitz, R.J., Arnold, S., Claßen, J., Benecke, R., & Freund, H.-J. (1996). Thalamic metabolism and integrity of the pyramidal tract determine motor recovery in stroke. *Annals of Neurology, 39*, 460–470.

Binkofski, F., & Seitz, R. J. (2004). Modulation of the BOLD-response in early recovery from sensorimotor stroke. *Neurology, 63*, 1223–1229.

Blondin, D., Seitz, R. J., Rusch, O., Janssen, H., Andersen, K., Wittsack, H. J., et al. (2009). Clinical impact of MRI perfusion disturbances and normal diffusion in acute stroke patients. *European Journal of Radiology, 71*, 1–10.

Boake, C., Noser, E. A., Ro, T., Baraniuk, S., Gaber, M., Johnson, R., et al. (2008). Constraint-induced movement therapy during early stroke rehabilitation. *Neurorehabilitation and Neural Repair, 21*, 14–24.

Boiten, J., & Lodder, J. (1991). Lacunar infarcts. Pathogenesis and validity of the clinical syndromes. *Stroke, 22*, 1374–1378.

Brodtmann, A., Puce, A., Darby, D., & Donnan, G. (2009). Serial functional imaging poststroke reveals visual cortex reorganization. *Neurorehabilitation and Neural Repair, 23*, 150–159.

Bütefisch, C. M., Kleiser, R., Körber, B., Müller, K., Wittsack, H.-J., Homberg, V., et al. (2005). Recruitment of contralesional motor cortex in stroke patients with recovery of hand function. *Neurology, 64*, 1067–1069.

Bütefisch, C. M., Netz, J., Wessling, M., Seitz, R. J., & Hömberg, V. (2003). Remote changes in cortical excitability after stroke. *Brain, 126*, 470–481.

Bütefisch, C. M., Wessling, M., Netz, J., Seitz, R. J., & Hömberg, V. (2008). Excitability and of ipsi- and contralesional motor cortices and their relationship in stroke patients. *Neurorehabilitation and Neural Repair, 22*, 4–21.

Canedo, A. (1997). Primary motor cortex influences on the descending and ascending systems. *Progress in Neurobiology, 51*, 287–335.

Carey, L. M., & Seitz, R. J. (2007). Functional neuroimaging in stroke recovery and neurorehabilitation: conceptual issues and perspectives. *International Journal of Stroke, 2*, 245–264.

Carmichael, S. T., Wei, L., Rovainen, C. M., & Woolsey, T. A. (2005). Growth-associated gene expression after stroke: evidence for a growth-promoting region in the peri-infarct cortex. *Experimental Neurology, 193*, 291–311.

Celnik, P., Paik, N. J., Vandermeeren, Y., Dimyan, M., & Cohen, L. G. (2009). Effects of combined peripheral nerve stimulation and brain polarization on performance of a motor sequence task after chronic stroke. *Stroke, 40*, 1764–1771.

Centonze, D., Rossi, S., Tortiglione, A., et al. (2007). Synaptic plasticity during recovery from permanent oc of the middle cerebral artery. *Neurobiological Disorders, 27*, 44–53.

Chemmanam, T., Campbell, B. C., Christensen, S., Nagakane, Y., Desmond, P. M., Bladin, C. F., et al. (2010). Ischemic diffusion lesion reversal is uncommon and rarely alters perfusion-diffusion mismatch. *Neurology, 75*, 1040–1047.

Cincenelli, P., Pascualetti, P., Zaccagnini, M., Traversa, R., Oliveri, M., & Rossini, P. M. (2003). Interhemispheric asymmetries of motor cortex excitability in the postacute stroke stage: a paired-pulse transcranial magnetic stimulation study. *Stroke, 34*, 2653–2658.

Classen, J., Schnitzler, A., Binkofski, F., Werhahn, K. J., Kim, Y. S., Kessler, K. R., et al. (1997) The motor syndrome associated with exaggerated inhibition within the primary motor cortex of patients with hemiparetic. *Brain, 120* (4), 605–619.

Connell, L. A., Lincoln, N. B., & Radford, K. A. (2008). Somatosensory impairment after stroke: frequency of different deficits and their recovery. *Clinical Rehabilitation, 22*, 758–767.

Crafton, K. R., Mark, A. N., & Cramer, S. C. (2003). Improved understanding of cortical injury by incorporating measures of functional anatomy. *Brain, 126*, 1650–1659.

Cramer, S. C. (2008a). Repairing the human brain after stroke: I. Mechanisms of spontaneous recovery. *Annals of Neurology, 63*, 272–287.

Cramer, S. C. (2008b). Repairing the human brain after stroke: II. Restorative therapies. *Annals of Neurology; 63*; 549–560.

Cumming, T. B., Thrift, A. G., Collier, J. M., Churilov, L., Dewey, H. M., Donnan, G. A. et al. (2011). Very early mobilization after stroke fast-tracks return to walking: further results from the phase II AVERT randomized controlled trial. *Stroke, 42*, 153–158.

Dancause, N., Barbay, S., Frost, S. B., Plautz, E. J., Chen, D., & Zoubina, E. V. et al. (2005). Extensive cortical rewiring after brain injury. *Journal of Neuroscience, 25*, 10167–10179.

Davis, S. M., Donnan, G. A., Parsons, M. W., Levi, C., Butcher, K. S., Peeters, A., et al. (2008). Effects of alteplase beyond 3 h after stroke in the Echoplanar Imaging Thrombolytic Evaluation Trial (EPITHET): a placebo-controlled randomised trial. *Lancet Neurology, 7*, 299–309.

Delgado-Mederos, R., Rovira, A., Alvarez-Sabín, J., Ribo, M., Munuera, J., Rubiera, M., et al. (2007). Speed of tPA-induced clot lysis predicts DWI lesion evolution in acute stroke. *Stroke, 38*, 955–960.

Dewey, H.M., Sturm, J., Donnan, G. A., MacDonnel, R. A., McNeill, J. J., Thrift, A. G. (2003). Incidence and outcome of subtypes of ischaemic stroke: initial results from the North East Melbourne stroke incidence study (NEMESIS). *Cerebrovascular Diseases, 15*, 133–139.

Dihné, M., Seitz, R. J., & Hartung, H.-P. (2011). Cell therapy for stroke: neuronal functionality meets post-stroke plasticity. *Stroke, 42*, 2342–2350.

Dirnagl, U., Iadecola, C., & Moskowitz, M. A. (1999). Pathobiology of ischaemic stroke: An integrated view. *Trends in Neuroscience, 22*, 391–397.

Diserens, K., Ruegg, D., Kleiser, R., Hyde, S., Perret, N., Vuadens, P., et al. (2010). Effect of repetitive arm cycling following Botulinum toxin for post-stroke spasticity: evidence from fMRI. *Neurorehabilitation and Neural Repair, 24*, 753–762.

Dohle, C., Püllen, J., Nakaten, A., Küst, J., Rietz, C., & Karbe, H. (2009). Mirror therapy promotes recovery from severe hemiparesis: a randomized controlled trial. *Neurorehabilitation and Neural Repair, 23*, 209–217.

Dohmen, C., Sakowitz, O.W., Fabricius, M., Bosche, B., Reithmeier, T., Ernestus, R-I., et al. (2008). Spreading depolarizations occur in human ischemic stroke with high incidence. *Annals of Neurology, 63*, 720–728.

Donnan, G. A., Bladin, P. F., Berkovic, S. F., Longley, W. A., & Saling, M. M (1991). The stroke syndrome of striatocapsular infarction. *Brain, 114*, 51–70.

Donnan, G. A., Baron, J. C., Ma, M., & Davis, S.M. (2009). Penumbral selection of patients for trials of acute stroke therapy. *Lancet Neurology, 8*, 261–269.

Dong, Y., Winstein, C.J., Albestegui-DuBois, R., & Dobkin, B. H. (2007). Evolution of fMRI activation in the perilesional primary motor cortex and cerebellum with rehabilitation training-related motor gains after stroke: a pilot study. *Neurorehabilitation and Neural Repair, 21*, 412–428.

Dreier, J. P., Major, S., Manning, A., Woitzik, J., Drenckhahn, C., Steinbrink, J., et al. (2009). Cortical spreading ischaemia is a novel process involved in ischaemic damage in patients with aneurismal subarachnoid haemorrhage. *Brain, 132*, 1866–1881.

Duncan, P. W., Lai, S. M., & Keighley, J. (2000). Defining post-stroke recovery: implications for design and interpretation of drug trials. *Neuropharmacology, 39*, 835–841.

Ertelt, D., Small, S., Solodkin, A., Dettmers, C., McNamara, A., Binkofski, F., et al. (2007) Action observation has a positive impact on rehabilitation of motor deficits after stroke. *NeuroImage, 36*, Suppl 2, T164–T173.

Finelli, P.F. (2008). Neuroimaging in acute posterior cerebral artery infarction. *Neurologist, 14*, 170–180.

Fisher, C. M. (1982). Lacunar strokes and infarcts: a review. *Neurology, 32*, 871–876.

Floel, A., Nagorsen, U., Werhahn, K. J., Ravindran, S., Birbaumer, N., Knecht, S., et al. (2004). Influence of somatosensory input on motor function in patients with chronic stroke. *Annals of Neurology, 56*, 206–212.

Foltys, H., Krings, T., Meister, I. G., Sparing, R., Boroojerdi, B., Thron, A., et al. (2003). Motor representation in patients rapidly recovering after stroke: a functional magnetic resonance imaging and transcranial magnetic stimulation study. *Clinical Neurophysiology, 114*, 2404–2015.

Fornage, M., Debette, S., Bis, J. C., Schmidt, H., Ikram, A., Dufouil, C., et al. (2011). Genome-wide association studies of cerebral white matter lesion burden: the CHARGE consortium. *Annals of Neurology, 69*, 928–939.

Francis, H. P., Wade, D. T., Turner-Stokes, L., Kingswell, R. S., Dott, C. S., & Coxon, E.A. (2004). Does reducing spasticity translate into functional benefit? An exploratory meta-analysis. *Journal of Neurology, Neurosurgery and Psychiatry, 75*, 1547–1551.

Fregni, F., Boggio, P. S., Mansur, C. G., Wagner, T., Ferreira, M., Lima, M., et al. (2005) Transcranial direct current stimulation of the unaffected hemisphere in stroke patients. *Neuroreport, 16*, 1551–1555.

Fries, W., Danek, A., & Witt, T. N. (1991) Motor responses after transcranial electrical stimulation of cerebral hemispheres with a degenerated pyramidal tract. *Annals of Neurology, 29*, 646–650.

Frost, S. B., Barbay, S., Friel, K. M., Plautz, E. J., & Nudo, R. J. (2003). Reorganization of remote cortical regions after ischemic brain injury: a potential substrate for stroke recovery. *Journal of Neurophysiology, 89*, 3205–3214.

Gauthier, L. V., Taub, E., Perkins, C., Ortmann, M., Mark, U. W., & Uswatte, G. (2008). Remodelling the brain: plastic structural brain changes produced by different motor therapies after stroke. *Stroke, 39*, 1520–1525.

Glymour, M. M., Berkman, L. F., Ertel, K. A., Fay, M. E., Glass, T. A., & Furie, K. L. (2007). Lesion characteristics, NIH stroke scale, and functional recovery after stroke. *American Journal of Physical Medicine and Rehabilitation, 86*, 725–733.

Gosselin, S., Desrosier, J., Corriveau, H., Hebert, R., Rochette, A., Provencher, V., et al. (2008). Outcomes during and after inpatient rehabilitation: comparison between adults and older adults. *Journal of Rehabilitative Medicine, 40*, 55–60.

Grefkes, C., Nowak, D. A., Eickhoff, S. B., Dafotakis, M., Kust, J., Karbe, H., et al. (2008). Cortical connectivity after subcortical stroke assessed with functional magnetic resonance imaging. *Annals of Neurology, 63*, 236–246.

Guadagno, J. V., Jonas, P. S., Aigbirghio, F. I., et al. (2008). Selective neuronal loss in rescued penumbra relates to initial hypoperfusion. *Brain, 131*, 2666–2678.

Hacke, W., Donnan, G., Fieschi, C., Kaste, M., von Kummer, R., Broderick, J. P., et al. (2004). Association of outcome with early stroke treatment: pooled analysis of ATLANTIS, ECASS, and NINDS rt-PA stroke trials. *Lancet, 363*, 768–774.

Hacke, W., Kaste, M., Bluhmki, E., Brozman, M., Davalos, A., Guidetti, D., et al. (2008). Thrombolysis with alteplase 3 to 4.5 hours after acute ischemic stroke. *New England Journal of Medicine, 359*, 1317–1329.

Hamzei, F., Dettmers, C., Rijntjes, M., & Weiller, C. (2008). The effect of cortico-spinal tract damage on primary sensorimotor cortex activation after rehabilitation therapy. *Experimental Brain Research, 190*, 329–336.

Hamzei, F., Knab, R., Weiller, C., & Röther, J. (2003). The influence of extra- and intracranial artery disease on the BOLD signal in fMRI. *NeuroImage, 20*, 1393–1399.

Heiss, W. D., Huber, M., Fink, G. R., Herholz, K. M., Pietrzyk, U., Wagner, R., et al. (1992) Progressive derangement of periinfarct viable tissue in ischemic stroke. *Journal of Cerebral Blood Flow and Metabolism, 12*, 193–203.

Heiss, W. D., Grond, M., Thiel, A. von Stockhausen, H-M., Rudolf, J., Ghaemi, M., et al. (1998). Tissue at risk of infarction rescued by early reperfusion: a positron emission tomography study in systemic recombinant tissue plasminogen activator thrombolysis of acute stroke. *Journal of Cerebral Blood Flow and Metabolism, 18,* 1298–1307.

Heiss, W. D., Sobeski, J., Smekal, U., Kracht, L.W., Lehnhardt, F-G., Thiel, A., et al. (2004). Probability of cortical infarction predicted by flumazenil binding and diffusion-weighted imaging signal intensity: a comparative positron emission tomography/magnetic resonance imaging study in early ischemic stroke. *Stroke, 35,* 1892–1898.

Hermanns, S., Klapka, N., & Müller, H. W. (2001). The collagenous lesion scar — an obstacle for axonal regeneration in brain and spinal cord injury. *Restorative Neurology and Neuroscience, 19,* 139–148.

Hesse, S. (2008). Treadmill training with partial body weight support after stroke: a review. *Neurorehabilitation, 23,* 55–65.

Hillis, A. E., Gold, L., Kannan, V., Cloutman, L., Kleinman, J. T., Newhart, M., et al. (2008). Site of the ischemic penumbra as a predictor of potential for recovery of functions. *Neurology, 71,* 184–189.

Hömke, L., Amunts, K., Bönig, L., Fretz, C., Binkofski, F., Zilles, K., et al. (2009). Analysis of lesions in patients with unilateral tactile agnosia using cytoarchitectonic probabilistic maps. *Human Brain Mapping, 30,* 1444–1456.

Hossmann, K.A. (1994). Viability thresholds and the penumbra of focal ischemia. *Annals of Neurology, 36,* 557–565.

Hummel, F., Celnik, P., Giraux, P., Floel, A., Wu, W-H., Gerloff, C., et al. (2005). Effects of non-invasive cortical stimulation on skilled motor function in chronic stroke. *Brain, 128,* 490–499.

Hummel, F. C., Steven, B., Hoppe, J., Heise, K., Thomalla, G., Cohen, L. G., et al. (2009). Deficient intracortical inhibition (SICI) during movement preparation after chronic stroke. *Neurology, 19,* 1766–1772.

Intiso, D., Stampatore, P., Zarrelli, M. M., Guerra, G. L., Arpaia, G., Simone, P., et al. (2003). Incidence of first-ever ischemic and hemorrhagic stroke in a well-defined community of southern Italy, 1993–1995. *European Journal of Neurology, 10,* 559–565.

Jaillard, A., Martin, C. D., Garambois, K., Lebas, J. F., & Hommel, M. (2005). Vicarious function within the human primary motor cortex? A longitudinal fMRI stroke study. *Brain, 128,* 1122–1138.

Kang, S. Y., & Kim, J. S. (2008). Anterior cerebral artery infarction. Stroke mechanism and clinical-imaging study in 100 patients. *Neurology, 70,* 2386–2393.

Karnath, H. O., Fruhmann Berger, M., Kuker, W., & Rorden, C. (2004). The anatomy of spatial neglect based on voxelwise statistical analysis: a study of 140 patients. *Cerebral Cortex, 14,* 1164–1172.

Karnath, H. O., Rorden, C., & Ticini, L. F. (2009) Damage to white matter fibre tracts in acute spatial neglect. *Cerebral Cortex, 19,* 2331–2337.

Khedr, E. M., Abdel-Fadeil, M. R., Farghali, A., & Qaid, M. (2009). Role of 1 and 3 Hz repetitive transcranial magnetic stimulation on motor function recovery after acute ischaemic stroke. *European Journal of Neurology, 16,* 1323–1330.

Kennedy, P. R. (1990). Corticospinal, rubrospinal and rubro-olivary projections: a unifying hypothesis. Trends in Neuroscience 13: 474–479.

Kidwell, C. S., Saver, J. L., Starkman, S., Duckwiler, G., Jahan, R., Vespa, P., et al. (2002). Late secondary ischemic injury in patients receiving intraarterial thrombolysis. *Annals of Neurology, 52,* 698–703.

Kim, J. S. (2001). Predominant involvement of a particular group of fingers due to small, cortical infarction. *Neurology, 56,* 1677–1682.

Kim, Y. H., Kim, D. S., Hong, J. H., Park, C. H., Hua, N., Bickart, K. C., et al. (2008). Corticospinal tract location in internal capsule of human brain: diffusion tensor tractography and functional MRI study. *Neuroreport, 28,* 817–820.

Kimberley, T. J., Lewis, S. M., Strand, C., Rice, B. D., Hall, S., & Slivnik, P. (2008). Neural substrates of cognitive load changes during a motor task in subjects with stroke. *Journal of Neurology and Physical Therapy, 32,* 110–117.

Kleiser, R., Wittsack, H.-J., Bütefisch, C. M., Jörgens, S., & Seitz, R. J. (2005). Functional activation within the PI-DWI mismatch region in recovery from hemiparetic stroke: preliminary observations. *NeuroImage, 24,* 515–523.

Kokaia, Z., Thored, P., Arvidsson, A., & Lindvall, O. (2006). Regulation of stroke-induced neurogenesis in adult brain—recent scientific progress. *Cerebral Cortex, 16,* 162–167.

Krebs, H. I., Volpe, B., & Hogan, N. (2009). A working model of stroke recovery from rehabilitation robotics practitioners. *Journal of Neuroengineering and Rehabilitation, 25,* 6.

Kretschmann, H. J. (1988). Localisation of the corticospinal fibres in the internal capsule in man. *Journal of Anatomy, 160,* 219–225.

Kurada, S., & Houkin, K. (2008). Moyamoya disease: current concepts and future perspectives. *Lancet Neurology, 7,* 1056–1066.

Kwakkel, G., Wagenaar, R.C., Twisk, J.W., Lankhorst, G.J., & Koetsier, J.C. (1999). Intensity of leg and arm training after primary middle-cerebral-artery stroke: a randomised trial. *Lancet, 354,* 191–196.

Kwakkel, G., Kollen, B. J., van der Grond, J., & Prevo, A. J. (2003). Probability of regaining dexterity in the flaccid upper limb: impact of severity of paresis and time since onset in acute stroke. *Stroke, 34,* 2181–2186.

Lang, C. E., & Schieber, M. H. (2004). Reduced muscle selectivity during individuated finger movements in humans after damage to the motor cortex or corticospinal tract. *Journal of Neurophysiology, 91,* 1722–1733.

Lang, C. E., Dejong, S. L., & Beebe, J. A. (2009). Recovery of thumb and finger extension and its relation to grasp performance after stroke. *Journal of Neurophysiology, 102,* 451–459.

Lee, L. J., Kidwell, C. S., Alger, J., Starkman, S., & Saver, J. L. (2000). Impact on stroke subtype diagnosis of early diffusion-weighted magnetic resonance imaging and magnetic resonance angiography. *Stroke, 31,* 1081–1089.

Lewis, G. N., & Perreault, E. J. (2007). Side of lesion influences bilateral activation in chronic, post-stroke hemiparesis. *Clinical Neurophysiology, 118,* 2050–2062.

Li, F., Liu, K. F., Silva, M. D., Omae, T., Sotak, C. H., Fenstermacher, J. D., et al. (2000). Transient and permanent resolution of ischemic lesions on diffusion- weighted imaging after brief periods of focal ischemia in rats: correlation with histopathology. *Stroke, 31,* 946–954.

Liebeskind, D. S., Cotsonis, G. A., Saver, J. L., Lynn, M. J., Turan, T. N., Cloft, H. J., et al. (2011). Collaterals dramatically alter stroke risk in intracranial atherosclerosis. *Annals of Neurology, 69,* 963–974.

Liepert, J., Miltner, W., Bauder, H., Sommer, M., Dettmers, C., Taub, E., et al. (1998). Motor cortex plasticity during constraint-induced movement therapy in stroke patients. *Neuroscience Letters, 250,* 5–8.

Liepert, J., Storch, P., Fritsch, A., & Weiller, C. (2000). Motor cortex disinhibition in acute stroke. *Clinical Neurophysiology, 111,* 671–676.

Liepert, J., Haevernick, K., Weiller, C., & Barzel, A. (2006). The surround inhibition determines therapy-induced cortical reorganization. *NeuroImage, 32,* 1216–1220.

Lindberg, P. G., Schmitz, C., Engardt, M., Forssberg, H., & Borg, J. (2007). Use-dependent up- and down-regulation of sensorimotor brain circuits in stroke patients. *Neurorehabilitation and Neural Repair, 21,* 315–326.

Lindenberg, R., Renga, V., Zhu, L. L., Betzler, F., Alsop, D., & Schlaug, G. (2010a). Structural integrity of corticospinal motor fibres predict motor impairment in chronic stroke. *Neurology, 74,* 280–287.

Lindenberg, R., Renga, V., Zhu, L. L., Nair, D., & Schlaug, G. (2010b). Bihemispheric brain stimulation facilitates motor recovery in chronic stroke patients. *Neurology, 75,* 2176–2184.

Lindenberg, R., Zhu, L. L., Rüber, T., & Schlaug, G. (2011). Predicting functional motor potential in chronic stroke patients using diffusion tensor imaging. *Human Brain Mapping,* in press. DOI: 10.1002/hbm.21266.

Luft, A. R., Macko, R. F., Forrester, L. W., Villagra, F., Ivey, F., Sorkin, J. D., et al. (2008). Treadmill exercise activates subcortical neural networks and improves walking after stroke: a randomized controlled trial. *Stroke, 39,* 3341–3350.

Malouin, F., Richards, C. L., Durand, A., Descent, M., Poire, D., Fremont, P., et al. (2009). Effects of practice, visual loss, limb amputation, and disuse on motor imagery vividness. *Neurorehabiliation and Neural Repair, 23,* 449–463.

Manganotti, P., Acler, M., Zanette, G. P., Smania, N., & Fiaschi, A. (2008) Motor cortical disinhibition during early and late recovery after stroke. *Neurorehabilitation and Neural Repair, 22,* 396–403.

Marangolo, P., Rizzi, C., Peran, P., Piras, F., & Sabatini, U. (2009). Parallel recovery in a bilingual aphasic: a neurolinguistic and fMRI study. *Neuropsychology, 23,* 405–409.

Marshall, R. S., Perera, G. M., Lazar, R. M., Krakauer, J. W., Constantine, R. C., & DeLaPaz, R. L. (2000). Evolution of cortical activation during recovery from corticospinal tract infarction. *Stroke, 31,* 656–661.

Marshall, R. S., Zarahn, E., Alon, L., Minzer, B., Lazar, R. M., & Krakauer, J. W. (2009). Early imaging correlates of subsequent motor recovery after stroke. *Annals of Neurology, 65,* 596–602.

McCombe Waller, S., Forrester, L., Villagra, F., & Whitall, J. (2008). Intracortical inhibition and facilitation with unilateral dominant, unilateral nondominant and bilateral movement tasks in left- and right-handed adults. *Journal of Neurological Science, 269,* 96–104.

McCombe, P. A., & Read, S. J. (2008). Immune and inflammatory responses to stroke: good or bad? *International Journal of Stroke, 3,* 254–265.

Merino, J. G., Latour, L. L., An, L., Hsia, A. W., Kang, D. W., & Warach, S. (2008). Reperfusion half-life: a novel pharmacodynamic measure of thrombolytic activity. *Stroke, 39,* 2148–2150.

Mintzopoulos, D., Khanicheh, A., Konstas, A. A., Astrakas, L. G., Singhal, A. B., Moskowitz, M. A., et al. (2008). Functional MRI of rehabilitation in chronic stroke patients using novel MR-compatible hand robotics. *Open Neuroimaging J, 2,* 94–101.

Misawa, S., Kuwabara, S., Matsuda, S., Honma, K., Ono, J., & Hattori, T. (2008). The ipsilateral cortico-spinal tract is activated after hemiparetic stroke. *European Journal of Neurology, 15,* 706–711.

Moustafa, R. P., & Baron, J. C. (2008). Pathophysiology of ischaemic stroke: insights from imaging, and implications for therapy and drug discovery. *British Journal of Pharmacology, 153* Suppl 1, S44–S54.

Mudie, M.H., & Matyas, T.A. (2001) Responses of the densely hemiplegic upper extremity to bilateral training. *Neurorehabilitation and Neural Repair, 15,* 129–140.

Muehlbacher, W., Richards, C., Ziemann, U., & Hallett, M. (2002). Improving hand function in chronic stroke. *Archives of Neurology, 59,* 1278–1282.

Müller, K., Bütefisch, C. M., Seitz, R. J., & Hömberg, V. (2007). Mental practice improves hand function after hemiparetic stroke. *Restorative Neurology and Neuroscience, 25,* 501–511.

Nair, D. G., Hutchinson, S., Fregni, F., Alexander, M., Pascual-Leone, A., & Schlaug, G. (2007). Imaging correlates of motor recovery from cerebral infarction and their physiological significance in well-recovered patients. *NeuroImage, 34,* 253–263.

Nelles, G., Cramer, S., Schaechter, J., Kaplan, J., & Finklestein, S. (1998). Quantitative assessment of mirror movements after stroke. *Stroke, 29,* 1182–1187.

Neumann-Haefelin, T., Wittsack, H.-J., Wenserski, F., et al. (1999). Diffusion- and perfusion-weighted MRI. The DWI/PWI mismatch region in acute stroke. *Stroke, 30,* 1591–1597.

Neumann-Haefelin, T., du Mesnil de Rochemont, R., Fiebach, J. B., Gass, A., Nolte, C., Kucinski, T., et al. (2004). Effect of incomplete (spontaneous and postthrombolytic) recanalization after middle cerebral artery occlusion: a magnetic resonance imaging study. *Stroke, 35,* 109–114.

Nhan, H., Barquist, K., Bell, K., Esselman, P., Odderson, I., & Cramer, S. (2004). Brain function early after stroke in relation to subsequent recovery. *Journal of Cerebral Blood Flow and Metabolism, 24,* 756–763.

Nowak, D. A., Grefkes, C., Dafotakis, M., Eickhoff, S., Kust, J., Karbe, H., et al. (2008). Effects of low-frequency repetitive transcranial magnetic stimulation of the contralesional primary motor cortex on movement kinematics and neural activity in subcortical stroke. *Archives of Neurology, 65,* 741–747.

Nudo, R., Wise, B., SiFuentes, F., & Milliken, G. (1996). Neural substrates for the effects of rehabilitative training on motor recovery after ischemic infarct. *Science, 272,* 1791–1794.

Ohab, J. J., Fleming, S., Blesch, A., & Carmichael, S. T. (2006). A vascular niche for neurogenesis after stroke. *Journal of Neuroscience, 26,* 13007–13016.

Olivot, J. M., Mlynash, M., Thijs, V. N., Kemp, S., Lansberg, M. G., Wechsler, L., et al. (2008a). Optimal Tmax threshold for predicting penumbral tissue in acute stroke. *Stroke, 40,* 469–475.

Olivot, J. M., Mlynash, M., Thijs, V. N., Kemp, S., Lansberg, M. G., Wechsler, L., et al. (2008b). Relationships between infarct growth, clinical outcome, and early recanalization in diffusion and perfusion imaging for understanding stroke evolution (DEFUSE). *Stroke, 39,* 2257–2263.

Page, S. J., Szaflarski, J. P., Eliassen, J. C., Pan, H., & Cramer, S. C. (2009). Cortical plasticity following motor skill learning during mental practice in stroke. *Neurorehabilitation and Neural Repair, 23,* 382–388.

Pannek, K., Chalk, J. B., Finnigan, S., & Rose, S. E. (2009). Dynamic corticospinal white matter connectivity changes during stroke recovery: a diffusion tensor probabilistic tractography study. *Journal of Magnetic Resonance Imaging, 29,* 529–536.

Parsons, M. W., Barber, P. A., Desmond, P. M., Baird, T. A., Darby, D. G., Byrnes, G., et al. (2002). Acute hyperglycemia adversely affects stroke outcome: a magnetic resonance imaging and spectroscopy study. *Annals of Neurology, 52,* 20–28.

Pazzaglia, M., Smania, N., Corato, E., & Aglioti, S. M. (2008). Neural underpinnings of gesture discrimination in patients with limb apraxia. *Journal of Neuroscience, 28,* 3030–3041.

Perez, M. A., & Cohen, L.G. (2008) Mechanisms underlying functional changes in the primary motor cortex ipsilateral to an active hand. *Journal of Neuroscience, 28,* 5631–5640.

Platz, T., van Kaick, S., Mehrholz, J., Leidner, O., Eickhoff, C., & Pohl, M. (2009). Best conventional therapy versus modular impairment-oriented training for arm paresis after stroke: a single-blind, multicenter randomized controlled trial. *Neurorehabilitation and Neural Repair, 23,* 706–716.

Poggel, D. A., Mueller, I., Kasten, E., & Sabel, B. A. (2008). Multifactorial predictors and outcome variables of vision restoration training in patients with post-geniculate visual field loss. *Restorative Neurology and Neuroscience, 26,* 321–339.

Price, C. J., Wang, D., Menon, D. K., Guardagno, J. V., Cleij, M., Fryer, T., et al. (2006) Intrinsic activated microglia map to the peri-infarct zone in the subacute phase of ischemic stroke. *Stroke, 37,* 1749–1753.

Redecker, C., Luhmann, H. J., Hagemann, G., Fritschy, J. M., & Witte, O. W. (2000) .Differential downregulation of GABAA receptor subunits in widespread brain regions in the freeze-lesion model of focal cortical malformations. *Journal of Neuroscience, 20,* 5045–5053.

Reis, J., Schambra, H. M., Cohen, L. G., Buch, E. R., Fritsch, B., Zarahn, E., et al. (2009). Noninvasive cortical stimulation enhances motor skill acquisition over multiple days through an effect on consolidation. *Proceedings of the National Academy of Science USA, 106,* 1590–1595.

Rey, B., Frischknecht, R., Maeder, P., & Clarke, S. (2007). Patterns of recovery following focal hemispheric lesions: relationship between lasting deficit and damage to specialized networks. *Restorative Neurology and Neuroscience, 25,* 285–294.

Rohl, L., Ostergaard, L., Simonsen, C. Z., Vestergaard-Poulsen, P., Andersen, G., Sakoh, M., et al. (2001). Viability thresholds of ischemic penumbra of hyperacute stroke defined by perfusion-weighted MRI and apparent diffusion coefficient. *Stroke, 32,* 1140–1146.

Rother, J., Schellinger, P. D., Gass, A., et al. (2002). Effect of intravenous thrombolysis on MRI parameters and functional outcome in acute stroke <6 hours. *Stroke, 33,* 2438–2445.

Rusconi, E., Pinel, P., Eger, E., LeBihan, D., Thirion, B., Dehaene, S., et al. (2009). A disconnection account of Gerstmann syndrome: functional neuroanatomy evidence. *Annals of Neurology, 66,* 654–662.

Saleh, A., Schroeter, M., Jonkmanns, C., Hartung, H. P., Mödder, U., & Jander, S. (2004). In vivo MRI of brain inflammation in human ischaemic stroke. *Brain, 127,* 1670–1677.

Saleh, A., Schroeter, M., Ringelstein, A., Hartung, H-P., Siebler, M., Modder, U., et al. (2007). Iron oxide particle-enhanced MRI suggests variability of brain inflammation at early stages after ischemic stroke. *Stroke, 38,* 2733–2737.

Saqqur, M., Tsivgoulis, G., Molina, C. A., Demchuk, A. M., Shuaib, A., Alexandrov, A.V., CLOTBUST investigators. (2009). Residual flow at the site of intracranial occlusion on transcranial Doppler predicts response to intravenous thrombolysis: a multi-center study. *Cerebrovascular Diseases, 27,* 5–12.

Saur, D., Lange, R., Baumgaertner, A., Schraknepper, V., Willmes, K., Rijntjes, M., et al. (2006). Dynamics of language reorganization after stroke. *Brain, 129,* 1371–1384.

Sawaki, L., Butler, A.J., Leng, X., Wassenaar, P. A., Mohammad, Y. M., Blanton, S., et al. (2008). Constraint-induced movement therapy results in increased motor map area in subjects 3 to 9 months after stroke. *Neurorehabilitation and Neural Repair, 22,* 505–513.

Schäbitz, W. R., Steigleder, T., Cooper-Kuhn, C. M., Schwab, S., Sommer, C., Schneider, A., et al. (2007). Intravenous brain-derived neurotrophic factor enhances poststroke sensorimotor recovery and stimulates neurogenesis. *Stroke, 38,* 2165–2172.

Schaechter, J. D., Perdue, K. L., & Wang, R. (2008). Structural damage to the corticospinal tract correlates with bilateral sensorimotor cortex reorganization in stroke patients. *NeuroImage, 39,* 1370–1382.

Schaechter, J. D., Fricker, Z. P., Perdue, K. L., et al. (2009) Microstructural status of ipsilesional and contralesional corticospinal tract correlates with motor skill in chronic stroke patients. *Human Brain Mapping, 30,* 3461–3474.

Schäfer, R., Popp, K., Jörgens, S., Lindenberg, R., Franz, M., & Seitz, R. J. (2007). Alexithymia-like disorder in right anterior cingulate infarction. *Neurocase, 13,* 201–208.

Schepers, P., Ketelaar, M., Visser-Meily, A. J., de Groot, V., Twisk, J. W., & Lindeman, E. (2008) Functional recovery differs between ischaemic and haemorrhagic stroke patients. *Journal of Rehabilitative Medicine, 40,* 487–489.

Schiemanck, S. K., Kwakkel, G., Post, M. W., Kappelle, L. J., & Prevo, A. J. (2008). Impact of internal capsule lesions on outcome of motor hand function at one year post-stroke. *Journal of Rehabilitative Medicine, 40,* 96–101.

Schroeter, M., Saleh, A., Wiedermann, D., Hoehn, M., & Jander, S. (2004). Histochemical detection of ultrasmall superparamagnetic iron oxide (USPIO) contrast medium uptake in experimental brain ischemia. *Magnetic Resonance Medicine, 52,* 403–406.

Schwab, S., Steiner, T., Aschoff, A., Schwarz, S., Steiner, H. H., Jansen, O., et al. (1998). Early hemicraniectomy in patients with complete middle cerebral artery infarction. *Stroke, 29,* 1888–1893.

Schwerin, S., Dewald, J. P. A., Haztl, M., Jovanovich, S., Nickeas, M., & MacKinnon, C. (2008). Ipsilateral versus contralateral cortical motor projections to a shoulder adductor in chronic hemiparetic stroke: implications for the expression of arm synergies. *Experimental Brain Research, 185,* 509–519.

Seitz, R. J., Knorr, U., Azari, N. P., Herzog, H., & Freund, H.-J. (1999). Recruitment of a visuomotor network in stroke recovery. *Restorative Neurology and Neuroscience, 14,* 25–33.

Seitz, R. J., Meisel, S., Weller, P., Junghans, U., Wittsack, H.-J., & Siebler, M. (2005). The initial ischemic event: PWI and ADC for stroke evolution. *Radiology, 237,* 1020–1028.

Seitz, R. J., Sondermann, V., Wittsack, H.-J., & Siebler, M. (2009). Lesion patterns in successful and failed thrombolysis in middle cerebral artery stroke. *Neuroradiology, 51,* 865–871.

Seitz, R. J., & Donnan, G. A. (2010). Role of neuroimaging in promoting long-term recovery from ischemic stroke. *Journal of Magnetic Resonance Imaging, 32,* 756–772.

Seitz, R. J., Hildebold, T., & Simeria, K. (2011a). Spontaneous arm movement activity assessed with accelerometry is a marker for early recovery after stroke. *Journal of Neurology, 258,* 457–463.

Seitz, R. J., Oberstrass, H., Ringelstein, A., Wittsack, H.-J., & Siebler, M. (2011b). Failed recovery from thrombolysis is predicted by the initial DWI lesion. *Cerebrovascular Diseases, 31,* 580–587.

Sharma, N., Simmons, L. H., Jones, S., Day, D. J., Carpenter, A., Pomeroy, V. M., et al. (2009a). Motor imagery after subcortical stroke. A functional magnetic resonance imaging study. *Stroke, 40,* 1315–1324.

Sharma, N., Baron, J. C., Rowe, J. B. (2009b). Motor imagery after stroke: relating outcome to motor network connectivity. *Annals of Neurology, 66,* 604–616.

Shiber, J. R., Fontane, E., & Adewale, A. (2010). Stroke registry: hemorrhagic vs. ischemic strokes. *American Journal of Emergency Medicine, 28,* 331–333.

Sobesky, J., Weber, O. Z., Lehnhardt, F.-G., Hesselmann, V., Thiel, A., Dohmen, C., et al. (2004). Which time-to-peak threshold best identifies penumbral flow? A comparison of perfusion-weighted magnetic resonance imaging and positron emission tomography in acute ischemic stroke. *Stroke, 35,* 2843–2847.

Sobesky, J., Weber O. Z., Lehnhardt, F.-G., Hesselmann, V., Neveling, M., Jacobs, A., et al. (2005). Does the mismatch match the penumbra? magnetic resonance imaging and positron emission tomography in early ischemic stroke. *Stroke, 36,* 980–985.

Sprigg, N., Gray, L. J., Bath, P. M., Lindenstrom, E., Boysen, G., De Deyn, P. P., et al. (2007). Early recovery and functional outcome are related with causal stroke subtype: data from the tinzaparin in acute ischemic stroke trial. *Journal of Stroke and Cerebrovascular Disease, 16,* 180–184.

Stinear, C. M., Barber, P. A., Smale, P. R., Coxon, J. P., Fleming, M. K., & Byblow, W. D. (2007). Functional potential in chronic stroke patients depends on corticospinal tract integrity. *Brain, 130,* 170–180.

Stoeckel, M. C., Meisel, S., Wittsack, H. J., & Seitz, R. J. (2007). Pattern of cortex and white matter involvement in severe middle cerebral artery ischemia. *Journal of Neuroimaging, 17,* 131–140.

Surikova, I., Meisel, S., Siebler, M., Wittsack, H.-J., & Seitz, R.J. (2006). Significance of the perfusion-diffusion mismatch area in chronic cerebral ischemia. *Journal of Magnetic Resonance Imaging, 24,* 771–778.

Takahashi, C. D., Der-Yeghiaian, L., Le, V., Motiwala, R. R., Cramer, S. C. (2008). Robot-based hand motor therapy after stroke. *Brain, 131,* 425–437.

Talelli, P., Greenwood, R. J., & Rothwell, J. C. (2007). Exploring theta burst stimulation as an intervention to improve motor recovery in chronic stroke. *Clinical Neurophysiology, 118,* 333–342.

Taoufik, E., & Probert, L. (2008). Ischemic neuronal damage. *Current Pharmaceutical Design, 14,* 3565–3573.

Taub, E., Crago, J. E., Burgio, L. D., Groomes, T. E., Cook, E. W. 3rd, DeLuca, S. C., et al. (1994). An operant approach to rehabilitation medicine: overcoming learned nonuse by shaping. *Journal of the Experimental Analysis of Behavior, 61,* 281–293.

Taub, E., Uswatte, G., & Pidikiti, R. (1999). Constraint-induced movement therapy: a new family of techniques with broad application to physical rehabilitation—a clinical review. *Journal of Rehabilitation Research and Development, 36,* 237–251.

Tecchio, F., Zappasodi, F., Tombini, M., Caulo, M., Vernieri, F., & Rossini, P. M. (2007). Interhemispheric asymmetry of primary hand representation and recovery after stroke: a MEG study. *NeuroImage, 36,* 1057–1064.

Thiel, A., Aleksic, B., Klein, J.Ch., Rudolf, J., & Heiss, W. D. (2007). Changes in proprioceptive systems activity during recovery from post-stroke hemiparesis. *Journal of Rehabilitative Medicine, 39,* 520–525.

Thrift, A. G., Dewey, H. M., MacDonnell, R. A., McNeil, J. J., & Donnan, G. A. (2001). Incidence of the major stroke subtypes: initial findings from the North East Melbourne stroke incidence study (NEMESIS). *Stroke, 32,* 1732–1738.

Vitali, P., Abutalebi, J., Tettamanti, M., Danna, M., Ansaldo, A-I., Perani, D., et al. (2007). Training-induced brain remapping in chronic aphasia: a pilot study. *Neurorehabilitation and Neural Repair, 21,* 152–160.

von Kummer, R., Meyding-Lamadé, U., Forsting, M., Rosin, L., Rieki, K., Hacke, W., et al. (1994). Sensitivity and prognostic value of early CT in occlusion of the middle cerebral artery trunk. *American Journal of Neuroradiology, 15,* 9–15.

Wang, X., Lam, W. W., Fan, Y. H., Graham, C. A., Rainer, T. H., & Wong, K. S. (2006). Topographic patterns of small subcortical infarcts associated with MCA stenosis: a diffusion-weighted MRI study. *Journal of Neuroimaging, 16,* 266–271.

Welmer, A. K., Holmqvist, L. W., & Sommerfeld, D. K. (2008). Limited fine hand use after stroke and its association with other disabilities. *Journal of Rehabilitative Medicine, 40,* 603–608.

Wenzelburger, R., Kopper, F., Frenzel, A., Stolze, H., Klebe, S., Brossmann, A., et al. (2005). Hand coordination following capsular stroke. *Brain, 128,* 64–74.

Winhuisen, L., Thiel, A., Schumacher, B., Kessler, J., Rudolf, J., Haupt, W.F., et al. (2007). The right inferior frontal gyrus and poststroke aphasia: a follow-up investigation. *Stroke, 38,* 1286–1292.

Witte, O. W., Bidmon, H.-J., Schiene, K., Redecker, C., & Hagemann, G. (2000). Functional differentiation of multiple perilesional zones after focal cerebral ischemia. *Journal of Cerebral Blood Flow and Metabolism, 20,* 1149–1165.

Wittenberg, G. F., Chen, R., Ishii, K., Bushara, K. O., Taub, E., Gerber, L. H. et al. (2003). Constraint-induced therapy in stroke: Magnetic-stimulation motor maps and cerebral activation. *Neurorehabilitation and Neural Repair, 16,* 1–10.

Wittsack, H. J., Ritzl, A., Fink, G. R., Wenserski, F., Siebler, M., Seitz, R. J., et al. (2002). MR Imaging in Acute Stroke: Diffusion-weighted and Perfusion Imaging Parameters for Predicting Infarct Size. *Radiology, 222,* 397–403.

Wolf, S. L., LeCraw, D. E., Barton, L. A., & Jann, B. B. (1989). Forced use of hemiplegic upper extremities to reverse the effect of learned nonuse among chronic stroke and head-injured patients. *Experimental Neurology, 104,* 125–132.

Yavuzer, G., Selles, R., Sezer, N., Sutbeyaz, S., Bussman, J. B., Koseoglu, F., et al. (2008). Mirror therapy improves hand function in sub-acute stroke: a randomized controlled trial. *Archives of Physical Medicine and Rehabilitation, 89,* 393–398.

Zhang, L., Butler, A. J., Sun, C. K., Sahgal, V., Wittenberg, G. F., & Yue, G. H. (2008). Fractional dimension assessment of brain white matter structural complexity post stroke in relation to upper-extremity motor function. *Brain Research, 1228,* 299–240.

PART C | STROKE REHABILITATION: CREATING THE RIGHT LEARNING CONDITIONS FOR REHABILITATION

7 | ORGANIZATION OF CARE

DOMINIQUE A. CADILHAC, TARA PURVIS, JULIE BERNHARDT, and NICOL KORNER-BITENSKY

7.1 INTRODUCTION

The global annual incidence of stroke is estimated at 15 million (Australian Bureau of Statistics, 2008; American Heart Association, 2010). About one-third of patients are left with permanent neurological damage resulting in loss of function after stroke (Senes, 2006; American Heart Association, 2010). The economic cost and societal impact of stroke is large in contrast to other diseases (Evers et al., 2004; Cadilhac, Carter, Thrift, & Dewey, 2009; Saka, McGuire, & Wolfe, 2009; Heidenreich et al., 2011). Indeed, it is rare to find an individual who is not affected by stroke either directly or indirectly (Dewey et al., 2003). Despite lower hospitalization rates over the past 10 years suggesting that stroke may be on the decline, the aging population and an increased prevalence of risk factors, such as obesity and diabetes, will likely result in a greater number of stroke events in populations over the next two decades (Public Health Agency of Canada, 2009, www.phac-aspc.gc.ca/publicat/2009/cvd-avc/summary-resume-eng.php).

The face of stroke is changing, and with this change comes a need to rethink approaches for rehabilitation after stroke. For one thing, improved early management of stroke over the last 20 years has resulted in a marked decline in mortality in high-income countries, with a concomitant increase in the numbers of individuals internationally who survive a stroke and who are alive long after stroke. The improvements in survival may be associated with a range of factors related to better management after stroke, as well as the effects of possible declines in stroke incidence or stroke severity from greater use of prevention interventions. Stroke is also becoming a leading cause of disability in low-income countries. We need to reposition stroke management from the traditional thinking that stroke is an acute condition treated with a short inten-

sive effort, usually for several months, to one that requires sophisticated chronic disease management over many years. Worldwide there are now more than 900 randomized clinical trials related to stroke management (Teasell et al., 2009) and a proliferation of reputable national and international best practice guidelines for stroke rehabilitation that clinicians can use to make informed best practice decisions. Making sure that these evidence-based interventions are adopted in the clinic is a key challenge in health service delivery.

As we face many new and exciting challenges in stroke rehabilitation, it is time to reflect on where we have been and where we are going. Thus, the aims of this chapter are to provide clinicians, policymakers, and other interested stakeholders with a broad overview of how stroke rehabilitation care is currently organized; to highlight the changing models of care delivery that optimize patient outcomes; and to discuss efforts that are needed to improve care and monitor quality. Barriers and facilitators to changing how care is organized are raised, along with a brief review of recent innovations in rehabilitation care and the implementation challenges that come along with innovation. This chapter concludes with a summary of the main messages from this overview related to the organization of stroke rehabilitation services.

What do we mean by the "organization of care"? Fundamentally, we are interested in looking at who delivers stroke care, how care is organized, or where care is delivered and how this relates to the ability of healthcare professionals to deliver effective rehabilitation services as efficiently as possible. Continuing education, quality assurance, informatics, and financial, organizational, and regulatory interventions can all influence healthcare delivery (for further information see http://epoc.cochrane.org/), and we will touch on most of these areas in this chapter.

7.2 MODELS OF STROKE REHABILITATION SERVICES

7.2.1 INPATIENT CARE

Rehabilitation is an expensive component of care in the first year after stroke (Moon, Moise, Jacobzone, & Group, 2003; Cadilhac et al., 2009), but one that is recognized as making a major contribution to improving outcomes after stroke (Stroke Unit Trialists' Collaboration, 2007). There is strong evidence that how and when rehabilitation is delivered matters. The most effective stroke rehabilitation services are those that manage all patients with stroke in a single geographical location or "stroke unit," with care coordinated and delivered by a specialized, interdisciplinary team (D'Amour, Ferrada-Videla, Rodriquez, & Beaulieu, 2005; Petri, 2010). This team is to be differentiated from a "multidisciplinary" team where different disciplines assess and treat the patient and then share the information among themselves, but do not necessarily coordinate patient assessment and care (Sorrells-Jones, 1997). When stroke management is provided within an organized stroke unit, with a skilled stroke team, rather than on a general medical ward, there is on average a 20% to 30% reduction in mortality and reduced need for long-term institutional care (Stroke Unit Trialists' Collaboration, 2007). Randomized controlled trials conducted in many countries with different healthcare systems have consistently demonstrated the benefits of stroke unit care, and these benefits extend to all patients with stroke regardless of stroke severity. Treatment within an organized stroke unit provides a greater overall benefit to patient outcome than any single intervention.

Explanations for why organized stroke unit care provides such large benefits to patients is described within the context of having effective stroke unit teams that focus on prevention and early management. This includes the provision of early rehabilitation therapy; participation in regular, ongoing professional education and training; having regular team meetings; and actively encouraging patients and carers to be involved in the rehabilitation process (Langhorne & Pollack, 2002). Stroke units may differ in their structure and have been described as:

- **Acute**, which accept patients acutely but discharge early (usually within 7 days).

- **Comprehensive**, which accept patients acutely but also provide rehabilitation if necessary. Both the rehabilitation unit (see below) and comprehensive unit models offer prolonged periods of rehabilitation.

- **Rehabilitation** stroke units which accept patients after a delay, usually of 7 days or more, and focus on rehabilitation

- **Mixed** rehabilitation units, a multidisciplinary team including specialist nursing staff in a ward providing a generic rehabilitation service, but not exclusively caring for patients with stroke.

Is one model superior to another? This topic has been explored by the Stroke Unit Trialists' Collaboration (2007) and extended with a specific focus on rehabilitation by Foley and colleagues (2007). In a meta-analysis conducted by Foley and colleagues, the units that provided several weeks of rehabilitation on a comprehensive unit or standalone stroke rehabilitation unit appeared to have the strongest benefits for reducing death and having an impact on disability (Foley, Salter, & Teasell, 2007). Although rehabilitation is an implicit component in each model, the timing associated with the commencement of rehabilitation varies and detailed information is often lacking about the actual type, dose, and intensity of rehabilitation delivered in each. This makes it difficult to determine the relative contribution of rehabilitation to the improved patient outcomes demonstrated with stroke unit care.

While much of the literature supporting the inclusion of early rehabilitation has been conducted during the subacute period (after 7 days) using descriptive study designs, there is growing evidence that commencing mobility-focused rehabilitation (early mobilization) within day(s) of stroke onset may help increase the number of patients recovering walking ability and the speed with which they recover (Cumming et al., 2011). This intervention is currently the subject of an international randomized clinical trial (A Very Early Rehabilitation Trial (AVERT); (Bernhardt et al., 2006)). Trials of early-onset aphasia therapy within the first week of stroke (ACTnow (Assessing Communication Therapy in the North West); http://www.psych-sci.manchester.ac.uk/actnow/), and upper limb training (Very Early Constraint-Induced Movement during Stroke Rehabilitation (VECTORS); Dromerick et al., 2009) have also been undertaken with mixed results. While the optimal moment to commence specific rehabilitation interventions may be uncertain, the body of evidence in support of earlier (rather than delayed) rehabilitation has led to a number of clinical guidelines all recommending that rehabilitation therapy be initiated as early as possible, which is usually within the first 24 to 72 hours (Adams et al., 2007; Intercollegiate Stroke Working Party, 2008; Lindsay et al., 2008; National Stroke Foundation, 2010a).

In the current healthcare system, the primary focus of the acute stroke unit is typically on early assessment and discharge planning to enable patient flow through the continuum of care (Purvis, 2009). Rehabilitation interventions may not commence until patients are transferred to a dedicated rehabilitation unit. If the growing body of literature continues to suggest that early rehabilitation is critical for maximal patient outcome, it will be important to address the need for early rehabilitation with the same rigor and international attention that other acute stroke strategies, such as intravenous thrombolysis have been afforded. These issues are discussed further in section 7.3.

7.2.2 COMMUNITY-BASED REHABILITATION AS AN ALTERNATIVE TO INPATIENT REHABILITATION

Stroke survivors may need weeks or even months of assistance from rehabilitation professionals before they feel ready to take over the planning and management of their ongoing recovery. How best to support survivors and meet both their short-term and long-term needs is an issue of considerable importance. An increased focus on patient-driven (or centered) care (rather than provider-driven care) and the increased numbers of stroke survivors being discharged directly home from the acute hospital (Cadilhac et al., 2011) has combined to foster a growing interest in early post-stroke home-based or community-based (day center) therapy models as alternatives to inpatient rehabilitation. Unfortunately, the option for further access to rehabilitation services beyond the first year after stroke is not common, but is desired by some survivors several years after stroke (National Stroke Foundation, 2007b). Current models of funding stroke rehabilitation services in Australia, and in many other countries with universal healthcare funding, are not well established for providing stroke rehabilitation years after an initial stroke event. This is an area that may grow in focus over the coming years as consumer demand for additional therapy input grows. Presently, health systems have adapted to providing greater alternate options for rehabilitation within the first months of stroke. These are outlined below.

A systematic review examining delivering rehabilitation care in the community has shown a small but worthwhile effect when compared to conventional inpatient rehabilitation or no care (Outpatient Service Trialists, 2003). Early supported discharge (ESD) as a model of care delivery appears to be effective for select individuals. ESD is designed to accelerate discharge home by providing appropriate rehabilitation and nursing services within the community (Teasell, Foley, Bhogal, & Speechley, 2003; Langhorne, Holmqvist, & for the Early Supported Discharge Trialists, 2007). The concept of ESD arose out of concern that inpatient stroke rehabilitation may not always result in optimal outcomes, particularly in establishing skills that are important for reintegration to the home environment and to the community. Furthermore, it is thought that patients generally prefer to be at home, if possible, rather than in the hospital. ESD interventions have been studied in comparison to conventional inpatient care, to determine their effectiveness in achieving optimal patient outcomes including activities of daily living, risk of death, cost-effectiveness, patient satisfaction, and perceived emotional, social, and physical health status. The ESD model has the potential to reduce inpatient length of stay, improve functional outcomes and survi-

vor satisfaction, and be cost effective when compared to conventional care (Brady, McGahan, & Skidmore, 2005; Early Supported Discharge Trialists, 2005; Langhorne et al., 2005) . This model has only been shown to be effective in patients with mild to moderate disability (Langhorne, et al., 2005), and requires a structured system of access to adequate community services for rehabilitation and carer support. These factors generally make it difficult to implement or provide this care option in hospitals that admit <100 strokes per year, or in rural communities where there are few specialized stroke rehabilitation professionals.

More recent innovations in the community rehabilitation sector include Telehealth to improve care of patients living in the community (Schmid et al., 2011). Telehealth rehabilitation is particularly useful in increasing patient and carer access to interdisciplinary stroke team members, especially for those who live in rural regions where rehabilitation professionals are often few in number, and those with specialized training in stroke are even rarer.

Whether Telehealth or ESD models are able to support the long-term rehabilitation needs of survivors is unknown. Despite the growing evidence that rehabilitation interventions commenced months after stroke can be effective in improving functional outcome and quality of life (e.g., sensory retraining, constraint induced movement therapy—CIMT, fitness training), many individuals fail to benefit because current services rarely extend beyond the first weeks or months after stroke.

Models of care that address the longer-term needs of patients with stroke and their families are becoming an increasing focus of attention (Murray, Young, Forster, Herbert, & Ashworth, 2006).

7.2.3 CURRENT PERSPECTIVES ON THE WAY FORWARD FOR PROVIDING STROKE REHABILITATION

It has been recognized that the biomedical model commonly used in the management of patients with stroke may contribute to frustration for patients and rehabilitation service providers alike (Siebens, 2011). Alternate models of healthcare have been proposed to bridge the boundaries between healthcare and individuals' experiences of chronic illness and health conditions (Siebens, 2011). Some authors have advocated for models of rehabilitation to move to a chronic disease management model that incorporates outcomes that are meaningful to patients, and do not assume the needs or outcomes as defined by rehabilitation professionals (Cott, Wiles, & Devitt, 2007). Others have designed trials to determine the efficacy of goal-directed practice that reflects the patient's valued activities (Graven et al., 2011). These proposed models recognize the patient as an important partner in the process of recovery. Indeed, these models are in sharp contrast to earlier models of care, such as stroke care pathways, that have failed to deliver the promised results. When first proposed, stroke care pathways—defined as goal-oriented, high-quality plans of care based on evidence/best practice guidelines—were touted as a way of enhancing the quality and consistency of stroke rehabilitation. Yet, they have not had the desired effects on mortality rates, frequency of institutionalization, or length of hospitalization (Sulch & Kalra, 2000; for a review of the evidence for care pathways see www.strokengine.ca). It is not clear why care pathways have not been as successful as anticipated. Some have suggested that imposing a blueprint of care, rather than individualizing treatment to the specific needs and sequelae of the patient, does not improve outcomes. Thus, models of care that focus on client-centered goals and individuals' goal-directed interventions may well be the optimal way to maximize patient recovery and increase patient satisfaction with the healthcare system. Further research is needed to evaluate the net benefits to patients, as well as how to support the implementation of these approaches in practice if they are highly effective.

The impact of the carer role is another consideration in providing rehabilitation services. The involvement of carers, not only in the decision-making process, but also in order to equip them with the skills to competently manage relatives or friends after stroke, is often "overlooked" in rehabilitation (McCullagh, Brigstocke, Donaldson, & Kalra, 2005; Rochette, Korner-Bitensky, & Desrosiers, 2007). Yet, it has been estimated that 25%–74% of stroke survivors require assistance with activities of daily living (e.g., dressing, showering, cooking) from informal caregivers, often family (Kalra et al., 2004) and that a carer training program can be effective in reducing carer burden and stress, improving quality of life of both the patient and the carer, and in improving patient function (Kalra, et al., 2004). Stress of family carers places them at risk for developing poor quality of life and health problems (Cumming, Cadilhac, Rubin, Crafti, & Pearce, 2008; Saban, Sherwood, DeVon, & Hynes, 2011). Authors have suggested that a mixed-methods model using domiciliary care and day hospital care could provide carers with the benefits of education, convenience, and opportunities for respite (Low, Roderick, & Payne, 2004). The evidence that combined counseling and education are more effective than conventional therapy for improving key outcomes in both the patient and the carer suggests that all rehabilitation programs should include carer interventions (see www.strokengine.ca for a review of the effectiveness of family intervention in the acute phase, as well as the subacute and chronic phases). Of importance is addressing how one might assist those who live in remote regions where access to counseling and education is challenging. Currently, there is a Canadian RCT being undertaken to investigate the effect of a remote multimodal intervention for patients and carers who never receive inpatient rehabilitation, but rather are discharged home directly from acute care (Rochette et al., 2010).

7.2.4 CHARACTERISTICS OF STROKE REHABILITATION SERVICES

Very few studies have been conducted that are designed to characterize in detail rehabilitation services for stroke. The most comprehensive recent data comes from Australia. Australia has a health system similar to the United Kingdom and Canada, whereby health insurance is universally available through a public Medicare program and individuals may also choose to have private health insurance. Australians may elect to have private insurance so that they have greater choices in which specialist treats them, and to ensure more timely treatment (e.g., not having to go on a public hospital waiting list for surgery). Overall, government is the main funder and provider of healthcare services in Australia. There are three levels of government: federal, state, and local councils, which each have responsibility for providing and funding different health and community care services. Rehabilitation services for stroke come under various jurisdictions, thus creating a risk of fragmentation in care as patients make their way through the continuum. The problem of cost-shifting between providers is a related issue, but is not discussed here.

In Australia, approximately 90% of people who experience a stroke present to a hospital (Thrift, Dewey, Macdonell, McNeil, & Donnan, 2000), and over a third will then receive further rehabilitation service input (National Stroke Foundation, 2007a). According to national data, of all patients who attend rehabilitation services, stroke patients represent the third largest group after rehabilitation for orthopedic and reconditioning admissions (Simmonds, 2009).

The most recent national audit of stroke services in Australia provides evidence that 39% of hospitals treating patients with acute stroke had established a stroke unit (National Stroke Foundation, 2011). In Canada, the 2011 National Stroke Audit on 38,210 cases of stroke admitted in 2008–2009 found that only 23% were admitted to a stroke unit (http://www.canadianstrokenetwork.ca/index.php5/news/the-quality-of-stroke-care-in-canada-2011/).

In the rehabilitation sector, only 22% of patients in Australia received treatment in a dedicated stroke rehabilitation unit (National Stroke Foundation, 2010b), in spite of the strong evidence that patients have better outcomes when treated on a unit. The audit findings suggest the need for improvements in the organization of stroke services for people requiring rehabilitation in Australia. Indeed, the Canadian context is similar and as such, the Canadian Stroke Network, within the context of a Canadian Stroke Strategy, has published a practical "hands-on" manual entitled, *A Guide to the Implementation of Stroke Unit Care*, in recognition of the importance of increasing the number of patients who are managed on a stroke unit (http://strokebestpractices.ca/wp-content/uploads/2010/11/CSS-Stroke-Unit-Resource_EN-Final2-for-print.pdf).

Expert opinion has suggested that, wherever possible, acute and rehabilitation services should be linked to facilitate a seamless transition through the health system for the person with stroke (National Stroke Foundation, 2010a), thus improving communication and reducing delays and costs associated with repeat assessments, and so on. Therefore, a greater emphasis on providing comprehensive stroke units may be logical. The majority of inpatient rehabilitation services within Australia are provided in a rehabilitation ward, onsite in the same building but separate from the acute ward (Table 7.1). While some mixed-methods research has been conducted that explores how the organization of care influences the provision of rehabilitation (Purvis, Cadilhac, & Bernhardt, 2010), further research is needed to understand how these various models of care enhance or impede communications and processes of care for patients.

Variable and limited access to community rehabilitation services within Australia and the United Kingdom, in both rural and urban areas, have been reported (National Stroke Foundation, 2008, 2010b; Intercollegiate Stroke Working Party, 2011) . In Australia, 97% of hospitals that responded to the organizational survey reported having access to at least one form of community-based rehabilitation option. In the United Kingdom, community-based services appear less frequently available, with only 55% of hospitals having a community rehabilitation service nearby. Only a quarter of Australian acute care hospitals had links with an ESD service, significantly lower than the 44% of hospitals reported to have access to the service in the United Kingdom.

Timelines in accessing rehabilitation services is an issue (Intercollegiate Stroke Working Party, 2011). In Australia, one in ten rehabilitation units reported that access to day hospital or outpatient services required wait times of 4 or more weeks (National Stroke Foundation, 2008). This highlights the importance of regular reviews of services in order to be able to identify and address capacity issues within the health system. These issues are further described below.

7.3 FACTORS AFFECTING ACCESS TO ORGANIZED STROKE REHABILITATION

The way in which stroke rehabilitation is organized and delivered is often dependent on the local services and resources that are available (Outpatient Service Trialists, 2003). In recent times, innovative approaches to the provision of stroke rehabilitation have been developed to address a number of system-based issues, such as access to services because of geographical location (see section 7.2.2).

Access to rehabilitation, infrastructure, and staffing resources varies worldwide (De Wit et al., 2005; Rudd, Hoffman, Irwin, Pearson, & Lowe, 2005; National Stroke Foundation, 2008, 2010b). It has been well documented that poor access to best practice stroke care affects outcomes (Cadilhac et al., 2004; Cadilhac, Pearce, Levi, & Donnan, 2008; Ingeman, Andersen, Hundborg, Svendsen, & Johnsen, 2011). There is evidence that the geographical location of hospitals may influence mortality and morbidity, with patients treated in rural hospitals more likely to have poorer outcomes (Joubert et al., 2008; Cadilhac, et al., 2011). Consequently, specific barriers are evident for rural, remote, and smaller services, where not only might resources be limited (such as access to specialist staff and equipment), but essential elements of organized stroke care may be lacking. In these circumstances, other service delivery models, based as much as possible on evidence-based care, are recommended (National Stroke Foundation, 2010a). For example, in Canada use of Telehealth has been used to increase access to intravenous thrombolysis (http://www.canadianstrokenetwork.ca/index.php5/news/the-quality-of-stroke-care-in-canada-2011/).

TABLE 7.1 Characteristics of Rehabilitation Services offered in Australia According to Location

CHARACTERISTICS OF REHABILITATION SERVICE	OVERALL (N=107)	URBAN (N=95)	RURAL (N=12)
INPATIENT SERVICES (PREDOMINANTLY MIXED REHABILITATION UNITS)			
Freestanding rehabilitation hospital not located on the same hospital site where acute care is provided	34 (32%)	31 (33%)	3 (25%)
Rehabilitation ward; same building of same health campus	54 (50%)	46 (48%)	8 (67%)
Rehabilitation ward; separate building of same health campus	17 (16%)	17 (18%)	0 (0%)
Rehabilitation service within acute hospital without designated beds within the same hospital site	2 (2%)	1 (1%)	1 (8%)
COMMUNITY-BASED SERVICES*			
Outpatient rehabilitation	87 (81%)	77 (81%)	10 (83%)
Early supported discharge teams	27 (25%)	24 (25%)	3 (25%)
Community-based rehabilitation (provided in the home)	74 (69%)	68 (72%)	6 (50%)
Day hospital	32 (30%)	2 (17%)	22 (24%)

SOURCE: Adapted from the Australian National Stroke Foundation, National Stroke Rehabilitation Services report 2010. *Sites may have reported one or more services.

Recognition of the importance of closing the gap in stroke service provision between urban and rural sectors led one state government in Australia to fund a program to enhance provision of evidence-based stroke care in rural areas of New South Wales. This initiative was referred to as the *Rural Stroke Project*. The main components of the enhancement program included improving clinical care processes within regional sites, and then creating a "hub and spoke" system of care between a regional "hub" center and smaller rural (spoke) sites (Cadilhac et al., 2011). These changes were facilitated by the appointment of a Rural Stroke Care Coordinator at each site. Following on from these initiatives, a review of services found that there was evidence of increased access to stroke unit care, more timely assessment by allied health within 24 hours, and that patients had an 87% greater odds of being discharged to a home setting rather than to a rehabilitation or aged care setting (Cadilhac et al., 2011). The positive results achieved were primarily attributed to the provision of a Rural Stroke Care Coordinator. A Cochrane systematic review provides evidence that having a stroke coordinator can positively help reduce the length of hospital stay after stroke and reduce emergency department representations (Kwan & Sandercock, 2004). There is no clear evidence that stroke care coordinators help improve patient outcome post-stroke. Nevertheless, the role seemingly aids in enhancing the organization of care and should be considered an important attribute of a health service to ensure a coordinated and evidence-based approach to delivering stroke care. Presently, only 22% of rehabilitation services across Australia had access to a stroke care coordinator (National Stroke Foundation, 2010b).

7.3.1 STAFFING RESOURCES AND THE INTERDISCIPLINARY APPROACH TO REHABILITATION

The complex process of stroke rehabilitation requires an interdisciplinary approach (D'Amour, et al., 2005), with a specialized team of health professionals who together provide a coordinated program of care. This program of care encompasses individualized assessment, tailored therapy, regular reviews, discharge planning, and follow-up (National Stroke Foundation, 2010b). Given that stroke affects many areas of human performance resulting in multiple impairments, no single discipline has the skills, resources, and expertise required to manage the full spectrum of physical, psychological, emotional, and social needs of patients. The diversity of clinical expertise involved in clinical decision making on behalf of and with patients and families is considered largely responsible for improvements in patient care and overall organizational effectiveness (Lemieux-Charles & McGuire, 2006).

Although interdisciplinary practices are often well established among "formally" organized stroke teams, with usually dedicated (funded) allocations to stroke, benchmarking of services and the development of generalizable staffing ratios across services is often difficult because patient characteristics and local organizational factors influence care requirements. Results from international organizational surveys examining staffing structures provide evidence that, in reality, the interdisciplinary team staffing ratios differ not only between but also within countries. These variations make it very difficult to benchmark or recommend a minimum complement of staff (Langhorne & Pollack, 2002). Often, staffing ratios are driven by hospital directors in response to local priorities, service arrangements, and budgetary constraints rather than consideration of how many and what mix of staff are necessary to ensure evidence-based care. Additional constraints to staffing include workforce availability, which can be particularly challenging in rural areas (Cadilhac et al., 2011).

Staffing ratios have not been shown to be directly related to rehabilitation intensity. The rehabilitation environment, organizational culture, and the focus of the unit also affect the amount of therapy received by patients (De Wit, et al., 2005; Purvis, 2009). In a comparison of stroke rehabilitation units across four settings in Europe, De Wit and colleagues demonstrated that while the United Kingdom setting had almost double the allied health resources available (approximately 70 hours/week across all disciplines), patients received the least amount of therapy input (1 hour/day) compared to almost 3 hours/day in Switzerland. This was attributed to the therapists in the United Kingdom spending a greater proportion of their time on administrative and nontherapy activities, while centers with structured and strictly timed therapy input had significantly more time spent with patients, resulting in improved health outcomes (De Wit, et al., 2005).

Interestingly, inability to access an extended interdisciplinary stroke team is not necessarily a barrier to providing good quality rehabilitation care, particularly in the first weeks after stroke. For example, a comparison of an acute stroke service in Norway with proven efficacy (Indredavik et al., 1991) that exhibits a strong rehabilitation culture and fosters an "enriched environment" (see Chapter 8 for further discussion of enrichment) provides significantly more time in therapy and fosters higher levels of physical activity in patients with only a small interdisciplinary team (nursing, physicians, physiotherapists) compared to an Australian acute stroke service with a full complement of team members (Bernhardt, Chitravas, Meslo, Thrift, & Indredavik, 2008). Skilled rehabilitation nursing underpins the care provided in this Norwegian model (Bernhardt, Chitravas, Meslo, Thrift, & Indredavik, 2008), as well as extended interdisciplinary training opportunities and a strong culture of teamwork (Purvis, 2009; Purvis, et al., 2010).

Within the interdisciplinary team, nurses are available 24 hours a day and, as such, play a vital role in rehabilitation, as well as in delivering other aspects of care. While there is some uncertainty about what the specific role of nurses in stroke rehabilitation should entail (Kirkevold, 1997; O'Connor, 2000), few studies have directly examined the effect of rehabilitation nursing on patient outcomes. This is an obvious topic warranting further research.

7.4 ENSURING THE QUALITY OF CARE

To optimize patient outcome derived from rehabilitation we need to ensure that the care provided is evidence-based, and that there is routine monitoring of the quality of care. This includes assessing not only the achievement of health outcomes and the processes of care that led to those outcomes, but also a consideration of the value of the interventions provided for the outcomes achieved. Assessment of the cost-effectiveness of the care provided is important, since resources are scarce and priority-setting in health care is necessary but is not often undertaken (Gloede, Cadilhac, & Dewey, 2010).

Research to date has largely been designed to focus on examining the quality of care delivered in the acute sector. Hospitals that provide organized "acute" stroke care adhere to a larger number of important processes of care indicators than general medical wards, and there is a strong relationship between total adherence to process of care indicators and survival following hospitalization for stroke (Cadilhac et al., 2004). Overall, the immense effort on audit and feedback focused on the acute medical management of stroke is providing evidence of an impact on clinical practice. Unfortunately, as the patient continues through the process of care there is less reliable information collected systematically about the quality of inpatient and outpatient rehabilitation services. What little we know supports the value of conducting quality assessment of rehabilitation services. For example, in the United States, Duncan and colleagues determined that greater adherence to 26 clinical care guidelines resulted in better functional outcomes post-stroke (Duncan et al., 2002). More recently, using data from Australian national audits of rehabilitation services, Hubbard and colleagues showed that rehabilitation units that deliver clinical management in accordance with national clinical guidelines achieved better outcomes, including more patients discharged home and greater improvement in function (Hubbard et al., 2011). Given the persuasive findings to date that the use of rehabilitation best practices improve patient outcome, it would be important to place emphasis on collecting and regularly reviewing data on rehabilitation processes and structures.

7.4.1 MONITORING AND IMPROVING THE QUALITY OF CARE IN REHABILITATION FOR STROKE

A number of models have been used to monitor and improve the quality of stroke care. Throughout Europe, Canada, the United States, and more recently in Australia, registries are becoming recognized as important contributors to quality improvement (AuSCR, Australian Stroke Clinical Registry; Riks-Stroke, Swedish Stroke Registry; Registry of the Canadian Stroke Network). Most current data collection programs only capture features of acute care, but there is increasing recognition that it is also critical to measure the processes of care related to rehabilitation (Purvis, Cadilhac, Donnan, & Bernhardt, 2009). Stroke registries provide a means to better understand clinical care and health outcomes, develop interventions and policies to improve the quality and safety of stroke care delivery, and assess change in clinical practice and health outcomes over time. Extending this concept, the European Registers of Stroke Collaborative group has developed and field tested a Stroke Quality Assessment Tool to be used as a framework to assess the quality of stroke care, including rehabilitation and long-term management (Wellwood et al., 2011). While further validation of the approach is required to test reliability and link the findings to patient outcomes, it forms an evidence-based tool with which to assess quality of stroke care. More specifically, a generic rather than stroke-specific rehabilitation data collection program has been established by the Australasian Rehabilitation Outcomes Centre (AROC). AROC is a joint initiative of the Australian rehabilitation sector, including providers, funders, regulators, and consumers (http://ahsri.uow.edu.au/aroc/index.html). The efficacy of rehabilitation interventions can be examined through the functional outcomes and impairment data collected. AROC is regarded as an important resource for national benchmarking in rehabilitation, and provides the opportunity to monitor clinical rehabilitation outcomes in both the public and private sectors.

Although a stroke-specific registry for rehabilitation is not maintained in Australia, there is a biennial national audit specifically focused on rehabilitation services that was established by the National Stroke Foundation in 2008. Process of care performance indicators were developed to measure whether recommendations in national guidelines for stroke rehabilitation were being adhered to in clinical practice (National Stroke Foundation, 2008, 2010a). The Australian audit was modeled on the Sentinel Stroke Audit Program run in the United Kingdom (Intercollegiate Stroke Working Party, 2002). The audit program comprises two components: an organizational survey to characterize the nature of the service providers, and a clinical audit of patients' medical records to describe the actual management provided.

At the end of each audit cycle, each hospital receives its audit results compared to the national average results as part of a feedback process. Audit and feedback has been shown to be highly effective in changing clinician behavior, achieving a 7% improvement when implemented as a single initiative (systematic review of 5 cluster trials; Grimshaw et al., 2004).

Where large-scale audits are not possible, a local or regional cross-sectional audit in a sample of patients (e.g., 40 consecutive patients per hospital) can be an efficient alternative to maintaining a prospective clinical registry that captures data on all patients. The use of clinical audit and feedback is not only important for benchmarking, but provides essential information to develop programs for improving clinical care by providing evidence of where resources should be directed for future areas of service development. Indeed, in 2010, Canada undertook a national audit of patient records, supplemented with data from national health databases, to produce the first ever report on the quality of stroke care in Canada (http://www.canadianstrokenetwork.ca/index.php5/news/the-quality-of-stroke-care-in-canada-2011/). The objectives of this assessment of the quality of stroke care in Canada included:

- to compare the current practice with best practice recommendations;

- to identify gaps in stroke care and levels of coordination;

- to describe economic and societal impacts of improved stroke care delivery; and

- to make recommendations for improving stroke care.

Some of the main findings from this Canadian audit included the need for stroke risk factors to be controlled better; that patients need to be treated more quickly when they arrive at the hospital; that Telestroke should be more widely used; that patients need greater access to stroke units; and that access to appropriate rehabilitation is vital, yet not well monitored (http://www.canadianstrokenetwork.ca/index.php5/news/the-quality-of-stroke-care-in-canada-2011/).

7.4.2 WHAT CLINICAL AUDITS TELL US ABOUT QUALITY OF REHABILITATION?

Despite the fact that many countries have developed clinical stroke guidelines with recommendations that are based on the most comprehensive review of the evidence for stroke care, their translation into clinical practice may not be as widespread as desired. While many aspects of acute care are improving because there are guidelines and data-monitoring systems to support efforts to improve clinical practice, advances in post-acute rehabilitation services remain limited. This can be attributed, in part, to the fact that monitoring of clinical care and outcome in rehabilitation is not routinely undertaken.

Serial audits in the United Kingdom (Irwin, Hoffman, Lowe, Pearson, & Rudd, 2005) and Australia (National Stroke Foundation, 2010b) have highlighted an increased proportion of patients accessing earlier specialist therapy services and better organization of stroke rehabilitation over time. However, the suggested standards of care are not being met consistently. Important benchmarks that were not being met were identified in national clinical audits in Australia (National Stroke Foundation, 2010b), Japan (Jeong, Kondo, NShiraishi, & Yusuke, 2010), the United Kingdom (Hammond et al., 2005), and Canada (Korner-Bitensky et al., 2004). In Canada, a national audit of the practices of 1800 stroke rehabilitation clinicians treating patients with stroke found large variations in practice and major gaps in best versus actual practice (Korner-Bitensky, et al., 2004; Dumoulin, Korner-Bitensky, & Tannenbaum, 2007). In specialist rehabilitation settings in the United Kingdom, the recommended care practices were met in only 20%–60% of patients (Hammond, et al., 2005). Although direct comparisons are not possible, Table 7.2 provides a summary of the results of the Australian and United Kingdom audits of rehabilitation services for a range of recommended clinical management criteria.

TABLE 7.2 Comparison of Rehabilitation Services Audit Results of Select Clinical Management Recommendations from Australia and the United Kingdom

CLINICAL MANAGEMENT CRITERIA	AUSTRALIA*	UNITED KINGDOM^
Team meetings at least once/week	99% hospitals	97% rehabilitation units
Targeted continuing education for staff	55% hospitals	69% rehabilitation units
Allied Health assessment - Physiotherapy - Occupational therapy	Median time to assessment 0 (0–1) days 1 (0–2) days	Assessment <72 hrs. 66% Assessment <7 days 50%
Home assessment completed	74%	87%
Carer training provided	74%	73%

*SOURCE: adapted from National Stroke Audit Rehabilitation Services 2010, National Stroke Foundation

^SOURCE: adapted from Hammond et al., 2005, no more recent rehabilitation data available

7.4.3 ESTABLISHING PROGRAMS TO INCREASE THE UPTAKE OF EVIDENCE INTO CLINICAL PRACTICE

Improving compliance with clinical guidelines and building a culture for the uptake of evidence in clinical practice are imperative to improve quality of care. Obstacles to change include personal experience and preferences, and engrained practices in existing units. A qualitative study by Pollack and colleagues showed that clinicians felt that a lack of time to keep up to date with literature, difficulties relating to the implementation of research findings, and the need for training in the interpretation of study results were major barriers to the implementation of evidence-based stroke rehabilitation (Pollock, Legg, Langhorne, & Sellars, 2000). Considering the reported issues, it is somewhat concerning that targeted stroke education for staff is not commonplace at many sites. In Australia, just over half the sites provided a regular program of continuing education for staff related to stroke management (National Stroke Foundation, 2010b). This is below the 69% reported in other rehabilitation units in the United Kingdom (Hammond, et al., 2005).

In an attempt to close the gap between research and clinical practice, a range of initiatives in various countries have been developed. For example, various strategies are evolving in the area of rehabilitation that seek to establish programs to improve the quality of care where deficiencies have been quantified, including the introduction of local champions to foster best practice research within sites, conferences, websites, and so forth. A recent systematic review on the effectiveness of these various strategies specific to rehabilitation professionals suggests that while this research area is still in its infancy, the evidence available to date supports introduction of multimodal interventions (Menon, Korner-Bitensky, Kastner, McKibbon, & Straus, 2009). Petzold and colleagues suggest the use of the "Knowledge to Action" translation model as a comprehensive blueprint for improving best practices at the local and national levels. This model provides a sequence of phases for researchers and clinicians to follow in order to optimize knowledge translation across various fields of practice, and to incite change in patient care with the goal of achieving better health outcomes (Petzold, Korner-Bitensky, & Menon, 2011). These phases include performing audits to identify actual clinician practices and to identify gaps between actual and best practices. As well, it encourages understanding of the local context, and barriers and facilitators specific to new knowledge uptake for a specific condition and setting; ongoing monitoring of practices; and the creation and use of learning tools to sustain and encourage easy access to the latest best practice information.

Other authors explain the move toward "pay-for-performance" models, whereby financial incentives are provided for rehabilitation centers to achieve the best outcomes possible for their patients but do not create additional costs for the insurance funds (Doran, Fullwood, & Gravelle, 2006; Gerdes et al., 2009; Jeong, et al., 2010). The system is conceived as a "quality competition" that is organized by the participating sites with a scientific institute acting as a "referee." Sites with outcomes above average receive a bonus financed by sites achieving below average results (Gerdes, et al., 2009). This form of incentive can be especially disadvantageous in stroke management, where often the patient who is going to change the least in terms of functional outcomes is the patient who most needs intensive interdisciplinary rehabilitation. When sites are compared on "patient outcomes" (e.g., change in Functional Independence Measure scores) we potentially bias sites to admit only those patients deemed most likely to exhibit large changes (those with no cognitive impairment, etc).

Determining what system-level versus patient-level factors can be modified is difficult when focusing attempts to monitor and improve the quality of care. The Cerebrovascular Consortium in the United States has reported significant disparities in the delivery of stroke care across the eight-state region in the northeast of the country. A multistate regional collaboration was established to address these disparities, as a viable process for developing specific regional recommendations (Gropen, Magdon-Ismail, Day, Melluzzo, & Schwamm, 2009). These authors suggest the need for the *Stroke Systems of Care Model* as a framework for implementing a regional approach to stroke across the continuum of care, whereby recommendations to address variations in care delivery can be systematically addressed. These recommendations include: the use of a common stroke data collection system; unified community education criteria; improvements to emergency medical services dispatch and training; adoption of prehospital care measures; creation of a web-based central repository of acute stroke protocols and order sets; a regional atlas of stroke resources and capabilities; a stroke patient "report card" to promote adherence to secondary prevention strategies; and explicit standards for rehabilitation services (Gropen, et al., 2009).

In Canada, a national initiative was launched in 2005 by the Canadian Stroke Network and the Heart and Stroke Foundation of Canada to improve stroke care in all parts of Canada. Modeled on a successful provincial effort in Ontario, the Canadian Stroke Strategy mobilized people (health ministers, clinicians, researchers, policymakers and patient stakeholders) with the goal of ensuring that the best stroke research findings were being moved into practice within each health system. At a national level, working groups were formed and given the mandate to develop tools and programs that could be used to help improve quality of stroke care. These efforts led to the creation of the Canadian Best Practice Recommendations for Stroke Care 2008, 2010, training programs for health professionals to enhance capacity-building specific to stroke, and the creation of a set of key performance measures to monitor quality of care and enable the setting of benchmarks of care. At a provincial and territorial level, each was encouraged to identify funding for best practice stroke implementation and to set up systems of care that would work well within existing healthcare structures. This was deemed a unique approach to improving stroke care by address-

ing differing provincial needs within the context of their resources and health priorities.

Others have nominated to establish international "communities of practice" via the development of websites that summarize the evidence base for stroke rehabilitation interventions. One example is StrokEngine (http://www.strokengine.ca/), which provides clinicians with access to

TABLE 7.3 Examples of New Rehabilitation Approaches and Challenges with Implementation

REHABILITATION APPROACH	SUMMARY OF EVIDENCE	LEVEL OF EVIDENCE*	CHALLENGES WITH IMPLEMENTATION
Constraint-induced movement therapy	Viable option to improve upper limb arm function in a select population, although results are more significant immediately after intervention (Langhorne, Coupar, & Pollock, 2009; Sirtori, Corbetta, Moja, & Gatti, 2009)	A, B	There are few current service models that support uptake in the "chronic" phase of care.
Art therapy	Consistent creative exploration of participants' goals through art therapy prompted therapists to enable participants to achieve their goals, particularly in areas of socialization, independence, inclusion, and integrity (Sainsbury & Lee, 2011)	C	
Electrical Stimulation (ES)	Variability in results of current literature; however, more advanced ES applications have been developed to promote upper limb recovery. Presents exciting opportunities for application into clinical practice and research in the future.	B	Equipment costs, late-stage access to services.
Task-oriented circuit class (versus individual therapy)	Means of increasing the amount of practice while making efficient use of therapist time. One systematic review found that circuit class training improved walking distance and speed (Wevers, van de Port, Vermue, Mead, & Kwakkel, 2009)	B	Minimal equipment or additional training required. May reduce resources required while not cutting service provision. Can involve a therapy assistant.
Video self-modeling	Involves videoing the exercise performance with subsequent feedback from a therapist using the video footage. RCT found it to be an effective and efficient way of increasing amount of practice and standing performance (McClellan & Ada, 2004).	B	Minimal equipment costs and training.
Communication and language	Early aphasia therapy (Godecke, Hird, Lalor, Rai, & Phillips, 2011).	B	Potentially will require more speech pathologists to be able to deliver the therapy.
Oral feeding early interventions	An early intervention program for oral feeding, consisting of intensive oral care and early behavioral interventions, has demonstrated that a high proportion of patients can tolerate oral feeding with no increase in complication rates. Positive results but an area justifying further investigation (Takahata, Tsutsumi, Baba, Nagata, & Yonekura, 2011).	C	
Robotics	Overall conflicting results, with methodological inconsistencies. Cochrane review found improved motor function and strength with electromechanical and robotic assisted training, but did not improve ADLs (Mehrholz, Platz, Kugler, & Pohl, 2008).	A, B	Significant equipment and technology costs.
Virtual reality training	Interventions and outcomes are mixed. Although methodological inconsistencies, RCTs have demonstrated positive results. Area where future research is required.	C	Significant equipment and technology costs and specialized space required.

*LEVELS OF EVIDENCE: A – based on robust information from randomized trials (RCT); B – based on less robust information (e.g., experimental studies); C – based on less robust studies, and care should be taken in its application; D – based on consensus or expert opinion.

systematic reviews on interventions and assessments that are applicable in stroke rehabilitation.

7.5 INNOVATIONS IN REHABILITATION AND APPLICATION IN CLINICAL PRACTICE

Major advances have occurred in the past 20 years in the development and testing of interventions for stroke rehabilitation, but there are still gaps and shortcomings in the evidence to inform clinical practice (Langhorne, Bernhardt, & Kwakkel, 2011). Outstanding rehabilitation questions that need answers if we are to optimize current care practices relate to (i) dose (e.g., how much rehabilitation is needed?); (ii) timing of rehabilitation (e.g., at what point after injury? And for how long should it continue?); (iii) who should provide rehabilitation services; and (iv) what is the best environment to provide rehabilitation given a range of geographical, workforce, and other constraints. For example, researchers in Japan have recently reported that greater input from rehabilitation specialists and more frequent therapy sessions resulted in improved functional outcomes, with patients more likely to be discharged home (Jeong, et al., 2010). However, applying these research findings within the reality of clinical practice may be problematic if there is not the capacity to provide more therapy sessions.

In this chapter, we have focused on the issues that influence how rehabilitation care is organized for people with stroke, and related factors that influence the efficiency and efficacy of services. It is worth considering, however, some of the recent innovations in stroke rehabilitation interventions (Table 7.3) and the potential implications for implementing these interventions in future models of rehabilitation care.

7.6 SUMMARY OF KEY MESSAGES

Increased demand for rehabilitation services will have important implications for the healthcare workforce and the organization and options for care delivery given the limited resources that are available. Therefore, policymakers, health administrators, clinicians, and researchers need to work together in determining the priorities for rehabilitation services. This will ensure resources are used to their greatest potential and provide patients with the best opportunity for recovery. In this chapter we have highlighted the attributes of organized care for stroke rehabilitation that help delivery of evidence-based care, and the importance of collecting data on the quality of care. Examples of quality improvement programs and innovations in rehabilitation practice were outlined. In summary,

- Organized stroke care provides better outcomes, and more could be done to improve access to organized stroke care in rehabilitation settings and throughout the stroke recovery pathway.

- Various models of organized care exist in hospitals and the community, and further research is needed to quantify the impact on patients and their caregivers, as well as the resource implications of the various options.

- Routine monitoring of care practices is needed to provide evidence for and prioritize quality improvement initiatives in stroke rehabilitation.

- Research is urgently needed in a number of areas to inform policy and practice with consideration of implementation issues.

REFERENCES

Adams, H. P., del Zoppo, G., Alberts, M. J., Bhatt, D. L., Brass, L., Furlan, A., et al. (2007). Guidelines for the early management of adults with ischemic stroke—A guideline from the American Heart Association/American Stroke Association Stroke Council, Clinical Cardiology Council, Cardiovascular Radiology and Intervention Council, and the Atherosclerotic Peripheral Vascular Disease and Quality of Care Outcomes in Research Interdisciplinary Working Groups (Reprinted from *Stroke*, Vol. 38, pp. 1655–1711, 2007). *Circulation, 115*(20), E478–E534.

American Heart Association. (2010). Heart disease and stroke statistics—2010 update. A report from the American Heart Association. *Circulation, 121*, e46–e215.

Australian Bureau of Statistics. (2008). *3303.0 Causes of death 2206: Australia.* (No. 3303.0). Canberra: ABS.

Bernhardt, J., Dewey, H., Collier, J., Thrift, A., Lindley, R., Moodie, M., et al. (2006). A Very Early Rehabilitation Trial (AVERT). *International Journal of Stroke, 1(3)*, 169–171.

Bernhardt, J., Chitravas, N., Meslo, I. L., Thrift, A. G., & Indredavik, B. (2008). Not all stroke units are the same: a comparison of physical activity patterns in Melbourne, Australia, and Trondheim, Norway. *Stroke, 39*(7), 2059–2065.

Brady, B., McGahan, L., & Skidmore, B. (2005). Systematic review of economic evidence on stroke rehabilitation services. *International Journal of Technology Assessment in Health Care, 21*(1), 15–21.

Cadilhac, D. A., Carter, R., Thrift, A. G., & Dewey, H. M. (2009). Estimating the long-term costs of ischemic (IS) and hemorrhagic (ICH) stroke for Australia: new evidence derived from the North East Melbourne Stroke Incidence Study (NEMESIS). *Stroke, 40*, 915–921.

Cadilhac, D. A., Ibrahim, J., Pearce, D. C., Ogden, K. J., McNeill, J., Davis, S. M., et al. (2004). Multicenter comparison of processes of care between Stroke Units and conventional care wards in Australia. *Stroke, 35*(5), 1035–1040.

Cadilhac, D. A., Kilkenny, M., Longworth, M., Pollack, M., Levi, C., & on behalf of Greater Metropolitan Clinical Taksforce and Stroke Services New South Wales Coordinating Committee. (2011). Metropolitan-rural divide for stroke outcomes: do stroke units make a difference? *Internal Medicine Journal, 41*(4), 231–236.

Cadilhac, D. A., Pearce, D. C., Levi, C. R., & Donnan, G. A. (2008). Improvements in the quality of care and health outcomes with new Stroke Care Units following implementation of a clinician-led, health-system redesign programme in New South Wales, Australia. *Quality and Safety in Health Care, 17,* 329–333.

Cadilhac, D. A., Purvis, T., Moss, K., Paice, K., Longworth, M., Pollack, M., et al. (2011). *Evaluation of rural New South Wales stroke services: New South Wales Rural Stroke Project (Phase III).* Melbourne: National Stroke Research Institute.

Cott, C. A., Wiles, R., & Devitt, R. (2007). Continuity, transition and participation: preparing clients for life in the community post-stroke. *Disability and Rehabilitation, 29*(20–21), 1566–1574.

Cumming, T. B., Cadilhac, D. A., Rubin, G., Crafti, N., & Pearce, D. (2008). Psychological distress and social support in informal caregivers of stroke survivors. *Brain Impairment, 9*(2), 152–160.

Cumming, T. B., Thrift, A. G., Collier, J. M., Churilov, L., Dewey, H. M., Donnan, G. A., et al. (2011). Very early mobilization after stroke fast-tracks return to walking: further results from the phase II AVERT randomized controlled trial. *Stroke, 42*(1), 153–158.

D'Amour, D., Ferrada-Videla, M., Rodriguez, L., & Beaulieu, M. (2005). The conpcetual basis for interprofessional collaboration: Core concepts and theoretical frameworks. *Journal of Interprofessional Care, 5*(Suppl. 1), 116–131.

De Wit, L., Putman, K., Dejaeger, E., Baert, I., Berman, P., Bogaerts, K., et al. (2005). Use of time by stroke patients: a comparison of four European rehabilitation centers. *Stroke, 36*(9), 1977–1983.

Dewey, H. M., Thrift, A. G., Mihalopoulos, C., Carter, R., Macdonell, R. A., McNeil, J. J., et al. (2003). Lifetime cost of stroke subtypes in Australia: findings from the North East Melbourne Stroke Incidence Study (NEMESIS). *Stroke, 34*(10), 2502–2507.

Doran, T., Fullwood, C., & Gravelle, H. (2006). Pay-for-performance programs in family practices in the United Kingdom. *New England Journal of Medicine, 355*(4), 375–384.

Dromerick, A. W., Lang, C. E., Birkenmeirer, R. L., Wagner, J. M., Miller, J. P., Videen, T. O., et al. (2009). Very Early Constraint-Induced Movement during Stroke Rehabilitation (VECTORS): A single-centre RCT. [RCT]. *Neurology, 73,* 195–201.

Dumoulin, C., Korner-Bitensky, N., & Tannenbaum, C. (2007). Urinary incontinence after stroke: identification, assessment, and intervention by rehabilitation professionals in Canada. *Stroke, 38*(10), 2745–2751.

Duncan, P., Horner, R., Reker, D., Samsa, G., Hoenig, H., Hamilton, B., et al. (2002). Adherence to post-acute rehabilitation guidelines is associated with functional recovery in stroke. *Stroke, 33,* 167–178.

Early Supported Discharge Trialists. (2005). Services for reducing duration of hospital care for acute stroke patients. *Cochrane Database of Systematic Reviews, 2,* CD000443.

Evers, S., Struijs, J. N., Ament, A., van Genugten, M. L. L., Jager, C., & van den Bos, G. A. M. (2004). International comparison of stroke cost studies. *Stroke, 35*(5), 1209–1215.

Foley, N., Salter, K., & Teasell, R. (2007). Specialized stroke services: a meta-analysis comparing three models of care. *Cerebrovascular Diseases, 23*(2–3), 194–202.

Gerdes, N., Funke, U. N., Schuwer, U., Kunze, H., Walle, E., Kleinfeld, A., et al. (2009). [Pay for performance in rehabilitation after stroke—results of a pilot project 2001–2008]. *Rehabilitation (Stuttg), 48*(4), 190–201.

Gloede, T., Cadilhac, D. A., & Dewey, H. M. (2010). Chapter 9: Cost and socioeconomic implications. *Clinical Guidelines for Stroke Management 2010* (pp. 119–126). Melbourne: National Stroke Foundation.

Godecke, E., Hird, K., Lalor, E., Rai, T., & Phillips, M. (2011). Very early post stroke aphasia therapy: A pilot randomised controlled efficacy trial. *International Journal of Stroke,* published online 6 October DOI: 10.1111/j.1747-4949.2011.00631.x

Graven, C., Brock, K., Hill, K., Ames, D., Cotton, S. & Joubert, L. (2011). From rehabilitation to recovery: protocol for a randomised controlled trial evaluating a goal-based intervention to reduce depression and facilitate participation post-stroke. *BMC Neurology, 11,* 73.

Grimshaw, J. M., Thomas, R. E., MacLennan, G., Fraser, C., Ramsay, C. R., Vale, L., et al. (2004). Effectiveness and efficiency of guideline dissemination and implementation strategies. *Health Technology Assessments, 8*(6), iii–iv, 1–72.

Gropen, T., Magdon-Ismail, Z., Day, D., Melluzzo, S., & Schwamm, L. H. (2009). Regional implementation of the stroke systems of care model: recommendations of the northeast cerebrovascular consortium. *Stroke, 40*(5), 1793–1802.

Hammond, R., Lennon, S., Walker, M., Hoffman, A., Irwin, P., & Lowe, D. (2005). Changing occupational therapy and physiotherapy practice through guidelines and audit in the United Kingdom. *Clinical Rehabilitation, 19*(4), 365–371.

Heidenreich, P., Trogdon, J., Khavjou, O., Butler, J., Dracup, K., Ezekowitz, M., et al. (2011). Forcasting the future of cardiovascular disease in the United States: A policy statement from the American Heart Association. *Circulation, 123*(8), 933–944.

Hubbard, I., Harris, D., Kilkenny, M. F., Faux, S., Pollack, M., & Cadilhac, D. A. (2012). Australian clinical practice of inpatient stroke rehabilitation and its relationship with patient outcomes. *Archives of Physical Medicine and Rehabilitation,* accepted 3 January.

Indredavik, B., Bakke, F., Solberg, R., Rokseth, R., Haaheim, L., & Holme, I. (1991). Benefit of a stroke unit: a randomized controlled trial. *Stroke, 22,* 1026–1031.

Ingeman, A., Andersen, G., Hundborg, H., Svendsen, M., & Johnsen, S. (2011). Processes of care and medical complications in patients with stroke. *Stroke, 42,* 167–172.

Intercollegiate Stroke Working Party. (2002). *National clinical guidelines for stroke.* London: Royal College of Physicians.

Intercollegiate Stroke Working Party. (2008). *National clinical guidelines for stroke* (3rd edition). London: Clinical Effectiveness and Evaluation Unit. Royal College of Physicians.

Intercollegiate Stroke Working Party. (2011). *National sentinel stroke clinical audit 2010 (Round 7).* London: Royal College of Physicians.

Irwin, P., Hoffman, A., Lowe, D., Pearson, M., & Rudd, A. (2005). Improving clinical practice in stroke through audit: results of three rounds of National Stroke Audit. *Journal of Evaluation in Clinical Practice, 11*(4), 306–314.

Jeong, S., Kondo, K., NShiraishi, N., & Yusuke, I. (2010). An evaluation of the quality of post-stroke rehabilitation in Japan. *Clinical Audit, 2,* 59–66.

Joubert, J., Prentice, L., Moulin, T., Liaw, S., Joubert, L., & Preux, P. (2008). Stroke in rural areas and small communities. *Stroke, 39,* 1920–1928.

Kalra, L., Evans, A., Perez, I., Melbourn, A., Patel, A., Knapp, M., et al. (2004). Training care givers of stroke patients: randomised controlled trial. *British Medical Journal, 328,* 1099–1101.

Kirkevold, M. (1997). The role of nursing in the rehabilitation of acute stroke patients: Toward a unified theoretical perspective. *Advances in Nursing Science, 19*(4), 55–64.

Korner-Bitensky, N., Wood-Dauphinee, S., Teasell, R., Hanley, J., Desrosiers, J., Kaizer, F., et al. (2004). The Canadian national survey on rehabilitatian practices for stroke: Preliminary findings. *Stroke, 35*(6), E191–E191.

Kwan, J., & Sandercock, P. (2004). In-hospital care pathways for stroke. *Cochrane Database of Systematic Reviews*(4), CD002924.

Langhorne, P., Bernhardt, J., & Kwakkel, G. (2011). Stroke rehabilitation. *Lancet, 377,* 1693–1702.

Langhorne, P., Coupar, F., & Pollock, A. (2009). Motor recovery after stroke: a systematic review. *Lancet Neurology, 8*(8), 741–754.

Langhorne, P., Holmqvist, L., & for the Early Supported Discharge Trialists. (2007). Early supported discharge after stroke. *Journal of Rehabilitative Medicine, 39,* 103–108.

Langhorne, P., & Pollack, A. (2002). What are the components of effective stroke unit care? *Age and Ageing, 31*(5), 365–371.

Langhorne, P., Taylor, G., Murray, G., Dennis, M., Anderson, C., & Bautz-Holter, E. (2005). Early supported discharge services for stroke patients: a meta-analysis of individual patient's data. *Lancet, 365*(9458), 591–506.

Lemieux-Charles, L., & McGuire, W. (2006). What do we know about health care team effectiveness? A review of the literature. *Medical Care Research and Review, 63*, 263.

Lindsay, M., Bayley, M., McDonald, A., Graham, I., Warner, G., & Phillips, S. (2008). Toward a more effective approach to stroke: Canadian best practice recommendations for stroke care. *Canadian Medical Association, 178*(11), 1418–1425.

Low, J. T., Roderick, P., & Payne, S. (2004). An exploration looking at the impact of domiciliary and day hospital delivery of stroke rehabilitation on informal carers. *Clinical Rehabilitation, 18*(7), 776–784.

McClellan, R., & Ada, L. (2004). A six-week, resource-efficient mobility program after discharge from rehabilitation improves standing in people affected by stroke: placebo controlled, randomised trial. *Australian Journal of Physiotherapy, 50*(3), 163–167.

McCullagh, E., Brigstocke, G., Donaldson, N., & Kalra, L. (2005). Determinants of caregiving burden and quality of life in caregivers of stroke patients. *Stroke, 36*, 2181–2186.

Mehrholz, J., Platz, T., Kugler, J., & Pohl, M. (2008). Electomechanical and robotic-assisted arm training for improving arm function and activities of daily living after stroke. *Cochrane Database of Systematic Reviews* (Issue 4), CD006876.

Menon, A., Korner-Bitensky, N., Kastner, M., McKibbon, K. A., & Straus, S. (2009). Strategies for rehabilitation professionals to move evidence-based knowledge into practice: A systematic review. *Journal of Rehabilitation Medicine, 41*(13), 1024–1032.

Moon, L., Moise, P., Jacobzone, S., & Group, a. t. A.-S. E. (2003). *Stroke care in OECD countries: A comparison of treatment, costs and outcomes in 17 countries.* Paris: Directorate for Employment, Labour and Social Affairs.

Murray, J., Young, J., Forster, A., Herbert, G., & Ashworth, R. (2006). Feasibility study of a primary care-based model for stroke aftercare. *British Journal of General Practice, 56*(531), 775–780.

National Stroke Foundation. (2007a). *National stroke audit clinical report: Acute services.* Melbourne: National Stroke Foundation.

National Stroke Foundation. (2007b). *Walk in our shoes. Stroke survivors and carers report on support after stroke.* Melbourne: National Stroke Foundation.

National Stroke Foundation. (2008). *National stroke audit clinical report: Post acute services.* Melbourne: National Stroke Foundation.

National Stroke Foundation. (2010a). *Clinical guidelines for stroke management 2010.* Melbourne: National Stroke Foundation.

National Stroke Foundation. (2010b). *National stroke audit rehabilitation services 2010.* Melbourne.

National Stroke Foundation. (2011). *National Stroke Audit-Acute Services Organizational Survey Report 2011.* Melbourne: National Stroke Foundation.

O'Connor, S. (2000). Mode of care delivery in stroke rehabilitation nursing: a development of Kirkevold's Unified Theoretical Perspective of the role of the nurse. *Clinical Effectiveness in Nursing, 4*(4), 180–188.

Outpatient Service Trialists. (2003). Therapy-based rehabilitation services for stroke patients at home. *Cochrane Database of Systematic Reviews, 1*(CD003585).

Petri, L. (2010). Concept analysis of interdisciplinary collaboration. *Nursing Forum, 45*(2), 73–82.

Petzold, A., Korner-Bitensky, N., & Menon, A. (2011). Using the knowledge to action process model to incite clinical change. *Journal of Continuing Education in the Health Professions, 30*(3), 167–171.

Pollock, A., Legg, L., Langhorne, P., & Sellars, C. (2000). Barriers to achieving evidence-based stroke rehabilitation. *Clinical Rehabilitation, 14*, 611–617.

Purvis, T. (2009). *Determining differences in stroke unit care: Melbourne versus Trondheim.* The University of Melbourne, Melbourne.

Purvis, T., Cadilhac, D., & Bernhardt, J. (2010). Not all stroke units are the same: early rehabilitation practices in Melbourne, Australia and Trondheim, Norway: O56. [Abstract]. *International Journal of Stroke, 1*(5 SUPPLEMENT), 10–11.

Purvis, T., Cadilhac, D. A., Donnan, G. A., & Bernhardt, J. (2009). A systematic review of process indicators, including early rehabilitation interventions, used to measure quality of acute stroke care. *International Journal of Stroke, 4*(2), 72–80.

Rochette, A., Korner-Bitensky, N., Bishop, D. S., Teasell, R., White, C., Bravo, G., et al. (2010). Study protocol of The YOU CALL—WE CALL TRIAL Impact of a multimodal support intervention after a "mild" stroke. *BMC Neurology, 10*, 3.

Rochette, A., Korner-Bitensky, N., & Desrosiers, J. (2007). Actual vs best practice for families post-stroke according to three rehabilitation disciplines. *Journal of Rehabilitative Medicine, 39*(7), 513–519.

Rudd, A. G., Hoffman, A., Irwin, P., Pearson, M., & Lowe, D. (2005). Stroke units: research and reality. Results from the National Sentinel Audit of Stroke. *Quality and Safety in Health Care, 14*(1), 7–12.

Saban, K. L., Sherwood, P. R., DeVon, H. A., & Hynes, D. M. (2011). Measures of psychological stress and physical health in family caregivers of stroke survivors: a literature review. *Journal of Neuroscience and Nursing, 42*(3), 128–138.

Sainsbury, S., & Lee, K. (2011). *Art therapy post stroke: helping participants find future direction through creative self-expression [abstract].* Paper presented at the Smart Strokes.

Saka, O., McGuire, A., & Wolfe, C. (2009). Cost of stroke in the United Kingdom. *Age and Ageing, 38*, 27–32.

Schmid, A. A., Kapoor, J. R., Miech, E. J., Kuehn, D., Dallas, M. I., Kerns, R. D., et al. (2011). A multidisciplinary stroke clinic for outpatient care of veterans with cerebrovascular disease. *Journal of Multidisciplinary Healthcare, 4*, 111–118.

Senes, S. (2006). *How we manage stroke in Australia. AIHW cat no CVD 31.* Canberra: Australian Institute of Health and Welfare.

Siebens, H. C. (2011). Proposing a practical clinical model. *Topics in Stroke Rehabilitation, 18*(1), 60–65.

Simmonds, F. (2009). *The AROC Annual Report: the state of rehabilitation in Australia in 2008:* Centre for Health Service Development, University of Woollongong.

Sirtori, V., Corbetta, D., Moja, L., & Gatti, R. (2009). Constraint induced movement therapy for upper extremities in stroke patients. *Cochrane Database of Systematic Reviews*(Issue 4), CD004433.

Sorrells-Jones, J. (1997). The challenge of making it real: interdisciplinary practices in a "seamless"organisation. *Nursing Administration Quarterly, 21*(2), 20–30.

Stroke Unit Trialists' Collaboration. (2007). Organised inpatient (stroke unit) care for stroke. *Cochrane Database of Systematic Reviews, Art. No.: CD000197*(Issue 4.).

Sulch, D., & Kalra, L. (2000). Integrated care pathways in stroke management. *Age and Ageing, 29*(4), 349–352.

Takahata, H., Tsutsumi, K., Baba, H., Nagata, I., & Yonekura, M. (2011). Early intervention to promote oral feeding in patients with intracerebral hemorrhage: a retrospective cohort study. *BMC Neurology, 11*, 6.

Teasell, R., Foley, N., Bhogal, S., & Speechley, M. (2003). Early supported discharge in stroke rehabilitation *Topics in Stroke Rehabilitation, 10*(2), 19–33.

Teasell, R., Foley, N., Salter, K., Bhogal, S., Jutai, J., & Speechley, M. (2009). Evidence-based review of stroke rehabilitation: Executive summary, 12th edition. *Topics in Stroke Rehabilitation, 16*(6), 463–488.

Thrift, A. G., Dewey, H. M., Macdonell, R. A., McNeil, J. J., & Donnan, G. A. (2000). Stroke incidence on the east coast of Australia: the North East Melbourne Stroke Incidence Study (NEMESIS). *Stroke, 31*(9), 2087–2092.

Wellwood, I., Wu, O., Langhorne, P., McKevitt, C., Di Carlo, A., Rudd, A., et al. (2011). Developing a tool to assess quality of stroke care across European populations. The EROS Quality Asssessment Tool. *Stroke, 42*, 1207–1211.

Wevers, L., van de Port, I., Vermue, M., Mead, G., & Kwakkel, G. (2009). Effects of task-orientated cicruit class training on walking competency after stroke: a systematic review. *Stroke, 40*(7), 2450–2459.

8 | MOTIVATION, MOOD, AND THE RIGHT ENVIRONMENT

THOMAS K. A. LINDEN, LEEANNE M. CAREY, and MICHAEL NILSSON

8.1 INTRODUCTION

Annually, 15 million people suffer a stroke. Of these, 5 million die and another 5 million are left disabled for life, placing a burden on the family and society (Donnan, Fisher, Macleod, & Davis, 2008). Yet, the consequence of stroke on physical function is just one side of the coin when it comes to consequences. When asked, patients place cognitive and psychiatric consequences on top of the list as their main problem after the stroke, and so do their close relatives (Haley et al., 2009; Haley, Roth, Kissela, Perkins, & Howard, 2010). One of the commonest and most problematic neuropsychiatric consequences is depression, which is substantially increased after stroke. While the World Health Organization (WHO) ranks cerebrovascular diseases in themselves as number six in the league of causes of burden of disease (Lopez, 2006), expressed as loss of disability-adjusted life years (DALYs), depression is placed as number three.

Depressed people have feelings of sadness, anxiety, and emptiness beyond what they can control. They often feel hopeless, guilty, worthless, irritable, and restless. They may experience disturbance of natural functions like sleep, appetite, initiative, and will (Linden, Blomstrand, & Skoog, 2007; Kouwenhoven, Kirkevold, Engedal, & Kim, 2011). A special obstacle in rehabilitation is that motivation is reduced and the patient may be difficult to engage in treatment activities.

For a long time, there was no strong notion that depression was at all increased after stroke. Findings of stroke sufferers with depressive symptomatologies were explained away with the idea that sadness and apathy were completely normal psychological reactions to sudden illness and loss of functions.

In a classic paper from 1977, Folstein et al. compared 20 stroke patients with 10 patients with equal functional loss but from orthopedic illness (Folstein, Maiberger, & McHugh, 1977) and reported that 45% of the stroke patients were classified as depressed, compared to 10% of the orthopedic patients. They concluded that, as the levels of functional disability were similar in both groups, mood disorder must be a specific complication of stroke rather than a simple response to motor disability. The finding that depression was increased in stroke convinced many that post-stroke depression may exist after all.

8.1.1 FREQUENCY AND NATURE OF POST-STROKE DEPRESSION

Since that time, depression has been meticulously charted in numerous studies (Finklestein et al., 1982; Robinson & Price, 1982; Wade, Legh-Smith, & Hewer, 1987; Astrom, Adolfsson, & Asplund, 1993; Pohjasvaara et al., 1998; Linden et al., 2007), finding high but a wide range of frequency estimates.

A systematic review in 2005 by Hackett and Anderson that pooled available studies of post-stroke depression occurrence (Hackett, Yapa, Parag, & Anderson, 2005), found that about one-third of stoke patients were depressed at various time points after stroke. Comparisons were difficult, however, because of differences in background populations, selection criteria, and diagnostic instruments. Lack of methodological uniformity between studies has been a specific problem when it comes to comparing and pooling the results. Further, it is likely to be a conservative estimate, given that high-risk groups, such as those with communication difficulties, are underestimated or not included in most incidence studies (Hackett, Yapa, Parag, & Anderson, 2005). Up to 70% of stroke survivors with aphasia are reported to fulfill diagnostic criteria of depression at 3 months (Kauhanen et al., 2000). Important depressive symptoms may also be experienced in stroke survivors with subthreshold scores on depression measures (Hackett, Hill, Hewison, Anderson, & House, 2010).

Time from stroke, assessment instruments, and diagnostic systems are far from uniform between the studies, making the results difficult to interpret. There are also differences in study populations and selection of patients (Rao, 2000; Provinciali & Coccia, 2002). Patients in stroke studies are often younger and, although it is generally recognized that depression is common after stroke, few studies have examined whether depression prevalence is increased in elderly stroke patients compared to age and gender matched controls. Only a few studies have used population-based control groups. One study (House, 1991) used general practitioner records for selecting controls, but these were not matched for gender. A Danish study (Robinson, Kubos, Starr, Rao, & Price, 1984) that made diagnosis by cut-off values used population-based controls, but did not publish risk estimates.

In order to investigate the frequency of long-term depression in patients, as they appear in the clinic, one group examined a stroke cohort in Gothenburg, 1.5 years after their strokes (Linden et al., 2007). The patients were part of a naturalistic randomized study set up by Blomstrand et al. (Fagerberg, Claesson, Gosman-Hedstrom, & Blomstrand, 2000) to evaluate the effects of stroke unit care. All 243 patients in this sub-study (Linden, Skoog, Fagerberg, Steen, & Blomstrand, 2004) were at least 70 years old at inclusion. The 149 patients that could be examined at 1.5 years were compared to a sample from the same background population, investigated with the same instruments, the comprehensive psychopathological rating scale of which the Montgomery-Åsberg Depression Rating Scale (Montgomery & Åsberg, 1979) is a derivative.

The authors found an age-dependent prevalence of depression, just as has been shown in the general population. The prevalence of depression in the stroke patients was 34% at that time point, half being diagnosed with major depressive disorder and half with milder forms (Linden et al., 2007). In the population sample the prevalence was 13%, giving an odds ratio for depressive disorders after stroke of 3.4. The prevalence was higher in the older than in the younger groups and higher in women than in men, both in stroke patients and controls. The increase in risk for depression after stroke was, however, higher for the younger stroke patients compared to controls.

8.1.2 IMPACT OF POST-STROKE DEPRESSION

The recognition and diagnosis of depression in stroke patients is important, as it has been associated with worse outcome in numerous studies (Monga, Lawson, & Inglis, 1986; Cushman, 1988; Parikh et al., 1990; Schubert, Taylor, Lee, Mentari, & Tamaklo, 1992; Morris, Robinson, Andrzejewski, Samuels, & Price, 1993; Kotila, Numminen, Waltimo, & Kaste, 1999). Depression is associated with an increased incidence of first and recurrent stroke, and greater mortality, with greater than 3 times the risk of dying in 10 years (Bos et al., 2008). Depressed stroke patients have, for example, more cognitive impairments, more days in the hospital, utilize more care, have poorer rehabilitation outcome (Hadidi, Treat-Jacobson, & Lindquist, 2009), and are more often institutionalized than the nondepressed (Linden, Blomstrand, & Skoog, 2007). They have reduced independence in activities of daily living, reduced participation in previous life activities, and an increased failure to return to work (Cully et al., 2005; Edwards, Hahn, Baum, & Dromerick, 2006; Hommel et al., 2009). Even those with relatively mild stroke return to fewer household, social/educational, leisure, and work activities when depressed (Edwards et al., 2006).

Nevertheless, depression after stroke is often underdiagnosed (Williams et al., 2011) despite that effective treatment seems to exist (de Man-van Ginkel, Gooskens, Schuurmans, Lindeman, & Hafsteinsdottir, 2010; Bueno, Brunoni, Boggio, Bensenor, & Fregni, 2011; Herrmann et al., 2011; Price et al., 2011). To date there is no quantitative estimation of the probably vast magnitude of how this impacts healthcare delivery systems (Provinciali & Coccia, 2002). In health economy studies of stroke, complications such as depression are not added to costs attributable to stroke but are regarded as an independent comorbidity, thus underestimating the societal costs for stroke.

8.1.3 ETIOLOGY OF DEPRESSION AFTER STROKE

The etiology of depression after stroke is debated. Some authors put focus on biological factors; particularly disruption of tracts such as aminergic corticostriatal, frontostriatal or left-sided prefrontal-subcortical pathways, or infarcts in strategic locations such as right hemisphere strokes, left anterior lesions, left-sided basal ganglia lesions, and inferior frontal lesions (Folstein et al., 1977; Robinson, Kubos, Starr, Rao, & Price, 1984; Bogousslavsky et al., 1988; Robinson, Starkstein, & Price, 1988; Starkstein, Robinson, Berthier, Parikh, & Price, 1988; Starkstein et al., 1989; Starkstein & Robinson, 1990; Starkstein, Fedoroff, Price, Leiguarda, & Robinson, 1992; Berthier, Kulisevsky, Gironell, & Fernandez Benitez, 1996; Alexopoulos et al., 1997;. Beblo, Wallesch, & Herrmann, 1999; Vataja et al., 2001; Singh, Omiccioli, Hegge, & McKinley, 2009). Other studies emphasize the impact of sudden disability and loss of autonomy as a cause of reactive depression after stroke (Gainotti, Azzoni, & Marra, 1999; Kneebone & Dunmore, 2000), and yet others try to join the two perspectives (Katz, 1996).

Interestingly, the relationship between stroke and depression seems to work both ways. Depression is increased after stroke, but depression does also increase the risk for stroke. The Rotterdam group investigated for depressive symptoms prospectively, within their large population-based cohort study, a general population sample initially free of stroke (Bos et al., 2008). They found increased risk for stroke in those with previous depressive symptoms. Men with symptoms of depression also had an increased risk for ischemic stroke. Specifically, males with depressive symptoms but not fulfilling all criteria for depression were at higher risk of stroke and ischemic stroke than were the women of the same study. For ischemic stroke, the study showed a hazard ratio over 4, placing "depressive symptoms" among the relative strong risk factors for stroke. Another study investigating a Swedish population-based sample of elderly people gave similar results (Liebetrau, Steen, & Skoog, 2003), with a hazard rate of 2.7 for the 3-year incidence of first-ever strokes in those with clinical depression at baseline. These findings give some support to the hypothesis of "vascular depression" by Alexopolous and others (Alexopoulos et al., 1997), which postulates that a single larger or several smaller cerebrovascular damages disrupting prefrontal systems or their connecting pathways give rise to depressive symptoms, mainly in geriatric populations.

8.2 IS POST-STROKE DEPRESSION A SPECIFIC DISORDER?

Many studies have focused on the specific problems in diagnosing depression in patients with somatic illnesses, not the least in stroke. It is a problem that physical illnesses of different kinds produce some of the symptoms that comprise the depression diagnosis. For instance, the symptoms increased—including crying, lethargy, appetite change, sleep disturbances, and apathy—are very common symptoms in stroke and depressive disorders alike.

Some authors even suggested that common stroke symptoms may lead to overdiagnosis of psychiatric illnesses; for example, as Calvert and colleagues (Calvert, Knapp, & House, 1998) suggested in the case of affect incontinence, or emotionalism, and as Staub and Bogousslavsky (2001) proposed for fatigue, or lethargy, or loss of energy in commentary on a research article by van der Werf and coworkers (van der Werf, van den Broek, Anten, & Bleijenberg, 2001).

Spalletta (Spalletta, Bria, & Caltagirone, 2005) and Gainotti (Gainotti & Marra, 2002) have studied the phenomenology of post-stroke depression, as have some other researchers, which has led to the question of whether depression after stroke and depression in other people really are etiologically the same. This is an interesting question, not least because we largely have to deduct conclu-

sions from studies in general depression on how to treat post-stroke depression.

One study (Cumming, Churilov, Skoog, Blomstrand, & Linden, 2010) examined the symptom profile in depressed stroke patients and compared it to the profile in depressed patients without stroke. The only items that differed significantly between stroke patients and controls were sleep disturbances and anhedonia (loss of interest). But the scores for these two items were higher for controls than stroke patients, leading them to conclude that depression is not overestimated in stroke patients due to somatic symptoms, and also that there is no reason to doubt that what is proven effective for depression is also effective in post-stroke depression. Absence of evidence is not, however, evidence of absence! They also did a factor analysis of the ten symptoms in the diagnostic algorithm, which grouped into two clusters, but again without differences in the two groups.

We can thus conclude that there *seems* to be no support for the notion that post-stroke depression is a psychopathological entity different from depression in people without a prior stroke. We still do not know, however, why some stroke survivors get depression and others do not. A reliable prognostic instrument or predictor would have the utility of making it possible to direct special attention, treatment, or rehabilitative efforts to patients more prone to develop this complication.

8.3 PREDICTORS OF POST-STROKE DEPRESSION

Despite the large number of clinical and social markers that have been investigated, meta-analysis revealed that more severe stroke was the only common variable associated with depression (Hackett & Anderson, 2005). Evidence for a relationship between lesion location and post-stroke depression is unresolved. Depression does not seem to correlate very well with stroke lesion location, despite laborious efforts to find those associations. Nor does it appear to be correlated with stroke size. This is despite many hypotheses to the contrary and despite what is common in other neurologic conditions.

Systematic review and meta-analysis did not find an association between brain infarct localization and depression (Singh, Herrmann, & Black, 1998; Carson et al., 2000a; Carson et al., 2000b). It has been suggested that this may be impacted by imaging methods and their ability to detect vascular changes and their locations within gray and white matter structures (Vataja et al., 2004). Using a standardized MRI protocol to detail side, site, type, and extent of the brain infarct, as well as severity of white matter lesions and brain atrophy in 70 stroke patients at 3 months, it was found that brain infarcts that affected structures of the frontal-subcortical circuits (i.e., the pallidum and caudate) predisposed stroke patients to depression (Vataja et al., 2004). A further meta-analysis that specifically investigated the correlation between severity of post-stroke depression and proximity of the lesion to the frontal pole found a negative association (Narushima, Kosier, & Robinson, 2003), despite the fact that previous meta-analyses failed to show evidence for this association (Singh et al., 1998; Carson et al., 2000b). In a prospective longitudinal study, an association was reported between size of lesion in putative limbic-cortical regions and depression (Terroni et al., 2011). Further focused investigation is warranted.

To date there have not been very many interesting genetic risk factors identified as predictors of post-stroke depression. One, however, is a polymorphism in a gene coding for a serotonin transporter. Serotonin, or 5-hydroxytryptophane (5-HT) is one of the major, or even the key neurotransmitters in regulation of mood on which Ramasubbu and coworkers have elaborated (Ramasubbu, Tobias, Buchan, & Bech-Hansen, 2006). One hypothesis involving this polymorphism is that people with certain allele combinations have enough serotonin transport capacity for the ordinary situation, but are less resilient to stress and more prone to react with depression on psychological or physiological stress, as in stroke.

Biochemical and genetic markers related to inflammation may also be candidate predictors of depression (Maes, 1995). Inflammatory cytokines are implicated in the pathophysiology of depression (Dinan, 2009). Major depression is associated with a prolonged proinflammatory response, as indexed by elevation in C-reactive protein and cytokines such as interleukin 6 and tumor necrosis factor-α (Dantzer, O'Connor, Freund, Johnson, & Kelley, 2008; Maes, 2008; Dinan, 2009). Systematic review has identified the common pattern of upregulation in proinflammatory cytokines, glutamate, nitric oxide, and apoptosis, and downregulation of interleukin 10, in clinical depression and ischemic stroke (Pascoe, Crewther, Carey, & Crewther, 2011). These changes in inflammation and stress following stroke highlight that post-stroke depression is theoretically more likely to be the norm rather than the exception. Further, the review summarizes evidence that reduction of inflammation reduces depression. The critical need has been highlighted for research to include measurement of combined candidate biochemical, genetic, and imaging biomarkers currently established as relating to clinical depression (Monroe, 2008).

8.4 FUNCTIONAL AND STRUCTURAL BRAIN CHANGES WITH DEPRESSION

Clinical depression has been associated with changes in structure and function in key brain regions, including limbic and cortical regions—regions that may be directly or indirectly impacted by the stroke infarct. Mayberg (1997) proposed a working model of clinical depression that implicates failure of the "coordinated interactions of a distributed network of limbic-cortical pathways." This model was systematically developed from lesion-deficit correlation studies, functional activation studies, clinical, biochemical, and electrophysiological evidence, and related animal studies. It considers the range of symptoms experienced with depression, as well as the attention and cognitive changes. The model provides strong support for depressive illness being associated with decreases in dorsal limbic (anterior and posterior cingulate) and neocortical (especially prefrontal) regions, and increases in ventral paralimbic areas (subgenual cingulate, anterior insula, hypothalamus, caudate). A more focused investigation of changes in brain structure and function associated with post-stroke depression may be informed by this literature, as discussed below. This may contribute to identification of novel imaging markers of depression post-stroke, potentially using more advanced neuroimaging techniques.

8.4.1 FUNCTIONAL BRAIN CHANGES

Findings from studies of resting-state functional connectivity (see Chapter 4) in clinical depression and major depressive disorder are consistent with the limbic-cortical model proposed. Decreased limbic-cortical functional connectivity was commonly found in different types of mood disorders (Anand, Li, Wang, Lowe, & Dzemidzic, 2009), and included subgenual cingulate and thalamus in major depression. (Greicius et al., 2007). Changes in central nodes of cortical networks have been identified, with altered nodal centralities in the left hippocampus and the left caudate nucleus being correlated with disease duration and severity (Zhang et al., 2011).

A recent review of interconnected brain regions highlighted the role of anterior cingulate cortex, amygdala, and hippocampus as part of an interconnected prefrontal and limbic network that is dysregulated in major depressive disorders (MDD; Bennett, 2011). Brain regions most consistently identified across imaging studies can be determined using meta-analysis and the statistical activation likelihood estimate method (ALE). This method quantitatively models reported brain coordinates and analyzes the locations where individual peak coordinates converge in a standard brain space (Eickhoff et al., 2009). The method was used to investigate functional activation changes in MDD at rest, after treatment, and during emotion induction (Fitzgerald, Laird, Maller, & Daskalakis, 2008). The most consistently identified regions included areas of the anterior cingulate, dorsolateral, medial and inferior prefrontal cortex, insula, superior temporal gyrus, basal ganglia, and cerebellum, although there was limited overlap between the different designs.

8.4.2 MORPHOLOGICAL BRAIN CHANGES

Increasing evidence has revealed gross morphological cerebral changes in (non-stroke) patients with depression, involving generalized and localized atrophy of areas including the prefrontal cortex, caudate nucleus, anterior cingulate gyrus, amygdala, and hippocampus; areas that are implicated in regulation of stress responsiveness and in mood and emotion (Koolschijn, van Haren, Lensvelt-Mulders, Pol, & Kahn, 2009; Lorenzetti, Allen, Fornito, & Yucel, 2009; Sacher et al., 2011). Hypercortisolemia has been postulated to lead to hippocampal neuronal loss, which in turn has been posited to be involved in pathogenesis of depression (Sapolsky, Romero, & Munck, 2000). A reduction in hippocampal volume, observed with MRI, is consistently shown in people with depression relative to age and gender matched controls, with evidence supported by a number of meta-analyses (Campbell, Marriott, Nahmias, & MacQueen, 2004; Videbech & Ravnkilde, 2004). Moreover, the magnitude of reduction in hippocampal volume is related to frequency and duration of depressive episodes (MacQueen et al., 2003). A reduction of 19% in patients with major depression has been reported relative to case matched controls (Bremner et al., 2000).

A meta-analysis of changes in volume of gray matter in patients with MDD found the largest decrease in grey matter in anterior cingulate cortex (11.5%), a 9% decline in the gray matter of the orbitofrontal cortex, and a 5% loss of gray matter in the hippocampus (Koolschijn et al., 2009). This change may be accommodated by the reported loss of synapses in the hippocampus (Eastwood & Harrison, 2000). Sacher (Sacher et al., 2011) reported a convergent change in the limbic-cortical brain circuit in depression compared to controls that included lower gray matter volumes in the amygdala, the dorsal frontomedian cortex, and the right paracingulate cortex, as well as increases in glucose metabolism in the right subgenual and pregenual anterior cingulate cortices. An association has been observed between depression and amygdala volume in depressed and nondepressed stroke patients (Sachdev, Chen, Joscelyne, Wen, & Brodaty, 2007).

Cerebrovascular burden, indicated by increased white matter hyperintensity (WMH) volume, is also shown to have a role in late-onset depression (Herrmann, Le Masurier, & Ebmeier, 2008). After stroke, severe deep WMHs remained an independent predictor of post-stroke depression in a multivariate analysis, with an odds ratio of 13.8 (p = 0.016; Tang et al., 2010). White matter hyperintensities may independently predict future depression in healthy elderly (Teodorczuk et al., 2010), late-life depression (Herrmann et al., 2008; Baune, Schmidt, Roesler, & Berger, 2009), and post-stroke, (Tang et al., 2010) and are associated with gene expression, oxidative stress, and inflammation (Xu et al., 2010).

8.4.3 DEPRESSION, COGNITION, AND BRAIN NETWORKS

The relations between emotion, affect, and cognition have been extensively studied (Pessoa, 2008) in animal models, in imaging studies, and in other diseases. While the current view of brain organization supports functional specialization of brain regions as either "affective" or "cognitive," it is argued that this view is problematic and that these behaviors have their basis in "dynamic coalitions of networks of brain areas" (Pessoa, 2008). For example, executive function involves making decisions that are influenced by the value of the goal or action, and thus involves a broader cognitive–affective control circuit (see Chapter 15). Further, the architecture of the proposed circuit suggests that cognitive, emotional, and affective contributions cannot be separated. Central to these cognitive–emotional–affective interactions are brain areas with a high degree of connectivity, called *hubs* (Sporns, Honey, & Kotter, 2007), which are critical for regulating the flow and integration of information between regions (Pessoa, 2008). Areas considered hubs are the lateral prefrontal cortex and amygdala; (with involvement of anterior cingulate cortex, hippocampus, and orbitofrontal cortex). The amygdala is associated with cognitive impairment and increased vulnerability to depression (Sachdev et al., 2007). It is proposed that complex mood/cognitive changes after stroke are linked with interruption to networks of brain areas, with increased likelihood of developing depression when "connector-hub" regions are interrupted.

8.5 TREATMENT OF DEPRESSION IN STROKE PATIENTS

So what is there to do in response to depression? There is vast evidence of the efficacy of pharmacological and psychological interventions in ordinary depression. Not, surprisingly, so much for post-stroke depression.

Hackett and Anderson conducted two systematic reviews (Anderson, Hackett, & House, 2004; Hackett, Anderson, House, & Xia, 2008) in the field of post-stroke depression. In the first they found a small effect of psychotherapy on preventing post-stroke depression, but not of serotonin reuptake inhibitors (SSRIs), which is the commonest drug for non-stroke clinical depression. Later, they could not even see a convincing effect of SSRIs in treating manifest depression in stroke patients. This was contrary to clinical experience and was received with scepticism. In addition, the authors' first interpretation of the findings was that it was due to study heterogeneity rather than lack of efficacy. Individual well-designed studies have shown effect on post-stroke depression of SSRIs and the question is still open.

Side effects of commonly used antidepressant pharmaceuticals (e.g., SSRIs) include initial worsening of symptoms, confusion, and lowered seizure threshold, and this is a particular concern in stroke patients. Nonpharmacological treatment methods are therefore sought as an alternative way of treating post-stroke depression.

8.5.1 NONPHARMACOLOGICAL TREATMENT OPTIONS

There are indeed examples of the demonstrated success also of nonpharmacological interventions. Within the FINNSTROKE study by Kotila, Kaste, and others (Kotila, Numminen, Waltimo, & Kaste, 1998), stroke patients were relieved of depression at 3 and 12 months by a program promoting social interaction within a patient organization framework. The intervention was built on a backbone of physiotherapy-based extra rehabilitation and curative help in adapting to life after stroke. The odds ratio for patients in the intervention group being depressed was 0.59 at 3 months and 0.55 at 12 months. The authors emphasize the importance of social interaction, but the results seem to emphasize that multimodal stimulation should be the focus of investigation, as the intervention program integrates physical activity, social interaction, and promotion of sense-of-coherence.

8.5.2 ENRICHED ENVIRONMENT

In experimental paradigms, physical activity, sensory stimulation, and social interaction have been strongly suggested to exert strong effects on brain plasticity and regeneration as well as on functional improvement (Johansson, 1996; Nilsson, Perfilieva, Johansson, Orwar, & Eriksson, 1999; Komitova, Zhao, Gido, Johansson, & Eriksson, 2005). It is not far-fetched to see these investigated as novel nonpharmacological interventions for post-stroke depression as well.

The brain strongly responds to environmental stimuli, physiological modifications, and different experiences, and, as a result, it restructures itself in several measurable ways (see Chapter 3). In animals and humans, some regions in the normal adult brain, particularly the cortex, can alter their biochemistry, structure, and function—for example, during learning or in response to an enriched environment (EE). First described by Donald Hebb (Hebb, 1959), the experimental paradigm of EE is the most widely used animal model of experience-induced plasticity. The term refers to an environment that provides greater possibilities for physical and social stimulation and/or interaction than standard housing conditions. EE is defined as "a combination of complex inanimate and social stimulation," indicating that the interaction of several factors is the essential feature of the EE.

The therapeutic potential of EE has been evaluated in animal models of various neurological conditions, including stroke and traumatic brain injury. For example, EE enhances the recovery of motor function after focal brain ischemia induced by middle cerebral artery occlusion (Grabowski, Sorensen, Mattsson, Zimmer, & Johansson, 1995). It also has beneficial effects on cognitive functions, such as memory and learning (Bouet, Freret, Dutar, Billard, & Boulouard, 2011). Further, EE has been demonstrated to have beneficial physiological and behavioral effects in animal models of psychiatric disorders including depression (Sifonios et al., 2009). Interestingly, EE might ameliorate emotional disturbances induced by psychological stress (Wright & Conrad, 2008; Ilin & Richter-Levin, 2009). It is shown that EE can rescue the submissive phenotype and depressive-like behaviors adopted in response to chronic psychosocial stress (Wright & Conrad, 2008; Ilin & Richter-Levin, 2009), suggesting that EE increases stress resilience and promotes adaptive coping. However, these results should be interpreted with caution, since existing models mimicking depression have several limitations. Complex cognitive/emotional behavior is underpinned by dynamic interactions between cellular networks in the brain and EE may interfere with them at multiple levels, making the effects hard to interpret. Nevertheless, EE has, in different models of depression, been suggested effective and this potential therapeutic effect must be studied further.

8.5.3 CORTICAL STIMULATION AND DEPRESSION

One emerging therapy paradigm for depression in stroke patients is repetitive transcranial magnetic stimulation (rTMS). Cortical electrical activity and neuronal excitability seems to be lowered in depressive disorders and these parameters can be modulated by transcranial magnetic stimulation (Fitzgerald, Fountain, & Daskalakis, 2006), which provides a rationale for treatment effect. The neural excitability can be increased or decreased depending on stimulation pulse frequency. It has been shown to have antidepressant effects in depressive patients without stroke (Pascual-Leone, Rubio, Pallardo, & Catala, 1996). The method was studied by Jorge, Robinson, Chemerinski (Jorge et al., 2004) and others in a 2004 clinical trial in 20 stroke patients beyond the acute phase after stroke. Outcomes were evaluated, as in many depression intervention trials, with scoring on the Hamilton Rating Scale for Depression showing about half the symptom scores as sham-treated patients. This should be interpreted as a strong indication of the efficacy of rTMS in depressed stroke patients.

Similar effects to those in rTMS can be achieved by transcranial direct current stimulation (tDCS) of the cerebral cortex (Been, Ngo, Miller, & Fitzgerald, 2007), which is occasionally somewhat carelessly described as a milder current form of electroconvulsive therapy. Depressive disorders may be associated with decreased brain activity and cortical excitability, constituting a rationale for electrophysiological treatment. Nitsche, Pascual-Leone and others did an informative review (Nitsche, Boggio, Fregni, & Pascual-Leone, 2009) of tDCS, finding such alterations in a distributed cortico-subcortical network across both hemispheres. They summarized a few promising pilot studies using tDCS in the treatment of depression, but also concluded that larger studies are needed. Rigonatti et al. conducted a study on tDCS and fluoxetine (Rigonatti et al., 2008). Their results show lowered Beck Depression Inventory (BDI) scores at different time points up to 6 weeks after DCS compared to both sham treatment and antidepressant therapy (Rigonatti et al., 2008).

8.5.4 PHYSICAL ACTIVITY

Pulse-raising physical activity has also been shown to improve depressive symptoms. In a study from Smith and Thompson (2008), stroke survivors were randomized to walking on a treadmill or, as control group, receiving a phone call. The intervention group did improve during the training period in depressive symptoms measured by the Beck Depression Index. An interesting finding was that the improvement continued after the end of the training period.

A recent French study (Chollet et al., 2011) compared the SSRI fluoxetine or placebo, given to 118 stroke patients with or without signs of depression before physiotherapy, and succeeded in showing significantly better motor recovery after 3 months in the patients that received the drug. They suggested that the SSRIs may be exerting their effect through promoting plasticity, and that this effect may also be used for boosting rehabilitation also in patients that are not depressed.

In this highly dynamic field of stroke recovery, more research is needed into finding effective treatment paradigms for depressive disorders in stroke patients, pharmaceutical as well as non-pharmaceutical. Many of these treatments seem to work synergistically and finding the right mix of treatments, along with their dosing and optimal timing, is a challenge in itself. Succeeding in this would increase the rehabilitation potential for the at least third of stroke patients that are struck by this devastating complication on top of the tremendous rehabilitation challenges they already face. It may also lead to better rehabilitation paradigms for stroke patients that are not depressed.

REFERENCES

Alexopoulos, G. S., Meyers, B. S., Young, R. C., Campbell, S., Silberswieg, D., & Charlson, M. (1997). "Vascular depression" hypothesis [see comments]. *Archives of General Psychiatry, 54*(10), 915–922.

Anderson, C. S., Hackett, M. L., & House, A. O. (2004). Interventions for preventing depression after stroke. *Cochrane Database of Systematic Reviews* (2), CD003689.

Anand, A., Li, Y., Wang, Y., Lowe, M. J., & Dzemidzic, M. (2009). Resting state corticolimbic connectivity abnormalities in unmedicated bipolar disorder and unipolar depression. *Psychiatry Research, 171* (3), 189–198.

Astrom, M., Adolfsson, R., & Asplund, K. (1993). Major depression in stroke patients. A 3-year longitudinal study. *Stroke, 24*(7), 976–982.

Baune, B. T., Schmidt, W. P., Roesler, A., & Berger, K. (2009). Functional consequences of subcortical white matter lesions and MRI-defined brain infarct in an elderly general population. *Journal of Geriatric Psychiatry and Neurology, 22*(4), 266–273.

Beblo, T., Wallesch, C. W., & Herrmann, M. (1999). The crucial role of frontostriatal circuits for depressive disorders in the post-acute stage after stroke. *Neuropsychiatry, Neuropsychology and Behavioural Neurology, 12*(4), 236–246.

Been, G., Ngo, T. T., Miller, S. M., & Fitzgerald, P. B. (2007). The use of tDCS and CVS as methods of non-invasive brain stimulation. *Brain Research Reviews, 56*(2), 346–361.

Bennett, M. R. (2011). The prefrontal-limbic network in depression: Modulation by hypothalamus, basal ganglia and midbrain. *Progress in Neurobiology, 93*, 468–487.

Berthier, M. L., Kulisevsky, J., Gironell, A., & Fernandez Benitez, J. A. (1996). Poststroke bipolar affective disorder: clinical subtypes, concurrent movement disorders, and anatomical correlates. *Journal of Neuropsychiatry and Clinical Neuroscience, 8*(2), 160–167.

Bogousslavsky, J., Ferrazzini, M., Regli, F., Assal, G., Tanabe, H., & Delaloye-Bischof, A. (1988). Manic delirium and frontal-like syndrome with paramedian infarction of the right thalamus. *Journal of Neurology, Neurosurgery and Psychiatry, 51*(1), 116–119.

Bos, M. J., Linden, T., Koudstaal, P. J., Hofman, A., Skoog, I., Breteler, M. M., et al. (2008). Depressive symptoms and risk of stroke: the Rotterdam Study. *Journal of Neurology, Neurosurgery, and Psychiatry, 79*(9), 997–1001.

Bouet, V., Freret, T., Dutar, P., Billard, J. M., & Boulouard, M. (2011). Continuous enriched environment improves learning and memory in adult NMRI mice through theta burst-related-LTP independent mechanisms but is not efficient in advanced aged animals. *Mechanics of Ageing and Development, 132*(5), 240–248.

Bremner, J. D., Narayan, M., Anderson, E. R., Staib, L. H., Miller, H. L., & Charney, D. S. (2000). Hippocampal volume reduction in major depression. *American Journal of Psychiatry, 157*(1), 115–118.

Bueno, V. F., Brunoni, A. R., Boggio, P. S., Bensenor, I. M., & Fregni, F. (2011). Mood and cognitive effects of transcranial direct current stimulation in post-stroke depression. *Neurocase, 17*(4), 318–322.

Campbell, S., Marriott, M., Nahmias, C., & MacQueen, G. M. (2004). Lower hippocampal volume in patients suffering from depression: a meta-analysis. *American Journal of Psychiatry, 161*(4), 598–607.

Calvert, T., Knapp, P., & House, A. (1998). Psychological associations with emotionalism after stroke. *Journal of Neurology, Neurosurgery and Psychiatry, 65*(6), 928–929.

Carson, A. J., MacHale, S., Allen, K., Lawrie, S. M., Dennis, M., House, A., et al. (2000a). Depression after stroke and lesion location: a systematic review. *Lancet, 356*(9224), 122–126.

Chollet, F., Tardy, J., Albucher, J. F., Thalamas, C., Berard, E., Lamy, C., et al. (2011). Fluoxetine for motor recovery after acute ischaemic stroke (FLAME): a randomised placebo-controlled trial. *Lancet Neurology, 10*(2), 123–130.

Cully, J. A., Gfeller, J. D., Heise, R. A., Ross, M. J., Teal, C. R., & Kunik, M. E. (2005). Geriatric depression, medical diagnosis, and functional recovery during acute rehabilitation. *Archives of Physical Medicine and Rehabilitation, 86*(12), 2256–2260.

Cumming, T. B., Churilov, L., Skoog, I., Blomstrand, C., & Linden, T. (2010). Little evidence for different phenomenology in poststroke depression. *Acta Psychiatrica Scandinavia, 121*(6), 424–430.

Cushman, L. A. (1988). Secondary neuropsychiatric complications in stroke: implications for acute care. *Archives of Physical Medicine and Rehabilitation, 69*(10), 877–879.

Dantzer, R., O'Connor, J. C., Freund, G. G., Johnson, R. W., & Kelley, K. W. (2008). From inflammation to sickness and depression: when the immune system subjugates the brain. *Nature Reviews Neuroscience, 9*(1), 46–56.

Dinan, T. G. (2009). Inflammatory markers in depression. *Current Opinions in Psychiatry, 22*(1), 32–36.

de Man-van Ginkel, J. M., Gooskens, F., Schuurmans, M. J., Lindeman, E., & Hafsteinsdottir, T. B. (2010). A systematic review of therapeutic interventions for poststroke depression and the role of nurses. *Journal of Clinical Nursing, 19*(23–24), 3274–3290.

Donnan, G. A., Fisher, M., Macleod, M., & Davis, S. M. (2008). Stroke. *Lancet, 371*(9624), 1612–1623.

Eastwood, S.L., & Harrison, P.J. (2000). Hippocampal synaptic pathology in schizophrenia, bipolar disorder and major depression: a study of complexin mRNAs. *Molecular Psychiatry, 5*(4), 425–432.

Edwards, D. F., Hahn, M., Baum, C., & Dromerick, A. W. (2006). The impact of mild stroke on meaningful activity and life satisfaction. *Journal of Stroke and Cerebrovascular Diseases, 15*(4), 151–157.

Eickhoff, S. B., Laird, A. R., Grefkes, C., Wang, L. E., Zilles, K., & Fox, P. T. (2009). Coordinate-based activation likelihood estimation meta-analysis of neuroimaging data: a random-effects approach based on empirical estimates of spatial uncertainty. *Human Brain Mapping, 30*(9), 2907–2926.

Fagerberg, B., Claesson, L., Gosman-Hedstrom, G., & Blomstrand, C. (2000). Effect of acute stroke unit care integrated with care continuum versus conventional treatment: a randomized 1-year study of elderly patients. The Goteborg 70+ Stroke Study. *Stroke, 31*(11), 2578–2584.

Finklestein, S., Benowitz, L. I., Baldessarini, R. J., Arana, G. W., Levine, D., Woo, E., et al. (1982). Mood, vegetative disturbance, and dexamethasone suppression test after stroke. *Annals of Neurology, 12*(5), 463–468.

Fitzgerald, P. B., Fountain, S., & Daskalakis, Z. J. (2006). A comprehensive review of the effects of rTMS on motor cortical excitability and inhibition. *Clinical Neurophysiology, 117*(12), 2584–2596.

Fitzgerald, P. B., Laird, A. R., Maller, J., & Daskalakis, Z. J. (2008). A meta-analytic study of changes in brain activation in depression. *Human Brain Mapping, 29*(6), 683–695.

Folstein, M.F., Maiberger, R., & McHugh, P.R. (1977). Mood disorder as a specific complication of stroke. *Journal of Neurology, Neurosurgery and Psychiatry, 40*(10), 1018–1020.

Gainotti, G., Azzoni, A., & Marra, C. (1999). Frequency, phenomenology and anatomical-clinical correlates of major post-stroke depression. *British Journal of Psychiatry, 175*, 163–167.

Gainotti, G., & Marra, C. (2002). Determinants and consequences of post-stroke depression. *Current Opinions in Neurology, 15*(1), 85–89.

Grabowski, M., Sorensen, J. C., Mattsson, B., Zimmer, J., & Johansson, B. B. (1995). Influence of an enriched environment and cortical grafting on functional outcome in brain infarcts of adult rats. *Experimental Neurology, 133*(1), 96–102.

Greicius, M. D., Flores, B. H., Menon, V., Glover, G. H., Solvason, H. B., Kenna, H., et al. (2007). Resting-state functional connectivity in major depression: abnormally increased contributions from subgenual cingulate cortex and thalamus. *Biological Psychiatry, 62*(5), 429–437.

Hackett, M. L., & Anderson, C. S. (2005). Predictors of depression after stroke: a systematic review of observational studies. *Stroke, 36*(10), 2296–2301.

Hackett, M. L., Anderson, C. S., House, A., & Xia, J. (2008). Interventions for treating depression after stroke. *Cochrane Database of Systematic Reviews* (4), CD003437.

Hackett, M. L., Hill, K. M., Hewison, J., Anderson, C. S., & House, A. O. (2010). Stroke survivors who score below threshold on standard depression measures may still have negative cognitions of concern. *Stroke, 41*, 478–481.

Hackett, M. L., Yapa, C., Parag, V., & Anderson, C. S. (2005). Frequency of depression after stroke: a systematic review of observational studies. *Stroke, 36*(6), 1330–1340.

Hadidi, N., Treat-Jacobson, D.J., & Lindquist, R. (2009). Poststroke depression and functional outcome: A critical review of literature. *Heart & Lung, 38*(2), 151–162.

Haley, W. E., Allen, J. Y., Grant, J. S., Clay, O. J., Perkins, M., & Roth, D. L. (2009). Problems and benefits reported by stroke family caregivers: results from a prospective epidemiological study. *Stroke, 40*(6), 2129–2133.

Haley, W. E., Roth, D. L., Kissela, B., Perkins, M., & Howard, G. (2010). Quality of life after stroke: a prospective longitudinal study. *Quality of Life Research, 20*(6), 799–806.

Hebb, D. O. (1959). Intelligence, brain function and the theory of mind. *Brain, 82*, 260–275.

Herrmann, L. L., Le Masurier, M., & Ebmeier, K. P. (2008). White matter hyperintensities in late life depression: a systematic review. *Journal of Neurology Neurosurgery and Psychiatry, 79*(6), 619–624.

Herrmann, N., Seitz, D., Fischer, H., Saposnik, G., Calzavara, A., Anderson, G., et al. (2011). Detection and treatment of post stroke depression: results from the registry of the Canadian stroke network. *International Journal of Geriatric Psychiatry, 26*(11), 1195–1200.

Hommel, M., Trabucco-Miguel, S., Joray, S., Naegele, B., Gonnet, N., & Jaillard, A. (2009). Social dysfunctioning after mild to moderate first-ever stroke at vocational age. *Journal of Neurology, Neurosurgery and Psychiatry, 80*(4), 371–375.

House, A. (1991). Mood disorders in the first year after stroke. *Nursing Times, 87*(15), 53–54.

Ilin, Y., & Richter-Levin, G. (2009). Enriched environment experience overcomes learning deficits and depressive-like behavior induced by juvenile stress. *PLoS One, 4*(1), e4329.

Johansson, B. B. (1996). Functional outcome in rats transferred to an enriched environment 15 days after focal brain ischemia. *Stroke, 27*(2), 324–326.

Jorge, R. E., Robinson, R. G., Tateno, A., Narushima, K., Acion, L., Moser, D., et al. (2004). Repetitive transcranial magnetic stimulation as treatment of poststroke depression: a preliminary study. *Biological Psychiatry, 55*(4), 398–405.

Katz, I. (1996). On the inseparability of mental and physical health in aged persons: Lessons from depression and medical comorbidity. *American Journal of Geriatric Psychiatry, 4*(1), 1–16.

Kauhanen, M.L., Korpelainen, J.T., Hiltunen, P., Maatta, R., Mononen, H., Brusin, E., et al. (2000). Aphasia, depression, and non-verbal cognitive impairment in ischaemic stroke. *Cerebrovascular Diseases, 10*(6), 455–461.

Kneebone, II, & Dunmore, E. (2000). Psychological management of post-stroke depression. *British Journal of Clinical Psychology, 39* (Pt 1), 53–65.

Komitova, M., Zhao, L. R., Gido, G., Johansson, B. B., & Eriksson, P. (2005). Postischemic exercise attenuates whereas enriched environment has certain enhancing effects on lesion-induced subventricular zone activation in the adult rat. *European Journal of Neuroscience, 21*(9), 2397–2405.

Koolschijn, P., van Haren, N. E. M., Lensvelt-Mulders, G., Pol, H. E. H., & Kahn, R. S. (2009). Brain volume abnormalities in major depressive disorder: A meta-analysis of magnetic resonance imaging studies. *Human Brain Mapping, 30*(11), 3719–3735.

Kotila, M., Numminen, H., Waltimo, O., & Kaste, M. (1998). Depression after stroke: results of the FINNSTROKE Study. *Stroke, 29*, 368–372.

Kotila, M., Numminen, H., Waltimo, O., & Kaste, M. (1999). Post-stroke depression and functional recovery in a population-based stroke register. The Finnstroke study. *European Journal of Neurology, 6*(3), 309–312.

Kouwenhoven, S. E., Kirkevold, M., Engedal, K., & Kim, H. S. (2011). Depression in acute stroke: prevalence, dominant symptoms and associated factors. a systematic literature review. *Disability Rehabilitation, 33*(7), 539–556.

Liebetrau, M., Steen, B., & Skoog, I. (2003). Stroke in 85-year-olds: prevalence, incidence, risk factors, and relation to mortality and dementia. *Stroke, 34*(11), 2617–2622.

Linden, T., Blomstrand, C., & Skoog, I. (2007). Depressive disorders after 20 months in elderly stroke patients: a case-control study. *Stroke, 38*(6), 1860–1863.

Linden, T., Skoog, I., Fagerberg, B., Steen, B., & Blomstrand, C. (2004). Cognitive impairment and dementia 20 months after stroke. *Neuroepidemiology, 23*(1–2), 45–52.

Lopez A. D., Mathers, C. D., Ezzati, M., Jamison, D. T., Murray, C. J. L. (2006). *Global burden of disease: 2004 update*. Geneva: World Health Organization.

Lorenzetti, V., Allen, N. B., Fornito, A., & Yucel, M. (2009). Structural brain abnormalities in major depressive disorder: A selective review of recent MRI studies. *Journal of Affective Disorders, 117*(1–2), 1–17.

MacQueen, G. M., Campbell, S., McEwen, B. S., Macdonald, K., Amano, S., Joffe, R. T., et al. (2003). Course of illness, hippocampal function, and hippocampal volume in major depression. *Proceedings of the National Academy of Science U S A, 100*(3), 1387–1392.

Maes, M. (1995). Evidence for an immune response in major depression: a review and hypothesis. *Progress in Neuropsychopharmacology and Biological Psychiatry, 19*(1), 11–38.

Maes, M. (2008). The cytokine hypothesis of depression: inflammation, oxidative & nitrosative stress (IO&NS) and leaky gut as new targets for adjunctive treatments in depression. *Neuro Endocrinology Letters, 29*(3), 287–291.

Mayberg, H. S. (1997). Limbic-cortical dysregulation: A proposed model of depression. *Journal of Neuropsychiatry and Clinical Neurosciences, 9*(3), 471–481.

Monga, T. N., Lawson, J. S., & Inglis, J. (1986). Sexual dysfunction in stroke patients. *Archives of Physical Medicine and Rehabilitation, 67*(1), 19–22.

Monroe, S.M. (2008). Modern approaches to conceptualizing and measuring human life stress. *Annual Review of Clinical Psychology, 4*, 33–52.

Montgomery, S., & Åsberg, M. (1979). A new depression scale designed to be sensitive to change. *British Journal of Psychiatry, 134*, 382–389.

Morris, P. L., Robinson, R. G., Andrzejewski, P., Samuels, J., & Price, T. R. (1993). Association of depression with 10-year poststroke mortality. *American Journal of Psychiatry, 150*(1), 124–129.

Narushima, K., Kosier, J. T., & Robinson, R. G. (2003). A reappraisal of poststroke depression, intra- and inter-hemispheric lesion location using meta-analysis. *Journal of Neuropsychiatry and Clinical Neurosciences, 15*(4), 422–430.

Nilsson, M., Perfilieva, E., Johansson, U., Orwar, O., & Eriksson, P. S. (1999). Enriched environment increases neurogenesis in the adult rat dentate gyrus and improves spatial memory. *Journal of Neurobiology, 39*(4), 569–578.

Nitsche, M. A., Boggio, P. S., Fregni, F., & Pascual-Leone, A. (2009). Treatment of depression with transcranial direct current stimulation (tDCS): a review. *Experimental Neurology, 219*(1), 14–19.

Parikh, R. M., Robinson, R. G., Lipsey, J. R., Starkstein, S. E., Fedoroff, J. P., & Price, T. R. (1990). The impact of poststroke depression on recovery in activities of daily living over a 2-year follow-up. *Archives of Neurology, 47*(7), 785–789.

Pascoe, M., Crewther, D., Carey, L., & Crewther, S. (2011). Inflammation and depression: why post-stroke depression may be the norm and not the exception. *International Journal of Stroke, 6*(2), 128–135.

Pascual-Leone, A., Rubio, B., Pallardo, F., & Catala, M. D. (1996). Rapid-rate transcranial magnetic stimulation of left dorsolateral prefrontal cortex in drug-resistant depression. *Lancet, 348*(9022), 233–237.

Pessoa, L. (2008). On the relationship between emotion and cognition. *Nature Reviews Neuroscience, 9*(2), 148–158.

Price, A., Rayner, L., Okon-Rocha, E., Evans, A., Valsraj, K., Higginson, I. J., et al. (2011). Antidepressants for the treatment of depression in neurological disorders: a systematic review and meta-analysis of randomised controlled trials. *Journal of Neurology, Neurosurgery and Psychiatry, 82*, 914–923.

Pohjasvaara, T., Leppavuori, A., Siira, I., Vataja, R., Kaste, M., & Erkinjuntti, T. (1998). Frequency and clinical determinants of poststroke depression. *Stroke, 29*(11), 2311–2317.

Provinciali, L., & Coccia, M. (2002). Post-stroke and vascular depression: a critical review. *Neurological Science, 22*(6), 417–428.

Ramasubbu, R., Tobias, R., Buchan, A. M., & Bech-Hansen, N. T. (2006). Serotonin transporter gene promoter region polymorphism associated with poststroke major depression. *Journal of Neuropsychiatry and Clinical Neuroscience, 18*(1), 96–99.

Rao, R. (2000). Cerebrovascular disease and late life depression: an age old association revisited. *International Journal of Geriatric Psychiatry, 15*(5), 419–433.

Rigonatti, S. P., Boggio, P. S., Myczkowski, M. L., Otta, E., Fiquer, J. T., Ribeiro, R. B., et al. (2008). Transcranial direct stimulation and fluoxetine for the treatment of depression. *European Psychiatry, 23*(1), 74–76.

Robinson, R. G., Kubos, K. L., Starr, L. B., Rao, K., Price, T. R. (1984). Mood disorders in stroke patients. Importance of location of lesion. *Brain, 107*(Pt 1), 81–93.

Robinson, R. G., & Price, T. R. (1982). Post-stroke depressive disorders: a follow-up study of 103 patients. *Stroke, 13*(5), 635–641.

Robinson, R. G., Starkstein, S. E., & Price, T. R. (1988). Post-stroke depression and lesion location. *Stroke, 19*(1), 125–126.

Sachdev, P. S., Chen, X., Joscelyne, A., Wen, W., & Brodaty, H. (2007). Amygdala in stroke/transient ischemic attack patients and its relationship to cognitive impairment and psychopathology: the Sydney Stroke Study. *American Journal of Geriatric Psychiatry, 15*(6), 487–496.

Sacher, J., Neumann, J., Funfstuck, T., Soliman, A., Villringer, A., & Schroeter, M. L. (2011). Mapping the depressed brain: a meta-analysis of structural and functional alterations in major depressive disorder. *Journal of Affective Disorders,* DOI: http://dx.doi.org/10.1016/j.jad.2011.08.001.

Sapolsky, R. M., Romero, L. M., & Munck, A. U. (2000). How do glucocorticoids influence stress responses? Integrating permissive, suppressive, stimulatory, and preparative actions. *Endocrine Reviews, 21*(1), 55–89.

Schubert, D. S., Taylor, C., Lee, S., Mentari, A., & Tamaklo, W. (1992). Physical consequences of depression in the stroke patient. *General Hospital Psychiatry, 14*(1), 69–76.

Sifonios, L., Trinchero, M., Cereseto, M., Ferrero, A., Cladouchos, M. L., Macedo, G. F., et al. (2009). An enriched environment restores normal behavior while providing cytoskeletal restoration and synaptic changes in the hippocampus of rats exposed to an experimental model of depression. *Neuroscience, 164*(3), 929–940.

Singh, A., Herrmann, N., & Black, S. E. (1998). The importance of lesion location in poststroke depression: a critical review. *Canadian Journal of Psychiatry, 43*(9), 921–927.

Singh, R., Omiccioli, A., Hegge, S. G., & McKinley, C. A. (2009). Can community surgeons perform laparoscopic colorectal surgery with outcomes equivalent to tertiary care centers? *Surgery Endoscopy, 23*(2), 283–288.

Smith, P. S., & Thompson, M. (2008). Treadmill training post stroke: are there any secondary benefits? A pilot study. *Clinical Rehabilitation, 22*(10–11), 997–1002.

Spalletta, G., Bria, P., & Caltagirone, C. (2005). Sensitivity of somatic symptoms in post-stroke depression (PSD). *International Journal of Geriatric Psychiatry, 20*(11), 1103–1104; author reply 1104–1105.

Sporns, O., Honey, C. J., & Kotter, R. (2007). Identification and classification of hubs in brain networks. *Public Library of Science One, 2*(10), e1049.

Starkstein, S. E., Fedoroff, J. P., Price, T. R., Leiguarda, R., & Robinson, R. G. (1992). Anosognosia in patients with cerebrovascular lesions. A study of causative factors. *Stroke, 23*(10), 1446–1453.

Starkstein, S. E., & Robinson, R. G. (1990). Depression following cerebrovascular lesions. *Seminars in Neurology, 10*(3), 247–253.

Starkstein, S. E., Robinson, R. G., Berthier, M. L., Parikh, R. M., & Price, T. R. (1988). Differential mood changes following basal ganglia vs thalamic lesions. *Archives of Neurology, 45*(7), 725–730.

Starkstein, S. E., Robinson, R. G., Honig, M. A., Parikh, R. M., Joselyn, J., & Price, T. R. (1989). Mood changes after right-hemisphere lesions. British Journal of Psychiatry, 155, 79-85.

Staub, F., & Bogousslavsky, J. (2001). Post-stroke depression or fatigue. *European Neurology, 45*(1), 3–5.

Tang, W. K., Chen, Y. K., Lu, J. Y., Chu, W. C. W., Mok, V. C. T., Ungvari, G. S., et al. (2010). White matter hyperintensities in post-stroke depression: a case control study. *Journal of Neurology Neurosurgery and Psychiatry, 81*(12), 1312–1315.

Teodorczuk, A., Firbank, M. J., Pantoni, L., Poggesi, A., Erkinjuntti, T., Wallin, A., et al. (2010). Relationship between baseline white-matter changes and development of late-life depressive symptoms: 3-year results from the LADIS study. *Psychological Medicine, 40*(4), 603–610.

Terroni, L., Amaro, E., Iosifescu, D. V., Tinone, G., Sato, J. R., Leite, C.C., et al. (2011). Stroke lesion in cortical neural circuits and post-stroke incidence of major depressive episode: A 4-month prospective study. *World Journal of Biological Psychiatry, 12*(7), 539–548.

van der Werf, S. P., van den Broek, H. L., Anten, H. W., & Bleijenberg, G. (2001). Experience of severe fatigue long after stroke and its relation to depressive symptoms and disease characteristics. *European Neurology, 45*(1), 28–33.

Vataja, R., Leppavuori, A., Pohjasvaara, T., Mantyla, R., Aronen, H. J., Salonen, O., et al. (2004). Poststroke depression and lesion location revisited. *Journal of Neuropsychiatry and Clinical Neurosciences, 16*(2), 156–162.

Vataja, R., Pohjasvaara, T., Leppavuori, A., Mantyla, R., Aronen, H. J., Salonen, O., et al. (2001). Magnetic resonance imaging correlates of depression after ischemic stroke. *Archives of General Psychiatry, 58*(10), 925–931.

Videbech, P., & Ravnkilde, B. (2004). Hippocampal volume and depression: a meta-analysis of MRI studies. *American Journal of Psychiatry, 161*(11), 1957–1966.

Wade, D. T., Legh-Smith, J., & Hewer, R. A. (1987). Depressed mood after stroke. A community study of its frequency. *British Journal of Psychiatry, 151,* 200–205.

Williams, L. S., Ofner, S., Yu, Z., Beyth, R. J., Plue, L., & Damush, T. (2011). Pre-post evaluation of automated reminders may improve detection and management of post-stroke depression. *Journal of General Internal Medicine, 26*(8), 852–857.

Wright, R. L., & Conrad, C. D. (2008). Enriched environment prevents chronic stress-induced spatial learning and memory deficits. *Behavioral Brain Research, 187*(1), 41–47.

Xu, H. C., Stamova, B., Jickling, G., Tian, Y. F., Zhan, X. H., Ander, B. P., et al. (2010). Distinctive RNA expression profiles of white matter hyperintensities in the blood of human subjects using genome wide microarray analyses. *Stroke, 41*(4), E214–E214.

Zhang, J. R., Wang, J. H., Wu, Q. Z., Kuang, W. H., Huang, X. Q., He, Y., et al. (2011). Disrupted brain connectivity networks in drug-naive, first-episode major depressive disorder. *Biological Psychiatry, 70*(4), 334–342.

9 | TRAINING PRINCIPLES TO ENHANCE LEARNING-BASED REHABILITATION AND NEUROPLASTICITY

PAULETTE VAN VLIET, THOMAS A. MATYAS, and LEEANNE M. CAREY

9.1 INTRODUCTION

This chapter will focus on some of the core principles underlying learning-based rehabilitation and relate these to neuroscience and neuroimaging research. In particular, we focus on task-specific training, intensity and repetition, and training for transfer. The term *task-specific training* is used to describe different constructs in the literature, including task-oriented training, repetitive training, and a combination of both of these. Task-oriented training has been described as "practicing real-life tasks (such as answering a telephone) with the intention of acquiring or reacquiring a skill (defined by consistency, flexibility and efficiency). The tasks are required to be challenging and progressively adapted and involve active participation. In contrast, repetitive training, describes the situation where a task is usually divided into component parts and then reassembled into an overall task once each component is learned. Repetitive training is usually considered a bottom-up approach, and is missing the end-goal of acquiring a skill" (SCORE, 2011). For the purpose of this chapter, "task-specific" training is defined as a combination of task-oriented training and repetitive training, using the definitions of those above. So the goal is to improve a real-life task by a combination of practice of the whole task, which can be progressively adapted, and practice of the component parts, which are reassembled into the whole task once some improvement in the performance of component parts has occurred. Examples will be provided primarily in relation to motor and perceptual learning, as these have been extensively studied. In each section of the chapter we draw implications for retraining movements in people with stroke, and the chapter finishes with a list of main messages for clinical practice.

9.2 TASK-SPECIFIC ACTIVATION OF BRAIN REGIONS

Research has indicated that the functional organization of the primary motor cortex, rather than being fixed, can change in response to practice of tasks (Elbert, Pantev, Wienruch, Rockstroh, & Taub, 1995; Karni et al., 1995; Hayashi, Hasegawa, & Kasai, 2002) One commonly used method to investigate this change is to measure the motor evoked potentials (MEPs) occurring in response to transcranial magnetic stimulation (TMS). TMS is noninvasive and works by delivering an electrical current through a magnetic coil placed near the skull, which causes cortical neurons to fire. By systematically moving the coil to different locations over the skull and recording the resultant MEPs, a cortical map can be constructed, indicating cortical representation of muscles or movements (see Chapter 5 for further details of TMS).

The literature on cortical plasticity contains many examples of activation of brain regions and networks according to task requirements. One study compared muscle representations in both hemispheres in people skilled at a volleyball "strike" movement and in runners (Tyc, Boyadjian, & Devanne, 2005). MEPs were recorded from the proximal medial deltoid and distal extensor carpi radialis muscles during magnetic stimulation, while subjects were seated and either aiming to hit a target or to perform static wrist extension. In the volleyball group, the size of the cortical map for middle deltoid was larger than for the runners. Furthermore, the total size representation of dominant arm muscles in the volleyball group was larger than that of nondominant for both medial deltoid and extensor carpi radialis. This finding supports the hypothesis that activity drives cortical plasticity, since there is different cortical organization between two groups with different types of skill.

There is also evidence that functional organization of somatosensory cortex may change dynamically according to and during task requirements. Braun et al. (2001) compared organization of somatosensory cortex when subjects were performing the well-learned task of writing compared to being at rest. During the two conditions a tactile sensation with force of 1.6 N was delivered to the 1st and 5th digits. Cortical representations of the stimulated fingers were measured. The cortical representations of each finger were farther apart during writing than at rest, indicating functional reorganization related to the task. The authors proposed that there are different preexisting maps, and the somatosensory cortex switches rapidly between them according to task requirements. This idea is supported by other studies of cortical plasticity and learning (e.g., Karni et al., 1998).

Neurophysiological studies using single cell recordings from primates performing specific tasks, and from humans with well-defined brain lesions, also reveal that different brain regions and neural networks are activated for these different tasks. For example, for reach-to-grasp movements, specific neural pathways exist for processing of visual and motor information for different components of the movement. For transporting the hand to the object, visual information about object location is carried in a neural circuit from primary visual cortex to posterior parietal cortex (Sakata, Taira, Kusunoki, Murata, & Tanaka, 1997), and a medial parietofrontal circuit, from the superior parietal lobule to dorsal premotor area 6, carries motor information for transport (Fattori et al., 2009). Grasp-related information, such as size and shape of an object, is communicated via a lateral parietofrontal circuit, from the inferior parietal lobule to ventral premotor area 6, and visual information is transported in a circuit from primary visual cortex to the inferotemporal lobe (Sakata et al., 1997). More recent studies have found that there is partial overlap of these pathways, so that medial and lateral parietofrontal circuits are partially involved in both processes, but they remain largely segregated (Tanne-Gariepy, Rouiller, & Boussaoud, 2002). Studies have also demonstrated selective cortical activation for different types of grasp (Rizzolatti et al., 1988).

Findings from these and similar studies suggest that therapy may not engage activation of neural networks in a normal manner if training does not incorporate task requirements into the movements patients are asked to practice. Certain types of practice are likely to elicit appropriate neural networks more than others. Practice of the entire action required for task completion is likely to activate appropriate networks more than practice of component parts of movements. Where the patient is only able to perform part component practice, the clinician can make the activation of appropriate networks more likely by utilizing part movements that resemble the whole movement on key parameters. For example, plantar flexor activity at the end of stance phase of walking could be practiced without stepping, but using similar amounts of force and range of movement as those used in walking itself. Where part practice occurs, there is a need to maximize transfer of learning to performance of the whole movement. Transfer of learning is discussed in section 9.9 in this chapter.

Another point of relevance for clinicians is the question of which brain regions and networks might be activated when passive movements are employed in therapy. For example, a common practice is for the therapist to perform passive trunk movements in a sitting position, in order to normalize muscle tone, or to guide the person's arm toward an object to indicate how various joint movements are coordinated. Performance of passive movements has been found to activate similar brain regions to those activated when voluntary movements are performed (Mima et al., 1999; Guzetta et al., 2007). However, this is not as effective a means for cortical activation as active movement (Hummelsheim, Hauptmann, & Neumann, 1995). For example, a positron emission tomography (PET) activation study compared passive and active finger movements and found that active movement was associated with activation of multiple areas, including contralateral primary sensorimotor cortex, premotor cortex, supplementary motor area, bilateral secondary sensorimotor areas, basal ganglia, and ipsilateral cerebellum. In contrast, passive finger movement elicited activity only in contralateral primary and secondary somatosensory areas (Mima et al., 1999). This is supported by a functional MRI study that found behavioral correlates of the differential brain activation for passive versus active movements. In this study, voluntary and passively elicited wrist extension movements were performed during active and passive motor training, respectively. Active training resulted in better motor performance, better motor response to TMS, and significantly higher activation in contralateral primary motor cortex than passive training (Lotze, Braun, Birbaumer, Anders, & Cohen, 2003). Therefore, if the goal of passive movement is to activate brain areas that will be used in active performance, this is unlikely to be the most effective way of accomplishing it.

There are situations in which passive movement may occur for other legitimate reasons; for example, where observational learning is being employed. This is discussed in a later section on enhancing motor learning with structured practice and feedback.

9.3 INFLUENCE OF TASK CHARACTERISTICS ON SENSORIMOTOR PERFORMANCE

Measures of motor performance, such as those obtained by 3-dimensional motion analysis to reveal detailed kinematics of movements, are also informative about motor control, as they provide a window into how the nervous system organizes, executes, and adjusts movements. There is also ample evidence from these studies that the motor control of everyday actions is task-specific. Here we will discuss, using the reach-to-grasp movement as an example, how the intended action to be performed with an object and the characteristics of the object (size, orientation) each influence the motor planning for task performance. First, the timing of grasp is adjusted for different size of objects. When grasping a smaller object, requirements for spatial precision increase and this causes a longer movement duration, a longer deceleration phase, allowing for more time for on-line adjustments for potential spatial error (Bootsma, Marteniuk, MacKenzie, & Zaal, 1994; Zoia et al., 2006), and the maximum grasp aperture occurs earlier to enable more precision with hand shaping (Cope & Trombly, 1998). Thus the object size determines the kinematics of the movement and, by inference, the force commands that produce the kinematics. People with stroke have an impaired ability to adjust timing of grasp for different sized objects (Wu et al., 2008). In one study stroke participants, in contrast to healthy controls, did not demonstrate an earlier maximum grip aperture (expressed as percentage of movement duration) when reaching for a smaller object (Wu et al., 2008). Another study noted that the temporal coupling between the start of hand transport and the start of hand opening was weaker when reaching for a large cup in people with stroke compared to healthy participants (van Vliet & Sheridan, 2007).

Interestingly, it is not only the object itself that determines kinematics of reach-to-grasp, but also the person's intended action to be performed with the object. Healthy participants, when presented with the same horizontal bar in the same location, will choose an overhand grip if required to stand the bar on one of its ends, or an underhand grip if required to stand the bar up on the other end (Rosenbaum & Jorgensen, 1992), and demonstrate a longer deceleration phase in reach-to-grasp when required to grasp a small disc to put it into a tight-fitting well compared to throwing the small object into a larger container (Marteniuk, Leavitt, MacKenzie, & Athenes, 1990). People with stroke also execute movements differently if presented with a different subsequent action. For example two studies have shown that when participants reached to grasp a cup or can of beverage to drink from it, their movement duration was shorter when the intention was to drink as opposed to just moving the cup (van Vliet, Kerwin, Sheridan, & Fentem, 1995) or taking a can to the mouth without drinking (Wu, Wong, Lin, & Chen, 2001). Stroke participants have also demonstrated better performance of reaching kinematics when reaching forward to an object, in this case to coins to scoop the coins off the table, compared to doing the same scooping action without the coins being present (Wu, Trombly, Lin, &

Tickle-Degnen, 2000). Together, this research shows that object affordances—the qualities of an object that suggests how it might be used, and the action to be performed with the object—are influential in determining movement organization.

What can be concluded from this literature on the effect of task parameters on performance? First, it consolidates the suggestion that motor control depends very much on task goal and contextual information. Second, there is an important therapeutic implication. People with stroke have been found to lack the skill exhibited by healthy participants in adjusting the kinematics of reach-to-grasp for different task requirements. Therefore, improving the ability to make these adjustments is an important part of the clinician's rehabilitation approach. By systematically varying task parameters and intended actions during practice, patients are given the opportunity to attempt adjustments to the force commands that produce the kinematics. In this way, they have the opportunity to learn the subtleties that produce the skilled movements required in varying contexts in everyday life. Dean and Shepherd (1997) have demonstrated that varying task parameters during practice can improve performance of seated reaching tasks. Further systematic, controlled studies are needed to examine the effects of varying task parameters and intended actions during practice.

9.4 TASK-SPECIFIC NATURE OF MOTOR LEARNING

Motor learning in rehabilitation requires a change in behavior that is relatively permanent, in contrast to a temporary change in motor performance (Schmidt & Wrisberg, 2000). Motor performance can be defined as "the observable attempt of an individual to produce a voluntary action" (Magill, 2007), whereas motor learning is "a set of processes associated with practice/experience leading to relatively permanent changes in the capability for producing skilled action" (Schmidt, 1988). One of the challenges for clinicians working in rehabilitation is to create the right conditions for motor learning to ensure that the improved performance achieved at the end of one training session is still intact at the following session.

Motor learning is enabled by neuroplastic changes in the nervous system, and these changes are what clinicians aim to effect with the interventions they employ. Neuroplastic changes can either consist of short-term neuronal changes, such as changes to synaptic efficiency of neurons, or long-term changes, such as changes to the structural organization of the nervous system (see Chapter 3). Short-term changes could be regarded as representing a change in motor performance. Even a small amount of practice can cause cortical changes. Hayashi et al. (2002) found that the amplitudes of motor-evoked potentials and the size of the cortical map increased dramatically after 100 repetitions of simple index finger abduction. Such quick changes are likely to be due to changes in synaptic efficiency from a strengthening of existing synapses (Hayashi et al., 2002). With larger amounts of practice, however, changes in the balance of excitation and inhibition may induce anatomical changes in synaptic organization. For example, people with stroke who participated in a neurorehabilitation program showed an increase in the number of cortical sites from where an MEP of the paretic hand could be elicited (Wittenberg et al., 2003). Such neuroplastic changes underlie the more permanent changes in motor behavior that occur in motor learning. For these to occur, many repetitions are required.

Neurophysiological and neuroanatomical evidence points to task-specific training and intensity of repetition as being key strategies for facilitating neuroplastic changes after stroke. A systematic review and meta-analysis of TMS and functional MRI (fMRI) evidence suggests that brain activation patterns after stroke are influenced by targeted motor rehabilitation, primarily involving task-specific training (Richards, Stewart, Woodbury, Senesac, & Cauraugh, 2008). For example, a task-oriented training intervention consisting of intensive finger movement tracking led to both improvement in finger control and change in activation from contralesional to the expected ipsilesional hemisphere and involved supplementary motor area, sensorimotor cortex, and premotor cortex as demonstrated with fMRI (J. R. Carey et al., 2002). The meta-analysis revealed a large overall effect for changes in the lesioned sensorimotor cortex associated with functional gains in the upper extremity and rehabilitation (Richards et al., 2008). These neural plastic changes occurred in individuals who were primarily in the chronic stage of recovery (>1 year post-stroke).

9.5   TASK COMPLEXITY

Task complexity can influence neuroplasticity. A recent systematic review (Muir & Jones, 2009) compared complex tasks, such as a numerical keypad sequencing task or moving a matchstick back and forth between fingers of the left hand, to simpler activities, such as squeezing a sponge or pressing a number of buttons. Both short-term neuronal changes, such as changes to synaptic efficiency of neurons, and long-term changes, such as changes to the structural organization of the nervous system, were found to be better enhanced by the more complex motor tasks in healthy subjects. Additionally, comparisons of expert versus novice groups in this review showed a positive correlation between neuroplasticity and amount of experience in performing a complex motor task (Muir & Jones, 2009). Together, these results imply that complex tasks enhance motor learning, and that longer-term practice of a task

results in an increase in neuroplasticity. Further research is needed to ascertain whether increased task complexity is positively correlated with neuroplasticity in people with stroke.

Performing complex tasks can be difficult initially after stroke. Complex task performance can be assisted, however, by the learning of movement segments which form part of these complex movements. Several studies have shown that the benefit of practicing movement segments, such as wrist flexion or extension (Butefisch, Hummelsheim, Denzler, & Mauritz, 1995), can improve performance of more complex tasks in people with stroke (Butefisch, Kleiser, & Seitz, 2006). Therefore, clinicians needing to teach complex tasks to their patients can initially teach movement segments and move on to more complex tasks when the patient is able to practice them. Transfer of skill between tasks is discussed further in section 9.9 of this chapter.

9.6   BEHAVIORAL EVIDENCE FOR TASK-SPECIFIC TRAINING

Stroke guidelines in several countries now recommend that task-specific or task-oriented training be utilized in stroke rehabilitation, including the Canadian Score stroke best practice recommendations (SCORE, 2011), the American Heart Association (Miller et al., 2010), the Australian National Stroke Foundation (Australian National Stroke Foundation, 2010), the Stroke Unit Network of New Zealand (Stroke Unit Network of New Zealand, 2003), the Royal College of Physicians UK National Clinical Guideline for Stroke (Intercollegiate Stroke Working Party, 2008), and the Scottish Intercollegiate Guidelines Network (Scottish Intercollegiate Guidelines Network, 2010). Several of these cite as evidence the Cochrane review of repetitive task-oriented training (French et al., 2007), which found a significant effect on short-term measures of walking distance, walking speed, sit-to-stand, functional ambulation, and activities of daily living. There was insufficient evidence to make any recommendations for upper limb task-specific training, partly due to the fact that intensity of treatment in the studies was low, with only three studies including more than 20 hours of training. They also point out that there is a lack of evidence for long-term effects of repetitive task-oriented training.

Studies have been undertaken to assess the effectiveness of delivering task-specific motor training to neurologically impaired patients. For example, in one well-designed randomized controlled trial, stroke patients' sitting balance was trained using systematically varied reaching tasks such as changing the speed, direction, object weight, seat height, and amplitude of the movement (Dean & Shepherd, 1997). The program resulted in significantly better performance compared to a placebo control group who received sham training. Other studies in patients with stroke have also demonstrated the positive effect of task-specific training (Richards et al., 1993; Dean, Richards, & Malouin, 2000; Blennerhassett & Dite, 2004). Two weeks of repetitive task practice at an intensity of 1.5–4.5 hours per day with constraint (CIMT), a padded mitt worn on the unaffected arm for 90% of waking hours, resulted in a significantly greater improvement in Wolf Motor Function Test performance time, Motor Activity Log amount of use, and Motor Activity Log quality of movement compared to usual care (Wolf et al., 2006). There is also evidence of positive outcomes associated with task-specific training of somatosensory functions involving discrimination of textured surfaces and limb positions, and recognition of common objects through touch (L. M. Carey, Matyas, & Oke, 1993; L. M. Carey, 2006; L. M. Carey, Macdonell & Matyas, 2011).

Implementing task-specific practice is not difficult. The key points are: (i) to work out how whole tasks and components of whole tasks can be practiced to enhance task performance in particular contexts; (ii) to vary task parameters in a systematic way; and (iii) if component practice is done, to facilitate this practice into the whole movement as soon as possible. Below are some examples of the parameters that may be varied in task-specific practice for reach-to-grasp:

- Amplitude of the movement required (e.g., the distance to be reached by extension of elbow and flexion of the shoulder)

- Direction of movement (e.g., shoulder flexion in a medial direction with adduction, or in a lateral direction with abduction)

- Load (e.g., weight of object being carried)

- Size/dimensions of object

- Height of the target (e.g., shoulder flexion required could start with enough to reach an object on a small stool on the floor and progress to a higher shelf)

- Degrees of freedom being used (e.g., shoulder flexion with or without elbow extension or external rotation included)

- Type of muscle contraction required—concentric, eccentric, isometric

- Speed of muscle contraction (utilizing fast or slow twitch muscle fibers)

- Joint range (e.g., practice in stronger or weaker part of joint range)

- Relationship to gravity

- Amount of friction to overcome (e.g., sliding arm along a table, could use powder, slippery material, or skate underneath arm to lessen friction to make movement easier)

- Using both arms together if appropriate to the task

- Using physical (e.g., seatbelt) or environmental restraint (object to discourage particular movements)

An accurate and detailed analysis of the biomechanics of task performance underpins the success of task-specific practice. If the main movement problems have been incorrectly diagnosed, the task-specific practice will be misdirected and result in low effectiveness of treatment. Analysis requires an intimate knowledge of the normal biomechanics, and the ability to systematically compare the patient's sensorimotor performance with this normal model. It also requires accurate sifting of the information gathered in the analysis, in order to identify the most important movement problem(s) to be trained.

9.7 MENTAL PRACTICE OF TASKS TO ENHANCE MOTOR LEARNING

Frequently patients are unable to perform tasks that need to be learned. In this situation, mental practice and observational learning can be employed. Mental practice is defined as "the cognitive rehearsal of a physical skill in the absence of overt physical movements" (Magill, 2007; p. 423). Mental practice combined with physical practice of bimanual, functional upper limb tasks has been shown to be more effective than relaxation combined with physical practice in a randomized controlled trial of 32 people with chronic stroke (Page, Levine, & Leonard, 2007). The same neural structures are activated when movements are mentally practiced as when they are actually physically practiced (Decety, 1996).

Observational learning, where a skill is learned by watching a person performing the skill, can also be useful. It has been discovered that specific neurons called *mirror neurons* exist in the primate premotor cortex, which were activated when the monkey performed goal-oriented actions such as grasping food but also when the monkey observed someone else doing the same action (Rizzolatti, Fadiga, Gallese, & Fogassi, 1996). A recent study using fMRI to explore the function of the mirror neurons in humans found that observing actions embedded in contexts that revealed the intention of grasping objects, such as drinking or cleaning, was associated with more activation in certain parts of the premotor cortex than observing grasping actions without a context (Iacoboni et al., 2005). It is proposed that these neurons are involved in understanding the actions of others, as well as in action recognition.

Mental practice, therefore, can be usefully employed in rehabilitation where the person is unable to manage the physical practice of the task, or to enhance physical practice. When a patient observes someone else performing a task, such as the therapist or another patient, this may facilitate brain areas that would be active in actual physical performance of the task. People with right-sided lesions have demonstrated difficulties with visual encoding in a short-term memory task (figure recognition), so it has been suggested that observational learning may aid motor learning in these patients (Campos, Barroso, & Menezes, 2010). When implementing observational learning, a pattern of several demonstrations of a task followed by physical practice, with further demonstrations interspersed into the physical practice at regular intervals, has been found in a sporting context to be superior to doing all the demonstration beforehand (Weeks & Anderson, 2000).

9.8 INCREASING REPETITIONS TO ENHANCE MOTOR LEARNING

Beginning with findings from early studies on motor learning in primates (Karni et al., 1995; Nudo, Milliken, Jenkins, & Merzenich, 1996), it has become increasingly clear that a higher degree of neuroplasticity occurs with greater amounts of repeated practice of a task. For lasting changes to occur to neural connections in the central nervous system, hundreds of repetitions of the task are necessary in primates. Studies investigating motor learning in healthy humans have also engaged participants in as many as 300–800 repetitions to bring about motor learning (J. R. Carey et al., 2002; Boyd & Winstein, 2006).

Following stroke, greater amounts of practice has also been shown to yield better results. In a systematic review (van der Lee et al., 2001) of 13 randomized controlled trials, which contrasted amount or duration of therapy for the upper limb after stroke, six showed a positive short-term result on an arm function test. In five of these six studies, there was an increased amount or duration of exercise in the most improved group. A further meta-analysis demonstrated that additional exercise therapy has a favorable effect on activities of daily living, particularly if routine amounts of therapy are increased by at least 16 hours in the first 6 months after stroke (Kwakkel et al., 2004). In a study comparing amounts of movement therapy received by stroke patients in four different European countries, therapy amount ranged from 1 hour per day in the United Kingdom up to 3 hours per day in Switzerland (Lincoln, Willis, Philips, Juby, & Berman, 1996). In countries with more therapy, outcomes were better for stroke patients (DeWit et al., 2005).

The actual number of repetitions needed to bring about motor learning in people with stroke, for particular tasks and in particular contexts, is not known. However, the above information gives an indication of how much more practice might be needed to increase motor learning. For example, in the review by van der Lee, the treatments showing significantly better outcomes on an arm function test contained up to 40 minutes of additional upper limb therapy per day compared to control groups. As a cautionary note, a recent study reported an inverse dose–response relationship between degree of improvement and higher doses of CIMT (3 hours per day) in the early stages after stroke, finding that a standard amount of CIMT (2 hours per day) or traditional therapy (2 hours per day) yielded better results at this stage (Dromerick et al., 2009).

Since one cannot be certain how much extra practice is actually occurring within a time period in these studies, it is more useful to know the actual number of movement repetitions. An example of current numbers of repetitions for different tasks has been presented by Lang, MacDonald, and Gnip (2007), who observed 36 sessions of outpatient physiotherapy and occupational therapy and identified an average 39 active exercise movements, 34 passive exercise movements, and 12 purposeful movements for the upper limb and 33 active-exercise movements, 6 passive exercise movements, and 8 purposeful movements for the lower limb, plus an average 292 steps for gait training. This number falls well below the number of repetitions required in the abovementioned studies in primates and humans to demonstrate evidence of motor learning. The same research group has since investigated the possibility of translating animal doses of task-specific training to people with chronic stroke, with encouraging results (Birkenmeier, Pragar, & Lang, 2010). Stroke participants were able to perform a mean 322 repetitions per 1-hour session, 3 times a week for 6 weeks. Moreover, attendance was 97% and there were low ratings of pain and fatigue. This demonstrates just how many more repetitions are possible compared to routine practice.

In routine neurorehabilitation, it is probable that the amount of practice falls short of the number required to enhance motor learning most effectively; therefore, ways of increasing practice could be explored. Engaging in greater amounts of self-monitored practice, group practice, or using an apparatus that allows increased repetitions of movements in a controlled environment, such as robotic rehabilitation or virtual reality training with or without telerehabilitation, are some of the ways in which amount of practice may be increased.

9.9 TRANSFER OF TRAINING EFFECTS

Attempts to restore motor function in an impaired adult necessarily contain transfer issues, whether it is because initial movement may not be adequate for practicing a targeted functional action or because the therapeutic setting permits supervised practice of only a limited number of tasks. Part–whole training sequences, "shaping" routines, transitions from mental to physical practice, from virtual reality practice to real tasks, from stimulation-facilitated practice to unstimulated performance, or from robotically assisted practice to unassisted action, all depend on the extent to which gains from the practice conditions produce improvements in either the performance of target actions or savings in the subsequent training required to achieve the target action. Improvement in the practiced task is typically not considered a sufficient measure of outcome. Rather, an improvement on criterion tasks combined to form standardized tests of upper or lower limb function is commonly employed. Transfer of training phenomena are thus critical to the enterprise of movement and sensory rehabilitation after stroke.

Despite the significance of transfer phenomena, and despite the availability of some transfer data from most studies employing stroke samples, the rehabilitation literature does not appear to have so far provided much *systematic* analysis of transfer effects across methods of training, nor a systematic, theoretically driven program of investigation of transfer effects. The study of transfer of motor training in unimpaired performers, however, comprises over a century of data and debate (e.g., Schmidt & Lee, 2011). Nevertheless, even in this literature there has been little systematic review since the significant volume by Cormier and Hagman (1987). Schmidt and Young (1987) in that publication provided an analysis of the largely behavioral literature, extracting the following conclusions: transfer of training between completely different tasks (intertask transfer) is small or negligible; and intertask transfer depends on the similarity between the two tasks, although how similarity might be evaluated is still regarded as insufficiently clear (Schmidt & Lee, 2011).

Variability of practice, correctly handled, appears to be one of the few manipulations that enhance transfer. For unimpaired humans, practising variants of a task—for example, where key parameters such as overall timing or force are varied across trials—is superior to constant practice when circumstances require a novel value of that parameter to be executed (Shapiro & Schmidt, 1982). Not all reviews of the empirical literature agree (Van Rossum, 1990). Nevertheless, more recent analyses (Shea & Wulf, 2005) have confirmed the conclusion, but with an important caveat: the scheduling of practice variation is important in two ways. First, practising variants in a random order rather than in a sequence of blocks, the so-called *contextual interference* phenomenon, does seem to facilitate motor learning (Shea & Wulf, 2005). This phenomenon has also been observed when practising several different movements after stroke (Hanlon, 1996). However, a subsequent study that combined active neuromuscular stimulation with these two types of practice schedule found similar improvements in their two stroke samples (Cauraugh & Kim, 2003). Importantly, introduction of the variations too early in the practice sequence, before an action pattern is established, has been detrimental (Shea & Wulf, 2005). Second, the nature of the learning goal matters. In tasks where a relative timing pattern is being learned, vari-

able practice has been detrimental compared to consistent (blocked) practice (Lai & Shea, 1999; Lai, Shea, Wulf, & Wright, 2000). The emerging conclusion from this literature suggests a schedule comprising constant early practice to establish a basic motor program, followed by randomly scheduled variations in various movement scaling parameters (Shea & Wulf, 2005). Prima facie, this conclusion seems compatible with clinical programs, but further controlled investigations in stroke samples seem necessary.

The observation that positive transfer is small unless the tasks are identical, or nearly so, supports organized task-specific practice but presents challenges to motor reeducation programs. Some intervention methods employ a wider range of practice tasks (e.g., repetitive task practice and constraint-induced programs), whereas others (e.g., some forms of bilateral or mirror training methods) choose a narrower range of action patterns to practice (Bayona, Bitensky, Salter, & Teasell, 2005; French et al., 2007; Oujamaa, Relave, Froger, Mottet, & Pelissier, 2009). Investigations of rehabilitation interventions for upper limb function frequently employ standardized tests based on performance of multiple actions (e.g., Wolf Motor Function Test, Action Research Arm Test). The intertask transfer literature predicts poor transfer results unless training activities relate closely to the variety of actions contained in the standardized tests. Unfortunately, systematic controlled comparisons of changes in performance of the specific trained tasks against changes in different functional actions have not yet been provided to assist insights about the gradient of generalization. Nevertheless, practice of a wider repertoire of tasks seems more likely to increase the overlap between training tasks and the tasks used in functional outcome tests. A recent systematic review of repetitive task training (French et al., 2007) found superior primary outcomes on functional tests for lower limb interventions compared to those for upper limb interventions. Although not definitive given other differences between upper limb and lower limb trials, it is interesting to note that the functional actions of the lower limb appear to afford less variation than those for the upper limb. A possible speculation is that the reduced movement options create more overlap between the practiced tasks and the outcome tests for lower limbs. Finally, another potential advantage of practising a variety of tasks is the opportunity to use random scheduling to enable the contextual interference effect.

The impaired movement abilities of stroke patients tempt intervention strategies where simpler component actions of tasks are sometimes practiced first, followed by combining these into a more complex movement. Neurorehabilitation practice is not alone in considering this strategy. Part–whole training strategies have been used for a long time in the training of motor skills where brain damage is not an issue. A successful approach seems to be backward chaining, where the last component is practiced first, then the immediately previous component is added, and so on, until the full sequence is achieved. The associated behavioral investigations suggest that the nature of the task is critical to the value of part–whole training methods (Schmidt & Lee, 2011): in serial tasks, part–whole transfer can be effective; however, in rapid discrete tasks part–whole practice is not supported; in continuous tasks requiring coordinated action, part–whole practice does not appear beneficial. Schmidt and Lee (2011, p.385) suggest that the underlying issue is whether a skilled movement is controlled by a single program or a sequence of separate movement programs. Continuous, coordinated actions, such as walking or swimming, and rapid movements are likely to be governed by a single program, whereas tasks with serial components and natural micro-pauses, such as the tennis toss and serve action or picking up a cup, are likely to be governed by several programs.

In the absence of *systematic* investigations of transfer phenomena in impaired performers, the empirical principles and theoretical models obtained from neurologically healthy samples are a reasonable starting point but seem unlikely to suffice given the major alterations caused by brain insult. These principles and models will need to be reviewed as more information emerges about transfer of learning in people with stroke.

Transfer-specific neuroimaging results have begun to enter the literature. Seidler and Noll (2008) observed that brain regions involved in the early stages of motor skill acquisition tended to show reduced activity during transfer tests, in contrast to regions activated in the later stages of the acquisition phase. Activation in the regions associated with the earlier stages of practice correlated better with individual differences in acquisition rates, whereas the extent to which savings occurred during the transfer phase was better correlated with different regions, notably regions activated in the late stages of the acquisition phase. An increased reliance on the cerebellum was noted with transfer of learning. These differences may, at least in part, explain individual differences in ability to benefit from rehabilitation after interruption of different brain networks, and highlight potential targets for therapeutic interventions. Further, individual differences in motor learning have been associated with function and structure of specific brain regions (Tomassini et al., 2011).

An improved understanding of motor learning, with implications for transfer theory, is underway via neuroscientific investigations. Motor learning can be conceptualized as the refinement in motor control that occurs through practice. Older models such as schema theory and its conceptual child, the generalized motor program (GMP; see Schmidt and Lee, 2011 for a full description), envisage that the central nervous system (CNS) contains networks that control movement by encoding the key processes (e.g., sequence of action components, their relative phasing, their relative forces, selection of involved effectors) and parameters (e.g., overall force, overall duration). However, it is not yet clear whether these have been adequately identified or exactly what is encoded by the CNS (Summers & Anson, 2009). Nonlinear dynamic models of motor control dispute how much of the control occurs through CNS stored codes and how much of the coordination arises through self-organized biomechanical properties or physical task affordances (Summers & Anson, 2009). In addition, the GMP model does not address issues about the neuroanatomical structures and network functions that encode and execute the GMP, an important aspect for neurorehabilitation theory.

In an alternative approach, Willingham (1998) reviewed a broad range of studies employing ablation, natural lesions, neurostimulation, single-cell recordings, and neuroimaging methods to propose a neuropsychological theory of motor learning. He identified four key processes: the strategic, responsible for goal selection; perceptual-motor integration, responsible for controlling the spatial location to which an effector moves; sequencing, responsible for assembling a sequence of movement endpoints; and dynamic control, responsible for translating spatial location representations into muscle commands. The existence of these as separate but cooperative processes is supported with reviews of evidence to indicate the neuroanatomical separability of the CNS networks responsible for the processes, as well as the existence of different representation codes (allocentric versus egocentric) for different processes. A very large volume of neuroimaging and other neuroscientific data that permit verification or further development of such a model have appeared since. Review of this literature is beyond the scope of this chapter; however, the time does seem ripe for a better understanding of the separate but cooperative networks, including what they encode and how. Such insights should illuminate the problem of shared elements of action, with consequent benefits for transfer theory. In tandem with systematic empirical work employing brain damaged samples, this can be reasonably expected to produce advances in transfer of training for reeducation of movement after stroke.

9.10   IMPLICIT AND EXPLICIT LEARNING

The learning and performance of skilled movement comprises conscious as well as unconscious processes, implying inter alia the involvement of different neural structures, at least some of the time. In the early stages of practice, and particularly for more complex tasks with recurring patterns, such as those that involve repeated sequences of movement targets or recurring dynamic patterns (consider dancing), theorists have long recognized that attention demands are higher than in later stages of training (see review, Logan, 1985). Motor skills can involve learning a variety of *procedures* that often are not conscious and usually require large amounts of practice to master (c.f., bicycle riding). Such *implicit learning* contrasts with learning *declarative* (verbalizable), *explicit knowledge*, which is memorized relatively quickly, is accessible to consciousness, and reportable verbally. Cognitive psychology identifies these explicit and implicit learning processes as separable (Squire, 1987). Observation of amnesiacs with intact motor learning capacity has led to suggestions that the processes are separable neurally, as well as behaviorally (Cohen & Squire, 1980; Squire, 1992). More recently, Willingham et al, (2002) investigated neural systems mediating conscious and unconscious motor sequence learning using functional neuroimaging. They concluded that some structures were activated when motor learning occurred with or without awareness of the sequence pattern being taught. Learning with awareness activated a wide range of additional regions.

Motor learning can involve explicit as well as implicit processes, and verbal instructions are variously included among the conditions of task practice to facilitate movement reeducation after stroke. What guidance does the literature provide? The separate but interacting network components of procedural and declarative processes in motor learning raise the possibilities that the two processes might aid each other or compete for neural resources. Poldrack and Packard (2003) review evidence that suggests the latter. Wulf and her colleagues have conducted several studies investigating the learning effects of directing attention internally, to body movements and coordination, or externally to the task outcome (see Wulf & Shea, 2002 for a review). Wulf and Shea conclude that there is a detrimental effect from an internal focus, but a beneficial effect of attending to outcome.

In the last decade, studies have begun to investigate explicit and implicit motor learning with stroke samples. Pohl et al. showed that people with stroke are able to implicitly learn a perceptuomotor task requiring hand movements to be made in response to target lights (Pohl, McDowd, Filion, Ricjards, & Stiers, 2001). Boyd and Winstein found that explicit training, via instruction about the sequence pattern and recognition tests, interfered with implicit motor learning after strokes that affected the sensorimotor cortex (Boyd & Winstein, 2003) or the basal ganglia (Boyd & Winstein, 2004). This phenomenon occurred when training either continuous movement patterns or discrete action sequences (Boyd & Winstein, 2006). The deleterious effect in stroke samples contrasted with the beneficial effect of explicit instructions in healthy controls observed within the same training paradigms. Boyd and Winstein (2006) infer that the phenomenon may be a consequence of increased load on impaired working memory in the context of connectivity problems between the prefrontal and sensorimotor cortex. This contrast illustrates the caveat raised in the earlier section on transfer of training effects: motor learning studies in unimpaired performers are a reasonable starting point for developing principles of motor reeducation consequent to brain insult, but such studies need to be viewed as a source of hypotheses rather than a validation of principles of rehabilitation training.

9.11 KEY CLINICAL MESSAGES

Evidence from neuroscience, neuroimaging studies, learning theory, and neuropsychology support the following key clinical messages:

- Use of task-specific training of sufficient intensity, and using strategies to enhance transfer of training to real life contexts, will facilitate activation of brain regions and networks in order to enhance motor learning after stroke.

- Task requirements should be incorporated into training in order to facilitate activation of appropriate neural networks and brain regions.

- Active, attended movements will more successfully activate appropriate neural networks and brain regions than passive movements.

- Systematic variation of task parameters during task practice affords opportunity to learn skilled movements required in varying contexts in everyday life.

- Task-specific training and intensity or repetition are key strategies for enhancing neuroplastic changes.

- Strategies for increasing the amount of practice need to be employed to enhance neuroplastic changes associated with motor learning.

- To enhance transfer of learning, whole movements should be incorporated into practice.

- Introducing variability of practice at an appropriate time enhances transfer of learning.

REFERENCES

Bayona, N. A., Bitensky, J., Salter, K., & Teasell, R. (2005). The role of task-specific training in rehabilitation therapies. *Topics in Stroke Rehabilitation, 12*(3), 58–65.

Birkenmeier, R. L., Pragar, E. M., & Lang, C. E. (2010). Translating animal doses of task-specific training to people with chronic stroke in 1-hour therapy sessions: proof of concept study. *Neurorehabilitation and Neural Repair, 24*, 620–635.

Blennerhassett, J., & Dite, W. (2004). Additional task-related practice improves mobility and upper limb function early after stroke: a randomised controlled trial. *Australian Journal of Physiotherapy, 50*, 219–224.

Bootsma, R. J., Marteniuk, R. G., MacKenzie, C. L., & Zaal, F. T. J. M. (1994). The speed-accuracy trade-off in manual prehension: effects of movement amplitude, object size and object width on kinematic characteristics. *Experimental Brain Research, 98*, 535–541.

Boyd, L., & Winstein, C. (2006). Explicit information interferes with implicit motor learning of both continuous and discrete movement tasks after stroke. *Journal of Neurology and Physical Therapy, 30*, 46–57.

Boyd, L. A., & Winstein, C. J. (2003). Impact of explicit information on implicit motor-sequence learning following middle cerebral artery stroke. *Physical Therapy, 83*, 976–989.

Boyd, L. A., & Winstein, C. J. (2004). Providing explicit information disrupts implicit motor learning after basal ganglia stroke. *Learning and Memory, 11*, 388–396.

Braun, C., Heinz, U., Schweizer, R., Wiech, K., Birbaumer, N., & Topka, H. (2001). Dynamic organization of the somatosensory cortex induced by motor activity. *Brain, 124*, 2259–2267.

Butefisch, C., Hummelsheim, H., Denzler, P., & Mauritz, K.-H. (1995). Repetitive training of isolated movements improves outcome of motor rehabilitation of the centrally paretic hand. *Journal of Neurological Sciences, 130*, 59–68.

Butefisch, C. M., Kleiser, R., & Seitz, R. J. (2006). Post-lesional cerebral reorganisation: evidence from functional neuroimaging and transcranial magnetic stimulation. *Journal of Physiology—Paris, 99*, 437–454.

Campos, T. F., Barroso, M. T.M., & Menezes, A. A. d.L. (2010). Encoding, storage and retrieval processes of the memory and the implications for motor practice in stroke patients. *Neurorehabilitation, 26*, 135–142.

Carey, J. R., Kimberley, T. J., Lewis, S. M., Auerbach, E. J., Dorsey, L., Rundquist, P., et al. (2002). Analysis of fMRI and finger tracking training in subjects with chronic stroke. *Brain, 125*, 773–788.

Carey, L. M. (2006). Loss of somatic sensation. In M. E. Selzer, S. Clarke, L. G. Cohen, P. W. Duncan and F. H. Gage. (Ed.), *Textbook of Neural Repair and Rehabilitation. Vol II*. Medical Neurorehabilitation. (Vol II. pp. 231–247). Cambridge: Cambridge University Press.

Carey, L. M., Macdonnell, R., & Matyas, T. A. (2011). SENSe: Study of the Effectiveness of Neurorehabilitation on Sensation: a randomized controlled trial. *Neurorehabilitation Neural Repair, 25*, 304–313.

Carey, L. M., Matyas, T. A., & Oke, L. E. (1993). Sensory loss in stroke patients: effective tactile and proprioceptive discrimination training. *Archives of Physical Medicine and Rehabilitation, 74*, 602–611.

Cauraugh, J. H., & Kim, S. B. (2003). Stroke motor recovery: active neuromuscular stimulation and repetitive practice schedules. *Journal of Neurology, Neurosurgery and Psychiatry, 74*, 1562–1566.

Cohen, L. G., & Squire, L. R. (1980). Preserved learning and retention of pattern analyzing skill in amnesia: dissociation of know how and knowing that. *Science, 210*, 207–209.

Cope, S., & Trombly, C. A. (1998). Grasping in children with and without cerebral palsy: A kinematic analysis. *Scandinavian Journal of Occupational Therapy, 5*, 59–68.

Cormier, S. M., & Hagman, J. D. (1987). *Transfer of learning: Contemporary research applications*. New York: Academic Press.

Dean, C. M., Richards, C. L., & Malouin, F. (2000). Task-related circuit training improves performance of locomotor tasks in chronic stroke. *Archives of Physical Medicine and Rehabilitation, 81*, 409–417.

Dean, C. M., & Shepherd, R. B. (1997). Task-related training improves performance of seated reaching tasks after stroke. *Stroke, 28*(4), 722–728.

Decety, J. (1996). Do imagined and execute actions share the same neural substrate? *Cognitive Brain Research, 3*, 87–93.

DeWit, L., Putman, K., Dejaeger, E., Baert, I., Berman, P., Bogaerts, K., et al. (2005). Use of time by stroke patients: a comparison of four European rehabilitation centers. *Stroke, 36*, 1977–1983.

Dromerick, A. W., Lang, C. E., Birkenmeier, R. L., Wagner, J. M., Miller, J. P., Videen, T. O., et al. (2009). Very early constraint-induced movement during stroke rehabilitation (VECTORS). *Neurology, 73*, 195–201.

Elbert, T., Pantev, C., Wienruch, C., Rockstroh, B., & Taub, E. (1995). Increased cortical representation of the fingers of the left hand in string players. *Science, 270*, 305–307.

Fattori, P., Breveglieri, R., Marzocchi, N., Filippini, D., Bosco, A., & Galleti, C. (2009). Hand orientation during reach-to-grasp movements modulates neuronal activity in the medial posterior parietal area V6. *The Journal of Neuroscience, 29*(6), 1928–1936.

French, B., Thomas, L. H., Leathley, M. J., Sutton, C. J., McAdam, J., Forster, A., et al. (2007). Repetitive task training for improving functional ability after stroke (Review). *Cochrane Database of Systematic Reviews* Issue 4, Art. No.: CD006073. DOI: 10.1002/14651858.CD006073.pub2.

Guzetta, A., Staudt, M., Petacchi, E., Ehlers, J., Erb, M., Wilke, M., et al. (2007). Brain representation of active and passive hand movements in children. *Pediatric Research, 61*(4), 485–490.

Hanlon, R. E. (1996). Motor learning following unilateral stroke. *Archives of Physical Medicine and Rehabilitation, 77*, 811–815.

Hayashi, S., Hasegawa, Y., & Kasai, T. (2002). Transcranial magnetic stimulation study of plastic changes of human motor cortex after repetitive simple muscle contractions. *Perceptual and Motor Skills, 95*, 699–705.

Hummelsheim, H., Hauptmann, B., & Neumann, S. (1995). Influence of physiotherapeutic facilitation techniques on motor evoked potentials in centrally paretic hand extensor muscles. *Electroencephalography and Clinical Neurophysiology, 97*, 18–28.

Iacoboni, M., Molnar-Szakacs, I., Gallese, V., Buccino, G., Mazziotta, J.C., & Rizzolatti, G. (2005). Grasping the intetnions of others with one's own mirror neuron system. *Public Library of Science Biology, 3*(3), e79.

Intercollegiate Stroke Working Party. (2008). *National Clinical Guideline for Stroke* (3rd ed.). London: Royal College of Physicians.

Karni, A., Meyer, G., Jezzard, P., Adams, M. M., Turner, R., & Ungerleider, L. G. (1995). Functional MRI evidence for adult motor cortex plasticity during motor skill learning. *Nature, 377*, 155–158.

Karni, A., Meyer, G., Rey-Hiploito, C., Jezzard, P., Adams, M. M., & Turner, R. (1998). The acquisition of skilled motor performance: fast and slow experience-driven changes in primary motor cortex. *Proceedings of the National Academy of Science USA, 95*, 861–868.

Kwakkel, G., van Peppen, R., Wagenaar, R. C., Dauphinee, S. W., Richards, C., Ashburn, A., et al. (2004). Effects of augmented exercise therapy time after stroke: a meta-analysis. *Stroke, 35*, 2529–2536.

Lai, Q., & Shea, C. H. (1999). Bandwidth knowledge of results enhances generalized motor program learning. *Research Quarterly for Exercise and Sport, 70*, 79–83.

Lai, Q., Shea, C. H., Wulf, G., & Wright, D. L. (2000). Optimizing generalized motor program and parameter learning. . *Research Quarterly for Exercise and Sport, 71*, 10–24.

Lang, C. E., MacDonald, J. R., & Gnip, C. (2007). Counting repetitions: an observational study of outpatient therapy for people with hemiparesis post-stroke. *Journal of Neurologic Physical Therapy, 31*, 3–10.

Lincoln, N. B., Willis, S., Philips, S. A., Juby, L. C., & Berman, P. (1996). Comparison of rehabilitation practice on hospital wards for stroke patients. *Stroke, 27*, 18–23.

Logan, G. D. (1985). Skill and automaticity: relations, implications and future directions. *Canadian Journal of Psychology, 39*, 367–386.

Lotze, M., Braun, C., Birbaumer, N., Anders, S., & Cohen, L. G. (2003). Motor learning elicited by voluntary drive. *Brain, 126*, 866–872.

Magill, R. A. (2007). *Motor learning and control: concepts and applications* (9th ed.). New York: McGraw Hill.

Marteniuk, R. G., Leavitt, J. L., MacKenzie, C. L., & Athenes, S. (1990). Functional relationships between grasp and transport components in a prehension task. *Human Movement Science, 9*, 149–176.

Miller, E. L., Murray, L., Richards, L., Zorowitz, R. D., Bakas, T., Clark, P., et al. (2010). Comprehensive overview of nursing and interdisciplinary rehabilitation care of the stroke patient: a scientific statement from the American Heart Association. *Stroke, 41,* 2402–2448.

Mima, T., Sadato, N., Yazawa, S., Hankawa, T., Fukuyama, H., & Yonekura, Y. (1999). Brain structures related to active and passive finger movements in man. *Brain 122,* 1989–1997.

Muir, A. L., & Jones, A. M. (2009). Is neuroplastcity promoted by task complexity? *New Zealand Journal of Physiotherapy, 37*(3), 136–144.

National Stroke Foundation, (2010). *Clinical guidelines for stroke management.* Melbourne, Australia.

Nudo, R. J., Milliken, G. W., Jenkins, W. M., & Merzenich, M. M. (1996). Use dependent alterations of movement representations in primary motor cortex of adult squirrel monkeys. *Journal of Neuroscience, 16,* 785–807.

Oujamaa, L., Relave, I., Froger, J., Mottet, D., & Pelissier, J.-Y. (2009). Rehabilitation of arm function after stroke. Literature review. *Annals of Physical and Rehabilitation Medicine, 52,* 269–293.

Page, S. J., Levine, P., & Leonard, A. (2007). Mental practice in chronic stroke: results of a randomized, placebo-controlled trial. *Stroke, 38,* 1293–1297.

Pohl, P. S., McDowd, J. M., Filion, D. L., Ricjards, L. G., & Stiers, W. (2001). Implicit learning of a perceptuo-motor skill after stroke. *Physical Therapy, 81*(11), 1780–1780.

Poldrack, R. A., & Packard, M. G. (2003). Competition among multiple memory systems: converging evidence from animal and human brain studies. *Neuropsychologia, 41,* 245–251.

Richards, C. L., Malouin, F., Wood-Dauphinee, S., Williams, J. I., Bouchard, J.-P., & Brunet, D. (1993). Task-specific physical therapy for optimization of gait recovery in acute stroke patients. *Archives of Physical Medicine and Rehabilitation, 74,* 612–620.

Richards, L. G., Stewart, K. C., Woodbury, M. L., Senesac, C., & Cauraugh, J. H. (2008). Movement dependent stroke recovery: a systematic review and meta-analysis of TMS and fMRI evidence. *Neuropsychology, 46,* 3–11.

Rizzolatti, G., Camarda, R., Fogassi, G., Gentilucci, M., Lupping, G., & Matelli, M. (1988). Functional organisation of inferior area 6 in the macque monkey. II. Area F5 and the control of distal movements. *Experimental Brain Research, 71,* 491–507.

Rizzolatti, G., Fadiga, L., Gallese, V., & Fogassi, L. (1996). Premotor cortex and the recognition of motor actions. *Brain Research Cognition, 3,* 131–141.

Rosenbaum, D. A., & Jorgensen, M. J. (1992). Planning macroscopic aspects of manual control. *Human Movement Science, 11,* 61–69.

Sakata, H., Taira, M., Kusunoki, M., Murata, A., & Tanaka, Y. (1997). The TINS lecture. The parietal association cortex in depth perception and visual control of hand action. *Trends in Neuroscience, 20,* 350–357.

Schmidt, R. A. (1988). *Motor control and learning: a behavioural emphasis* (2nd ed.). Champaign, IL: Human Kinetics.

Schmidt, R. A., & Lee, D. T. (2011). *Motor Control and Learning: A Behavioral Emphasis* (4th ed.). Champaign, Illinois: Human Kinetics.

Schmidt, R. A., & Wrisberg, C. A. (2000). *Motor learning and performance: a problem-based learning approach.* (2nd ed.). Champaign, IL: Human Kinetics.

Schmidt, R. A., & Young, D. E. (1987). Transfer of movement control in motor learning. In S.M. Cormier and J.D. Hagman (Ed.), *Transfer of learning: Contemporary research applications.* (pp. 47–49). New York: Academic Press.

SCORE (2011). SCORE recommendations for upper limb and shoulder: management of the arm and hand. Summary of the evidence. Canadian best practice recommendations for stroke care: rehabilitation. From http://www.strokebestpractices.ca/index.php/stroke-rehabilitation/.

Scottish Intercollegiate Guidelines Network, (2010). *Management of patients with stroke: Rehabilitation, prevention, and management of complications, and discharge planning. A national clinical guideline.* Edinburgh, Scotland.

Seidler, R. D., & Noll, C. D. (2008). Neuroanatomical correlates of motor acquisition and motor transfer. *Journal of Neurophysiology, 99,* 1836–1845.

Shapiro, D. C., & Schmidt, R. A. (1982). The schema theory: recent evidence and developmental implications. In J. A. S. Kelso and J. E. Clark (Eds.), *The development of movement control and coordination.* (pp. 113–150). New York: Wiley.

Shea, C. H., & Wulf, G. (2005). Schema theory: A critical appraisal and re-evaluation. *Journal of Motor Behavior, 37*(2), 85–101.

Squire, L. R. (1987). *Memory and brain.* New York: Oxford University Press.

Squire, L. R. (1992). Memory and the hippocampus: a synthesis from findings with rats, monkeys and humans. *Psychological Review,, 99,* 195–231.

Stroke Foundation of New Zealand (2003). *Life after stroke: New Zealand guideline for management of stroke. New Zealand protocols for the management of stroke and ischemic attack.* Wellington, New Zealand: Stroke Foundation NZ Inc.

Summers, J., & Anson, J. G. (2009). Current status of the motor program: revisited. *Human Movement Science, 28,* 566–577.

Tanne-Gariepy, J., Rouiller, E. M., & Boussaoud, D. (2002). Parietal inputs to dorsal versus ventral premotor areas in the macaque monkey: evidence for largely segregated visuomotor pathways. *Experimental Brain Research, 145,* 91–103.

Tomassini, V., Jbabdi, S., Kincses, Z. T., Bosnell, R., Douaud, G., Pozzilli, C., et al. (2011). Structural and functional bases for individual differences in motor learning. *Human Brain Mapping, 32,* 494–508.

Tyc, F., Boyadjian, A., & Devanne, H. (2005). Motor cortex plasticity induced by extensive training revealed by transcranial magnetic stimulation in human. *European Journal of Neuroscience, 21,* 259–266.

Van der Lee, J. H., Snels, I. A., Beckerman, H., Lankhorst, G. J., Wagenaar, R. C., & Bouter, L. M. (2001). Exercise therapy for arm function in stroke patients: a systematic review of randomized controlled trials. *Clinical Rehabilitation, 15*(1), 20–31.

Van Rossum, J. (1990). Schmidt's schema theory: the empirical base of the variability of practice hypothesis. A critical analysis. *Human Movement Science, 9,* 387–435.

Van Vliet, P., Kerwin, D. G., Sheridan, M. R., & Fentem, P. H. (1995). A study of reaching movements in stroke patients. In M. A. Harrison (Ed.), *Physiotherapy in Stroke Management* (pp. 183–191). Singapore: Churchill Livingstone.

Van Vliet, P. M., & Sheridan, M. R. (2007). Coordination between reaching and grasping in patients with hemiparesis and normal subjects. *Archives of Physical Medicine and Rehabilitation, 88*(10), 1325–1331.

Weeks, D. L., & Anderson, L. P. (2000). The interaction of observational learning with overt practice: effects on motor skill learning. *Acta Psychologia, 104,* 259–271.

Willingham, D. B., Salidis, J., & Gabrieli, J. D. E. (2002). Direct comparison of neural systems mediating conscious and unconscious skill learning. *Journal of Neurophysiology,, 88,* 1451–1460.

Willingham, D. T. (1998). A neuropsychological theory of motor learning. *Psychological Review,, 105*(3), 558–584.

Wittenberg, G. F., Chen, R., Ishii, K., Bushara, K. O., Taub, E., Gerber, L. H., et al. (2003). Constraint-induced therapy in stroke: magnetic-stimulation motor maps and cerebral activation. *Neurorehabilitation and Neural Repair, 1*(4), 1–10.

Wolf, S. L., Winstein, C. J., Miller, J. P., Taub, E., Uswatte, G., Morris, D., et al. (2006). Effect of constraint-induced movement therapy on upper extremity function 3 to 9 months after stroke. *Journal of the American Medical Association, 296,* 2095–2104.

Wu, C.-Y., Wong, M.-K., Lin, K.-C., & Chen, H.-C. (2001). Effects of task goal and personal preference on seated reaching kinematics after stroke. *Stroke, 32,* 70–76.

Wu, C., Trombly, C. A., Lin, K., & Tickle-Degnen, L. (2000). A kinematic study of contextual effects on reaching performance in persons with and without stroke: influences of object availablility. *Archives of Physical Medicine and Rehabilitation, 81,* 95–101.

Wu, C.Y., Chou, S. H., Kuo, M. Y., Chen, C. L., Lu, T. W., & Fu, Y. C. (2008). Effects of object size on intralimb and interlimb coordination during a bimanual prehension task in patients with left cerebral vascular accidents. *Motor Control, 12*(4), 296–310.

Wulf, G., & Shea, C. H. (2002). Principles derived from the study of simple motor skills do not generalize to complex skill learning. *Pschonomic Bulletin and Review, 9,* 185–211.

Zoia, S., Pezzetta, E., Blason, L., Scabar, A., Carrozzi, M., Bulgheroni, M., et al. (2006). a comparison of the reach-to-grasp movement between children and adults: a kinematic study. *Developmental Neuropsychology, 30,* 719–738.

10 | ADJUNCTIVE THERAPIES

CHARLOTTE J. STAGG and HEIDI JOHANSEN-BERG

10.1   INTRODUCTION AND RATIONALE

The ability of training and physical activity to restore motor function after neural injury has long been appreciated, both from animal studies (Nudo, Milliken, Jenkins, & Merzenich, 1996) and in clinical practice. Intensive physical therapy, including both task-specific training and evidence-based movement interventions, is therefore currently the gold-standard intervention in stroke rehabilitation. However, in current practice around 50% of patients are left dependent on others for activities of daily living (NAO, UK, 2005). Therefore, a variety of putative adjunctive therapies have been suggested, all of which have the overall aim of enhancing response to more traditional interventions such as physiotherapy and occupational therapy.

The rationale for adjunctive therapies stems from the idea that the beneficial effects of a standard treatment, such as physical therapy, are mediated via brain plasticity. Interventions that modulate brain plasticity, such as drugs or brain stimulation, can therefore be used to enhance the effects of standard regimes. A number of possible adjunctive approaches have been tested in proof-of-principle studies, all of which are at relatively early stages of investigation and translation into clinical trials and then into clinical practice. Here, we will discuss the major pharmacological agents and transcranial stimulation approaches trialed to date, and briefly highlight some other emerging adjunctive therapies that may come to prominence over the next few years. The majority of the work has been performed on motor function; therefore, we will concentrate on that aspect of recovery after stroke, though many of the principles underlying the potential therapeutic options discussed here are applicable to other spheres of recovery.

It is important to note that although a number of therapies have been identified as promising from proof-of-principle

studies, translation of these into full-scale clinical trials has been limited. This "translational road block" (Endres et al., 2008) has arisen for many reasons, including the need to extrapolate approaches from animal models, to optimize parameters for pharmacological or stimulation interventions, and to identify patients most likely to respond to a given therapy. Further translational studies are therefore required to increase our understanding of the mechanisms underlying motor recovery after stroke, and how our interventions may interact with these. In addition, large-scale, multicenter randomized control trials are required to overcome the noise imparted by the inherent heterogeneity of patient populations and allow adequately powered studies to investigate the effects of adjunctive therapies in detail.

10.1.1   INSIGHTS FROM ANIMAL MODELS

The adjunctive therapies discussed in this chapter all have a rationale for their use based in our understanding of mechanisms of induction of plasticity from the animal literature (see Chapter 3). This raises two important considerations about their potential use in patients: (i) the need for multiple rather than single applications of an adjunctive therapy, and (ii) the necessity of combining adjunctive therapies with training interventions such as physical therapy.

10.1.1.1   THE NEED FOR MULTIPLE SESSIONS OF STIMULATION

Animal studies suggest that long-term plasticity (LTP)-like changes within the neocortex, where changes in excitability outlast the stimulation period by days to weeks, can only be induced in the awake, moving animal if multiple, spaced sessions of stimulation are used (Trepel & Racine, 1998; Froc, Chapman, Trepel, & Racine, 2000). By extension, multiple interventions or doses will probably be required to induce long-term clinical benefits in patients. A number of studies discussed here have used the response to a single session of an intervention to demonstrate proof-of-principle, with the suggestion that multiple sessions could reinforce and stabilize the outcomes seen. Although this is a reasonable hypothesis, it should be noted that it has not yet been determined whether response to a single session can be directly translated into long-term outcome after multiple sessions.

10.1.1.2 COMBINATION WITH PHYSICAL THERAPY

The primary rationale for the use of the adjunct therapies discussed here is that they promote plasticity. With the brain in a more receptive state, it may be that the acquisition of motor skills proceeds more easily. It has been hypothesized, based on this rationale, that adjunctive therapies are of most use in conjunction with intense rehabilitative therapy. In rats there is evidence that pharmacological interventions need to be paired with motor activity to be effective (Feeney, Gonzalez, & Law, 1982), and although it is likely that this argument follows for humans, it has yet to be directly tested.

10.2 PHARMACOLOGICAL STUDIES

Pharmacological treatment of stroke, as with other neurological disorders, is limited by the challenge of designing drugs capable of crossing the blood-brain barrier. Blood-brain barrier permeability is low for agents with low lipid solubility or for molecules with a large molecular weight, limiting the agents that can be used. Potential approaches to circumvent this problem include invasive methods, such as: intracisternal injections, which may be of concern in the stroke population; pharmacological modulation of the drug to increase lipid solubility; or physiological approaches, such as conjugating the drug with a ligand that is recognized and taken up by a membrane transporter (Gabathuler, 2009). It is to be hoped that these approaches will increase the number of potential pharmaceutical agents for the treatment of stroke.

To date, a number of pharmacological agents have been trialed in animal models of stroke and in proof-of-principle studies in humans, but the translation of these findings into larger-scale clinical studies and then into clinical practice has been slow. Some of these pharmacological agents have been selected in part based on their ability to facilitate neuronal plasticity—the most thoroughly investigated of these are discussed here.

10.2.1 AMPHETAMINES

Amphetamines are indirect sympathomimetic drugs that have a complex mode of action in the central nervous system (CNS). Their effects are mediated primarily by an increased release of endogenous noradrenaline (norepinephrine) as well as dopamine and probably serotonin. Dexamphetamine, the most widely used of the amphetamines, has relatively few effects in the periphery. Central nervous system effects in response to the usual therapeutic dose of 5–30mg in healthy subjects include appetite suppression, increased arousal, euphoria, and stereotyped behavior (Rang, Dale, Ritter, & Flower, 2007). Increased motor activity, improved learning, and increased use-dependent plasticity have also been demonstrated at similar doses in healthy subjects (Soetens, Casaer, D'Hooge, & Hueting, 1995; Kumari et al., 1997; Greenwald, Schuster, Johanson, & Jewell, 1998; Bütefisch et al., 2002; Sawaki, Cohen, Classen, Davis, & Bütefisch, 2002). An initial clinical trial in acute stroke patients combining a single-dose of dexamphetamine with one session of physical training demonstrated an improvement in the Fugl-Meyer (FM) score of motor impairment the day after the intervention (Crisostomo, Duncan, Propst, Dawson, & Davis, 1988). However, subsequent clinical trials showed mixed results and a Cochrane review concluded that there was insufficient evidence to draw conclusions on the benefit of amphetamines in stroke rehabilitation, and that more research was justified (Martinsson, Hårdemark, & Eksborg, 2007). A subsequent randomized controlled trial in 16 patients 14–60 days post-stroke showed a trend toward improvement in activities of daily living and arm motor function (assessed by the Chedoke-McMaster Stroke Assessment) in the treated group compared with placebo-controlled group, which was maintained for at least 6 months post-treatment (Schuster et al., 2011).

The inconsistency of effects across trials of amphetamine may reflect difficulties translating highly promising effects in animals into the human population, in particular in relation to the question of the optimal dose. The dose-effect of amphetamine-promoted motor recovery in animals is an inverted "U" shape, with both high and low doses proving relatively ineffective (Goldstein, 2009). In addition, it is not yet clear how to combine amphetamines and training for optimal effect. At the time of writing, the Amphetamine-Enhanced Stroke Recovery (AESR) trial, designed to evaluate the impact of timing and duration of amphetamine treatment, is ongoing.

There are some safety concerns about the use of amphetamines in the stroke patient population. Amphetamines are known to increase blood pressure, and therefore there is a theoretical increased risk of cardiovascular events, including stroke, with treatment. One study concluded that dexamphetamine "was safe and well tolerated" by patients with acute cerebral ischemia, although a subsequent Cochrane Review by the same group found that there is currently not enough evidence to draw a conclusion about the relative risk of treatments in this patient group (Martinsson & Wahlgren, 2003; Martinsson et al., 2007).

10.2.2 DOPAMINERGIC AGENTS

Experimental studies in healthy controls have demonstrated that increasing dopaminergic tone, either with levadopa or a dopamine agonist, enhanced motor cortical plasticity, while decreasing dopaminergic tone reduced plasticity (Flöel et al., 2005; Meintzschel & Ziemann, 2006). Dopaminergic modulation has also been trialed in the subacute recovery phase after stroke, and one study reported significantly better motor function with 3 weeks of levodopa and physiotherapy compared with placebo and physiotherapy (Scheidtmann, Fries, Müller, & Koenig, 2001). Two other studies demonstrated only a trend toward improvement, although with relatively small patient numbers (Sonde & Lokk, 2007; Lokk, Roghani, & Delbari, 2011). In the chronic phase of recovery, a single dose of levodopa also leads to an improvement in motor plasticity (Flöel, Hummel, Breitenstein, Knecht, & Cohen, 2005) and in procedural motor learning (Rosser et al., 2008). In a single Phase I trial, 5 weeks of levodopa given in the absence of physiotherapy improved walking speed and manual dexterity compared with a placebo (Acler, Fiaschi, & Manganotti, 2009).

10.2.3 CHOLINERGIC AGENTS

Drugs designed to increase cholinergic tone are commonly used in the management of patients with Alzheimer's disease, and their utility in improving memory retention in other domains is beginning to be investigated. In healthy subjects, increasing cholinergic signaling with donepezil, an acetylcholinesterase (AChE) inhibitor, enhanced use-dependent motor plasticity, whereas decreasing cholinergic signaling with a muscarinic antagonist reduced motor plasticity (Sawaki et al., 2002; Meintzschel & Ziemann, 2006). A single case study in a chronic stroke patient demonstrated dramatic improvements in function with an AChE inhibitor given for 16 weeks (Berthier et al., 2003), although a subsequent randomized clinical trial in chronic stroke patients showed only a trend toward greater behavioral gains in a group given donepezil combined with constraint-induced therapy (CIT) compared to a placebo group (Nadeau et al., 2004). An open-label study in patients with cognitive impairment in the acute stages of stroke recovery showed a 14-point greater improvement in outcome (Functional Independence Measure—motor subscale) with a 12-week treatment of donepezil compared to either patients treated with galantamine, another AChE inhibitor, or with historical controls (Whyte et al., 2008).

10.2.4 SEROTONINERGIC AGENTS

A number of small clinical trials of the selective serotonin reuptake inhibitors (SSRIs) have suggested that they may be beneficial in the recovery of motor function both in the acute (Dam et al., 1996; Pariente et al., 2001; Acler, Robol, Fiaschi, & Manganotti, 2009) and chronic stages of recovery (Zittel, Weiller, & Liepert, 2008). A subsequent large randomised controlled trial (RCT) in patients within 3 months of stroke (the FLAME study) compared outcomes in patients treated with fluoxetine for 90 days in combination with physiotherapy and standard care with a placebo-treated group, who also received physiotherapy and standard care. The authors demonstrated a significantly greater improvement in FM score at 90 days post-stroke in the treated group than in the control group (Figure 10.1; Chollet et al., 2011).

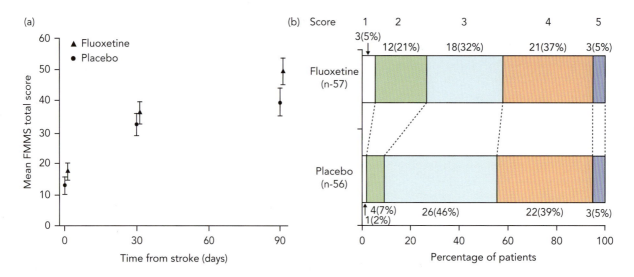

Figure 10.1 Improvement in motor function in patients in the acute stages of stroke recovery treated with the SSRI fluoxetine compared with placebo. A. Fugl-Meyer motor scores (FMMS) at days 0, 30, and 90, adjusted for center, age, history of stroke, and FMMS at inclusion. Points are mean ± 95% CI. B. Distribution of modified Rankin Score (mRS) at day 90. The proportion of independent patients (mRS ≤ 2), adjusted for center, age, history of stroke, and baseline mRS was significantly higher in the fluoxetine treated group than in the placebo group. Data are number (%). (Adapted from Figures 2 & 3 in Chollet et al., 2011).

10.3 TRANSCRANIAL STIMULATION TECHNIQUES

Therapies that directly or indirectly stimulate the central nervous system may enhance the potential for neuroplasticity in the post-stroke period and may therefore help patients overcome their residual motor impairments post-stroke. Transcranial stimulation approaches have a potential advantage over pharmacological interventions, in that they can be targeted specifically to localized brain regions. The most common target for recovery of upper limb function, considered here, is the primary motor cortex (M1). Transcranial stimulation methods, depending on the details of the protocols used, are capable of either increasing or decreasing cortical excitability.

10.3.1 ABNORMAL INTERHEMISPHERIC BALANCE

A consistent observation from neuroimaging studies of patients after stroke is the presence of overactivation of the motor areas in the contralesional hemisphere when a stroke patient moves their paretic hand compared with controls (see Chapter 4; Chollet et al., 1991; Weiller, Chollet, Friston, Wise, & Frackowiak, 1992; Liepert, Hamzei, & Weiler, 2000; Ward, Brown, Thompson, & Frackowiak, 2003a, 2003b).

There is conflicting evidence as to whether this increased contralesional activity is maladaptive in all patients. Converging evidence from a number of modalities suggests that this activity is greatest in patients who have made a poor recovery (Ward et al., 2003b), and longitudinal studies have demonstrated that activity in this region decreases as patients recover over time (Marshall et al., 2000; Ward et al., 2003a). In addition, Transcranial Magnetic Stimulation (TMS) studies demonstrate that poorly recovered patients exhibit abnormally high levels of interhemispheric inhibition between the M1s in the two hemispheres during movement (Murase, Duque, Mazzocchio, & Cohen, 2004).

However, there is also evidence that activity in the contralesional M1 may be supportive of function in some patients. A number of studies have demonstrated recruitment of the contralesional hemisphere even in well-recovered patients (Bütefisch, Netz, Wessling, Seitz, & Hömberg, 2003; Bütefisch et al., 2005), and disrupting activity in the contralesional premotor cortex using single pulses of TMS impairs motor responses in patients in the chronic phase of recovery (Johansen-Berg et al., 2002). Using repetitive TMS (rTMS) to disrupt activity has even more widespread effects: rTMS over contralesional premotor, primary motor, or superior parietal cortex resulted in a detriment in performance even in well-recovered patients (Lotze et al., 2006).

Overall, it seems likely that individual patient factors are likely to determine whether activity in the contralesional

M1 is adaptive or maladaptive. It could be hypothesized that, in patients who are able to rely on the ipsilesional M1 for the majority of function, contralesional M1 activity is maladaptive. In comparison, for patients in whom there is insufficient residual function in the ipsilesional M1, either in terms of cortex or residual output tracts, contralesional M1 activity is important in preserving function. However, it is not clear currently what biomarkers might be available to distinguish between these two groups of patients. A discussion of the evidence to support the debate of this controversial topic can be found in Chapter 5.

This increased inhibition from the contralesional M1, reflecting interhemispheric imbalance between the two motor cortices, leads to the hypothesis that "rebalancing" the hemispheres might have beneficial effects (see Figure 10.2). This rebalancing could be achieved either by directly increasing the activity within the ipsilesional motor cortex or by indirectly increasing activity in this region via a downregulation of the M1 in the contralesional hemisphere (Ward & Cohen, 2004).

Although this model informs many of the transcranial stimulation studies in the stroke population, it is important to note that there is evidence that the increased activity within the contralesional hemisphere may not be maladaptive in

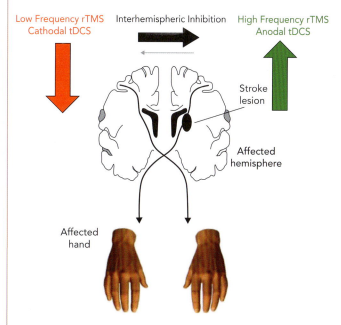

Figure 10.2 Schematic demonstrating the abnormal interhemispheric balance between the two primary motor cortices frequently reported after subcortical stroke. Decreased excitability within the ipsilesional M1 leads to a decreased inhibitory influence on the contralesional M1, therefore leading to increased activity within the contralesional M1. This increased contralesional activity exerts increased inhibition over the ipsilesional cortex, further decreasing the activity seen here. This model presents two potential targets for transcranial stimulation— either upregulating activity within the ipsilesional M1 with facilitatory transcranial stimulation protocols or downregulating the contralesional M1 with inhibitory protocols. (Adapted from Figure 1, Nowak et al., 2009).

all patients, and indeed may confer a behavioral advantage in some (Johansen-Berg et al., 2002; Gerloff et al., 2006; Lotze et al., 2006). It is not yet clear in which patients contralesional activity is adaptive and in which it is maladaptive, but it is important to bear in mind that a "one size fits all" approach is likely to be suboptimal.

10.3.2 INTRODUCTION TO THE TECHNIQUES

Two transcranial stimulation approaches are currently being investigated as potential adjunctive therapies in stroke rehabilitation: transcranial magnetic stimulation (TMS) and transcranial direct current stimulation (tDCS; Figure 10.3).

10.3.2.1 *TRANSCRANIAL MAGNETIC STIMULATION (TMS)*

TMS is described in detail in Chapter 5. In summary, TMS is a noninvasive stimulation technique that induces currents within the brain via the principles of electromagnetic induction. A brief current flowing through a coil of wire contained within a figure_of_eight coil placed on the scalp is used to generate a magnetic field, which in turn induces an electric current in the underlying brain tissue (see Chapter 5). When TMS is applied to the motor cortex it can elicit a muscle response, and so its effects can be measured via the study of electromyographic (EMG) recordings of affected muscles. TMS is typically targeted to the primary motor cortex (M1) by finding the "motor hotspot"—the scalp position at which the lowest intensity TMS pulse evokes a just-noticeable response, or a motor evoked potential (MEP), within the targeted muscle. The intensity of stimulation is then calibrated for an individual patient by modulating the intensity of the stimulation to elicit an MEP of a predefined size. The intensity of the TMS pulse that elicits an MEP of > 50 μV in 5 out of 10 pulses is known as the *resting motor threshold* (RMT),

and gives an index of the ease with which signals can pass from M1 to the muscles.

For therapeutic purposes, TMS is typically applied as a series of pulses, often called repetitive TMS (rTMS). The effect of rTMS protocols on cortical excitability is dependent on the frequency, the pattern, and the intensity of pulses (for a review see Classen & Stefan, 2008; see Figure 10.4). Effects of rTMS on excitability are assessed by measuring the amplitude of MEPs elicited by single TMS pulses applied before and after rTMS. Low-frequency stimulation, where TMS pulses are applied at 1Hz or less, is inhibitory in nature and reduces cortical excitability (Pascual-Leone, Valls-Sole, Wassermann, & Hallett, 1994). High-frequency stimulation, usually applied at 3Hz or more, is usually facilitatory to the cortex and increases cortical excitability (Pascual-Leone et al., 1994), although the precise effect on cortical excitability depends on the stimulation parameters used (Fitzgerald, Fountain, & Daskalakis, 2006). These protocols are typically applied continuously for 10–30 minutes, and should only be applied within the current safety guidelines (see below).

In addition to studying the effects of protocols consisting of regularly spaced pulses, recently more complex patterned protocols have been developed. Of these, theta burst stimulation (TBS) is the most studied. TBS was conceived to mimic experimental paradigms known to induce long-term excitability changes via synaptic modulation in animals. TBS delivers three TMS pulses at 50Hz, repeated every 200ms (the theta frequency; Huang, Edwards, Rounis, Bhatia, & Rothwell, 2005). Two protocols are in common use—(i) intermittent TBS (iTBS), in which a 2s train of TBS is repeated every 10s for a total of 190s (600 pulses), increases cortical excitability; whereas (ii) continuous TBS (cTBS), where an uninterrupted stream of 600 pulses is given over 40s, decreases cortical excitability (Huang et al., 2005).

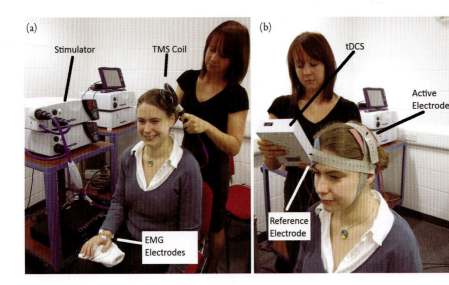

Figure 10.3 Transcranial stimulation techniques. a. Transcranial Magnetic Stimulation (TMS). The figure-eight coil is centered over the primary motor cortex. Stimulation is delivered via a large stimulator and muscle responses can be recorded via electromyography (EMG). b. Transcranial Direct Current Stimulation (tDCS). The active electrode is centered over the primary motor cortex and the reference over the contralateral supraorbital ridge. The tDCS stimulator is a handheld box that delivers a constant direct current in the milliampere range.

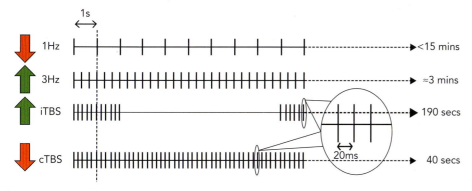

Figure 10.4 Schematic of the major rTMS protocols and their effects on cortical excitability. 1Hz rTMS, where pulses are given at 1s intervals is inhibitory, whereas 3Hz rTMS is excitatory. Theta burst TMS protocols consist of 3 pulses given at 50Hz every 200ms. Intermittent TBS (iTBS), where TBS is given for 2s with 8s inter-train intervals, is excitatory and continuous TBS (cTBS) is inhibitory.

The physiological changes induced by rTMS protocols are complex and are outside the scope of this chapter. Interested readers should consult a detailed review; for example, a recent consensus paper by Ziemann et al. (2008).

10.3.2.2 TRANSCRANIAL DIRECT CURRENT STIMULATION (tDCS)

Transcranial direct current stimulation (tDCS) is a neuromodulatory technique that is said to be "subthreshold," as it does not induce any measurable muscle responses. tDCS relies on a small electric current, in the order of 1–2mA, passed between two large (5x7cm) electrodes placed on the scalp and is targeted to the motor system by the placement of one electrode over M1, with the reference electrode commonly placed over the contralateral supraorbital ridge (Nitsche & Paulus, 2000). The current is gradually ramped up over 10s and is passed between the two electrodes for up to 20 minutes. The effects of tDCS on the underlying cortex are polarity-specific. Anodal tDCS, when the current passes from the M1 electrode to the reference, increases cortical excitability, whereas cathodal stimulation, when the current direction is reversed, is inhibitory (Nitsche & Paulus, 2000).

10.3.2.3 PLACEBO CONTROLS

For clinical trials, inclusion of a placebo control condition is critical and, ideally, both patient and therapist would be blind to experimental condition. This can be a challenge with brain stimulation interventions, where both patient and therapist are aware of certain aspects of the stimulation being delivered. Different approaches to this challenge have been taken.

For tDCS, it is more straightforward to design a placebo condition, as subjects are commonly only aware of the current being applied as it is ramped up. Therefore, the sham stimulation condition typically consists of ramping up the current over the first few tens of seconds as usual, but then switching it off for the remaining 20 minutes or so. Empirical studies suggest that subjects are unable to differentiate between real and sham stimulation with this approach (Gandiga, Hummel, & Cohen, 2006).

For TMS it is more difficult to design an appropriate control condition, as the subject can hear and feel the stimulation being applied throughout the protocol. Possibilities include selecting a control stimulation site or positioning the coil differently (e.g., angled away from the head); this can effectively blind the patient, but may not be effective in blinding therapists. Some TMS manufacturing companies now also construct sham coils that can typically be positioned in the same location as for real stimulation and recreate the sound of a pulse. It is more challenging to elicit tactile sensation without stimulating the brain tissue, but it is to be expected that technology for sham coils will advance, particularly as there is increasing need for well-matched conditions in the clinical trials setting.

10.3.3 rTMS TRIALS

A number of rTMS studies have been performed in patients in the acute, subacute, and chronic stages of recovery. "Excitatory" (i.e., high-frequency) stimulation to the ipsilesional motor cortex is applied according to the rationale that such stimulation should increase plasticity in the stimulated cortex (Ziemann et al., 2008) and so, when paired with physiotherapy, should enhance therapeutic effects. "Inhibitory" (i.e., low-frequency) stimulation to the contralesional hemisphere has been applied in line with the rationale for rebalancing motor cortical activity across the hemispheres.

10.3.3.1 ACUTE STROKE

Three studies to date have investigated the effects of daily sessions of excitatory rTMS protocols to the ipsilesional M1 in the acute or subacute phase post-stroke. Khedr and colleagues gave patients in the acute stages of stroke recovery 10 daily sessions of 3Hz rTMS applied to the ipsilesional hemisphere. Patients also had daily rehabilitation and the authors found that true rTMS led to a significantly greater improvement in motor function than a control group treated with sham rTMS. The group treated with true rTMS and physiotherapy continued to have better motor function than those treated with sham rTMS and physiotherapy for at least 10 days after the stimulation period (Khedr, Ahmed, Fathy, & Rothwellt, 2005).

A similar study showed motor improvements with daily sessions of subthreshold 10Hz rTMS that were greater in the treated group than in the control group after 3 months (Chang et al., 2010). A subsequent study, which compared the effects of 3Hz and 10Hz rTMS applied daily for 5 days to the ipsilesional M1, suggested that the rTMS groups improved more than the control group and that this additional improvement was maintained for at least a year after the end of the stimulation (Khedr, Etraby, Hemeda, Nasef, & Razek, 2010). There was no significant difference in response to the 3Hz or 10Hz stimulation.

A single session of 1Hz rTMS to the contralesional hemisphere led to an improvement in motor performance in patients with subcortical stroke in the subacute stages of recovery (Mansur et al., 2005; Liepert, Zittel, & Weiller, 2007; Dafotakis et al., 2008; Nowak et al., 2008). Multiple sessions of 1Hz rTMS have also been applied to the contralesional M1 in acute stroke patients. Patients within 1 week of stroke were given either 1Hz stimulation to the contralesional hemisphere or 3Hz stimulation to the ipsilesional hemisphere daily for 5 days. Patients received rehabilitation at another time during the day on each of the 5 days. Motor function in both treatment groups improved compared with the sham group, and the improvement was greater in the 1Hz group than in the 3Hz group (Khedr, Abdel-Fadeil, Farghali, & Qaid, 2009).

One study recruited patients who were at least 1 month after ischemic stroke. Patients were randomized to receive 10 daily sessions of either sham rTMS, 5 Hz rTMS to the ipsilesional M1, or 1Hz rTMS to the contralesional M1, immediately preceding standard physical therapy. Both treatment groups showed behavioral improvements compared with the sham treatment group that outlasted the stimulation period by at least 12 weeks (Emara et al., 2010).

10.3.3.2 CHRONIC STROKE

A number of studies have investigated the effects of single sessions of rTMS on motor function in the chronic stages of stroke recovery. One session of 10Hz stimulation to the ipsilesional hemisphere in chronic patients improved accuracy in performance of a complex, sequential motor task compared with sham stimulation (Kim et al., 2006). A subsequent study studied the effects of 20 minutes of 20Hz stimulation to the ipsilesional M1 in 20 patients, and demonstrated modest behavioral improvements that outlasted the stimulation by at least 1 week. No safety concerns were identified (Yozbatiran et al., 2009). However, a further study investigating the effects of a single session of suprathreshold 20 and 25 Hz rTMS to the ipsilesional hemisphere demonstrated no improvement in motor performance, but patients showed abnormal EMG activity that might be attributed to increased seizure risk (Lomarev, Kim, Richardson, Voller, & Hallett, 2007).

Two small studies have investigated the effects of a single session of iTBS to the affected hemisphere and showed an improvement in motor function compared with sham stimulation (Talelli, Greenwood, & Rothwell, 2007; Ackerley, Stinear, Barber, & Byblow, 2010).

A single session of 1Hz rTMS to the contralesional hemisphere led to an improvement in motor performance (Takeuchi, Chuma, Matsuo, Watanabe, & Ikoma, 2005; Takeuchi et al., 2008) and, when combined with motor training, the beneficial effects lasted at least 1 week (Takeuchi et al., 2008). One study showed that a single session of cTBS to the ipsilesional hemisphere modulated cortical excitability but did not change motor performance (Talelli et al., 2007). However, another did demonstrate improvement of motor performance (Ackerley et al., 2010). In addition, one study demonstrated that five sessions of 1Hz rTMS to the contralesional hemisphere performed at rest on consecutive days led to an improvement in reaction times and motor performance in the actively treated TMS group compared with the sham group, which outlasted the stimulation by at least 2 weeks (Fregni et al., 2006).

However, not all trials of daily rTMS interventions have shown an added benefit of stimulation over physical therapy intervention alone. One study investigated daily 20Hz rTMS to the ipsilesional M1 with constraint-induced therapy (CIT) compared with sham rTMS and CIT in chronic stroke patients and saw no added benefit of rTMS (Malcolm et al., 2007). A more recent study investigated both iTBS to the ipsilesional hemisphere or cTBS to the contralesional hemisphere paired with daily standardized physiotherapy for 10 working days in chronic stroke patients and saw no added benefit of TBS (Talelli et al., in review).

10.3.4 tDCS TRIALS

tDCS offers some practical advantages over TMS as an adjunctive therapy. The kit is less bulky and therefore is more portable; it can easily be transported to a bedside, or to a patient's home. It is also easier to use than TMS, meaning a therapist could be trained to give tDCS in a relatively short time. A basic set of tDCS equipment is also approximately ten times cheaper than a TMS kit. However, the key consideration in comparing the two approaches is efficacy and, as with TMS, evidence of effects of tDCS is mixed but promising, and large randomized controlled trials remain to be carried out.

The potential of tDCS in motor recovery post-stroke was first demonstrated when anodal tDCS was applied to the ipsilesional hemisphere of one chronic stroke patient (Hummel et al., 2005). Significant improvements in hand function were noted after a single session and this positive finding was subsequently supported by two small proof-of-principle studies showing significant reductions in the time taken to complete the Jebson-Taylor Task (JTT) in patients who had been treated with anodal tDCS to the ipsilesional M1 compared with a sham stimulation (Fregni et al., 2005; Hummel et al., 2005). An improvement in reaction times (Hummel et al., 2006; Stagg et al., 2012) and grip force (Hummel et al., 2006) have also been demonstrated with anodal tDCS to the ipsilesional M1.

Cathodal tDCS to the contralesional M1 has also been shown to be effective in reducing the time taken to perform the JTT (Fregni et al., 2005), although subsequent studies have not demonstrated significant improvements in reaction times (Stagg et al., 2012).

One novel approach that builds on the theory of interhemispheric imbalance is to simultaneously upregulate the ipsilesional M1 and downregulate the contralesional M1. In theory, this could be achieved by placing the anode over the ipsilesional M1 and the cathode over the contralesional M1, commonly referred to as *bilateral stimulation*. Although the neurophysiological effects of this stimulation paradigm have yet to be fully elucidated, clinical improvements have been demonstrated in chronic stroke patients after 5 consecutive daily sessions of bilateral tDCS combined with physiotherapy. Patients treated with bilateral tDCS showed a significantly greater improvement in Fugl-Meyer score than the sham stimulation–treated control group, improvements that outlasted the stimulation period by at least 1 week (Lindenberg, Renga, Zhu, Nair, & Schlaug, 2010). Direct comparisons of outcomes between the bilateral configuration and the more standard configurations have yet to be performed.

At the time of writing, only one study has investigated the long-term effects of daily tDCS in conjunction with occupational therapy in subacute stroke patients. Cathodal tDCS to the contralesional hemisphere led to greater improvements in motor function than sham stimulation. No improvement over the sham group was seen with anodal tDCS to the ipsilesional hemisphere (Kim et al., 2010). Ongoing studies registered with ClinicalTrials.gov include a large multicenter trial in Germany in acute stroke patients with motor impairment.

10.3.5 THE NECESSITY FOR INDIVIDUALLY TARGETED TREATMENTS

Stroke is a highly heterogeneous disease, both in terms of lesion location and in degree of motor impairment. As discussed above, it is likely that differences between patients will mean that some patients will respond to a given stimulation approach, whereas others will not. However, only limited attention has been paid to these intersubject differences. One study in patients from 1–88 weeks post-stroke investigated the effects of rTMS on patients with cortical and subcortical strokes and found that 10Hz rTMS to the ispilesional M1 improved motor function in patients with subcortical stroke but not those with cortical strokes, in 10/13 of whom it slightly decreased motor performance (Ameli et al., 2009). The reasons for these differences are not clear, but this finding highlights the need to stratify patients in order to maximize the chances of positive out-comes, necessitating an increase in the number of patients recruited for any given clinical trial.

10.3.6 SAFETY OF TRANSCRANIAL STIMULATION APPROACHES

All interventions that increase cortical excitability, whether pharmacological or transcranial stimulation approaches, have the potential to induce seizures. This is of particular relevance in stroke patients, who have a reduced seizure threshold. The risk of inducing a seizure with TMS in an individual patient (or healthy volunteer) is related to patient factors such as medications, prior personal history of seizures and family history of epilepsy, and to TMS factors including intensity, rate, and duration of the stimulation. Full safety guidelines for the use of rTMS, including its use in clinical trials, were developed by a consensus group of TMS experts and were published in 2009, and we encourage the interested reader to refer to these for further details (Rossi et al., 2009). This document reported that since the previous set of guidelines in 1998, only nine possible seizures in healthy subjects had been reported in the literature as a result of TMS. Six of these occurred in subjects taking drugs known to reduce seizure threshold or who were sleep deprived (which also decreases seizure threshold), and three of the cases may represent non-epileptic events (Rossi et al., 2009). Too few stroke patients have had rTMS to accurately assess seizure risk in this population.

In addition to seizure risk, TMS is absolutely contraindicated in patients with metallic hardware in close contact to the discharging coil, as TMS may induce malfunction of the device. Metal elsewhere in the head or neck is a relative contraindication and the inclusion of the patient in the study should be discussed with a TMS expert (Rossi et al., 2009).

10.4 NOVEL THERAPEUTIC APPROACHES

There are a number of potential therapeutic approaches that have shown promise in preclinical animal studies and are currently undergoing evaluation in humans. We concentrate on four of the most promising here, but many others have been suggested for which the rationale is perhaps less clear, including acupuncture and music therapy (see Langhorne, Bernhardt, & Kwakkel, 2011, for a review).

10.4.1 DIRECT CORTICAL STIMULATION

Direct cortical stimulation was initially investigated when patients with epidural stimulators implanted over the ipsilesional M1 for pain relief post-stroke reported improved motor function of the stroke-affected upper limb. A handful of small pilot studies investigating the potential of direct epidural stimulation of the hand area of the motor cortex coupled with simultaneous rehabilitative therapy showed promising results (Brown, Lutsep, Cramer, & Weinand, 2003; Huang et al., 2008; Levy et al., 2008).

A full scale, prospective, single-blind randomized clinical trial (the EVEREST trial) compared the safety and efficacy of targeted epidural stimulation in conjunction with intensive task-oriented rehabilitation compared with rehabilitation alone (Harvey et al., 2009). A stimulator was implanted over the ipsilesional motor cortex and was programmed to provide 250 μs electrical pulses at 50Hz at 50% of a threshold intensity that induced observable movements during physiotherapy. Ninety-one patients were recruited to the treatment arm and 55 to the control arm, but the study did not meet its primary efficiency endpoint at 4-week follow-up, with approximately 30% improvement in function seen in both the treatment and control groups (http://www.medscape.com/viewarticle/569229). While these results are disappointing, they should be treated with some caution. The inclusion criteria for the study were very broad, including patients who had had more than one stroke and patients with either cortical or subcortical strokes, and who were more than 4 months from stroke. The efficacy of direct cortical stimulation may well differ between patients with cortical and subcortical lesions, as has been demonstrated for rTMS (Ameli et al., 2009) and with time from stroke (Gerloff et al., 2006; Lotze et al., 2006), and therefore subgroup analysis is needed to define whether cortical stimulation may be a potentially useful adjunct therapy in some subgroups.

10.4.2 ROBOTIC THERAPY/ NEUROPROSTHETICS

Robotic therapy offers another alternative adjunctive approach. At its simplest, a robot in the context of stroke rehabilitation is a mechanical device that can move parts of the patient's body. Often they are able to provide feedback about the patients' performance, and some robots are additionally able to constrain unwanted motor activity in order to optimize a movement pattern. The rationale for most robotic therapy is that it provides a way for the patient to experience intensive, repetitive, "good" movements of a paretic limb, rather than falling into bad movement habits or into learned non-use. The complexity of a motor task can be controlled more precisely with robotics than with other conventional approaches, making optimization of motor training for an individual patient easier. The idea is that robot-based programs will help to reinforce these positive movement patterns so that patients will be more likely to execute them in activities of daily living. Other advantages of a robotic system are that detailed measures of performance can be taken, and that therapy can usually be provided within a highly motivating context, such as a computer game.

A variety of such robots have been designed and many are commercially available (Loureiro, Harwin, Nagai, &

Johnson, 2011). These vary widely in complexity, ranging from a simple computer-assisted joystick (Volpe et al., 1999) to a complex exoskeleton, providing 3-D assisted movement of the entire upper limb (Staubli, Nef, Klamroth-Marganska, & Riener, 2009). Although these devices are technically extremely impressive, the challenge is to establish that they are effective and feasible in the clinical setting (Brochard, Robertson, Medee, & Remy-Neris, 2010). Some proof-of-principle studies are encouraging. For example, with the MIT-MANUS robot, the patient moves a robotically controlled joystick to play video games. The robot is able to assist and correct the patient's movements interactively. Repeated training with this device resulted in improvements in motor performance that were retained at follow-up and even 3 years later (Volpe et al., 1999; Ferraro et al., 2003; Fasoli et al., 2004;). However, this same device was recently tested in a large multicenter randomized controlled study, the first of a robotic intervention (Lo et al., 2010). The study compared robot therapy with non-robot therapy of a similar intensity and with usual care. Results showed that although the robot therapy was significantly more effective than usual care, it did not differ from the intensive non-robot-based approach. Therefore, the key to successful outcomes was the intensity of the therapy rather than the nature of its delivery.

Sufficient numbers of randomized trials of robot-based approaches have now been conducted to allow for systematic review, though many of these trials include relatively small patient numbers. A Cochrane review of 11 randomized trials of robot-assisted upper limb training found good evidence for improvements in arm motor strength and function but little evidence that this transferred to activities of daily living (Mehrholz, Platz, Kugler, & Pohl, 2008). A Cochrane review of 17 trials of robotic-assisted gait training devices found that such training improved patients' chances of becoming independent in walking but did not have significant effects on walking velocity or capacity (Mehrholz, Werner, Kugler, & Pohl, 2007). In both these systematic reviews, there was wide variation between trials, and more work needs to be done to establish the optimal frequency, duration, and timing of these interventions. A further systematic review concluded that the absence of significant effects may in part reflect limitations of outcome measures that do not adequately assess the kinematics of recovered movements (Kwakkel, Kollen, & Krebs, 2008).

10.4.3 STEM CELL THERAPY

Stem cells have the ability to divide and differentiate into multiple different cell types, depending on the environmental milieu in which they are placed. Stem cells derived from an embryonic human teratocarcinoma (hNT), fetal porcine cells, and autologous bone marrow-derived mesenchymal stem cells (MSCs) have all shown promise in preclinical trials and have been tested in early Phase I and Phase II clinical trials (Bliss, Andres, & Steinberg, 2009). Although there remain safety concerns about tumor formation following injection of exogenous stem cells into the brain (Seminatore et al., 2010), two proof-of-principle studies investigated the effects of injecting exogenous hNT-derived neuronal cells (LBS neurons) into patients with chronic stroke (Kondziolka et al., 2000; Kondziolka et al., 2005). Neither study demonstrated any cell-related serologic or imaging-defined effects in the 6 months after treatment compared with baseline. Similarly, transplantation of MSCs did not result in any cell-related adverse effects in the 12 months post-injection (Bang, Lee, Lee, & Lee, 2005). However, injection of fetal porcine cells led to seizure development or worsening of motor deficits in 2/5 patients treated (Savitz et al., 2005) and the trial was terminated.

Injection of hNT cells into the striatum led to a small improvement in function in chronic patients compared with baseline (Kondziolka et al., 2000; Kondziolka et al., 2005), although only a trend toward improvement was noted when compared with the placebo-treated group (Kondziolka et al., 2005). A study of 30 acute stroke patients treated with either MSCs (n = 5) or a placebo injection demonstrated significantly greater function in the treated group than placebo at 12 months (Bang et al., 2005). A follow-up study investigated the effects of MSC injection in acute patients at 5 years post-treatment and showed no increased mortality or morbidity with stem cell treatment compared with the placebo-treated group. A modest improvement in outcome was also noted (Lee et al., 2011). A recent unblinded study in patients 1 month or more post-stroke also demonstrated a substantial and sustained improvement in motor function after MSC injection (Honmou et al., 2011).

A number of questions remain about how to optimize stem cell treatment in humans, including selecting the optimal window for therapy, patient selection, the route of cell delivery, and injected cell type (Bliss et al., 2009; Lindvall & Kokaia, 2011). At the time of writing there are a number of ongoing clinical trials, which it is to be hoped will address at least some of these questions.

10.4.4 GROWTH FACTORS

Growth factors are a diverse group of naturally occurring cytokines that are defined by their biological actions of stimulating cell growth, division, and differentiation. A large number of growth factors have neuronal effects, and levels naturally increase in the weeks after a stroke (Carmichael, 2003). The role of a number of exogenous growth factors has therefore been examined to aid recovery after stroke. A variety of growth factors have shown promise in preclinical studies (see Cramer, 2008, for a review), of which a few have gone into early stage proof-of-principle studies in humans.

One candidate growth factor is erythropoietin (EPO), a glycoprotein produced in the kidney known to cross the blood-brain barrier (Jelkmann, 1992; Brines et al., 2000). In a trial of 40 patients with hyperacute stroke (<8 hours), EPO was found to improve functional outcome at 30 days compared with a placebo-treated control group (Ehrenreich et al., 2002). However, a subsequent study in 522 patients treated within 6 hours of symptom onset showed no beneficial effect of EPO compared to placebo, and an increased death rate in patients also receiving thrombolysis, although the mechanism for this increase is unclear (Ehrenreich et al., 2009).

Another growth hormone that has been studied as a potential therapeutic adjunct is granulocyte–colony stimulating factor (G-CSF). G-CSF is a glycoprotein that has long been used to stimulate white blood cell production to address neutropenia and, more recently, G-CSF has been found to cross the blood-brain barrier and to affect neurons, reducing cell death and promoting neurogenesis (Schäbitz & Schneider, 2007). A recent placebo-controlled double-blind randomized control trial demonstrated the safety and tolerability of G-CSF in chronic patients (>4 months post stroke) but showed no additional improvement in hand function in the group treated with subcutaneous G-CSF daily for 10 days compared with placebo (Flöel et al., 2011). It should be noted, however, that the study was not powered as an efficacy study, and further large-scale studies are therefore warranted.

10.5 CONCLUSIONS

The possibility of augmenting recovery outcomes through supplementary interventions is an attractive one. Here we have reviewed several putative adjunct therapies for the recovery of motor function post-stroke. A number of pharmacological agents and transcranial stimulation approaches, as well as more invasive procedures such as stem cell therapy, have been shown to be effective in small proof-of-principle studies. However, quantifying the benefits of the majority of these therapies is difficult due to a lack of large-scale, adequately controlled clinical trial data from which to draw conclusions.

Stroke is a highly heterogeneous disease and the effects of therapy are likely dependent on many factors discussed here, such as time since stroke, lesion location and size, and degree of functional recovery, as well as many other factors such as genetic influences and age of the patient. For many of the adjunct therapies discussed, large-scale studies with adequate placebo controls and blinding are underway, and these will be invaluable to determine the efficacy of these treatments. In addition, detailed proof-of-principle studies to determine the optimal parameters for treatment on a patient-by-patient basis are also necessary if we are to take full advantage of the significant promise offered by adjunctive therapies in stroke recovery.

REFERENCES

Ackerley, S. J., Stinear, C. M., Barber, P. A., & Byblow, W. D. (2010). Combining theta burst stimulation with training after subcortical stroke. *Stroke, 41*, 1568–1572.

Acler, M., Fiaschi, A., & Manganotti, P. (2009). Long-term levodopa administration in chronic stroke patients. A clinical and neuro-physiologic single-blind placebo-controlled cross-over pilot study. *Restorative Neurology and Neuroscience, 27*, 277–283.

Acler, M., Robol, E., Fiaschi, A., & Manganotti, P. (2009). A double blind placebo RCT to investigate the effects of serotonergic modulation on brain excitability and motor recovery in stroke patients. *Journal of Neurology, 256*, 1152–1158.

Ameli, M., Grefkes, C., Kemper, F., Riegg, F., Rehme, A., Karbe, H., et al. (2009). Differential effects of high-frequency repetitive transcranial magnetic stimulation over ipsilesional primary motor cortex in cortical and subcortical middle cerebral artery stroke. *Annals of Neurology, 66*, 298–309.

Bang, O. Y., Lee, J., Lee, P., & Lee, G. (2005). Autologous mesenchymal stem cell transplantation in stroke patients. *Annals of Neurology, 57*, 874–882.

Berthier, M., Pujol, J., Gironell, A., Kulisevsky, J., Deus, J., Hinojosa, J., et al. (2003). Beneficial effect of donepezil on sensorimotor function after stroke. *American Journal of Physical Medicine & Rehabilitation, 82*, 725–729.

Bliss, T. M., Andres, R. H., & Steinberg, G. K. (2009). Optimizing the success of cell transplantation therapy for stroke. *Neurobiology of Disease, 37*, 275–283.

Brines, M. L., Ghezzi, P., Keenan, S., Agnello, D., de Lanerolle, N. C., Cerami, C., et al. (2000). Erythropoietin crosses the blood-brain barrier to protect against experimental brain injury. *Proceedings of the National Academy of Sciences of the United States of America, 97*, 10526–10531.

Brochard, S., Robertson, J., Medee, B., & Remy-Neris, O. (2010). What's new in new technologies for upper extremity rehabilitation? *Current Opinion in Neurology, 23*, 683–687.

Brown, J. A., Lutsep, H., Cramer, S. C., & Weinand, M. (2003). Motor cortex stimulation for enhancement of recovery after stroke: case report. *Neurological Research, 25(8)*, 815–818.

Bütefisch, C. M., Davis, B. C., Sawaki, L., Waldvogel, D., Classen, J., Kopylev, L., et al. (2002). Modulation of use-dependent plasticity by d-amphetamine. *Annals of Neurology, 51*, 59–68.

Bütefisch, C. M., Kleiser, R., Körber, B., Müller, K., Wittsack, H. J., Hömberg, V., et al. (2005). Recruitment of contralesional motor cortex in stroke patients with recovery of hand function. *Neurology, 64*, 1067–1069.

Bütefisch, C. M., Netz, J., Wessling, M., Seitz, R. J., & Hömberg, V. (2003). Remote changes in cortical excitability after stroke. *Brain, 126*, 470–481.

Carmichael, S. T. (2003). Gene expression changes after focal stroke, traumatic brain and spinal cord injuries. *Current Opinion in Neurology, 16*, 699–704.

Chang, W. H., Kim, Y., Bang, O. Y., Kim, S. T., Park, Y. H., & Lee, P. K. (2010). Long-term effects of rTMS on motor recovery in patients after subacute stroke. *Journal of Rehabilitative Medicine, 42*, 758–764.

Chollet, F., DiPiero, V., Wise, R., Brooks, D., Dolan, R. J., & Frackowiak, R. (1991). The functional anatomy of motor recovery after stroke in humans: a study with positron emission tomography. *Annals of Neurology, 29*, 63–71.

Chollet, F., Tardy, J., Albucher, J. F., Thalamas, C., Berard, E., Lamy, C., et al. (2011). Fluoxetine for motor recovery after acute ischaemic stroke (FLAME): a randomised placebo-controlled trial. *Lancet Neurology, 10*, 123–130.

Classen, J., & Stefan, K. (2008). Changes in TMS measures induced by repetitive TMS. In E. Wassermann, C. Epstein, U. Ziemann, V. Walsh, T. Paus, & S. Lisanby (Eds.), *The Oxford handbook of transcranial stimulation*. Oxford: Oxford University Press.

Cramer, S. C. (2008). Repairing the human brain after stroke. II. Restorative therapies. *Annals of Neurology, 63*, 549–560.

Crisostomo, E. A., Duncan, P. W., Propst, M., Dawson, D. V., & Davis, J. N. (1988). Evidence that amphetamine with physical therapy promotes recovery of motor function in stroke patients. *Annals of Neurology, 23*, 94–97.

Dafotakis, M., Grefkes, C., Eickhoff, S. B., Karbe, H., Fink, G. R., & Nowak, D. (2008). Effects of rTMS on grip force control following subcortical stroke. *Experimental Neurology, 211*, 407–412.

Dam, M., Tonin, P., De Boni, A., Pizzolato, G., Casson, S., Ermani, M., et al. (1996). Effects of fluoxetine and maprotiline on functional recovery in poststroke hemiplegic patients undergoing rehabilitation therapy. *Stroke, 27*, 1211–1214.

Ehrenreich, H., Hasselblatt, M., Dembowski, C., Cepek, L., Lewczuk, P., Stiefel, M., et al. (2002). Erythropoietin therapy for acute stroke is both safe and beneficial. *Molecular Medicine, 8*, 495–505.

Ehrenreich, H., Weissenborn, K., Prange, H., Schneider, D., Weimar, C., Wartenberg, K., et al. (2009). Recombinant human erythropoietin in the treatment of acute ischemic stroke. *Stroke, 40*, e647–e656.

Emara, T. H., Moustafa, R. R., Elnahas, N. M., Elganzoury, A. M., Abdo, T. A., Mohamed, S. A., et al. (2010). Repetitive transcranial magnetic stimulation at 1Hz and 5Hz produces sustained improvement in motor function and disability after ischaemic stroke. *European Journal of Neurology, 17*, 1203–1209.

Endres, M., Engelhardt, B., J., Koistinaho, J., Lindvall, O., Meairs, S., Mohr, J., et al. (2008). Improving outcome after stroke: overcoming the translational roadblock. *Cerebrovascular Journal, 25*, 268–278.

Fasoli, S. E., Krebs, H. I., Stein, J., Frontera, W. R., Hughes, R., & Hogan, N. (2004). Robotic therapy for chronic motor impairments after stroke: Follow-up results. *Archives of Physical Medicine Rehabilitation, 85*, 1106–1111.

Feeney, D. M., Gonzalez, A., & Law, W. A. (1982). Amphetamine, haloperidol, and experience interact to affect rate of recovery after motor cortex injury. *Science, 217*, 855–857.

Ferraro, M., Palazzolo, J. J., Krol, J., Krebs, H. I., Hogan, N., & Volpe, B. T. (2003). Robot-aided sensorimotor arm training improves outcome in patients with chronic stroke. *Neurology, 61*, 1604–1607.

Fitzgerald, P. B., Fountain, S., & Daskalakis, Z. J. (2006). A comprehensive review of the effects of rTMS on motor cortical excitability and inhibition. *Clinical Neurophysiology, 117*, 2584–2596.

Flöel, A., Breitenstein, C., Hummel, F., Celnik, P., Gingert, C., Sawaki, L., et al. (2005). Dopaminergic influences on formation of a motor memory. *Annals of Neurology, 58*, 121–130.

Flöel, A., Hummel, F., Breitenstein, C., Knecht, S., & Cohen, L. G. (2005). Dopaminergic effects on encoding of a motor memory in chronic stroke. *Neurology, 65*, 472–474.

Flöel, A., Warnecke, T., Duning, T., Lating, Y., Uhlenbrock, J., Schneider, A., et al. (2011). Granulocyte-colony stimulating factor (G-CSF) in stroke patients with concomitant vascular disease—a randomized controlled trial. *PloS One, 6*, e19767.

Fregni, F., Boggio, P., Mansur, C., Wagner, T., Ferreira, M., Lima, M., et al. (2005). Transcranial direct current stimulation of the unaffected hemisphere in stroke patients. *Neuroreport, 16*, 1551–1555.

Fregni, F., Boggio, P. S., Valle, A. C., Rocha, R. R., Duarte, J., Ferreira, M. J., et al. (2006). A sham-controlled trial of a 5-day course of repetitive transcranial magnetic stimulation of the unaffected hemisphere in stroke patients. *Stroke, 37*, 2115–2122.

Froc, D. J., Chapman, C. A., Trepel, C., & Racine, R. J. (2000). Long-term depression and depotentiation in the sensorimotor cortex of the freely moving rat. *Journal of Neuroscience, 20*, 438–445.

Gabathuler, R. (2009). Approaches to transport therapeutic drugs across the blood–brain barrier to treat brain diseases. *Neurobiology of Disease, 37*, 48–57.

Gandiga, P. C., Hummel, F. C., & Cohen, L. G. (2006). Transcranial DC stimulation (tDCS): A tool for double-blind sham-controlled clinical studies in brain stimulation. *Clinical Neurophysiology, 117*, 845–850.

Gerloff, C., Bushara, K., Sailer, A., Wassermann, E. M., Chen, R., Matsuoka, T., et al. (2006). Multimodal imaging of brain reorganization in motor areas of the contralesional hemisphere of well recovered patients after capsular stroke. *Brain, 129*, 791–808.

Goldstein, L. (2009). Amphetamine Trials and Tribulations. *Stroke, 40*, S133–S135.

Greenwald, M. K., Schuster, C. R., Johanson, C. E., & Jewell, J. (1998). Automated measurement of motor activity in human subjects: effects of repeated testing and d-amphetamine. *Pharmacology, Biochemistry, and Behavior, 59*, 59–65.

Harvey, R. L., Winstein, C. J., & Everest Trial Group. (2009). Design for the Everest randomized trial of cortical stimulation and rehabilitation for arm function following stroke. *Neurorehabilitation and Neural Repair, 23*, 32–44.

Honmou, O., Houkin, K., Matsunaga, T., Niitsu, Y., Ishiai, S., Onodera, R., et al. (2011). Intravenous administration of auto serum-expanded autologous mesenchymal stem cells in stroke. *Brain, 134*, 1790–1807.

Huang, M., Harvey, R. L., Stoykov, M., Ruland, S., Weinand, M., Lowry, D., et al. (2008). Cortical stimulation for upper limb recovery following ischemic stroke: A small phase II pilot study of a fully implanted stimulator. *Topics in Stroke Rehabilitation, 15*, 160–172.

Huang, Y. Z., Edwards, M. J., Rounis, E., Bhatia, K. P., & Rothwell, J. (2005). Theta burst stimulation of the human motor cortex. *Neuron, 45*, 201–206.

Hummel, F., Celnik, P., Giraux, P., Floel, A., Wu, W.-H., Gerloff, C., et al. (2005). Effects of non-invasive cortical stimulation on skilled motor function in chronic stroke. *Brain, 128*, 490–499.

Hummel, F. C., Voller, B., Celnik, P., Floel, A., Giraux, P., Gerloff, C., et al. (2006). Effects of brain polarization on reaction times and pinch force in chronic stroke. *Biology & Medicine Central Neuroscience, 7*, 73.

Jelkmann, W. (1992). Erythropoietin: structure, control of production, and function. *Physiological reviews, 72*, 449–489.

Johansen-Berg, H., Rushworth, M. F., Bogdanovic, M. D., Kischka, U., Wimalaratna, S., & Matthews, P. M. (2002). The role of ipsilateral premotor cortex in hand movement after stroke. *Proceedings of the National Academy of Sciences of the United States of America, 99*, 14518–14523.

Khedr, E., Abdel-Fadeil, M., Farghali, A., & Qaid, M. (2009). Role of 1 and 3 Hz repetitive transcranial magnetic stimulation on motor function recovery after acute ischaemic stroke. *European Journal of Neurology, 16*, 1323–1330.

Khedr, E. M., Ahmed, M. A., Fathy, N., & Rothwellt, J. C. (2005). Therapeutic trial of repetitive transcranial magnetic stimulation after acute ischemic stroke. *Neurology, 65*, 466–468.

Khedr, E. M., Etraby, A. E., Hemeda, M., Nasef, A. M., & Razek, A. A. (2010). Long-term effect of repetitive transcranial magnetic stimulation on motor function recovery after acute ischemic stroke. *Acta Neurologica Scandinavica, 121*, 30–37.

Kim, D. Y., Lim, J. Y., Kang, E. K., You, D. S., Oh, M. K., Oh, B. M., et al. (2010). Effect of transcranial direct current stimulation on motor recovery in patients with subacute stroke. *American Journal of Physical Medicine & Rehabilitation, 89*, 879–886.

Kim, Y., You, S. H., Ko, M., Park, J., Lee, K. H., Jang, S. H., et al. (2006). Repetitive transcranial magnetic stimulation-induced corticomotor excitability and associated motor skill acquisition in chronic stroke. *Stroke, 37*, 1471–1476.

Kondziolka, D., Steinberg, G. K., Wechsler, L., Meltzer, C. C., Elder, E., Gebel, J., et al. (2005). Neurotransplantation for patients with subcortical motor stroke: a phase 2 randomized trial. *Journal of Neurosurgery, 103*, 38–45.

Kondziolka, D., Wechsler, L., Goldstein, S., Meltzer, C., Thulborn, K. R., Gebel, J., et al. (2000). Transplantation of cultured human neuronal cells for patients with stroke. *Neurology, 55*, 565–569.

Kumari, V., Corr, P. J., Mulligan, O. F., Cotter, P. A., Checkley, S. A., & Gray, J. A. (1997). Effects of acute administration of d-amphetamine and haloperidol on procedural learning in man. *Psychopharmacology, 129*, 271–276.

Kwakkel, G., Kollen, B. J., & Krebs, H. I. (2008). Effects of robot-assisted therapy on upper limb recovery after stroke: a systematic review. *Neurorehabilitation and Neural Repair, 22*, 111–121.

Langhorne, P., Bernhardt, J., & Kwakkel, G. (2011). Stroke rehabilitation. *Lancet, 377*, 1693–1702.

Lee, J., Hong, J., Moon, G., Lee, P., Ahn, Y., Bang, O. Y., et al. (2011). A long-term follow-up study of intravenous autologous mesenchymal stem cell transplantation in patients with ischemic stroke. *Stem Cells, 28*, 1099–1106.

Levy, R., Ruland, S., Weinand, M., Lowry, D., Dafer, R., & Bakay, R. (2008). Cortical stimulation for the rehabilitation of patients with hemiparetic stroke: a multicenter feasibility study of safety and efficacy. *Journal of Neurosurgery, 108*, 707–714.

Liepert, J., Hamzei, F., & Weiler, C. (2000). Motor cortex disinhibition of the unaffected hemisphere after acute stroke. *Muscle Nerve, 23*, 1761–1763.

Liepert, J., Zittel, S., & Weiller, C. (2007). Improvement of dexterity by single session low-frequency repetitive transcranial magnetic stimulation over the contralesional motor cortex in acute stroke: a double-blind placebo-controlled crossover trial. *Restorative Neurology and Neuroscience, 25*, 461–465.

Lindenberg, R., Renga, V., Zhu, L., Nair, D., & Schlaug, G. (2010). Bihemispheric brain stimulation facilitates motor recovery in chronic stroke patients. *Neurology, 75*, 2176–2184.

Lindvall, O., & Kokaia, Z. (2011). Stem cell research in stroke: How far from the clinic? *Stroke, 42*, 2369–2375.

Lo, A. C., Guarino, P. D., Richards, L. G., Haselkorn, J. K., Wittenberg, G. F., Federman, D. G., et al. (2010). Robot-assisted therapy for long-term upper-limb impairment after stroke. *New England Journal of Medicine, 362*, 1772–1783.

Lokk, J., Roghani, R., & Delbari, A. (2011). Effect of methylphenidate and/or levodopa coupled with physiotherapy on functional and motor recovery after stroke—a randomized, double-blind, placebo-controlled trial. *Acta Neurologica Scandinavica, 123*, 266–273.

Lomarev, M. P., Kim, D. Y., Richardson, S. P., Voller, B., & Hallett, M. (2007). Safety study of high-frequency transcranial magnetic stimulation in patients with chronic stroke. *Clinical Neurophysiology, 118*, 2072–2075.

Lotze, M., Markert, J., Sauseng, P., Hoppe, J., Plewnia, C., & Gerloff, C. (2006). The role of multiple contralesional motor areas for complex hand movements after internal capsular lesion. *Journal of Neuroscience, 26*(22), 6096–6102.

Loureiro, R. C., Harwin, W. S., Nagai, K., & Johnson, M. (2011). Advances in upper limb stroke rehabilitation: a technology push. *Medicine, Biology & Engineering Computing* epub ahead of print.

Malcolm, M. P., Triggs, W. J., Light, K. E., Gonzalez Rothi, L. J., Wu, S., Reid, K., et al. (2007). Repetitive transcranial magnetic stimulation as an adjunct to constraint-induced therapy: an exploratory randomized controlled trial. *American Journal of Physical Medicine & Rehabilitation, 86*, 707–715.

Mansur, C., Fregni, F., Boggio, P. S., Riberto, M., Gallucci-Neto, J., Santos, C., et al. (2005). A sham stimulation-controlled trial of rTMS of the unaffected hemisphere in stroke patients. *Neurology, 64*, 1802–1804.

Marshall, R. S., Perera, G. M., Lazar, R. M., Krakauer, J. W., Constantine, R. C., & DeLaPaz, R. L. (2000). Evolution of cortical activation during recovery from corticospinal tract infarction. *Stroke, 31*, 656–661.

Martinsson, L., Hårdemark, H., & Eksborg, S. (2007). Amphetamines for improving recovery after stroke. *Cochrane Database of Systematic Reviews, 1*, CD002090.

Martinsson, L., & Wahlgren, N. G. (2003). Safety of dexamphetamine in acute ischemic stroke: a randomized, double-blind, controlled dose-escalation trial. *Stroke, 34*, 475–481.

Mehrholz, J., Platz, T., Kugler, J., & Pohl, M. (2008). Electromechanical and robot-assisted arm training for improving arm function and activities of daily living after stroke. *Cochrane Database of Systematic Reviews, 4*, CD006876.

Mehrholz, J., Werner, C., Kugler, J., & Pohl, M. (2007). Electromechanical-assisted training for walking after stroke. *Cochrane Database of Systematic Reviews, 4,* CD006185.

Meintzschel, F., & Ziemann, U. (2006). Modification of practice-dependent plasticity in human motor cortex by neuromodulators. *Cerebral Cortex, 16,* 1106–1115.

Murase, N., Duque, J., Mazzocchio, R., & Cohen, L. G. (2004). Influence of interhemispheric interactions on motor function in chronic stroke. *Annals of Neurology, 55,* 400–409.

Nadeau, S. E., Behrman, A. L., Davis, S. E., Reid, K., Wu, S. S., Stidham, B. S., et al. (2004). Donepezil as an adjuvant to constraint-induced therapy for upper-limb dysfunction after stroke: an exploratory randomized clinical trial. *Journal of Rehabilitation Research and Development, 41,* 525–534.

Nitsche, M., & Paulus, W. (2000). Excitability changes induced in the human motor cortex by weak transcranial direct current stimulation. *Journal of Physiology, 527,* 633–639.

Nowak, D., Grefkes, C., Dafotakis, M., Eickhoff, S., Küst, J., Karbe, H., et al. (2008). Effects of low-frequency repetitive transcranial magnetic stimulation of the contralesional primary motor cortex on movement kinematics and neural activity in subcortical stroke. *Archives of Neurology, 65,* 741–747.

Nowak, D., Grefkes, C., Ameli, M., & Fink G. (2009). Interhemispheric competition after stroke: brain stimulation to enhance recovery of function of the affected hand. *Neurorehabilitation and Neural Repair, 23,* 641–656.

Nudo, R. J., Milliken, G. W., Jenkins, W. M., & Merzenich, M. M. (1996). Use-dependent alterations of movement representations in primary motor cortex of adult squirrel monkeys. *Journal of Neuroscience, 16,* 785–807.

National Audit Office, UK Government (2005). *Reducing brain damage: Faster access to better stroke care.* Published online at http://www.nao.org.uk/publications/0506/reducing_brain_damage.aspx

Pariente, J., Loubinoux, I., Carel, C., Albucher, J. F., Leger, A., Manelfe, C., et al. (2001). Fluoxetine modulates motor performance and cerebral activation of patients recovering from stroke. *Annals of Neurology, 50,* 718–729.

Pascual-Leone, A., Valls-Sole, J., Wassermann, E. M., & Hallett, M. (1994). Responses to rapid-rate transcranial magnetic stimulation of the human motor cortex. *Brain, 117,* 847–858.

Rang, H., Dale, M., Ritter, J., & Flower, R. (2007). *Pharmacology* (6th ed.). Churchill Livingstone, Edinburgh, UK.

Rosser, N., Heuschmann, P., Wersching, H., Breitenstein, C., Knecht, S., & Flöel, A. (2008). Levodopa improves procedural motor learning in chronic stroke patients. *Archives of Physical Medicine & Rehabilitation, 89,* 1633–1641.

Rossi, S., Hallett, M., Rossini, P. M., Pascual-Leone, A., & Safety of TMS Consensus Group. (2009). Safety, ethical considerations, and application guidelines for the use of transcranial magnetic stimulation in clinical practice and research. *Clinical Neurophysiology, 120,* 2008–1039.

Savitz, S. I., Dinsmore, J., Wu, J., Henderson, G. V., Stieg, P., & Caplan, L. R. (2005). Neurotransplantation of fetal porcine cells in patients with basal ganglia infarcts: a preliminary safety and feasibility study. *Cerebrovascular Diseases, 20,* 101–107.

Sawaki, L., Boroojerdi, B., Kaelin-Lang, A., Burstein, A. H., Bütefisch, C. M., Kopylev, L., et al. (2002). Cholinergic influences on use-dependent plasticity. *Journal of Neurophysiology, 87,* 166–171.

Sawaki, L., Cohen, L. G., Classen, J., Davis, B. C., & Bütefisch, C. M. (2002). Enhancement of use-dependent plasticity by D-amphetamine. *Neurology, 59,* 1262–1264.

Schäbitz, W. R., & Schneider, A. (2007). New targets for established proteins: exploring G-CSF for the treatment of stroke. *Trends in Pharmacological Sciences, 28,* 157–161.

Scheidtmann, K., Fries, W., Müller, F., & Koenig, E. (2001). Effect of levodopa in combination with physiotherapy on functional motor recovery after stroke: a prospective, randomised, double-blind study. *Lancet, 358,* 787–790.

Schuster, C., Maunz, G., Lutz, K., Kischka, U., Sturzenegger, R., & Ettlin, T. (2011). Dexamphetamine improves upper extremity outcome during rehabilitation after stroke: A pilot randomized controlled trial. *Neurorehabilitation and Neural Repair, 25,* 749–755.

Seminatore, C., Polentes, J., Ellman, D., Kozubenko, N., Itier, V., Tine, S., et al. (2010). The postischemic environment differentially impacts teratoma or tumor formation after transplantation of human embryonic stem cell-derived neural progenitors. *Stroke, 41,* 153–159.

Soetens, E., Casaer, S., D'Hooge, R., & Hueting, J. E. (1995). Effect of amphetamine on long-term retention of verbal material. *Psychopharmacology, 119,* 155–162.

Sonde, L., & Lokk, J. (2007). Effects of amphetamine and/or l-dopa and physiotherapy after stroke? a blinded randomized study. *Acta Neurologica Scandinavica, 115,* 55–59.

Stagg, C., Bachtiar, V., O'Shea, J., Allman, C., Bosnell, R., Kischka, U., et al. (2011). Cortical activation changes underlying stimulation-induced behavioural gains in chronic stroke. *Brain,* (2012). Cortical activation changes underlying stimulation-induced behavioural gains in chronic stroke. *Brain,135,* 276–284.

Staubli, P., Nef, T., Klamroth-Marganska, V., & Riener, R. (2009). Effects of intensive arm training with the rehabilitation robot ARMin II in chronic stroke patients: four single-cases. *Journal of Neuroengineering & Rehabilitation, 6,* 46.

Takeuchi, N., Chuma, T., Matsuo, Y., Watanabe, I., & Ikoma, K. (2005). Repetitive transcranial magnetic stimulation of contralesional primary motor cortex improves hand function after stroke. *Stroke, 36,* 2681–2686.

Takeuchi, N., Tada, T., Toshima, M., Chuma, T., Matsuo, Y., & Ikoma, K. (2008). Inhibition of the unaffected motor cortex by 1 Hz repetitive transcranical magnetic stimulation enhances motor performance and training effect of the paretic hand in patients with chronic stroke. *Journal of Rehabilitative Medicine, 40,* 298–303.

Talelli, P., Greenwood, R. J., & Rothwell, J. C. (2007). Exploring theta burst stimulation as an intervention to improve motor recovery in chronic stroke. *Clinical Neurophysiology, 118,* 333–342.

Trepel, C., & Racine, R. (1998). Long-term potentiation in the neocortex of the adult, freely moving rat. *Cerebral cortex, 8,* 719–729.

Volpe, B. T., Krebs, H. I., Hogan, N., Edelsteinn, L., Diels, C. M., & Aisen, M. L. (1999). Robot training enhanced motor outcome in patients with stroke maintained over 3 years. *Neurology, 53,* 1874–1876.

Ward, N. S., Brown, M. M., Thompson, A. J., & Frackowiak, R. S. (2003a). Neural correlates of motor recovery after stroke: a longitudinal fMRI study. *Brain, 126,* 2476–2496.

Ward, N. S., Brown, M. M., Thompson, A. J., & Frackowiak, R. S. (2003b). Neural correlates of outcome after stroke: a cross-sectional fMRI study. *Brain, 126,* 1430–1448.

Ward, N. S., & Cohen, L. G. (2004). Mechanisms underlying recovery of motor function after stroke. *Archives of Neurology, 61,* 1844–1848.

Weiller, C., Chollet, F., Friston, C., Wise, R., & Frackowiak, R. (1992). Functional reorganization of the brain in recovery from striatocapsular infarction in man. *Annals of Neurology, 31,* 463–472.

Whyte, E., Lenze, E., Butters, M., Skidmore, E., Koenig, K., Dew, M., et al. (2008). An open-label pilot study of acetylcholinesterase inhibitors to promote functional recovery in elderly cognitively impaired stroke patients. *Cerebrovascular Diseases, 26,* 317–321.

Yozbatiran, N., Alonso-Alonso, M., See, J., Demirtas-Tatlidede, A., Luu, D., Motiwala, R. R., et al. (2009). Safety and behavioral effects of high-frequency repetitive transcranial magnetic stimulation in stroke. *Stroke, 40,* 309–312.

Ziemann, U., Paulus, W., Nitsche, M. A., Pascual-Leone, A., Byblow, W. D., Berardelli, A., et al. (2008). Consensus: Motor cortex plasticity protocols. *Brain Stimulation, 1,* 164–182.

Zittel, S., Weiller, C., & Liepert, J. (2008). Citalopram improves dexterity in chronic stroke patients. *Neurorehabilitation and Neural Repair, 22,* 311–314.

PART D | REHABILITATION OF COMMON FUNCTIONS

11 | MOVEMENT

CATHY STINEAR and ISOBEL J. HUBBARD

11.1 INTRODUCTION

The ability to live independently after stroke critically depends on the recovery of motor function (Schiemanck, Kwakkel, Post, Kappelle, & Prevo, 2006). About one-third of people diagnosed with stroke go home with minimal residual disability, but one-third to one-half must rely on others to manage their everyday activities (Schaechter, 2004). Motor rehabilitation is aimed at overcoming the impact of stroke on motor function. Stroke can cause a range of motor symptoms, including weakness, slowness, tremor, lack of coordination, and a loss of precision and dexterity, in isolation or combination (Pomeroy et al., 2011).

Currently, most studies investigating the neural mechanisms underlying improvements in motor function use functional magnetic resonance imaging (fMRI) and transcranial magnetic stimulation (TMS). Upper limb recovery receives more research attention, possibly because there are more technical challenges when applying TMS and fMRI to studying neural plasticity in the control of the lower limbs. There is also a bias toward studies investigating patients at the chronic stage of recovery, but this is beginning to change with more studies recruiting in the acute and subacute stages.

This chapter will review the behavioral effects and neural mechanisms of a selection of motor rehabilitation techniques. These techniques belong to the targeted/facilitated practice component of the learning-based rehabilitation model presented in Chapter 2. They have been selected based on the evidence for their effectiveness from systematic reviews and meta-analyses of the literature, and the extent to which they are used in clinical practice.

11.2 REPETITIVE TASK-SPECIFIC TRAINING

11.2.1 DESCRIPTION

Repetitive task-specific training (RTT) involves repeatedly practicing functional tasks that are relevant to activities of everyday living. This type of training combines elements of intensity and goal-directedness to promote motor learning, as detailed in Chapter 9.

11.2.2 BEHAVIORAL EFFECTS

While individual studies have shown some benefit of upper limb RTT, systematic reviews have found borderline (Langhorne, Coupar, & Pollock, 2009) or no evidence (French et al., 2007) for improved upper limb and hand function, and activities of daily living. There is stronger evidence for the benefits of RTT on lower limb function. Walking distance and speed, and sit-to-stand performance, are improved by RTT. However, there is no evidence that standing balance during reaching is improved by RTT (French et al., 2007; Langhorne et al., 2009). For the lower limb, mixed training appears to be more beneficial than training a single task in each session (French et al., 2007), in line with the principle of variation to promote motor learning (Chapter 9).

11.2.3 NEURAL MECHANISMS

The very few studies that have examined the neural effects of upper limb RTT have used neuroimaging to measure changes in cortical activity during paretic upper limb movement and are limited by small sample sizes. Jang et al. (2003) studied four chronic stroke patients who completed

4 weeks of RTT with the paretic upper limb. Grip strength and manual dexterity (measured with the Purdue pegboard) improved in all four patients. FMRI was used to measure cortical activity during finger tapping with the paretic hand, paced at 1 Hz. The authors found that in all patients, the balance of sensorimotor cortex activity across both hemispheres shifted toward greater activity in the ipsilesional hemisphere after the RTT intervention. Furthermore, this shift in sensorimotor cortex activity was related to improvements in manual dexterity. Similar results were reported by Askim et al. (2009), who studied 12 subacute stroke patients who received a comprehensive therapy package including early mobilization and task-specific training. These authors also report improved paretic hand function and an increase in ipsilesional sensorimotor cortical activity during self-paced finger tapping with the paretic hand, 3 months after stroke. They also observed bilateral increases in the activation of somatosensory association areas, indicating widespread reorganization in the sensorimotor network.

These studies indicate that RTT may improve upper limb function by promoting more normal patterns of motor cortex activity, presumably via use-dependent and/or learning-dependent plasticity mechanisms. However, the small sample sizes and lack of control groups means these studies can only provide weak, preliminary evidence.

Studies of RTT for the lower limb primarily test the neural effects of treadmill training, and have provided some preliminary evidence of neural plasticity at both cortical and subcortical levels of the motor network (Forrester, Wheaton, & Luft, 2008). An early study by Forrester et al. (2006) used TMS to measure corticomotor excitability before and after a single session of treadmill walking. Eight treadmill-naive chronic stroke patients were studied, and compared to three chronic stroke patients who had completed three months of progressive treadmill training. After a single session of treadmill walking, the excitability of the paretic quadriceps representation in the ipsilesional primary motor cortex (M1) was unchanged in the untrained patients, and tended to increase in the trained patients. This early study provided some proof-of-concept evidence that treadmill training may improve gait by promoting a cumulative increase of excitability in the ipsilesional motor cortex.

In a subsequent study, Yen et al. (2008) randomized 18 chronic stroke patients to receive either a 4-week general therapy program aimed at improving gait, or the same program with additional RTT for gait in the form of treadmill training. Walking speed improved in both groups of patients, with a greater increase in both walking speed and step length in the RTT group. TMS was used to measure corticomotor excitability of the paretic tibialis anterior and abductor hallucis muscle representations in the ipsilesional M1, before and after the 4-week program. The excitability of these represen-

tations increased to a greater extent in the RTT group than in the control group, probably due to use-dependent plasticity elicited by the treadmill training (Yen et al., 2008). A similar study conducted by Yang et al. (2010) also reported facilitation of the paretic abductor hallucis M1 representation after a 4-week program of general therapy plus treadmill training, compared to a general therapy program alone. This study of 18 chronic stroke patients found that those who completed additional RTT also experienced a greater reduction in lower limb impairment (Fugl-Meyer scale). Interestingly, these authors also report that the increases in corticomotor excitability tended to be greater in early-chronic patients (<6 months) than late-chronic patients (>12 months). This indicates that RTT for gait may elicit greater neural plasticity when delivered in the first few months of rehabilitation. While these results are promising, this study is limited by not having any outcome measures specifically related to gait.

A general limitation of studies using TMS is that they are largely confined to studying neural plasticity at the cortical level. One of the advantages of neuroimaging techniques is that they can detect changes in neural activity in other areas, such as the cerebellum and midbrain, which are known to play essential roles in walking. Luft et al. (2008) randomly assigned 71 chronic stroke patients to receive a 6-month program of either treadmill RTT or stretching. Walking speed and cardiovascular fitness increased to a greater extent in the RTT group than the control group. Fifteen RTT patients and 17 control patients also completed fMRI scans before and after the intervention. In this subset of patients, walking speed increased to a greater extent in the RTT group but only when tested on the treadmill rather than over ground. During scanning, patients actively extended their paretic knee, paced at 0.33 Hz. The authors report that activity in the posterior cerebellum and midbrain increased to a greater extent in the RTT group than the control group. The increase in cerebellar activity was related to the improvements observed in walking speed. This indicates that treadmill RTT may elicit use-dependent plasticity in key brain regions, such as the cerebellum, promoting better control of the paretic lower limb.

There is also evidence for a plastic response to treadmill RTT in sensorimotor cortex. Enzinger et al. (2009) used fMRI to study cortical activity during paretic foot movement, before and after treadmill RTT. Eighteen chronic stroke patients completed a 4-week intervention and exhibited improved walking speed and endurance. During scanning, patients were cued to perform active ankle dorsiflexion and plantar flexion at their self-selected comfortable pace, which was kept constant across scanning sessions. While there was no overall change in cortical activity during paretic ankle movement after training, the authors found that the extent of improvement in walking endurance was related to an increase in bilateral sensorimotor cortex activity during paretic ankle movement. While this study adds further support to the idea that treadmill RTT can promote neural plasticity in cortical representations, it is limited by a lack of control group.

11.2.4 SUMMARY

There is currently more evidence for the clinical benefits and neural mechanisms of RTT for the lower limb than upper limb. RTT is founded on well-accepted neuroscience principles (Chapter 9), emphasizing the need for repetition and task-orientation to promote neural plasticity; however, there are very few studies of the neural mechanisms of RTT in stroke patients. The few studies that have been conducted indicate that RTT facilitates activity in cortical and subcortical components of the ipsilesional motor network. Further work is needed to understand how to target RTT to suitable patients, with the optimal dose and timing, to promote neural plasticity and recovery of function.

11.3 CONSTRAINT-INDUCED MOVEMENT THERAPY

11.3.1 DESCRIPTION

Constraint-induced movement therapy (CIMT) involves restricting use of the nonparetic upper limb for most of the patient's waking hours, thereby forcing them to use the paretic upper limb, in combination with targeted massed practice prescribed by therapists using shaping techniques (Taub et al., 1993). Based on evidence from animal models of stroke, CIMT is aimed at overcoming learned non-use of the stroke-affected or paretic upper limb (Knapp, Taub, & Berman, 1958, 1963).

Traditionally, CIMT involves more than 3 hours per day of massed practice, where a therapist progressively shapes the patient's goal-directed movements toward the desired performance (Hakkennes & Keating, 2005). There are several modified versions of CIMT, including one that involves 3 hours or less of therapy per day (Hoare, Wasiak, Imms, & Carey, 2007); however, all CIMT is based on the principles of intensive practice of goal-directed tasks, with motivation and graded progression guided by the therapist, to promote motor learning. For the purposes of this chapter, the term CIMT will refer to all versions irrespective of modification.

11.3.2 BEHAVIORAL EFFECTS

Systematic reviews have found strong evidence for reduced upper limb impairment, improved upper limb function, and reduced disability when CIMT is employed with selected patients (Langhorne et al., 2009; Sirtori, Corbetta, Moja, & Gatti, 2009). However, there is conflicting evidence of the benefits of CIMT for hand function (Hakkennes & Keating, 2005; Langhorne et al., 2009), and a study of patients at the subacute stage of recovery found that CIMT is not superior to traditional therapy (Dromerick et al., 2009). CIMT is most likely to benefit patients who have at least 10 degrees active extension of the paretic wrist and/or fingers, with minimal pain or spasticity in the paretic upper limb, and who make limited use of this limb in everyday activities (Sirtori et al., 2009). Patients need residual voluntary movement of the distal paretic upper limb in order to engage in massed practice as part of CIMT.

11.3.3 NEURAL MECHANISMS

Constraint of the nonparetic upper limb is expected to reduce the excitability of contralesional M1 (e.g., Sawaki et al., 2008). This may reduce the suppression of ipsilesional M1 by contralesional M1, via transcallosal pathways. Massed practice with the paretic upper limb is expected to increase the excitability of the ipsilesional motor cortex and promote use-dependent plasticity. These combined effects are thought to promote more balanced excitability between the two hemispheres, which is related to more favorable outcomes (Talelli, Greenwood, & Rothwell, 2006). However, the few studies of the neural effects of CIMT are typically limited by small sample sizes and have produced mixed results.

Neurophysiological studies use TMS to assess the excitability of the corticomotor pathway in both hemispheres from M1 to the target muscles (see Chapter 10). Liepert et al. (2000) examined the effects of a 12-day CIMT intervention in 13 patients who had experienced stroke between 6 months and 17 years earlier. Use of the paretic upper limb was assessed with the Motor Activity Log, and TMS was used to measure corticomotor excitability and the size of the cortical representation of the abductor pollicis brevis muscle in each hemisphere. Patients used their paretic upper limb to a greater extent after the intervention, and there was a significant increase in the size of the abductor pollicis brevis representation in the ipsilesional M1. Furthermore, there was a significant decrease in the size of the abductor pollicis brevis representation in the contralesional M1, indicating an overall balancing and normalization of motor cortex maps. These results indicate that CIMT may benefit upper limb function by redressing the imbalance in corticomotor excitability commonly observed after stroke. However, the authors don't report whether there was a relationship between the neural effects and behavioral effects of CIMT, so a link can only be assumed. This study is also limited by its small sample size and lack of a control group.

In one of the larger studies conducted, Sawaki et al. (2008) randomly assigned 30 patients who had experienced stroke between 3 and 9 months earlier to either a treatment group, which received 14 days of CIMT, or a control group, which received usual and customary care. Patients in the CIMT group had a significant increase in paretic upper limb grip strength after treatment compared to the control group. The authors also used TMS to measure corticomotor excitability and the size of the cortical representation of the long finger extensors (extensor digitorum communis) before and after the intervention. There were no significant differences between the two groups in corticomotor excitability in either hemisphere, either before or after the treatment. Despite the observed increase in grip strength, this study did not detect any neural effects of CIMT. Similarly, Wittenberg et al. (2003) randomized 16 chronic stroke patients to receive 10 days of either CIMT or a less intense control therapy, and observed an increase in paretic upper limb use in the CIMT group. Both groups of patients exhibited a shift in the contralesional M1 map of the nonparetic extensor digitorum communis muscle detected with TMS, and a decrease in ipsilesional M1 activity during paretic hand movement detected with positron emission tomography (PET) scanning. There were no differences between the groups in these measures, and no clear evidence of an increase in ipsilesional excitability and/or a decrease in contralesional excitability that could support the observed behavioral effects.

Overall, neurophysiological studies provide little support for the idea that CIMT works by altering corticomotor excitability in one or both hemispheres, and it is unclear whether any observed effects are brought about by the constraint and/or massed practice components. Those studies showing modest effects are limited by small sample sizes (Liepert et al., 2000; Ro et al., 2006). The effects of CIMT on the excitability of intracortical interneurons within M1 have also been examined, but no consistent results have been reported (Wittenberg et al., 2003; Liepert, Hamzei, & Weiller, 2004; Liepert, 2006).

Neuroimaging studies have used fMRI to evaluate cortical activity before and after CIMT. However, many are limited by studying only two to six patients, and not having a control group (Levy, Nichols, Schmalbrock, Keller, & Chakeres, 2001; Schaechter et al., 2002; Y.H. Kim, Park, Ko, Jang, & Lee, 2004; Szaflarski et al., 2006; Wu et al., 2010), which prevents meaningful interpretation and generalization of the results. Dong et al. (2006) studied eight patients who had experienced stroke at least 3 months earlier, and used fMRI to evaluate motor cortex activity before, after one week, and after two weeks of CIMT. During scanning, patients repeatedly performed a pinch task with their paretic hand, paced with an auditory metronome at 75% of their maximum speed. Visual feedback was provided with a target force level of 50% of the patient's maximum pinch force. Setting the speed and force of the pinch task relative to each patient's capabili-

ties is a strength of this experimental design. Overall, the authors found a decrease in the blood oxygen level dependent (BOLD) signal of the contralesional M1 and dorsal premotor cortex during pinch task performance with the paretic hand, and this was related to improved paretic upper limb function after 2 weeks of CIMT. This result supports the idea that constraint of the nonparetic upper limb reduces activity in the contralesional motor cortex. However, there was no consistent increase in ipsilesional motor cortex activity during or after CIMT.

Contrasting results have been reported by Lin et al. (2010), who observed an increase in contralesional M1 BOLD signal after 3 weeks of CIMT. These authors randomized 13 chronic stroke patients, with 5 in the treatment group and 8 in the control group. While the inclusion of a control group is a strength of this study, the small number of patients in each group is a limitation. During scanning, patients repeatedly flexed and extended their fingers, paced with an auditory metronome at 0.67 Hz. The patients who completed 3 weeks of CIMT experienced a decrease in upper limb impairment and an increase in the use of their paretic upper limb compared to the control group. Imaging results showed that activation of cortical motor areas increased in both hemispheres after CIMT, particularly in the contralesional M1 during movement of either hand. There was no consistent increase in ipsilesional motor cortex activity after CIMT, in line with the findings of Dong et al. (2006).

Neuroimaging can also be used to measure changes in the volume of grey matter within specific cortical areas, which is thought to reflect increases or decreases in the number of synaptic inputs to the cortex (Bandettini, 2009). Some evidence for structural plasticity in the motor cortex after CIMT has been reported by Gauthier et al. (2008). These authors randomly assigned 36 chronic stroke patients to receive either CIMT, or CIMT plus a "transfer package," for 10 consecutive days. The transfer package involves therapists spending an extra 30 minutes per day with each patient, discussing how the paretic upper limb is being used in everyday life and identifying ways to increase its use. This is designed to facilitate the transfer of improvements made in the laboratory to the real world. Both groups experienced similar improvements in motor abilities after the intervention, while the patients who also received the transfer package made significantly more use of the paretic upper limb in everyday activities. The authors also used MRI to measure the volume of grey matter in the sensorimotor cortex of both hemispheres, before and after the intervention. They found that the volume of grey matter in the contralesional sensorimotor cortex increased to a greater extent in the patients who received CIMT plus the transfer package compared to the patients who received CIMT alone. This study provides some evidence of structural plasticity in response to a version of CIMT.

Together, these studies provide contrasting results for the neural effects of CIMT on contralesional motor cortex and no consistent evidence of an effect on ipsilesional motor cortex. The interindividual variability in the neural response to CIMT might be due to differences in the extent of damage to key connections within the motor system, such as the corticospinal tract. Hamzei and colleagues have conducted two studies of the effects of CIMT in chronic stroke patients and observed two patterns of neural effects on the ipsilesional sensorimotor cortex (Hamzei, Liepert, Dettmers, Weiller, & Rijntjes, 2006; Hamzei, Dettmers, Rijntjes, & Weiller, 2008). A total of 14 patients were assessed with fMRI and TMS before and after each intervention. FMRI was used to assess the cortical response to passive flexion and extension of each wrist, while TMS was used to test the integrity of the descending corticomotor pathway from the ipsilesional M1 to the abductor pollicis muscle of the paretic upper limb. In both studies, motor ability and amount of use of the paretic upper limb improved after therapy. The authors also found that the ipsilesional BOLD signal response to passive movement of the paretic wrist increased after therapy in patients with damaged corticomotor pathways, and decreased after therapy in patients with intact corticomotor pathways. Similar results have been reported by Rijntjes et al. (2011), who studied 12 chronic patients before and after 14 days of CIMT. These authors also report that the ipsilesional sensorimotor cortex response to passive movement of the paretic wrist increased after CIMT in patients with a lesioned corticomotor pathway (assessed with TMS), and decreased after CIMT in patients with an intact corticomotor pathway. Interestingly, Rijntjes et al. also report that while paretic upper limb function improved after CIMT in all patients, only those with an intact corticomotor pathway retained these improvements at 6-month follow-up (Rijntjes et al., 2011). These findings highlight the importance of this key connection between the motor cortex and the spinal cord in recovery of motor function.

Increased ipsilesional BOLD signal after CIMT could reflect a beneficial facilitation of cortical excitability in the ipsilesional hemisphere, which may promote neural plasticity and reorganization in chronic patients with more damage to corticomotor pathways. In contrast, decreased ipsilesional BOLD signal could reflect a focusing of neural activity and enhanced efficiency in patients with less damage to corticomotor pathways. These studies illustrate the idea that neural plasticity can result in various patterns of cortical activity, depending on the underlying functional connectivity of key elements of the motor network. Interindividual variability in the patterns of reorganization in response to CIMT may help to explain the lack of clear and consistent evidence of the neural mechanisms responsible for the clinical effects of CIMT.

11.3.4 SUMMARY

There is strong evidence that CIMT benefits motor ability and use of the paretic upper limb in selected patients. There is limited evidence that these clinical benefits are the result of neural plasticity and reorganization within the cortical motor network. Neurophysiological and neuroimaging studies have found both increases and decreases in motor cortex activity in both the ipsilesional and contralesional hemisphere. There is no consistent evidence for the recovery of ipsilesional neural function and balanced motor cortex activity as a result of CIMT. The clinical benefits of CIMT might stem from compensatory reorganization in both hemispheres, and the pattern of this reorganization in each patient may depend on the residual functional connectivity in the motor network. Further studies with larger samples are needed to gain a better understanding of the neural mechanisms underlying the clinical benefits of CIMT.

11.4 MENTAL PRACTICE

11.4.1 DESCRIPTION

Mental practice involves repeatedly imagining performing a specific movement or task. In healthy adults, imagining and actually performing movement activate similar cortical and subcortical elements of the sensorimotor network, with similar timing (Stinear, 2010). Mental practice can, therefore, be used to rehearse movements and facilitate their movement representations (Sharma, Pomeroy, & Baron, 2006). This can be a useful adjunct technique, particularly when actual practice is limited by fatigue or paresis. Mental practice can be repetitive, progressive, and include variation, in keeping with the principles of motor learning.

11.4.2 BEHAVIORAL EFFECTS

Systematic reviews have found that mental practice has a positive effect on paretic upper limb function, though the number of studies is small (Langhorne et al., 2009; Nilsen, Gillen, & Gordon, 2010). There have been no systematic reviews of mental practice for recovery of gait function after stroke. However, the few studies completed with small samples show a positive effect (Dickstein, Dunsky, & Marcovitz, 2004; Dunsky, Dickstein, Ariav, Deutsch, & Marcovitz, 2006; Dunsky, Dickstein, Marcovitz, Levy, & Deutsch, 2008; J. S. Kim, Oh, Kim, & Choi, 2011). Studies of mental practice are highly heterogeneous in terms of the amount and type of practice given and the outcome measures used. Most studies combine physical and mental practice and use auditory instructions to guide the patient through the imagined movements. The potential importance of combining mental practice with physical practice is highlighted by a recent randomized controlled trial of 121 chronic stroke patients, which found no benefit of mental practice alone on paretic upper limb movement (Ietswaart et al., 2011).

11.4.3 NEURAL MECHANISMS

The few studies investigating the neural mechanisms of mental practice in stroke patients have used fMRI to evaluate cortical activity before and after the mental practice intervention. While some case studies report facilitated ipsilesional cortical activity after a mental practice training intervention (Butler & Page, 2006; Johnson-Frey, 2004), the number of cases is too small to draw any conclusions. In a study of 10 chronic stroke patients, Page et al. (2009) evaluated the effects of a combined physical and mental practice intervention on paretic upper limb impairment (Fugl-Meyer scale) and function (Action Research Arm test). Patients completed three one-on-one therapy sessions per week for 10 weeks. Each session involved 30 minutes of physical practice of an activity of daily living with their paretic upper limb, followed by 20 minutes of mental practice of the same activity. After the intervention, paretic upper limb impairment decreased and function increased, and patients reported some improvements in their performance of both the practiced and related activities of daily living. FMRI data were also collected before and after the 10-week intervention. Patients performed paretic wrist flexion and extension during scanning, and the authors report an increase in the BOLD signal recorded from the contralesional parietal cortex, and the premotor and primary motor cortex bilaterally, after the intervention. While this study is limited by the small sample size and lack of a control group completing physical practice alone, it provides some preliminary evidence that combined mental and physical practice may improve paretic upper limb function in chronic stroke patients. However, the neural mechanisms are unclear, as the intervention seemed to produce a generalized facilitation of motor cortex activity during paretic upper limb movement, which was not specific to the ipsilesional hemisphere.

11.4.4 SUMMARY

Current evidence indicates that adding mental practice to a physical rehabilitation program may be useful, though more work is needed to identify patients most likely to benefit and to establish optimal dose parameters. Further work is also required to understand the neural effects of mental practice and how these relate to the observed improvements in motor function after stroke. While actual and imagined movement produce similar patterns of neural activity at the time of performance, it is not yet known whether mental practice can produce a cumulative effect on sensorimotor network activity after stroke.

11.5 ELECTROSTIMULATION AND EMG BIOFEEDBACK

11.5.1 DESCRIPTION

Electrostimulation (ES), neuromuscular ES, or functional ES, involves the application of a transcutaneous electrical current to activate a muscle or muscle group, usually in combination with voluntary effort by the patient (Peckham & Knutson, 2005). Positioning the electrodes on the skin over a particular nerve or muscle can elicit a contraction in the targeted muscle fibers. The characteristics of the contraction can be controlled by setting the intensity and frequency of the electrical current, its duration, and the rate it ramps up and down at the beginning and end of the stimulation. Some ES devices have the option of multiple electrodes and others, such as neuroprosthetic ES devices, are fitted to the upper limb much like a splint or prosthesis, with an array of surface electrodes that can be individually positioned. These types of devices allow the underlying muscles to be activated in a specific pattern.

Some ES devices can also detect voluntary activation of a muscle and provide stimulation to assist once the voluntary activation reaches a specified threshold. This EMG-triggered ES provides the patient with feedback on whether or not they have activated the target muscle to the required level. Biofeedback can also be provided by using an electromyogram (EMG) to record voluntary activity in individual muscles with recording electrodes on the surface of the skin. EMG biofeedback can, therefore, provide both the patient and therapist with visual or auditory feedback about the timing and strength of voluntary muscle activity and can be used alone or in combination with electrostimulation.

The various types of ES and EMG biofeedback are typically used as adjuncts to training of specific movements or tasks, consistent with the principles of repetition, progression, and feedback in motor learning. The amount of assistance provided by the ES device can be progressively decreased as tasks are repeated, and feedback on the amount and timing of voluntary muscle activation can be provided.

11.5.2 BEHAVIORAL EFFECTS

Systematic reviews have found that electrostimulation (ES) can improve some aspects of upper limb motor function and standing balance after stroke, but that there are insufficient data to support its clinical use in stroke rehabilitation (Pomeroy, King, Pollock, Baily-Hallam, & Langhorne, 2006; Langhorne et al., 2009). In a review of EMG biofeedback, Woodford and Price (2007) found little evidence supporting its effectiveness in stroke rehabilitation. However, they note that there are no known adverse effects of EMG biofeedback, and some individual studies have shown positive effects on strength and gait quality. Therefore, this approach could be usefully added to standard therapy for selected patients.

11.5.3 NEURAL MECHANISMS

The few studies of the neural effects of ES are of the upper limb in patients at the chronic stage of stroke. The afferent input produced by contraction of the electrically stimulated muscles is expected to facilitate motor neuron excitability at cortical and subcortical levels of the central nervous system, and thereby increase voluntary motor output to the paretic limb. Von Lewinski et al. (2009) investigated the effects of upper limb EMG-triggered ES in nine patients who completed 8 weeks of daily stimulation during a task that required stacking and moving plastic cups. They measured paretic upper limb function (Box and Block test and Action Research Arm test) and observed improvements in patients with higher baseline scores, but no change in the scores of the most severely affected patients. Before and after the 8-week intervention, TMS was used to measure corticomotor excitability of the paretic extensor digitorum communis and abductor pollicis representations in ipsilesional M1. FMRI was also used to measure the BOLD signal in ipsilesional sensorimotor cortex during active opening–closing of the paretic hand and passive extension of the paretic wrist and fingers, before and after the intervention. The authors report that improvements in paretic upper limb function were related to an increase in ipsilesional sensorimotor cortex BOLD signal during passive movement of the paretic wrist and fingers. Furthermore, the excitability of neurons within ipsilesional M1 increased after the intervention, measured with TMS. These results may reflect facilitation of ipsilesional cortical activity in response to the intervention, driven by the additional afferent input produced by ES during attempted voluntary motor activity. Interestingly, these positive effects were predicted by the presence of motor evoked potentials in response to TMS, highlighting the importance of the corticomotor pathway in the recovery of motor function after stroke.

In a similar study, Page et al. (2010) studied the effects of neuroprosthetic ES in eight patients who had no voluntary extension of the paretic wrist or fingers. A neuroprosthetic ES device was tailored to each patient and programmed to assist wrist extension and hand opening during a range of everyday activities. Patients engaged in repetitive task-specific training (RTT) with assistance from the neuroprosthetic ES device for 30 minutes each weekday for 8 weeks. After the intervention, most patients exhibited a decrease in upper limb impairment (Fugl-Meyer scale) and an increase in the amount of paretic upper limb use (Motor Activity Log); however, no statistical analyses of these clinical outcomes are reported. FMRI was used to measure the cortical BOLD signal during repeated attempts to actively flex the paretic wrist, before and after the intervention. The authors report an increase in ipsilesional cortical activity after the intervention, particularly in the primary sensory and motor cortices, inferior parietal lobule, and middle frontal gyrus. This indicates that RTT with neuroprosthetic ES may facilitate ipsilesional cortical activity. However, the relationship between increased ipsilesional BOLD signal and decreased paretic upper limb impairment was not explored. The fMRI component of this study is also limited by the lenient threshold for cortical activation and the use of a wrist flexion task during scanning, rather than active wrist extension, which was assisted by ES during the intervention.

Taken together, these studies provide some evidence that ES may facilitate ipsilesional cortical activity and promote recovery of upper limb function (von Lewinski et al., 2009; Page, Harnish, Lamy, Eliassen, & Szaflarski, 2010). However, both studies are limited by small sample sizes and a lack of control groups. The reported effects may also be observable after 8 weeks of daily task-oriented therapy without EMG-triggered or neuroprosthetic ES.

In a randomized, sham-controlled trial, Kimberley et al. (2004) studied 16 patients who completed 60 hours of paretic wrist and finger extension training over a 3-week period. For the eight patients in the treatment group, extension was assisted by EMG-triggered ES for half of each session and produced by the ES device without voluntary effort for the other half of each session. Patients in the control group were provided with a similar device and told that the stimulation strength might be too low to produce muscle contraction. They received the same instructions as the treatment group, and actively extended their paretic wrist and fingers for half of each session and remained relaxed for the other half of each session. The authors report that paretic upper limb function (Box and Block test) and daily use (Motor Activity Log) improved in the treatment group, while paretic finger extension strength improved in both groups. FMRI was used to measure the BOLD signal during a tracking task with the paretic index finger, and the authors report an increase in BOLD signal intensity in the contralesional M1 in the treatment group only. This is in contrast to the previously described studies of ES showing an increase in ipsilesional M1 after an 8-week intervention in patients with greater initial impairment (von Lewinski et al., 2009; Page et al., 2010). However, Kimberley et al. (2004) did not directly compare the outcomes for the treatment and control groups, which limits the interpretation of their results.

Shin et al. (2008) randomly assigned 14 chronic patients to complete either daily sessions of repeated paretic wrist extension with EMG-triggered ES, or low-intensity physical activity, for 10 weeks. Paretic upper limb function improved to a greater extent in the treatment group than in the control group (Box and Block test). FMRI was also used to measure the BOLD signal in sensory and motor areas of each hemisphere, before and after the intervention. During scanning, patients performed a tracking task with their paretic index finger, and a laterality index was calculated reflecting the balance of sensory and motor cortex activity across both hemispheres during the tracking task. After the intervention, there was a greater shift toward ipsilesional primary sensorimotor cortex activity in the treatment group than in the control group. Furthermore, this shift in the balance of cortical activity was related to improvement in the Box and Block test score (Shin et al., 2008). These results indicate that the EMG-triggered ES intervention facilitated ipsilesional sensorimotor cortex activity, which may have supported the observed improvement in paretic upper limb function. The direct comparisons between the treatment and control groups are a strength of this study. However, the authors do not describe the physical activity undertaken by the control group, making it difficult to evaluate whether there was adequate control for the effects of wrist extension training alone. Therefore, the potential benefits of adding EMG-triggered ES to a wrist extension training protocol remain unclear.

The effects of EMG-triggered ES and finger tracking training have also been compared. Bhatt et al. (2007) randomly assigned 20 chronic stroke patients to one of three groups. The first group practiced voluntary extension of the paretic wrist and fingers with EMG-triggered ES. The second group practiced a tracking task, where they flexed and extended their index fingers to move a cursor on a computer screen along a target line. The third group practiced both tasks in each session, in a combined intervention. All patients completed ten 1-hour sessions over a 3-week period. Paretic upper limb function was measured with the Box and Block test and Jebsen Taylor test before and after the 3-week intervention. FMRI was also used to determine a laterality index of cortical activity during a paretic index finger tracking task. The authors found that paretic upper limb function improved in the patients who received EMG-triggered ES alone, and in combination with the finger tracking task. Overall, there were no consistent changes in the pattern of cortical activity during paretic index finger tracking in any of the three groups of patients. However, in the combined training group there was a positive relationship between improvement on the Box and Block text and a shift toward greater ipsilesional cortical activity, particularly in the primary somatosensory cortex and the supplementary motor area. This indicates that the combination of EMG-triggered ES and finger tracking training may more effectively facilitate ipsilesional cortical activity than either in isolation. However, the small sample size allocated across three interventions

means that this study lacks the statistical power needed to draw firm conclusions, and further investigation is needed. The effects of tracking tasks with visual feedback are further described in a subsequent section.

11.5.4   SUMMARY

There is some evidence that the potential benefits of ES for paretic upper limb function relate to facilitation of ipsilesional sensorimotor cortex activity. However, firm conclusions are precluded by the range of study designs and ES interventions used in the few studies reported thus far. Further studies with sufficient sample sizes and suitable control groups are needed to understand the mechanisms involved for both the upper and lower limbs and at the acute stage of recovery. While it is promising that ES may be useful for patients with moderate to severe upper limb impairment, preliminary results indicate that patients with severe damage to corticomotor pathways are unlikely to benefit.

11.6   ROBOT-ASSISTED TRAINING

11.6.1   DESCRIPTION

Robot-assisted training involves the use of a mechanical device to passively move, or assist voluntary movement of, the paretic limb. Some devices are designed to produce isolated movement around a single joint, such as wrist flexion-extension, and others are designed for multi-joint movements that simulate real-world tasks, such as reaching or walking. Robotic devices for the upper limb typically produce movement at the shoulder and elbow joints; wrist and finger movement is less common. Robotic devices for the lower limb include electromechanical gait trainers and exoskeleton robotics that provide guidance and assistance to paretic leg movements.

Robot-assisted therapy has a number of potential advantages. A large number of movement repetitions can be performed to increase the intensity of therapy, and the quality of movement can be controlled. In some circumstances, movement repetitions can be completed with minimal therapist supervision, or independently. The level of assistance provided by the device can be gradually reduced, enabling progression of therapy. Robot-assisted training, therefore, combines elements of intensity and grading to promote motor learning.

11.6.2   BEHAVIORAL EFFECTS

Systematic reviews report good evidence that robot-assisted training can improve strength and reduce impairment in the paretic upper limb of selected patients who are without cognitive or communication impairments, unstable cardiovascular conditions, or limited ranges of motion in paretic arm joints (Mehrholz, Platz, Kugler, & Pohl, 2008; Langhorne et al., 2009). However, there is currently no evidence that robot-assisted training improves hand function (Langhorne et al., 2009) or activities of daily living (Kwakkel, Kollen, & Krebs, 2008; Mehrholz et al., 2008).

There is limited evidence that robot-assisted training can improve lower limb function. Two systematic reviews (Mehrholz, Werner, Kugler, & Pohl, 2007; Hesse, Mehrholz, & Werner, 2008) indicate that electromechanical gait training in tandem with conventional physiotherapy is more effective in increasing walking capacity than conventional physiotherapy alone. However, Mehrholz et al. (2007) found that electromechanical gait training did not improve gait velocity and Hesse et al. (2008) found no benefit from exoskeleton robotics.

11.6.3 NEURAL MECHANISMS

There are very few studies of the neural effects of robot-assisted training in stroke patients. Takahashi et al. (2008) randomly assigned 13 chronic stroke patients to receive one of two robotic training protocols to improve paretic hand function. All patients practiced opening and closing their paretic hand in training sessions lasting around 90 minutes, on 15 consecutive weekdays. The robot actively assisted hand opening and closing in all sessions for seven patients. For the other six patients, the robot provided no assistance for the first 7.5 sessions, and then actively assisted hand movement in the remaining 7.5 sessions. Both groups of patients experienced a reduction in upper limb impairment and increase in upper limb function, and these gains were greater in the group that received active assistance from the robot throughout the training period. Neither group experienced an improvement in manual dexterity (9-hole peg test). The neural effects of training were assessed with fMRI by scanning patients before and after training. During scanning, patients opened and closed their paretic hand, and pronated and supinated their paretic forearm. This allowed the researchers to examine whether the neural effects of the robotic therapy were specific to the trained task (hand opening–closing) or generalized to other untrained tasks (pronation–supination). FMRI data from all patients were pooled for analysis and revealed a significant increase in the volume of ipsilesional sensorimotor cortex activated during paretic hand opening–closing, but not during forearm pronation–supination. This task-specific expansion of ipsilesional cortical activation was most likely due to use-dependent or learning-dependent plasticity in response to the robotic training. However, the lack of control group in this study makes it difficult to evaluate the importance of the robotic device compared to a similar therapy dose with no robotic assistance. The authors point out that at the midpoint of training, the patients who had received robotic assistance had already made greater improvements than those who trained with no assistance for the first 7.5 sessions. This indicates that the active assistance of the robotic device was beneficial. However, the neural effects of training with or without robotic assistance were not evaluated at the midpoint of training. Despite this limitation, this is a useful study demonstrating ipsilesional neural plasticity in response to robot-assisted training.

A subsequent study from the same laboratory evaluated the response of 23 chronic stroke patients to a similar active assistance training protocol (Riley et al., 2010). Overall, there was a significant reduction in impairment (Fugl-Meyer scale) and improvement in function (Action Research Arm test, Box and Blocks test) in the paretic upper limb after robot-assisted training. However, as there was no control group, it's impossible to know whether the robot assistance was necessary or whether these improvements could have been observed with other forms of physical therapy. Interestingly, this study also found that the reduction in upper limb impairment depended on the extent of damage to the corticospinal tract, evaluated with diffusion-weighted MRI. Patients with more damage to the corticospinal tract made the smallest improvements. This again highlights the importance of the corticospinal tract as a key pathway in the motor system.

11.6.4 SUMMARY

While there is good evidence that robot-assisted training can benefit upper limb impairment and function, there is almost no evidence of its neural effects. For the lower limb, evidence indicates that only electromechanical gait training in tandem with conventional physiotherapy can benefit walking capacity and that there is no benefit from exoskeleton robotics. Further studies are needed to more fully understand the mechanisms responsible for the observed clinical benefits, particularly in the lower limb. Some studies combine robot-assisted training with virtual reality environments (Merians, Tunik, Fluet, Qiu, & Adamovich, 2009), and the evidence for virtual reality in stroke rehabilitation is described below.

11.7 VIRTUAL REALITY AND VISUOMOTOR TRACKING TRAINING

11.7.1 DESCRIPTION

Virtual Reality (VR) training is an attractive option to therapists and researchers in this computer technology and Internet era. The term *virtual reality* refers to a computer-based technology that generates a novel environment. The degree of immersion experienced in the VR environment depends on the extent to which the VR technology isolates the patient from his or her physical surroundings. Greater immersion is typically achieved by providing a completely artificial visual environment via a set of goggles. VR usually provides real-time visual feedback of at least some of the patient's movements. Auditory and text feedback can also provide the patient with information about many aspects of their performance, such as the number of times they have attempted and/or completed a task, and their accuracy. While some laboratory-based VR environments include multiple cameras to capture the patients' movements, and robotics to provide proprioceptive feedback, some researchers are investigating and adapting non-immersive VR technologies, such as Nintendo Wii™ and Xbox Kinect™ games.

Virtual reality training is thought to promote motor learning by enhancing the repetitive performance of goal-oriented tasks with salient feedback and progressive increases in difficulty and intensity. VR training provides an opportunity to increase practiced movement repetitions while at the same time reducing therapist-to-patient treatment contact time. VR software can be designed to instruct patients on the task requirements, record the number of tasks or actions completed, monitor how well the tasks are achieved, and alter what's required of the patient on the basis of data from previous attempts. These augmented feedback functions make VR technology a potentially useful adjunct to stroke rehabilitation therapies.

Augmented visual feedback can also be used to improve control of paretic limb movements. A number of studies have investigated the effects of a visuomotor finger tracking intervention on paretic hand and arm function. During the intervention, patients flex and extend their index finger to control the position of a cursor on a computer screen. Their task is to move the cursor so that it traces a target line presented on the screen, which can take the form of a sine wave or square wave, for example. This visuomotor control task can also be performed with the paretic ankle or knee, but to date very little is known about the effects of tracking training on lower limb function after stroke. While tracking training doesn't take place in a novel virtual environment, it does provide real-time visual feedback of the patient's movements and is thought to promote motor learning through repetition, progression, and salient feedback.

11.7.2 BEHAVIORAL EFFECTS

VR training may improve motor abilities in stroke patients (Saposnik & Levin, 2011), but the evidence is biased toward chronic stroke patients and upper limb interventions. In 2009, Lucca found that there was insufficient evidence to conclude that VR training was superior to conventional therapy, and noted the heterogeneity of VR interventions between studies (Lucca, 2009). In a more recent meta-analysis of 12 studies, Saposnik and Levin (2011) report that while only five had a randomized and controlled study design, they provided strong evidence of reduced upper

limb motor impairment after VR training when compared to placebo. Across the remaining seven observational studies, they found a 15% decrease in upper limb motor impairment and a 20% improvement in upper limb motor function (Saposnik & Levin, 2011). While the evidence in favor of upper limb VR training is accumulating, there is very little known about the potential benefits of lower limb VR training, or the benefits of adding VR training to a standard rehabilitation program. There are currently no reported systematic reviews or meta-analyses of tracking training; however, individual studies have shown some positive effects of index finger and ankle tracking training on upper limb function and gait, respectively.

11.7.3 NEURAL MECHANISMS

Very little is known about the neural effects of VR training or tracking training after stroke. In a preliminary study by Jang et al. (2005), 10 chronic stroke patients were randomly assigned to either a VR training group or a control group. The treatment group completed five daily VR training sessions per week for 4 weeks. Each session lasted an hour and used semi-immersive VR technology to train the patients in reaching, lifting, and grasping with their paretic upper limb. The training program was tailored to each patient by the treating therapist and included visual and text feedback. The control group did not participate in any therapy or training. After the intervention, the VR training group had less impairment (Fugl-Meyer scale), better function (Box and Block test), and greater use (Motor Activity Log) of the paretic upper limb than the control group. FMRI was also used to determine a laterality index of cortical activity during paretic elbow movement, before and after the intervention. The authors report that the balance of sensorimotor cortex activity shifted towards the ipsilesional hemisphere in the VR training group, but do not report any imaging data for the control group. It's therefore not clear whether the shift in laterality index was due to the VR training or whether it was related to the observed improvements in upper limb function. The effects of the VR training weren't compared to any other kind of training or therapy, also limiting the interpretation of these results. Further studies are needed to understand whether VR training has any unique neural effects compared to other rehabilitation techniques or no rehabilitation.

In an early study of finger tracking training, Carey et al. (2002) randomly assigned 10 chronic stroke patients to either tracking training with their paretic index finger or a control group that received no therapy or training. The intervention group completed 18–20 training sessions, each lasting up to an hour. Paretic upper limb function improved in the intervention group (Box and Block test) but not in the control group; however, the two groups were not directly compared. FMRI was also used to determine a laterality index of cortical activity during finger tracking, before and after the intervention. The authors report a shift toward greater activity in the ipsilesional primary sensory cortex after tracking training. When the control group crossed over to tracking training, their Box and Block scores also improved. Furthermore, when their post-training fMRI data were combined with the treatment group, it was found that the balance of M1 activity for the total trained group also shifted toward the ipsilesional side. This study indicates that tracking training with the paretic index finger can improve upper limb function and facilitate ipsilesional sensorimotor cortex activity during a visuomotor tracking task with the paretic hand. However, one of the limitations of this study is that the effect of the visual feedback provided by the tracking task wasn't separated from the effect of repeatedly moving the paretic index finger.

This was addressed in a subsequent study by the same authors, where they compared tracking training with performing the same movements without visual feedback (Carey et al., 2007). Twenty chronic stroke patients were randomly assigned to perform either tracking training with the paretic index finger, or repeated movement of the paretic index finger through its full active range without tracking a visual cue and without any feedback. After the 2-week intervention, index finger range of motion improved in the treatment group. Both groups had a similar improvement in Jebsen Taylor test score, while the Box and Block test score improved to a greater extent in the control group than the treatment group. On balance, there was no consistent evidence that tracking training had greater clinical benefits that performing similar movements without tracking and visual feedback. FMRI data collected before and after the intervention also produced mixed results, with no consistent effects on the intensity, extent, or lateralization of cortical activity after the intervention in either group. This study indicates that the visuomotor demands of tracking training may not translate into clinical or neurophysiological benefits over and above those produced by repetitive movement without specific visual feedback.

In an early case study of tracking training with the paretic ankle, Carey et al. (2004) found that self-reported lower limb function improved in a single chronic stroke patient after 16 sessions of ankle tracking training. M1 activity during paretic ankle tracking increased in both hemispheres after training; however, walking speed and ankle range of motion did not improve. A subsequent study by Cho et al. (Cho et al., 2007) randomly allocated 10 chronic stroke patients to complete either paretic knee tracking training or to a control group that received no therapy or training. The treatment group completed around 40 minutes of tracking training every weekday for 4 weeks. Walking speed increased in the treatment group, but not the control group; however, the groups were not directly compared. FMRI was used to calculate a laterality index of cortical activity during flexion and extension of the paretic knee, before and after the intervention period,

in all patients. The balance of cortical activity during voluntary paretic knee movement shifted toward the ipsilesional sensorimotor cortex in the treatment group but not the control group, although there was no direct comparison between the groups. While this study is limited by its small sample size, it does provide preliminary evidence that knee tracking training may improve gait function, possibly via facilitation of the paretic knee representations in ipsilesional sensorimotor cortex. However, as in the early finger tracking study by Carey et al. (2002), the lack of active control group means that the effect of the visuomotor tracking task wasn't separated from the effect of repetitive movement.

11.7.4 SUMMARY

Both VR and tracking training provide augmented feedback during visuomotor tasks. While the evidence for tracking training is inconclusive, there is growing evidence that VR training may be a useful adjunct to motor rehabilitation after stroke. The advantages of VR training include its capacity to increase the intensity of therapy and improve monitoring of practice and progress. However, further work is required to establish its efficacy, particularly for the lower limb. Further research is also required to investigate the neural mechanisms underlying any therapeutic benefits. While VR training is in its infancy from a clinical perspective, this intervention should remain on the research agenda, particularly as technological advances are likely to increase the availability of VR and its use in the home and workplace.

11.8   OTHER APPROACHES

This chapter has focused on movement interventions that are clinically proven and have a neuroscience basis. However, there are other rehabilitation techniques in clinical practice that as yet do not have the evidence to meet these criteria. For example, bilateral practice was not included because the one meta-analysis of this specific approach (Stewart, Cauraugh, & Summers, 2006) included a heterogeneous group of studies—some combined bilateral training with peripheral stimulation, others used bilateral training as a "priming" technique prior to therapy. This makes it very difficult to draw conclusions about the potential efficacy of this approach. A more recent review (Langhorne et al., 2009) concluded that there is currently no evidence that bilateral training is beneficial for arm or hand function after stroke.

11.9   CONCLUSIONS

The rehabilitation techniques described in this chapter are based on the neuroscience principles underpinning the learning-based rehabilitation model presented in Chapter 2, and the core principles of training discussed in Chapter 9. They all include elements of repetitive practice and the elements of goal-directed tasks, intensity, variation, and progression in different combinations. The therapeutic benefits of these techniques are being actively investigated, and more evidence has accumulated in favor of some techniques than others. The effects of these learning-based rehabilitation techniques on neural function are starting to be explored. While TMS and fMRI techniques have been used to shed light on the neural correlates of learning in healthy adults, their application to studies of recovery after stroke is more challenging. To date, most studies using these techniques to study neural plasticity in response to specific rehabilitation techniques have recruited small cohorts of patients at the chronic stage of recovery, and primarily focused on the paretic upper limb. Despite these limitations, the general theme emerging is that learning-based rehabilitation techniques can alter the neural control of movement of the paretic limbs, presumably via neural plasticity mechanisms. This plastic reorganization is not limited to a simple increase in ipsilesional motor cortex activity, and can produce widespread effects in the sensorimotor network in both hemispheres. The pattern of reorganization may depend, in part, on the residual connectivity within the sensorimotor network, and therefore be quite variable between patients. Interestingly, there is some evidence that patients with more severe damage to the corticospinal tract are less likely to benefit from CIMT, electrostimulation, and robot-assisted training. This could also be the case for other techniques, such as repetitive task-specific training, mental practice, and VR training. Future studies may need to stratify patients according to the residual functional connectivity between key nodes in the motor network, such as between M1 and the spinal cord. Stratification of larger cohorts is likely to produce a clearer understanding of which patients are most likely to benefit from a given rehabilitation technique, and the neural mechanisms underlying those benefits. This issue is discussed further in Chapter 17 of this book. In conclusion, future studies will need to be randomized and controlled, shift toward the subacute stage of recovery, and recruit larger cohorts of patients. This will develop our understanding of the neural mechanisms responsible for the clinical benefits of learning-based rehabilitation techniques, so that they can be selected and optimized for individual patients to promote the best possible motor outcomes.

REFERENCES

Askim, T., Indredavik, B., Vangberg, T., & Haberg, A. (2009). Motor network changes associated with successful motor skill relearning after acute ischemic stroke: a longitudinal functional magnetic resonance imaging study. *Neurorehabilitation and Neural Repair, 23*(3), 295–304.

Bandettini, P. A. (2009). What's new in neuroimaging methods? *Annals of the New York Academy of Science, 1156*, 260–293.

Bhatt, E., Nagpal, A., Greer, K. H., Grunewald, T. K., Steele, J. L., Wiemiller, J. W., et al. (2007). Effect of finger tracking combined with electrical stimulation on brain reorganization and hand function in subjects with stroke. *Experimental Brain Research, 182*(4), 435–447.

Butler, A .J., & Page, S. J. (2006). Mental practice with motor imagery: evidence for motor recovery and cortical reorganization after stroke. *Archives of Physical Medicine and Rehabilitation, 87*(12 Suppl 2), S2–S11.

Carey, J. R., Anderson, K. M., Kimberley, T. J., Lewis, S. M., Auerbach, E. J., & Ugurbil, K. (2004). fMRI analysis of ankle movement tracking training in subject with stroke. *Experimental Brain Research, 154*(3), 281–290.

Carey, J. R., Durfee, W. K., Bhatt, E., Nagpal, A., Weinstein, S. A., Anderson, K. M., et al. (2007). Comparison of finger tracking versus simple movement training via telerehabilitation to alter hand function and cortical reorganization after stroke. *Neurorehabilitation and Neural Repair, 21*(3), 216–232.

Carey, J. R., Kimberley, T. J., Lewis, S. M., Auerbach, E. J., Dorsey, L., Rundquist, P., et al. (2002). Analysis of fMRI and finger tracking training in subjects with chronic stroke. *Brain, 125*(Pt 4), 773–788.

Cho, S. H., Shin, H. K., Kwon, Y. H., Lee, M. Y., Lee, Y. H., Lee, C. H., et al. (2007). Cortical activation changes induced by visual biofeedback tracking training in chronic stroke patients. *NeuroRehabilitation, 22*(2), 77–84.

Dickstein, R., Dunsky, A., & Marcovitz, E. (2004). Motor imagery for gait rehabilitation in post-stroke hemiparesis. *Physical Therapy, 84*(12), 1167–1177.

Dong, Y., Dobkin, B. H., Cen, S. Y., Wu, A. D., & Winstein, C. J. (2006). Motor cortex activation during treatment may predict therapeutic gains in paretic hand function after stroke. *Stroke, 37*(6), 1552–1555.

Dromerick, A. W., Lang, C.E., Birkenmeier, R. L., Wagner, J. M., Miller, J. P., Videen, T. O., et al. (2009). Very early constraint-induced movement during stroke rehabilitation (VECTORS): A single-center RCT. *Neurology, 73*(3), 195–201.

Dunsky, A., Dickstein, R., Ariav, C., Deutsch, J., & Marcovitz, E. (2006). Motor imagery practice in gait rehabilitation of chronic post-stroke hemiparesis: four case studies. *International Journal of Rehabilitation Research, 29*(4), 351–356.

Dunsky, A., Dickstein, R., Marcovitz, E., Levy, S., & Deutsch, J. E. (2008). Home-based motor imagery training for gait rehabilitation of people with chronic poststroke hemiparesis. *Archives of Physical Medicine and Rehabilitation, 89*(8), 1580–1588.

Enzinger, C., Dawes, H., Johansen-Berg, H., Wade, D., Bogdanovic, M., Collett, J., et al. (2009). Brain activity changes associated with treadmill training after stroke. *Stroke, 40*(7), 2460–2467.

Forrester, L. W., Hanley, D. F., & Macko, R. F. (2006). Effects of treadmill exercise on transcranial magnetic stimulation-induced excitability to quadriceps after stroke. *Archives of Physical Medicine and Rehabilitation, 87*(2), 229–234.

Forrester, L. W., Wheaton, L.A., & Luft, A. R. (2008). Exercise-mediated locomotor recovery and lower-limb neuroplasticity after stroke. *Journal of Rehabilitation Research and Development, 45*(2), 205–220.

French, B., Thomas, L. H., Leathley, M. J., Sutton, C. J., McAdam, J., Forster, A., et al. (2007). Repetitive task training for improving functional ability after stroke. *Cochrane Database of Systematic Reviews* (4), CD006073.

Gauthier, L. V., Taub, E., Perkins, C., Ortmann, M., Mark, V. W., & Uswatte, G. (2008). Remodeling the brain: plastic structural brain changes produced by different motor therapies after stroke. *Stroke, 39*(5), 1520–1525.

Hakkennes, S., & Keating, J. L. (2005). Constraint-induced movement therapy following stroke: A systematic review of randomised controlled trials. *Australian Journal of Physiotherapy, 51*, 221–231.

Hamzei, F., Dettmers, C., Rijntjes, M., & Weiller, C. (2008). The effect of cortico-spinal tract damage on primary sensorimotor cortex activation after rehabilitation therapy. *Experimental Brain Research, 190*(3), 329–336.

Hamzei, F., Liepert, J., Dettmers, C., Weiller, C., & Rijntjes, M. (2006). Two different reorganization patterns after rehabilitative therapy: an exploratory study with fMRI and TMS. *NeuroImage, 31*(2), 710–720.

Hesse, S., Mehrholz, J., & Werner, C. (2008). Robotic-assisted upper and lower limb rehabilitation after stroke: walking and arm/hand function. *Deutsches Arzteblatt International, 105*(18), 330–336.

Hoare, B. J., Wasiak, J., Imms, C., & Carey, L. (2007). Constraint-induced movement therapy in the treatment of the upper limb in children with hemiplegic cerebral palsy. *Cochrane Database of Systematic Reviews* (2), CD004149.

Ietswaart, M., Johnston, M., Dijkerman, H. C., Joice, S., Scott, C. L., MacWalter, R. S., et al. (2011). Mental practice with motor imagery in stroke recovery: randomized controlled trial of efficacy. *Brain, 134*(Pt 5), 1373–1386.

Jang, S. H., Kim, Y. H., Cho, S. H., Lee, J. H., Park, J. W., & Kwon, Y. H. (2003). Cortical reorganization induced by task-oriented training in chronic hemiplegic stroke patients. *Neuroreport, 14*(1), 137–141.

Jang, S. H., You, S. H., Hallett, M., Cho, Y. W., Park, C. M., Cho, S. H., et al. (2005). Cortical reorganization and associated functional motor recovery after virtual reality in patients with chronic stroke: an experimenter-blind preliminary study. *Archives of Physical Medicine and Rehabilitation, 86*(11), 2218–2223.

Johnson-Frey, S. H. (2004). Stimulation through simulation? Motor imagery and functional reorganization in hemiplegic stroke patients. *Brain Cognition, 55*(2), 328–331.

Kim, J. S., Oh, D. W., Kim, S. Y., & Choi, J. D. (2011). Visual and kinesthetic locomotor imagery training integrated with auditory step rhythm for walking performance of patients with chronic stroke. *Clinical Rehabilitation, 25*(2), 134–145.

Kim, Y. H., Park, J. W., Ko, M. H., Jang, S. H., & Lee, P. K. (2004). Plastic changes of motor network after constraint-induced movement therapy. *Yonsei Medical Journal, 45*(2), 241–246.

Kimberley, T. J., Lewis, S. M., Auerbach, E. J., Dorsey, L. L., Lojovich, J. M., & Carey, J. R. (2004). Electrical stimulation driving functional improvements and cortical changes in subjects with stroke. *Experimental Brain Research, 154*(4), 450–460.

Knapp, H., Taub, E., & Berman, A. (1958). Effect of deafferentiation on a conditioned avoidance response. *Science, 128*, 842–843.

Knapp, H., Taub, E., & Berman, A. (1963). Movement in monkeys with deafferented forelimbs. *Experimental Neurology, 7*, 305–315.

Kwakkel, G., Kollen, B. J., & Krebs, H. I. (2008). Effects of robot-assisted therapy on upper limb recovery after stroke: a systematic review. *Neurorehabilitation and Neural Repair, 22*(2), 111–121.

Langhorne, P., Coupar, F., & Pollock, A. (2009). Motor recovery after stroke: a systematic review. *Lancet Neurology, 8*(8), 741–754.

Levy, C. E., Nichols, D. S., Schmalbrock, P. M., Keller, P., & Chakeres, D. W. (2001). Functional MRI evidence of cortical reorganization in upper-limb stroke hemiplegia treated with constraint-induced movement therapy. *American Journal of Physical Medicine and Rehabilitation, 80*(1), 4–12.

Liepert, J. (2006). Motor cortex excitability in stroke before and after constraint-induced movement therapy. *Cognitive and Behavioral Neurology, 19*(1), 41–47.

Liepert, J., Bauder, H., Wolfgang, H. R., Miltner, W. H., Taub, E., & Weiller, C. (2000). Treatment-induced cortical reorganization after stroke in humans. *Stroke, 31*(6), 1210–1216.

Liepert, J., Hamzei, F., & Weiller, C. (2004). Lesion-induced and training-induced brain reorganization. *Restorative Neurology and Neuroscience, 22*(3–5), 269–277.

Lin, K. C., Chung, H. Y., Wu, C. Y., Liu, H. L., Hsieh, Y. W., Chen, I. H., et al. (2010). Constraint-induced therapy versus control intervention in patients with stroke: a functional magnetic resonance imaging study. *American Journal of Physical Medicine and Rehabilitation, 89*(3), 177–185.

Lucca, L. F. (2009). Virtual reality and motor rehabilitation of the upper limb after stroke: a generation of progress? *Journal of Rehabilitative Medicine, 41*(12), 1003–1100.

Luft, A. R., Macko, R. F., Forrester, L. W., Villagra, F., Ivey, F., Sorkin, J. D., et al. (2008). Treadmill exercise activates subcortical neural networks and improves walking after stroke: a randomized controlled trial. *Stroke, 39*(12), 3341–3350.

Mehrholz, J., Platz, T., Kugler, J., & Pohl, M. (2008). Electromechanical and robot-assisted arm training for improving arm function and activities of daily living after stroke. *Cochrane Database of Systematic Reviews* (4), CD006876.

Mehrholz, J., Werner, C., Kugler, J., & Pohl, M. (2007). Electromechanical-assisted training for walking after stroke. *Cochrane Database of Systematic Reviews* (4), CD006185.

Merians, A. S., Tunik, E., Fluet, G. G., Qiu, Q., & Adamovich, S. V. (2009). Innovative approaches to the rehabilitation of upper extremity hemiparesis using virtual environments. *European Journal of Physical Rehabilitative Medicine, 45*(1), 123–133.

Nilsen, D. M., Gillen, G., & Gordon, A. M. (2010). Use of mental practice to improve upper-limb recovery after stroke: a systematic review. *American Journal of Occupational Therapy, 64*(5), 695–708.

Page, S. J., Harnish, S. M., Lamy, M., Eliassen, J. C., & Szaflarski, J. P. (2010). Affected arm use and cortical change in stroke patients exhibiting minimal hand movement. *Neurorehabilitation and Neural Repair, 24*(2), 195–203.

Page, S. J., Harnish, S. M., Lamy, M., Eliassen, J. C., & Szaflarski, J. P. (2010). Affected arm use and cortical change in stroke patients exhibiting minimal hand movement. *Neurorehabilitation and Neural Repair, 24*(2), 195–203.

Page, S. J., Szaflarski, J. P., Eliassen, J. C., Pan, H., & Cramer, S. C. (2009). Cortical plasticity following motor skill learning during mental practice in stroke. *Neurorehabilitation and Neural Repair, 23*(4), 382–388.

Peckham, P. H., & Knutson, J. S. (2005). Functional electrical stimulation for neuromuscular applications. *Annual Review of Biomedical Engineering, 7*, 327–360.

Pomeroy, V., Aglioti, S. M., Mark, V. W., McFarland, D., Stinear, C., Wolf, S. L., et al. (2011) Neurological principles and rehabilitation of action disorders: rehabilitation interventions. *Neurorehabilitation and Neural Repair, 25*(5 Suppl), 33S–43S.

Pomeroy, V. M., King, L. M., Pollock, A., Baily-Hallam, A., & Langhorne, P. (2006). Electrostimulation for promoting recovery of movement or functional ability after stroke. Systematic review and meta-analysis. *Stroke. 37*(7) 2441–2442.

Rijntjes, M., Hamzei, F., Glauche, V., Saur, D., & Weiller, C. (2011). Activation changes in sensorimotor cortex during improvement due to CIMT in chronic stroke. *Restorative Neurology and Neuroscience, 29*(5) 299–310.

Riley, J. D., Le, V., Der-Yeghiaian, L., See, J., Newton, J. M., Ward, N.S ., et al. (2010). Anatomy of stroke injury predicts gains from therapy. *Stroke, 42*(2), 421–426.

Ro, T., Noser, E., Boake, C., Johnson, R., Gaber, M., Speroni, A., et al. (2006). Functional reorganization and recovery after constraint-induced movement therapy in subacute stroke: case reports. *Neurocase, 12*(1), 50–60.

Saposnik, G., & Levin, M. (2011). Virtual reality in stroke rehabilitation: a meta-analysis and implications for clinicians. *Stroke, 42*(5), 1380–1386.

Sawaki, L., Butler, A. J., Leng, X., Wassenaar, P. A., Mohammad, Y. M., Blanton, S., et al. (2008). Constraint-induced movement therapy results in increased motor map area in subjects 3 to 9 months after stroke. *Neurorehabilitation and Neural Repair, 22*(5), 505–513.

Schaechter, J. D. (2004). Motor rehabilitation and brain plasticity after hemiparetic stroke. *Progress in Neurobiology, 73*(1), 61–72.

Schaechter, J. D., Kraft, E., Hilliard, T. S., Dijkhuizen, R. M., Benner, T., Finklestein, S. P., et al. (2002). Motor recovery and cortical reorganization after constraint-induced movement therapy in stroke patients: a preliminary study. *Neurorehabilitation and Neural Repair, 16*(4), 326–338.

Schiemanck, S. K., Kwakkel, G., Post, M. W., Kappelle, L. J., & Prevo, A. J. (2006). Predicting long-term independency in activities of daily living after middle cerebral artery stroke: does information from MRI have added predictive value compared with clinical information? *Stroke, 37*(4), 1050–1054.

Sharma, N., Pomeroy, V. M., & Baron, J. C. (2006). Motor imagery: a backdoor to the motor system after stroke? *Stroke, 37*(7), 1941–1952.

Shin, H. K., Cho, S. H., Jeon, H. S., Lee, Y. H., Song, J. C., Jang, S. H., et al. (2008). Cortical effect and functional recovery by the electromyography-triggered neuromuscular stimulation in chronic stroke patients. *Neuroscience Letters, 442*(3), 174–179.

Sirtori, V., Corbetta, D., Moja, L., & Gatti, R. (2009). Constraint-induced movement therapy for upper extremities in stroke patients. *Cochrane Database of Systematic Reviews* (4), CD004433.

Stewart, K. C., Cauraugh, J. H., & Summers, J. J. (2006). Bilateral movement training and stroke rehabilitation: a systematic review and meta-analysis. *Journal of Neurological Science, 244*(1–2), 89–95.

Stinear, C. M. (2010). Corticospinal facilitation during motor imagery. In A. Guillot & C. Collet (Eds.), *The neurophysiological foundations of mental and motor imagery* (pp. 47–61). Oxford: Oxford University Press.

Szaflarski, J. P., Page, S. J., Kissela, B. M., Lee, J. H., Levine, P., & Strakowski, S. M. (2006). Cortical reorganization following modified constraint-induced movement therapy: a study of 4 patients with chronic stroke. *Archives of Physical Medicine and Rehabilitation, 87*(8), 1052–1058.

Takahashi, C. D., Der-Yeghiaian, L., Le, V., Motiwala, R. R., & Cramer, S. C. (2008). Robot-based hand motor therapy after stroke. *Brain, 131*(Pt 2), 425–437.

Talelli, P., Greenwood, R. J., & Rothwell, J. C. (2006). Arm function after stroke: Neurophysiological correlates and recovery mechanisms assessed by transcranial magnetic stimulation. *Clinical Neurophysiology, 117*(8), 1641–1659.

Taub, E., Miller, N. E., Novack, T. A., Cook, E. W., 3rd, Fleming, W. C., Nepomuceno, C. S., et al. (1993). Technique to improve chronic motor deficit after stroke. *Archives of Physical Medicine and Rehabilitation, 74*(4), 347–354.

von Lewinski, F., Hofer, S., Kaus, J., Merboldt, K. D., Rothkegel, H., Schweizer, R., et al. (2009). Efficacy of EMG-triggered electrical arm stimulation in chronic hemiparetic stroke patients. *Restorative Neurology and Neuroscience, 27*(3), 189–197.

Wittenberg, G. F., Chen, R., Ishii, K., Bushara, K. O., Eckloff, S., Croarkin, E., et al. (2003). Constraint-induced therapy in stroke: magnetic-stimulation motor maps and cerebral activation. *Neurorehabilitation and Neural Repair, 17*(1), 48–57.

Woodford, H. J., & Price, C. I. M. (2007). EMG biofeedback for the recovery of motor function after stroke. *Cochrane Database of Systematic Reviews, 2*, CD004585.

Wu, C. Y., Hsieh, Y. W., Lin, K. C., Chuang, L. L., Chang, Y. F., Liu, H. L., et al. (2010). Brain reorganization after bilateral arm training and distributed constraint-induced therapy in stroke patients: a preliminary functional magnetic resonance imaging study. *Chang Gung Medical Journal, 33*(6), 628–638.

Yang, Y. R., Chen, I. H., Liao, K. K., Huang, C. C., & Wang, R. Y. (2010). Cortical reorganization induced by body weight-supported treadmill training in patients with hemiparesis of different stroke durations. *Archives of Physical Medicine and Rehabilitation, 91*(4), 513–518.

Yen, C. L., Wang, R. Y., Liao, K. K., Huang, C. C., & Yang, Y. R. (2008). Gait training induced change in corticomotor excitability in patients with chronic stroke. *Neurorehabilitation and Neural Repair, 22*(1), 22–30.

12 | TOUCH AND BODY SENSATIONS

LEEANNE M. CAREY

12.1 SOMATOSENSORY FUNCTION

Somatosensory function is the ability to interpret bodily sensation (Puce & Carey, 2010). It refers to the detection, discrimination, and recognition of body (*somato*) sensations. It includes submodalities of touch sensation, such as light touch (on the surface of the skin), vibration, firm pressure, and texture discrimination; proprioception, involving sensing the location and movement of body parts; temperature sensation, and pain (nociception). The experience of sensing often involves a more complex integration of somatosensory inputs (e.g., haptic recognition of objects) or somatosensory and emotional components (e.g., pain) and may be influenced by emotional and social contexts (e.g., perception of tickle) (Dunn, Carey, Morrison, & Sabata, 2010).

Somatosensations are important for perception and for action (Dijkerman & de Haan, 2007). Sensation for perception involves characterizing and localizing touch and pain, sensing the position of different parts of the body with respect to one another, recognition of objects through the sense of touch, and memory of those perceptions (Dijkerman & de Haan, 2007). Sensory perception is part of our conscious experience of who we are in our environment. We want to feel objects and where our arm is for its own sake, and to interact with other people and our environment. We need our sensation to make sense of our environment and make quick adjustments. It allows us to explore and interact with the world and others, to experience pleasure, and be alerted to danger. Senses are part of the way we learn and adapt. Sensation is also important for action. It provides feedback for most movements and particularly affects the quality of motor control, including pinch grip (Johansson & Westling, 1984); ability to sustain and adapt appropriate force without vision (Jeannerod, Michel, & Prablanc, 1984); object manipulation (Johansson, 1996); combining component parts of movement (Gentilucci, Toni, Daprati, & Gangitano, 1997); and adjustment to sensory conflict conditions, for example, rough surface (Wing, Flanagan, & Richardson, 1997).

12.2 SOMATOSENSORY LOSS AFTER STROKE

One in two people after a stroke experience loss in ability to feel everyday objects through touch or know where their limbs are in space (Carey, 1995; Sullivan & Hedman, 2008; Carey & Matyas, 2011). Frequency of somatosensory loss is reported to be 50% to 60% in studies using quantitative measures and in independent reviews (Carey, 1995; Kim & Choi-Kwon, 1996; Yekutiel, 2000; Winward, Halligan, & Wade, 2002; Connell, Lincoln, & Radford, 2008; Sullivan & Hedman, 2008; Tyson, Hanley, Chillala, Selley, & Tallis, 2008; Carey & Matyas, 2011). Loss is evident across a range of modalities, with impaired discriminative sensibility reported in 85% in the acute setting (Kim & Choi-Kwon, 1996) and in 67% in a subacute rehabilitation sample after unilateral stroke (Carey & Matyas, 2011). Impaired touch sensation is reported in approximately half of patients tested (Winward et al., 2002; Tyson et al., 2008; Carey & Matyas, 2011) and impaired proprioception in 27% to 52% (Winward et al., 2002; Tyson et al., 2008; Carey & Matyas, 2011), with variation likely due to a combination of measures used, body parts tested, and samples investigated (Carey & Matyas, 2011). A clinically significant proportion, approximately 20%, experience impairment in the ipsilesional "unaffected" hand in addition to the contralateral deficit (Kim & Choi-Kwon, 1996; Carey & Matyas, 2011).

Clinically, somatosensory loss may range from complete loss of sensation (anesthetic syndrome) to impaired discrimination of particular body sensations (Head & Holmes, 1911; Carey, 1995; Bowsher, Brooks, & Enevoldson, 2004). Typically, the body half contralateral to the lesion is affected, although the loss is not usually evenly distributed. Impairment of the hand ipsilateral to the lesion is also reported, but is usually relatively mild (Kim & Choi-Kwon, 1996; Carey & Matyas, 2011). Impairment can vary from selective involvement of one somatosensory modality, such as tactile discrimination or proprioception, to all somatosensory modalities depending on the site and extent of the lesion (Carey, 1995; Connell et al., 2008). Severity ranges from quite mild to very severe impairment, and this pattern may vary across modalities such as touch and proprioception (Carey & Matyas, 2011). Impairment of discriminative sensibility is the more characteristic clinical scenario (Bowsher, 1993; Carey, 1995; Kim & Choi-Kwon, 1996), and may involve one or more of the following: localization of tactile stimuli; two-point discrimination; texture discrimination; appreciation of size, shape, and form of objects; discrimination of limb position; and weight discrimination (Head & Holmes, 1911; Bowsher, 1993; Carey, 1995; Carey & Matyas, 2011). Hypersensitivity (non-noxious stimuli are perceived as irritating) may be experienced early after stroke or develop with time (Carey, 2006). Neuropathic pain, in which pain occurs spontaneously and responses to noxious and innocuous stimuli are pathologically amplified, is an expression of maladaptive plasticity triggered by lesions of the somatosensory system and may occur in some individuals (Costigan, Scholz, & Woolf, 2009). Task-specific focal hand dystonia, also considered to be associated with maladaptive plasticity, can develop with time following somatosensory lesions (Schabrun, Stinear, Byblow, & Ridding, 2009).

Somatosensory loss impairs the ability to explore the environment through touch and to execute everyday tasks such as grasping and manipulating objects. Loss of the ability to perceive sensations has a significant impact in its own right. In the words of a stroke survivor, "I may look alright but I feel all left … and half lost" (Lyons, 2010). In relation to its role for action, the affected limb may not be used spontaneously, despite adequate movement abilities. This may contribute to a learned non-use of the limb and further deterioration of motor function (Dannenbaum & Dykes, 1988). Motor control in the upper limb, in particular the ability to sustain an appropriate level of force during grasp without vision (Nowak, Hermsdörfer, & Topka, 2003), precision grip (Blennerhassett, Matyas, & Carey, 2007), object manipulation (Hermsdörfer, Hagl, Nowak, & Marquardt, 2003) and reacquisition of skilled movements (Kusoffsky, Wadell, & Nilsson, 1982; Floel & Cohen, 2006; Schaechter, Moore, Connell, Rosen, & Dijkhuizen, 2006) may be affected.

Somatosensory loss can also have an ongoing and negative impact on individuals in their daily lives. It contributes to inferior results in level of function and independence, mobility, activity performance, quality of life, length of rehabilitation, and discharge destination (Carey, 1995, 2006; Patel, Duncan, Lai, & Studenski, 2000; Han, Law-Gibson, & Reding, 2002; Sommerfeld & von Arbin, 2004; Sullivan & Hedman, 2008; Tyson et al., 2008). Patient groups with hemiparesis, hemihypesthesia, and/or hemianopia compared to hemiparesis alone show significantly poorer function (Han et al., 2002) and time to maximal recovery (Reding & Potes, 1988; Dromerick & Reding, 1995). Loss of sensation also negatively impacts personal safety and return to sexual and leisure activities (Carey, 1995; Sullivan & Hedman, 2008).

The high prevalence of tactile and proprioceptive discrimination impairments, and the impact of these impairments on daily activities and rehabilitation outcome, reinforces the importance of adequately detecting these impairments and addressing the functional consequences in rehabilitation. Yet, despite the high prevalence and negative impact, there are relatively few studies of sensory recovery. The neural changes that underpin somatosensory impairment and recovery after stroke remain relatively unexplored.

12.3 CENTRAL PROCESSING OF SOMATOSENSORY INFORMATION

The somatosensory system allows us to interpret sensory messages received from the body, and consists of sensory receptors located in the skin, tissues and joints, the nerve cell tracts in the body and spinal cord, and brain centers that process and modulate incoming sensory information (Puce & Carey, 2010). The major brain regions involved in processing somatosensory information and their roles are outlined below. These core regions are part of a more distributed network involved in conscious processing of somatosensory information that includes attention and vision networks, and both hemispheres.

Primary Somatosensory Cortex (SI): Somatosensory information is processed in SI, located posterior to the central sulcus in anterior parietal cortex. SI includes Brodmann Areas (BA) 3a, 3b, 1 and 2. BA2 is known to have more bilateral connections (Naito et al., 2005). SI is primarily involved in feature detection and remains somewhat modality-specific. For example, BA3b, BA1, and BA2 receive information from skin receptors regarding texture (Burton & Sinclair, 2000; Carey, Abbott, Egan, & Donnan, 2008), size, and shape (Bodegard et al., 2000; Savini et al., 2010), while knowledge of limb position has been associated with processing in BA3a (Moore et al., 2000) and BA2 (Naito et al., 2005). Task-relevant somatosensory information leads to selective facilitation within the SI and this modulation may be regulated, at least in part, by the prefrontal cortex (Staines, Graham, Black, & McIlroy, 2002). Higher-level processing also begins to take place in SI, for example with the coordination of tactile and proprioceptive information as may be required for object recognition. Information from SI projects to secondary sensory cortex (SII). SI also has connections with motor cortex and supplementary motor area (SMA), with sensory perception studies showing activation in these areas (Carey et al., 2008).

Secondary Somatosensory Cortex (SII): SII has a role in discrimination and recognition of somatosensory stimuli and is located in the parietal operculum (Eickhoff, Grefkes, Zilles, & Fink, 2007). Neurons have less modality specificity than those in SI, and respond to bilateral stimuli (Ruben et al., 2001). SII is implicated in texture discrimination and tactile object recognition (Murray & Mishkin, 1984), and is considered to be specialized for tactile learning (Kandel, Schwartz, & Jessell, 2000) and tactile working memory (Burton, Sinclair, Wingert, & Dierker, 2008). SII has reciprocal connections with SI (Gardner & Kandel, 2000) and connections from the thalamus to SII (Bear, Connors, & Paradiso, 2007; D. Y. Zhang et al., 2008). SII also has projections to motor regions such as premotor cortex (Disbrow, Litinas, Recanzone, Padberg, & Krubitzer, 2003). Supramarginal gyrus (SMG), adjacent to SII (Eickhoff, Schleicher, Zilles, & Amunts, 2006), is reported to have a role in conscious proprioceptive perception and processing of spatial stimuli (Loubinoux et al., 2001; Ben-Shabat, Pell, Brodtmann, Matyas, & Carey, 2008).

Thalamus: The thalamus has a role in gating of sensory information. Touch information from the periphery is transferred via the ventroposterior thalamus to contralateral SI and SII cortices (Gardner & Kandel, 2000). Thalamocortical connections are part of the prefrontal-thalamic inhibitory system that is involved with optimizing the detection of novel or hard to sense stimuli (Nicolelis, 2005). Projections to the posterior parietal cortex and insula also exist (Dijkerman & de Haan, 2007). Interhemispheric connections between bilateral thalami occur via the anterior cingulate (Raos & Bentivoglio, 1993). The thalamus has strong correlations with bilateral cerebral hemispheres based on functional resting state connectivity (D. Y. Zhang et al., 2008).

Insula: The insula has a major role in perceptual recognition and learning (Dijkerman & de Haan, 2007). It is an association area, particularly involved in interoceptive information processing and salience of sensory information (Dijkerman & de Haan, 2007).

Posterior Parietal Cortex (PPC): The posterior parietal cortex processes information for perception and for action. It receives projections from SI and SII, as well as from thalamic nuclei. In turn, it projects back to SII and premotor cortex (Kaas & Pons, 2006; Dijkerman & de Haan, 2007). The PPC contains multiple representations of space with scope for functional interactions between somatosensory and visual systems (Reed, 2007). The PPC is identified as a key node for integration of somatosensory information with other senses, particularly vision, and for multisensory integration to guide motor action (Dijkerman & de Haan, 2007).

Cerebellum: The cerebellum also has a role in processing of somatosensory information (Molinari, Filippini, & Leggio, 2002) in addition to its role in modulating motor output, cognition (Molinari et al., 2008), and adaptive motor skill learning (Thach, 1998; Seidler, 2010). Of interest, it is active during anticipation of somatosensory events (Tesche & Karhu, 2000) and is involved in comparison of temporal and spatial information for detection of sequences (Molinari et al., 2008; Wu, Nestrasil, Ashe, Tuite, & Bushara, 2010). Evidence from functional connectivity studies show that regions of the cerebellum are connected to the contralateral somatosensory cortical network (O'Reilly, Beckmann, Tomassini, Ramnani, & Johansen-Berg, 2010).

12.3.1 A MODEL OF SOMATOSENSORY PROCESSING

A model of somatosensory information processing has been proposed by Dijkerman et al. (Dijkerman & de Haan, 2007) that relates to the *purpose* of the information processing: sensation for *perception* and sensation for *action*. The model involves parallel and serial processing. Sensation for conscious perception and memory of that perception involves a processing stream from SI via SII to posterior insula (ventral stream). Sensation for action (guidance of movements) primarily involves SI, SII, and PPC (dorsal stream). The model also distinguishes between information processing about the body (where you are touched) and about external stimuli (e.g., object edges; Dijkerman & de Haan, 2007) A summary of the key regions involved, their interconnections, and primary purpose are depicted in Figure 12.1.

Processing of information increases in complexity from feature detection, primarily involving SI, to higher-order recognition involving SII, insula, and PPC (Dijkerman & de Haan, 2007). The first level of processing for perception and memory involves feature detection; in other words, information on the location and duration of a stimulus. It may also involve features such as spatial and nonspatial features of an object, and primarily involves processing in SI and thalamus. The next level involves recognition of the stimulus and occurs in SII, insula, and PPC. The focus is on body-centered or internal sensations. Processing of information for action also involves feature processing at the level of the thalamus and SI, and includes detection and direction of the stimulus with a focus on object-centered,

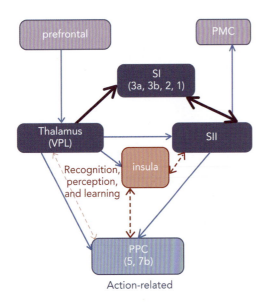

Figure 12.1 Summary of somatosensory information processing proposed by Dijkerman and deHann (2007). Core regions involved in processing for both perception and action are colored dark blue. Additional regions and connections involved in sensation for perception are in red, while regions related to processing for action are in light blue. Additional connected regions are in purple. SI = primary somatosensory cortex; SII = secondary somatosensory cortex; PPC = posterior parietal cortex; PMC = premotor cortex; 3a, 3b, 5, 7b refer to Brodmann areas; VPL = ventroposterior lateral area of the thalamus.

external stimulus. Information is then processed in PPC, which has reciprocal connections with the thalamus.

It is proposed that somatosensory processing for the guidance of action can be dissociated from the processing that leads to perception and memory (Dijkerman & de Haan, 2007). Tactile information processing in relation to external objects, versus the body itself, also appears to involve different regions. This has implication for networks involved, how they may be impacted following injury, and how they may be accessed and used in the process of recovery and rehabilitation. Thus, the importance of taking a network perspective in understanding brain function is highlighted.

12.3.2 KEY FEATURES OF CENTRAL PROCESSING OF SOMATOSENSORY INFORMATION

A few features of how somatosensory information is processed centrally are critical in understanding the nature of the somatosensory processing deficit experienced following stroke, and the potential for recovery and targeted rehabilitation, as outlined below.

Parallel and Serial Processing within the Somatosensory System: Somatosensory information is processed in the brain by a network of regions that feature modality-specific lines of communication, specific columnar organization, and submodality-specific neurons in SI and SII (Kaas, 1984; Mountcastle, 1997). This system supports a

high degree of specificity in information processing; for example, as required for topographical localization of a sensory stimulus. This serial line of information processing is complemented by parallel pathways (Kaas & Pons, 2006) that allow the opportunity for convergence of somatosensory information within the CNS (Mesulam, 1998). Parallel paths to the brain stem, thalamus, and cortex are functionally distinct but may partially substitute for each other (Kaas & Pons, 2006). For example, recent connectivity research has revealed 4 parallel networks involved in tactile exploration and discrimination of a series of parallelepipeds (Hartmann et al., 2008). This complexity provides a rich framework for neural plastic changes (Kaas & Pons, 2006) and has implications for stimulus-specific and transfer-enhanced modes of perceptual processing and learning.

Multiple and Multimodal Representations of Sensory Maps: There are several somatotopic representations of the body in sensory regions such as SI and SII (Shoham & Grinvald, 2001; Kaas & Pons, 2006; Eickhoff et al., 2007). In addition, specific brain regions and multisensory maps play a crucial role in sensorimotor information processing and integration (Driver & Noesselt, 2008; Friedel & van Hemmen, 2008). For example, in the superior colliculus the motor maps lie on top of the sensory input maps and are in spatial register, so that the sensory input can directly generate motor output (Friedel & van Hemmen, 2008). In multimodal maps, several sensory input modalities can merge so as to form a unified map of multisensory space, and multimodal neurons are responsive to sensory input from more than one modality. Matching of sensory map representations across modalities can show early influences in primary sensory areas (Driver & Noesselt, 2008). Involvement of multiple input modalities leads to an increase in firing rate and is a basic computational principle to improve input signal and thus object identification and localization (Becker, 1996). The transformation of sensory maps is dynamic and related to the goal of the task (Frey et al., 2011).

Interhemispheric Connections—Functional and Structural: There is evidence from neuroanatomical, neuroimaging, and electrophysiological studies of interhemispheric connections between SI–SI and SII–SII via the corpus callosum (Gardner & Martin, 2000; Fabri et al., 2005). The balance of activity between hemispheres and in relation to facilitation and inhibition is critical. For example, unilateral touch of fingers is associated, in addition to the well-known activation of the contralateral SI cortex, with deactivation of the ipsilateral SI cortex, suggested to be linked with transcallosal inhibition (Hlushchuk & Hari, 2006). Therapy may need to focus on removal of sources of inhibition across hemispheres and/or use of tasks and attention to prime the threshold for activation within the lesioned hemisphere.

Top-down and Bottom-up Influences on Information Processing: Thresholds in the somatosensory network may be influenced by the attention network and by multisensory processing of information. Sensory signals are buried in noise. Top-down influences can help to effectively find the relevant signal. Perceptual awareness occurs from an interaction between specialized sensory cortices and a higher-order frontoparietal attention network (Goldberg, Harel, & Malach, 2006; Boly et al., 2007) that has cortico-thalamic connections (Heidi Johansen-Berg et al., 2005). For example, the prefrontal-thalamic inhibitory system is involved with optimizing the detection of novel or hard to sense stimuli (Nicolelis, 2005). Attention operates across different sensory modalities to facilitate selection of relevant information and multisensory integration. Stimulus-driven, bottom-up mechanisms induced by cross-modal interactions can influence attention towards multisensory events (Talsma, Senkowski, Soto-Faraco, & Woldorff, 2010). There are strong links between sensory systems, in particular between touch and vision (Sathian, Zangaladze, Hoffman, & Grafton, 1997; Sathian, 2006). Viewing the body can modulate tactile receptive fields and is associated with enhancement in somatosensory perception (Haggard, Christakou, & Serino, 2007). In fact, visual cortical processing may be necessary for normal tactile perception (Zangaladze, Epstein, Grafton, & Sathian, 1999; Sathian, 2006).

12.4 NEURAL CORRELATES OF SENSORY RECOVERY AFTER STROKE

Relatively few studies have investigated the neural correlates of somatosensory recovery after stroke. A few neuroimaging studies have involved small samples (n ≤ 7), mostly of patients with sensory loss following thalamic lesions (Carey et al., 2002; Staines, Black, Graham, & McIlroy, 2002). These studies highlight relative sparing of activation in ipsilesional SI in those with mild impairment and return of activation in ipsilesional SI and bilateral SII with good recovery (Remy et al., 1999; Carey et al., 2002; Staines, Black et al., 2002; Rossini et al., 2007). With more severe impairment, reduced activation of ipsilesional SI was reported with preserved responsiveness of SII (Taskin et al., 2006) and distributed activation (Weder et al., 1994). More recently, patients with lesions primarily of the thalamus (n = 11) showed bilateral activation in secondary sensory areas, while those with lesions of SI and SII (n = 8) showed a more variable pattern with common deactivation in distributed regions at 1 month post-stroke (Carey et al., 2006; Carey et al., 2011). Baseline brain activity may also be important, based on evidence of selective hypoperfusion in ipsilesional SI at rest following thalamic lesions (Remy et al., 1999).

Disruption to interhemispheric activity has been demonstrated using magnetoencephalography. Following post-acute somatosensory deficit (n = 19), severe deficit was associated with absence of SI activity after affected-hand stimulation and a significant asymmetry in post-central spontaneous slow oscillatory activity toward the affected hemisphere (Castillo et al., 2008). Patients with moderate sensory loss showed asymmetry in their post-central MEG activity that was variable across subjects, but no atypical amplitudes in SI activation. Similarly, investigation of sensorimotor recovery (n = 17) has highlighted the role of interhemispheric differences in sensory hand areas, particularly in patients with subcortical lesions (Rossini et al., 2001).

Sites of brain activation have also been correlated with severity of impairment (Carey, Abbott et al., 2011). Touch discrimination of the affected hand was associated with activation in ipsilesional SI (adjacent to the SI hand area activated in age matched healthy controls), ipsilesional SII, contralesional thalamus, and in attention-related frontal and occipital regions in those with lesions of subcortical regions, primarily thalamus. The relationship with SI was inverse, such that those with better touch discrimination showed relatively reduced activity in the region surrounding the typically activated hand area of SI. It was argued that this may represent local inhibition, consistent with correlates of somatosensory processing in healthy subjects (Kastrup et al., 2008) and with evidence of task-relevant modulation of SI by the prefrontal cortex (Staines, Graham et al., 2002; Devor et al., 2007; Carey, Abbott, et al., 2011). By contrast, the subgroup of patients with SI and/or SII lesions did not show a common pattern of correlated activity, likely due to variation in lesion location. Contralesional thalamus was correlated with touch discrimination ability in the total group, highlighting that modulation of sensory inputs, rather than cortical representation alone, is important in sensory processing after stroke—a finding consistent with evidence from animal studies (Kaas, 1999; Jain, Qi, Collins, & Kaas, 2008).

These findings have implication for therapists. They suggest a role for local inhibition of ipsilesional SI and frontal attention regions in better processing of touch sensation following thalamic lesions. Top-down attentional modulation of bilateral SI may also be accessed via contralesional thalamus, irrespective of lesion location. Thus, interventional approaches that focus on training the ability to attentively discriminate sensory information, rather than stimulation-only approaches or bombardment, are recommended (Carey, Abbott, et al., 2011). The potential role of vision and multisensory processing in recovery is also highlighted. Lesion-specific mechanisms of brain adaption and different rehabilitative strategies to target specific brain regions are suggested.

Resting-state functional connectivity studies may also provide novel insight, especially in relation to the interhemispheric connectivity (see Chapter 4). In a pilot study we observed a relative lack of significant interhemispheric connectivity between homologous SI regions, when

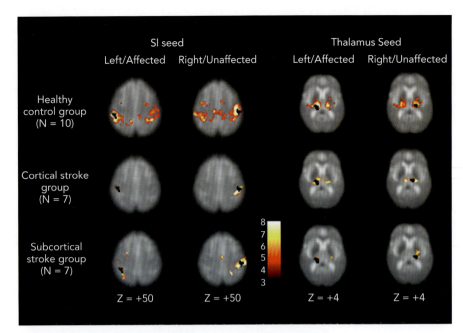

Figure 12.2 Functional connectivity maps with seed (black shape) placed in primary somatosensory cortex (SI) or thalamus of either hemisphere. Healthy controls showed extensive interhemispheric SI connections, which were absent for cortical (S/SII) and subcortical (thalamus) lesion groups (when seeded in either hemisphere). Interhemispheric thalamic connections were observed in healthy control and cortical groups, but were virtually absent in the subcortical group. Color scale indicates T scores for correlations. This figure is adapted from a figure presented by Bannister et al., 2010.

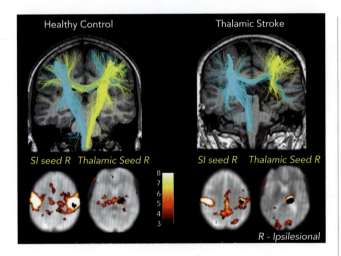

Figure 12.3 White matter structural (top) and resting state functional (bottom) connectivity maps for healthy control and patient with thalamic lesion. Note symmetrical pattern of probabilistic tractography results (top left) for healthy control when seeded in primary somatosensory cortex (SI) of each hemisphere (coronal projection). In contrast, following thalamic lesion there is a relative lack of interhemispheric SI and ipsilesional SI–thalamus fiber tract connections. Functional connections (seeded in the lesioned or right hemisphere, black shape) show a bilateral pattern for the healthy control for SI and thalamic seeds. The thalamic patient shows no connectivity to contralesional thalamus with thalamic seed but does show connections to contralesional SI and cingulate cortex when seeded in ipsilesional SI.

seeded in either the lesioned or nonlesioned hemisphere for patients with lesions of SI/SII (cortical) or thalamus (subcortical) (Bannister, Gavrilescu, Crewther, & Carey, 2010). Connectivity from the thalamic seeds was also lacking for the subcortical group and reduced for the cortical group. These observations contrasted those of age matched healthy controls who demonstrated robust interhemispheric connectivity (see Figure 12.2).

Changes in structural and functional connections in the somatosensory network may also be observed, as shown for a chronic stroke survivor with a right thalamic lesion who had been involved in sensory rehabilitation, as described by Carey et al. (Carey, Matyas, & Oke, 1993; Carey, Macdonnell, & Matyas, 2011; Figure 12.3). Despite a virtual lack of structural interhemispheric SI connections and ipsilesional SI–thalamus connections (0.2% in the patient compared to a mean of 6.24%, SD = 1.6%, in 6 healthy controls), we observed functional interhemispheric SI connections in this patient. There was, however, no interhemispheric thalamic functional connectivity. This finding highlights the importance of measuring functional and structural connectivity, and suggests the potential for significant changes in functional connectivity despite virtual lack of structural connectivity.

Changes in brain activation and resting state connectivity may also be observed following a perceptual learning approach to sensory rehabilitation. Figure 12.4 shows changes in brain activity in an individual before and after a 6-week period of SENSe discrimination training (Carey, Macdonnell et al., 2011) using a task-related somatosensory discrimination paradigm and resting state connectivity analysis.

12.5 TREATMENT PRINCIPLES AND STRATEGIES ARISING FROM NEUROSCIENCE

Review of the literature on perceptual learning and neural plasticity reveals core principles/conditions of learning that have potential for use in a rehabilitation setting. Three key principles arising from neuroscience and the evidence

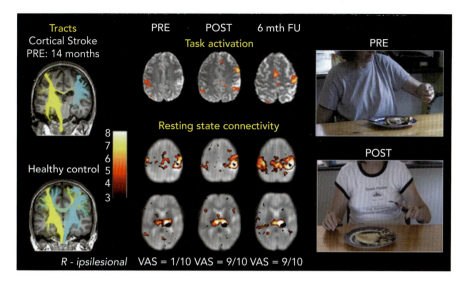

Figure 12.4 Probability fiber tracts of stroke survivor with primary somatosensory cortex (SI) lesion show a relative lack of interhemispheric SI connectivity and reduced connectivity from ipsilesional thalamus to SI. Task-related activation maps show activation in the contralesional hemisphere pre-intervention and activation in perilesional regions post-intervention. At the 6-month follow-up, activation was present in SI and bilateral supplementary motor area (SMA). Functional connectivity maps show reduced interhemispheric SI connectivity before and immediately following training. An increase in interhemispheric SI connectivity was observed at the follow-up study together with an increase in connectivity in SMA. A potential increase in interhemispheric thalamic connectivity was observed immediately following training. VAS = visual analogue scale of client's self-rated ability to perceive touch stimulus during MRI scanning.

supporting them are discussed in the context of sensation and perceptual learning. They are: goal-directed attention and deliberate anticipation, calibration across modality and within modality, and graded progression within and across sensory attributes and tasks. Examples of training strategies that directly use these principles are provided from the sensory training program described by Carey et al. (Carey et al., 1993; Carey, 2006; Carey, Macdonnell, et al., 2011). This training program has demonstrated effectiveness in randomized controlled trial (Carey, Macdonnell, et al., 2011) and meta-analysis of 30 single-case experiments (Carey, 2006).

12.5.1 GOAL-DIRECTED ATTENTION AND DELIBERATE ANTICIPATION

Goal-directed attentive processing of somatosensory information and deliberate use of anticipation have potential application on the basis that attention has been shown to preferentially bias processing of somatosensory information, attentive information processing can be manipulated via the goal of the task, and similar brain regions are involved in perception and anticipation of a stimulus. Use of these strategies may facilitate links to the somatosensory network via distributed regions or networks that may not be directly affected by the sensory lesion.

Attention is critical to processing of any sensory information and to learning (Jagadeesh, 2006; Lewis, Baldassarre, Committeri, Romani, & Corbetta, 2009; see also Chapter 14). Tactile attention biases processing in the somatosensory cortex, through amplification of responses to relevant features of selected stimuli (Burton & Sinclair, 2000; Boly et al., 2007; Kiesel et al., 2010).

Heightening the response to sensory features of relevance can occur at multiple levels of the somatosensory network. At the level of the thalamus there is "gating" of sensory information that is relevant to the task (Castro-Alamancos, 2002; Staines, Black, et al., 2002). Thalamic thresholds may be selectively heightened, influencing the selection and intensity of signals that are relayed to cortical regions (Krupa, Ghazanfar, & Nicolelis, 1999). Prefrontal attention regions have a top-down influence on thresholds within the thalamus (Krupa et al., 1999) and SI (Staines, Graham et al., 2002). Bilateral SII and insula also have a major role in modulation of sensory information and are influenced by attention (Burton et al., 1999; Johansen-Berg, Christensen, Woolrich, & Matthews, 2000). Enhanced activity is also evident in SI (Johansen-Berg et al., 2000; Staines, Graham, et al., 2002), highlighting the role of top-down processes on early sensory information processing. Brain activity at rest (Deco & Corbetta, 2011) and prior to task-related activation (Boly et al., 2007) appears important and may be influenced by attention. For example, a positive relationship was observed between conscious perception of low-intensity somatosensory stimuli and immediately preceding levels of baseline activity in medial thalamus and the lateral frontoparietal network, which are thought to relate to vigilance and "external monitoring." (Boly et al., 2007). Computational neuroscience highlights the role of adaptive sensory processing (Friston & Dolan, 2010; Roberts & Leen, 2010) and larger-scale neural networks in gating of sensory information (Gisiger & Boukadoum, 2011). Thus, manipulation of attention may lead to top-down and/or bottom-up influences on the network.

Deliberate use of anticipation also has potential to access key regions in the sensory network and to make new connections that may have been interrupted. Evidence indicates that brain regions typically involved in processing a touch stimulus may also be active in anticipation of that stimulus (Roland, 1981). This occurred when the subject was asked to imagine the stimulus immediately after the experience of feeling the actual stimulus. These findings are consistent with an increasing body of knowledge from neuroimaging studies that have investigated brain activation under actual and imagined conditions, and with the potential use of motor imagery after stroke (Sharma, Baron, & Rowe, 2009; Butler & Page, 2006). Thus, directed attention and deliberate anticipation may be used in therapy to preselect and tune into stimulus attributes relevant to the goal of the task.

In the sensory training program described by Carey et al., directed attention is facilitated by requiring the subject to give a response; for example, to discriminate if a stimulus pair are the same or different (Carey et al., 1993; Carey, 2006; Carey, Macdonnell, et al., 2011). The goal of the task is made explicit with reference to the sensory attribute that is being trained; for example, the spatial feature of roughness. The difference is manipulated according to the trained sensory attribute and is applied in the context of textured surfaces, limb positions, and everyday objects. The therapist helps direct the patient's attention to the salient features of the task and distinctive features of difference, with less noticing of irrelevancies. The goal of the task and sensory discrimination is also linked with exploratory movements that are most optimal in processing the particular sensory attribute. Lederman et al. (Lederman & Klatzky, 1993) have defined optimal exploratory procedures related to the purpose of the task. For example, to discriminate or recognize texture attributes of a task, lateral motion of the fingertip over the surface is most optimal. In comparison, to discriminate the hardness of an object such as a crushable cup, application of controlled pressure is the most optimal exploratory procedure. The client is cued to use the most optimal exploratory procedures relevant to the goal of the task.

Anticipation trials are interspersed in the sequence of training whereby after an initial experience of a particular training set, the client is cued that the sensory task they are about to experience will be similar to that which they have just experienced and received feedback on (Carey et al., 1993; Carey, 2006; Carey, Macdonnell, et al., 2011). The client is instructed to anticipate the sensory attribute or perceptual judgment required based on immediate prior experience, thus limiting the response choices and heightening the salience of the sensory attribute to be judged. The patient is also directed to imagine what a stimulus is supposed to feel like by reference to what it actually feels like with the "unaffected" hand and with reference to immediate prior experience.

12.5.2 CALIBRATION ACROSS MODALITY AND WITHIN MODALITY

Use of calibration as a treatment strategy is supported by evidence that matching of sensory map representations improves signal input and is important in early information processing (Becker, 1996), and that cross-modal plasticity may facilitate new neural connections (Sathian, 2006). The potential for tactile–visual matching is highlighted.

Our senses are interpreted with cross-reference to each other and immediate prior experience. Matching sensory map representations is important in early information processing (Driver & Noesselt, 2008). For example, functional representation of a touch stimulus in SI can be matched with the brain map of a touch experienced just prior, or with the visual representation in the visual cortex of what was touched (Kaas & Pons, 2006). Computational neural models indicate that when two modalities are trained at the same time and provide feedback for each other, a higher level of performance is possible than if they had remained independent (Becker, 1996). Similarly, temporally and spatially aligned sensory inputs across different modalities are more likely to be attended to and undergo further information processing than nonaligned stimuli (Talsma et al., 2010). Sensory maps can be decoupled (or misaligned), requiring the nervous system to actively realign the sensory maps and perceptual templates. This may be facilitated by matching within and across modalities when the information is congruent. Transformation of sensory maps is dynamic and related to function. This provides an opportunity for modulation of maps via other senses and attention.

Cross-modal plasticity in sensory systems may facilitate alternate and new neural connections, particularly when one sensory modality is deprived (Sathian, 2006). There is strong evidence that visual cortical activity is regularly associated with the neural processing of tactile inputs (Sathian, 2005), providing support for calibration across these modalities. Processing of touch and visual information is often congruent, for example, in processing the spatial dimensions of a textured stimulus or the size and shape of an object. Tactile discrimination of grating orientation involves a region in parieto-occipital cortex, an area known to process visuospatial information (Sathian et al., 1997). Similarly, a network of occipital, parietal, and prefrontal areas was identified in visuotactile recognition of objects in humans (Tal & Amedi, 2009). Further, there is evidence of effective connectivity of parietal and occipital cortical regions during haptic shape perception (Peltier et al., 2007). Tactile perception recruits multiple visual cortical areas in a task-specific manner (Sathian, 2006). Visual and tactile signals are combined in the brain to ensure appropriate interactions with the space around the body (Macaluso & Maravita, 2010). Evidence of cross-modal interactions in sensory systems provides a strong foundation for rehabilitation.

An example of how calibration may be used in neurological rehabilitation and therapy is provided by Carey et al. (Carey et al., 1993; Carey, 2006; Carey, Macdonnell, et al., 2011). After initial exposure to a stimulus set without vision, the stroke patient is guided to recalibrate his/her altered sensation by reference to a more normal sensation experienced through the other hand and vision. The stimulus sets used have clearly defined differences, such as differences in the spatial features of texture grids, which may be interpreted in a congruent way using vision and touch. The person feels the surface with the affected hand, views the texture in terms of spatial roughness, and is guided to match in the "mind's eye" what the texture should feel like in terms of roughness. The sensation is also calibrated with reference to actually feeling the texture with their other hand. The stimulus is felt by the affected hand and then, immediately after, by the unaffected hand with the same goal, and then repeated a few times in a sequence. The clients are guided to match the important *feature*/s of the stimulus they are feeling (e.g., spatial roughness) as well as the salient *difference* within a stimulus set.

12.5.3 GRADED PROGRESSION WITHIN SENSORY ATTRIBUTES AND ACROSS SENSORY ATTRIBUTES AND TASKS

Evidence from perceptual learning demonstrates that a better level of perceptual differentiation can be achieved when that level is progressively approximated versus repeated exposure at the same level (Ahissar & Hochstein, 1997; Goldstone, 1998). This is consistent with evidence that neural plastic changes associated with learning are enhanced when the system is progressively challenged (Selzer, Clarke, Cohen, Duncan, & Gage, 2006). However, there are limits to the transfer of perceptual learning (Lewis et al., 2009). It is suggested that transfer should be more prominent where the stimuli are more complex and potentially share a number of distinctive features (Goldstone, 1998).

Functions are distributed in interconnected networks, with gradients of separation between them (Frey et al., 2011). Knowledge of these networks and levels of processing may be used to enhance information processing in areas that are deficient. Graded progression facilitates perceptual differentiation, as presentation of an easy discrimination first allows the subject to allocate attention to the relevant dimension (Goldstone, 1998). This is consistent with the evidence that perceptual learning is stimulus-dependent and enhances processing in regions implicated in attention-gated learning (J. X. Zhang & Kourtzi, 2010). Further, learning-induced changes are reported to be distributed throughout the sensory network (Op de Beeck & Baker, 2010).

In therapy we also need to train for transfer to novel, untrained stimuli. To achieve transfer to novel stimuli and tasks, graded progression should be across sensory attributes and tasks. Perceptual learning (Goldstone, 1998) and neurophysiological (Johnson & Hsiao, 1992) evidence propose that "distinctive features of difference" are learned and form the basis of transfer of training. This hypothesis is supported in a recent fMRI study that showed that learning is transferred to novel objects that share parts with the trained objects (Song, Hu, Li, Li, & Liu, 2010). This highlights that the perceptual processing strategy by which objects are encoded during learning is important. Transfer of learning to novel tasks is best achieved when the conditions of training and stimuli used are varied (Goldstone, 1998). It may also be facilitated with multimodal training (Olsson, Jonsson, & Nyberg, 2008). Neural correlates of sensorimotor adaptation suggest that transfer of learning involves an increased reliance on the cerebellum (Seidler, 2010).

Application may be seen in the stimulus-specific (Carey et al., 1993) and transfer-enhanced (Carey & Matyas, 2005; Carey, Macdonnell, et al., 2011) programs of sensory discrimination retraining. For example, stimulus-specific training of texture gratings involves progressive presentation of surface sets that vary in the dimension of spatial roughness. Training commences with the largest texture differences, followed by medium and progressively smaller differences. This helps to highlight the most salient feature of the task in the early stages when the client is having difficulty searching for and perceiving the sensation that is important. The client is asked to respond if the surfaces are the same or different and is then guided in identifying the distinctive feature of difference. In the transfer-enhanced program of sensory retraining, stimuli used in training are organized in a matrix according to difficulty of stimulus difference to be discriminated and type of stimulus difference (Carey & Matyas, 2005). The patient is trained both in the process of discriminating large, then medium and fine differences, through to recognizing the different types of sensory attributes. For example, patients are trained on large differences in surface features such as roughness and friction, followed by medium differences in these and medium differences in novel stimulus sets with attributes they have not been previously trained on, such as contour differences. In this way, the person can get feedback on the process of transfer. Through this matrix of tasks, clients are also guided to efficiently build up their repertoire of perceptual experiences. The same principles are used when training limb position sense, object recognition, and during training of everyday tasks.

12.6 CURRENT APPROACHES TO SENSORY REHABILITATION

A number of approaches to sensory rehabilitation have been proposed over the years. These approaches will be grouped according to the major principles of training underlying them and reviewed in the context of current neuroscience evidence and empirical foundations. To date, only a few interventions are supported by empirical evidence and strong science foundations.

12.6.1 PASSIVE STIMULATION AND BOMBARDMENT

Early approaches used sensory bombardment and passive stimulation and did not demonstrate a positive outcome (Van Deusen Fox, 1964) or showed limited effect (De Jersey, 1979). Training involved passive stimulation of the limb using high-intensity, nonspecific stimulation such as rubbing the limb with a texture, icing, vibration, clapping, and brisk toweling for 1–5 minutes each. The overall aim of sensory rehabilitation, informed by neuroscience, is to better interpret altered somatosensory information after stroke. A bombardment/passive stimulation approach would appear to be opposed to this outcome based on current neuroscience evidence. Sensory processing involves attended processing with differentiation and modulation relative to the task goal. Passive bombardment protocols do not facilitate attentive processing of information relative to a goal; it does not allow sensory matching or calibration and does not provide graded progression of stimulation. It potentially competes for attention to relevant stimuli and has an unknown effect on interhemispheric balance of activity. Patients frequently report that the approach is "frustrating," "confusing," (Lyons, 2010) and that being asked to retrieve objects from bowls of rice (another form of bombardment) "feels like putting your hand into shards of glass." Some studies have used transient passive somatosensory stimulation to achieve short-term outcomes for motor recovery. These should not be confused with interventions designed to rehabilitate sensory functions (Carey, Blennerhassett, & Matyas, 2010). The purpose of passive stimulation for motor recovery is different and was not intended for individuals with somatosensory impairment, despite the fact that they have been included in reviews of sensory rehabilitation.

12.6.2 ATTENDED STIMULATION OF SPECIFIC BODY SITES

Dannenbaum and Dykes (1988) piloted a sensory retraining program founded on neurophysiology and rules governing cortical reorganization in a case study. The program involved presentation of high-intensity stimuli to relevant body sites and in a manner that is attentive. Stimulation was also provided in actions in which the sensation may be used (e.g., Velcro knife). Although the study was limited to a single case and did not deliberately incorporate principles of perceptual learning, the approach was based on sound therapeutic rationale with positive outcomes.

12.6.3 GRADED SENSORY EXERCISES WITH FEEDBACK

Yekuteil and Guttman (1993) founded their approach on principles of training derived from peripheral nerve injury training programs with contributions from psychology. They included focus on the hand, attention and motivation, guided exploration of the tactics of perception, and use of the "good" hand. Sensory tasks included: identification of number of touches or letters drawn on the arm; "find your (plegic) thumb" blindfolded; discrimination of weight, shape, and texture of objects; and passive drawing with the finger. Training was conducted 3 times a week for 6 weeks. Twenty chronic stroke survivors participated in the controlled trial. A control group (n = 19) was tested but received no intervention. There was no randomization to groups. Significant gains of approximately 8% to 25% on four sensory measures were reported following sensory training. Variation in results was observed across individuals and the authors noted that the method may still be "too peripheral." Patients with right hemisphere stroke did more poorly than those with left hemisphere stroke.

Lynch et al. (Lynch, Hillier, Stiller, Campanella, & Fisher, 2007) conducted a pilot randomized control trial of sensory retraining of the lower limb after acute stroke in 21 patients with sensory deficits in the feet. Principles were reportedly similar to those used in previous perceptual learning training. The intervention involved sensory retraining of the more affected lower limb versus relaxation (sham intervention). Training was conducted over 10×30-minute sessions involving education, practice in detection and touch on soles of the feet, discrimination of hardness, temperature, and texture of different floor surfaces, and proprioception training of the big toe. Significant improvement was reported over time with sensory retraining, but there were no significant between-group effects. It was noted that this was likely due to the poor power due to small sample size.

12.6.4 ECLECTIC APPROACH INVOLVING SENSORIMOTOR EXERCISES

The approach by Byl et al. (2003) uses sensory-motor exercises to achieve outcomes of improved accuracy and speed in relation to sensorimotor function. Sensory training involved use of the hand in functional activities, sensory exercises with and without vision, tasks to "quiet the nervous system," and reinforcement with mental rehearsal and imagery using a mirror. Sensory exercises included playing board games and learning to read Braille books; retrieving objects from a box filled with rice; exercises in graphesthesia, localization, stereognosis, and kinesthesia; and use of Velcro on objects. Use of the hand in functional activities and mental rehearsal were common to the sensory and motor training programs. In addition, patients were educated regarding the potential for neural plasticity and the unaffected limb was constrained using a glove. Supervised sensory training was conducted for 1.5 h/week over 4 weeks and reinforced with constraint of the unaffected limb and task practice at home. Principles of training were derived from theories of neural plasticity (Byl & Merzenich, 2000) and included matching tasks to ability of the patient, use of attention, repetition, feedback on performance, and progression in difficulty. Training was investigated in 18 chronic stroke survivors. Order of sensory or motor training was crossed. The design was a crossover design (sensory and motor training) with blinded assessors and random assignment (method not specified). It was conducted as a single group, repeated measures design, with no control group and no between-group comparisons for sensory retraining; thus, it was not possible to determine the effectiveness of sensory training alone.

Smania et al. (2003) conducted a study of sensory-motor exercises in four case studies. Focus was on sensory *and* motor functions and incorporated practice of functional tasks. Principles of training were consistent with learning and neural plasticity and included graded exercises and feedback on accuracy and execution of the task for each trial. Exercises included tactile discrimination of textured surfaces, object recognition, joint position sense, weight discrimination, blindfolded motor tasks involving reach and grasp of different objects, and practice of seven daily activities. Assessment of sensory and motor functions was conducted before and after intervention and at 6-month follow-up. All patients showed improvement in one or more of the sensory tasks and three showed increased use of the limb in daily activities.

12.6.5 PERCEPTUAL LEARNING AND NEUROSCIENCE-BASED APPROACH: STIMULUS-SPECIFIC AND TRANSFER-ENHANCED TRAINING

The sensory discrimination training approach by Carey et al. is based on perceptual learning, principles of neural plasticity, and theories of recovery following brain injury (Carey et al., 1993; Carey & Matyas, 2005; Carey, 2006; Carey, Macdonnell, et al., 2011). It is consistent with "learning-dependent" neural plasticity theory (Selzer et al., 2006) and is designed to facilitate interhemispheric communication and cross-modal plasticity (Carey, 2006; Sathian, 2006). The individual calibrates his/her impaired touch sensation internally by reference to more normal touch sensation experienced through the "unaffected" hand and via vision. Anticipation trials, attentive exploration, and feedback are also used to modulate and enhance sensory attributes. The approach has been operationalized and evaluated in the context of two different training protocols with positive results.

Stimulus-specific training (Carey et al., 1993; Carey, 2006) involves graded and repeated learning-based discrimination training of specific sensory stimuli, such as texture grids and limb positions (Carey et al., 1993). Outcomes are clinically and statistically effective in improving sensory tasks trained, based on meta-analysis of 30 controlled single case experiments (z = −8.6, p <.0001; Carey, 2006).

Transfer-enhanced training (Carey & Matyas, 2005; Carey, Macdonnell, et al., 2011) involves learning-based discrimination training of a variety of sensory attributes, such as roughness, across a matrix of sensory tasks including common textures, limb positions, and everyday objects. A variety of stimuli and learning conditions, tuition of training principles, and feedback on the act of transfer to novel stimuli are used to facilitate transfer (Carey & Matyas, 2005). Transfer-enhanced training significantly improved transfer to novel stimuli not trained (z = −5.7; p < .0001) (Carey & Matyas, 2005; Carey, 2006).

Transfer-enhanced training has been incorporated into a clinical training package and tested in our randomized controlled trial, **S**tudy of the **E**ffectiveness of **N**eurorehabilitation on **Se**nsation (**SENSe**), with positive outcomes (Carey, Macdonnell, et al., 2011). Principles of training were applied to three types of sensory tasks: texture discrimination, limb position sense, and tactile object recognition. Texture discrimination training used graded stimuli with varying surface characteristics. Limb position sense was trained across a wide range of limb positions of the upper limb. Tactile object recognition training focused on discrimination of shape, size, weight, texture, hardness, and temperature using a range of multidimensional, graded objects. Between-group comparisons revealed a significantly greater improvement in sensory capacity following sensory discrimination training and improvements were maintained at 6-week and 6-month follow-ups (Carey, Macdonnell, et al., 2011). Improvements in upper limb function were also observed (Mastos & Carey, 2010; Carey, Macdonnell, et al., 2011). Investigation of individual differences revealed improvement with varying characteristics, including side of lesion and age (Carey, Matyas, Walker, & Macdonell, 2010). Both stimulus-specific and transfer-enhanced approaches have clinical application.

In summary, attentive exploration of stimuli, use of motivating and meaningful tasks, use of stimulus discriminations ranging from easy to difficult, and provision of feedback have been shown under controlled and quasi-experimental conditions to be features of successful retraining approaches (Carey et al., 1993; Yekutiel & Guttman, 1993; Byl et al., 2003; Carey & Matyas, 2005; Carey, 2006; Carey, Macdonnell, et al., 2011). Additional principles of deliberate use of anticipation, calibration within and across modalities, and graded progression within and across sensory attributes have strong foundations in neuroscience and are associated with positive outcomes (Carey, 2006; Carey, Macdonnell, et al., 2011). A few novel approaches are currently being investigated at a proof-of-principle stage (Voller et al., 2006; Haggard et al., 2007).

However, these will require systematic development and testing in clinical settings.

12.7 TOWARD A NEUROSCIENCE-BASED MODEL OF SENSORY REHABILITATION

Developing a neuroscience-based model of sensory rehabilitation involves a number of interrelated steps. The first step is to identify brain networks that have potential to be accessed for goal-directed sensory information processing. This includes:

Identification of core sensory networks involved in processing goal-directed somatosensory information. In the somatosensory system the distinction of information processing according to its purpose of "sensation for perception" or "sensation for action" has been highlighted (Dijkerman & de Haan, 2007). Common processing occurs from SI to SII, then to posterior insula (ventral stream) for perception and memory of that perception, or to posterior parietal cortex (dorsal stream) for action and guidance of movement. While this core is an obvious simplification, it does remind us of the importance of the goal of the task and the likely impact of interruption to particular parts of the network.

Identification of related networks that have a role in processing sensory information under certain conditions but may not be necessary under all circumstances. Knowledge of these networks and the conditions under which they may facilitate processing of somatosensory information will contribute to building a model of interconnected networks that may be targeted in therapy. Two key networks are the attention and visual networks. These may be targeted via set-up of conditions that facilitate their involvement in therapy, or may be accessed via augmented therapies if necessary. A model of these networks requires systematic development.

The second step is to identify the impact of a lesion on functional and anatomical networks and the likely information-processing deficit. It is proposed that we should look beyond the local lesion and identify the extent to which the lesion interrupts white matter tracts and overlaps regions known from activation studies to have a role in somatosensory processing. Remote effects on functionally connected regions and interhemispheric balance of activity should also be assessed, using activation and/or connectivity studies. Resting state functional connectivity studies may be of particular value, given their low impact on the patient and suggested value in predicting outcome across different functions (Carter et al., 2010).

The third step is identification and manipulation of brain networks and conditions of training designed to facilitate learning following brain damage. Conditions of training that may be of particular value in rehabilitation of somatosensory functions, based on neuroscience evidence, include: goal-directed attention and deliberate anticipa-

tion; calibration across modality and within modality; and graded progression of training task within and across sensory attributes (see section 12.5). Examples of how they may be operationalized in the context of a sensory retraining program have been provided. These principles may be used in conjunction with core principles of training outlined in Chapter 2. The additional impact of the damaged brain needs to be accounted for.

Finally, it may be beneficial for therapy to be individually targeted based on viable brain networks with capacity for plasticity. This may help clinicians to select the most optimal therapy for an individual based on knowledge of residual brain networks that can be accessed in therapy to achieve the known demands of the task. Based on evidence to date, it may be hypothesized that response to sensory rehabilitation will vary according to structural connectivity of white matter tracts between somatosensory nodes prior to intervention, particularly interhemispheric SI–SI and ipsilesional SI–thalamus connections. The relative integrity of these networks can be identified within an individual to guide more targeted rehabilitation.

REFERENCES

Ahissar, M., & Hochstein, S. (1997). Task difficulty and the specificity of perceptual learning. *Nature, 387*, 401–406.

Bannister, L. C., Gavrilescu, M., Crewther, S. C., & Carey, L. M. (2010). *Resting state functional connectivity of sensory networks after cortical and subcortical lesions.* Paper presented at the 16th Annual Meeting of the Organization for Human Brain Mapping, Barcelona, Spain.

Bear, M. F., Connors, B. W., & Paradiso, M. A. (2007). *Neuroscience: Exploring the brain* (3rd ed.). Philadelphia: Lippincott Williams & Wilkins.

Becker, S. (1996). Mutual information maximization: models of cortical self-organization. *Network Computation in Neural Systems, 7*, 7–31.

Ben-Shabat, E., Pell, G., Brodtmann, A., Matyas, T., & Carey, L. M. (2008). *Proprioceptive perception, an fMRI study of brain alateralization and its relationship with behavioural measures.* Paper presented at the 14th Annual Meeting of the Organization for Human Brain Mapping, Melbourne, Australia.

Blennerhassett, J. M., Matyas, T. A., & Carey, L. M. (2007). Impaired discrimination of surface friction contributes to pinch grip deficit after stroke. *Neurorehabilitation and Neural Repair, 21*(3), 263–272.

Bodegard, A., Ledberg, A., Geyer, S., Naito, E., Zilles, K., & Roland, P. E. (2000). Object shape differences reflected by somatosensory cortical activation. *Journal of Neuroscience, 20*(1) RC51.

Boly, M., Balteau, E., Schnakers, C., Degueldre, C., Moonen, G., Luxen, A., et al. (2007). Baseline brain activity fluctuations predict somatosensory perception in humans. *Proceedings of the National Academy of Sciences U S A, 104*(29), 12187–12192.

Bowsher, D. (1993). Sensory consequences of stroke. *Lancet, 341*(8838), 156.

Bowsher, D., Brooks, J., & Enevoldson, P. (2004). Central representation of somatic sensations in the parietal operculum (SII) and insula. *European Neurology, 52*(4), 211–225.

Burton, H., Abend, N.S., MacLeod, A. M. K., Sinclair, R.J., Snyder, A. Z., & Raichle, M.E. (1999). Tactile attention tasks enhance activation in somatosensory regions of parietal cortex: A positron emission tomography study. *Cerebral Cortex, 9*(7), 662–674.

Burton, H., & Sinclair, R. (2000). Attending to and remembering tactile stimuli: a review of brain imaging data and single-neuron responses. *Journal of Clinical Neurophysiology, 17*(6), 575–591.

Burton, H., Sinclair, R. J., Wingert, J. R., & Dierker, D. L. (2008). Multiple parietal operculum subdivisions in humans: tactile activation maps. *Somatosensory and Motor Research, 25*(3), 149–162.

Butler, A., & Page, S. (2006). Mental practice with motor imagery: evidence for motor recovery and cortical reorganization after stroke. *Archives of Physical Medicine and Rehabilitation, 87*(12 Suppl 2), S2–S11.

Byl, N., Roderick, J., Mohamed, O., Hanny, M., Kotler, J., Smith, A., et al. (2003). Effectiveness of sensory and motor rehabilitation of the upper limb following the principles of neuroplasticity: patients stable poststroke. *Neurorehabilitation and Neural Repair, 17*, 176–191.

Byl, N. N., & Merzenich, M. M. (2000). Principles of neuroplasticity: implications for neurorehabilitation and learning. In E. S. Gonzalez, S. Myers, J. Edelstein, J. S. Liebermann & J. A. Downey (Eds.), *Downey and Darling's physiological basis of rehabilitation medicine* (pp. 609–628). Boston: Butterworth-Heinemann.

Carey, L. M. (1995). Somatosensory loss after stroke. *Critical Reviews in Physical Rehabilitation and Medicine, 7*(1), 51–91.

Carey, L. M. (2006). Loss of somatic sensation. In M. E. Selzer, S. Clarke, L. G. Cohen, P. W. Duncan & F. H. Gage (Eds.), *Textbook of Neural Repair and Rehabilitation. Vol II. Medical neurorehabilitation* (Vol. II, pp. 231–247). Cambridge: Cambridge Uni Press.

Carey, L. M., Abbott, D. F., Egan, G. F., & Donnan, G. A. (2008). Reproducible activation in BA2, 1 and 3b associated with texture discrimination in healthy volunteers over time. *NeuroImage, 39*(1), 40–51.

Carey, L. M., Abbott, D. F., Harvey, M. R., Puce, A., Seitz, R. J., & Donnan, G. A. (2011). Relationship between touch impairment and brain activation after lesions of subcortical and cortical somatosensory regions. *Neurorehabilitation and Neural Repair, 25*(5), 443–457.

Carey, L. M., Abbott, D. F., Puce, A., Jackson, G. D., Syngeniotis, A., & Donnan, G. A. (2002). Reemergence of activation with poststroke somatosensory recovery: a serial fMRI case study. *Neurology, 59*(5), 749–752.

Carey, L. M., Abbott, D. F., Puce, A., Seitz, R. J., Harvey, M., & Donnan, G. A. (2006). IN_Touch: Imaging Neuroplasticity of Touch post-stroke with moderate and severe touch impairment. *NeuroImage, 31*(Suppl 1), e1.

Carey, L. M., Blennerhassett, J., & Matyas, T. (2010). Evidence for the retraining of sensation after stroke remains limited. [Critically Appraised Papers. Commentary.]. *Australian Occupational Therapy Journal, 57*(3), 200–202.

Carey, L. M., Macdonnell, R., & Matyas, T. A. (2011). SENSe: Study of the Effectiveness of Neurorehabilitation on Sensation: a randomized controlled trial. *Neurorehabilitation and Neural Repair, 25*(4), 304–313.

Carey, L. M., Matyas, T., Walker, J., & Macdonell, R. (2010). *SENSe: Study of the Effectiveness of Neurorehabilitation on Sensation: Individual patient characteristics that predict favourable outcomes.* Paper presented at the 21st Annual Scientific Meeting of the Stroke Society of Australasia Melbourne, Australia.

Carey, L. M., & Matyas, T. A. (2005). Training of somatosensory discrimination after stroke: facilitation of stimulus generalization. *American Journal of Physical Medicine and Rehabilitation, 84*(6), 428–442.

Carey, L. M., & Matyas, T. A. (2011). Frequency of discriminative sensory loss in the hand after stroke. *Journal of Rehabilitation Medicine, 43*(3), 257–263.

Carey, L. M., Matyas, T. A., & Oke, L. E. (1993). Sensory loss in stroke patients: effective training of tactile and proprioceptive discrimination. *Archives of Physical Medicine and Rehabilitation, 74*(6), 602–611.

Carter, A. R., Astafiev, S. V., Lang, C. E., Connor, L. T., Rengachary, J., Strube, M. J., et al. (2010). Resting interhemispheric functional magnetic resonance imaging connectivity predicts performance after stroke. *Annals of Neurology, 67*(3), 365–375.

Castillo, E. M., Boake, C., Breier, J. I., Men, D. S., Garza, H. M., Passaro, A., et al. (2008). Aberrant cortical functionality and somatosensory deficits after stroke. *Journal of Clinical Neurophysiology, 25*(3), 132–138.

Castro-Alamancos, M. A. (2002). Role of thalamocortical sensory suppression during arousal: focusing sensory inputs in neocortex. *Journal of Neuroscience, 22*(22), 9651–9655.

Connell, L. A., Lincoln, N. B., & Radford, K. A. (2008). Somatosensory impairment after stroke: frequency of different deficits and their recovery. *Clinical Rehabilitation, 22*(8), 758–767.

Costigan, M., Scholz, J., & Woolf, C. J. (2009). Neuropathic Pain: a maladaptive response of the nervous system to damage. *Annual Review of Neuroscience, 32*, 1–32.

Dannenbaum, R. M., & Dykes, R. W. (1988). Sensory loss in the hand after sensory stroke: therapeutic rationale. *Archives of Physical Medicine and Rehabilitation, 69*, 833–839.

De Jersey, M. C. (1979). Report on a sensory programme for patients with sensory deficits. *Australian Journal of Physiotherapy, 25*, 165–170.

Deco, G., & Corbetta, M. (2011). The dynamical balance of the brain at rest. *Neuroscientist, 17*(1), 107–123.

Devor, A., Tian, P., Nishimura, N., Teng, I. C., Hillman, E. M., Narayanan, S. N., et al. (2007). Suppressed neuronal activity and concurrent arteriolar vasoconstriction may explain negative blood oxygenation level-dependent signal. *Journal of Neuroscience, 27*(16), 4452–4459.

Dijkerman, H., & de Haan, E. (2007). Somatosensory processes subserving perception and action. *Behavioral Brain Science, 30*(2), 189–201.

Disbrow, E., Litinas, E., Recanzone, G. H., Padberg, J., & Krubitzer, L. (2003). Cortical connections of the second somatosensory area and the parietal ventral area in macaque monkeys. *Journal of Comparative Neurology, 462*(4), 382–399.

Driver, J., & Noesselt, T. (2008). Multisensory interplay reveals crossmodal influences on "sensory-specific" brain regions, neural responses, and judgments. *Neuron, 57*(1), 11–23.

Dromerick, A. W., & Reding, M. J. (1995). Functional outcome for patients with hemiparesis, hemihypesthesia, and hemianopia. Does lesion location matter? *Stroke, 26*(11), 2023–2026.

Dunn, W., Carey, L., Morrison, T., & Sabata, D. (2010). *Development of somatosensory measures for the NIH Neurological and Behavioral Toolbox: Findings from tryouts.* Paper presented at the American Occupational Therapy Association's 90th Annual Conference & Expo Orlando, Florida.

Eickhoff, S. B., Grefkes, C., Zilles, K., & Fink, G. R. (2007). The somatotopic organization of cytoarchitectonic areas on the human parietal operculum. *Cerebral Cortex, 17*(8), 1800–1811.

Eickhoff, S. B., Schleicher, A., Zilles, K., & Amunts, K. (2006). The human parietal operculum. I. Cytoarchitectonic mapping of subdivisions. *Cerebral Cortex, 16*(2), 254–267.

Fabri, M., Del Pesce, M., Paggi, A., Polonara, G., Bartolini, M., Salvolini, U., et al. (2005). Contribution of posterior corpus callosum, to the interhemispheric transfer of tactile information. *Cognitive Brain Research, 24*(1), 73–80.

Floel, A., & Cohen, L. G. (2006). Translational studies in neurorehabilitation: from bench to bedside. *Cognitive Behavioral Neurology, 19*(1), 1–10.

Frey, S. H., Leonardo, F., Grafton, S. T., Picard, N., Rothwell, J. C., Schweighofer, N., et al. (2011). Neurological principles and rehabilitation of action disorders: Computation, anatomy, and physiology (CAP) model. *Neurorehabilitation and Neural Repair, 5*(Suppl 1), 65–205.

Friedel, P., & van Hemmen, J. L. (2008). Inhibition, not excitation, is the key to multimodal sensory integration. *Biological Cybernetics, 98*(6), 597–618.

Friston, K. J., & Dolan, R. J. (2010). Computational and dynamic models in neuroimaging. *NeuroImage, 52*(3), 752–765.

Gardner, E. P., & Kandel, E. R. (2000). Touch. In E. R. Kandel, J. H. Schwartz & T. M. Jessell (Eds.), *Principles of neural science.* (4th ed., pp. 451–471). New York: McGraw-Hill.

Gardner, E. P., & Martin, J. H. (2000). Coding of sensory information. In E. R. Kandel, J. H. Schwartz & T. M. Jessell (Eds.), *Principles of neural science.* (pp. 412–429). New York: McGraw-Hill.

Gentilucci, M., Toni, I., Daprati, E., & Gangitano, M. (1997). Tactile input of the hand and the control of reaching to grasp movements. *Experimental Brain Research, 114*, 130–137.

Gisiger, T., & Boukadoum, M. (2011). Mechanisms gating the flow of information in the cortex: what they migt look like and what their uses may be. *Frontiers in Computational Neuroscience, 5*, 1–15.

Goldberg, I., Harel, M., & Malach, R. (2006). When the brain loses its self: prefrontal inactivation during sensorimotor processing. *Neuron, 50*(2), 329–339.

Goldstone, R. L. (1998). Perceptual learning. *Annual Reviews in Psychology, 49*, 585–612.

Haggard, P., Christakou, A., & Serino, A. (2007). Viewing the body modulates tactile receptive fields. *Experimental Brain Research, 180*(1), 187–193.

Han, L., Law-Gibson, D., & Reding, M. (2002). Key neurological impairments influence function-related group outcomes after stroke. *Stroke, 33*(7), 1920–1924.

Hartmann, S., Missimer, J. H., Stoeckel, C., Abela, E., Shah, J., Seitz, R. J., et al. (2008). Functional connectivity in tactile object discrimination–A principal component analysis of an event related fMRI study. *Public Library of Science One, 3*(12), e3861.

Head, H., & Holmes, G. (1911). Sensory disturbances from cerebral lesions. *Brain, 34*, 102–254.

Hermsdörfer, J., Hagl, E., Nowak, D., & Marquardt, C. (2003). Grip force control during object manipulation in cerebral stroke. *Clinical Neurophysiology, 114*, 915–929.

Hlushchuk, Y., & Hari, R. (2006). Transient suppression of ipsilateral primary somatosensory cortex during tactile finger stimulation. *Journal of Neuroscience, 26*(21), 5819–5824.

Jagadeesh, B. (2006). Attentional modulation of cortical plasticity. In M. E. Selzer, S. Clarke, L. G. Cohen, P. W. Duncan & F. H. Gage (Eds.), *Textbook of Neural Repair and Rehabilitation*: Vol 1. Neural repair and plasticity. (Vol. 1, pp. 194–206). Cambridge: Cambridge University Press.

Jain, N., Qi, H. X., Collins, C. E., & Kaas, J. H. (2008). Large-scale reorganization in the somatosensory cortex and thalamus after sensory loss in macaque monkeys. *Journal of Neuroscience, 28*(43), 11042–11060.

Jeannerod, M., Michel, F., & Prablanc, C. (1984). The control of hand movements in a case of hemianaesthesia following a parietal lesion. *Brain, 107*, 899–920.

Johansen-Berg, H., Behrens, T. E. J., Sillery, E., Ciccarelli, O., Thompson, A. J., Smith, S. M., et al. (2005). Functional-anatomical validation and individual variation of diffusion tractography-based segmentation of the human thalamus. *Cerebral Cortex, 15*(1), 31–39.

Johansen-Berg, H., Christensen, V., Woolrich, M., & Matthews, P. (2000). Attention to touch modulates activity in both primary and secondary somatosensory areas. *Neuroreport, 11*(6), 1237–1241.

Johansson, R. S. (1996). Sensory control of dexterous manipulation in humans. In A. M. Wing, P. Haggard, & J. R. Flanagan (Eds.), *Hand and brain: The neurophysiology and psychology of hand movements.* (pp. 381–414). San Diego: Academic Press.

Johansson, R. S., & Westling, G. (1984). Roles of glabrous skin receptors and sensorimotor memory in automatic control of precision grip when lifting rougher or more slippery objects. *Experimental Brain Research, 56*, 550–564.

Johnson, K. O., & Hsiao, S. S. (1992). Neural mechanisms of tactual form and texture perception. *Annual Review of Neuroscience, 15*, 227–250.

Kaas, J. H. (1984). The organization of somatosensory cortex in primates and other mammals *Somatosensory mechanisms. Proceedings of an International Symposium held at the Wenner-Gren Center, Stockholm, June 8–10, 1983* (pp. 51–59).

Kaas, J. H. (1999). Is most of neural plasticity in the thalamus cortical? *Proceedings of the National Academy of Sciences USA, 96*(14), 7622–7623.

Kaas, J. H., & Pons, T. P. (2006). Plasticity of mature and developing somatosensory systems. In M. E. Selzer, S. Clarke, L. G. Cohen, P. W. Duncan, & F. H. Gage (Eds.), *Textbook of neural repair and rehabilitation: Vol. I. Neural repair and plasticity* (Vol. 1, pp. 97–108). Cambridge: Cambridge University Press.

Kandel, E. R., Schwartz, J. H., & Jessell, T. M. (2000). *Principles of neural science.* (4th ed.). New York: McGraw-Hill.

Kastrup, A., Baudewig, J., Schnaudigel, S., Huonker, R., Becker, L., Sohns, J., et al. (2008). Behavioral correlates of negative BOLD signal changes in the primary somatosensory cortex. *NeuroImage, 41*(4), 1364–1371.

Kiesel, A., Wendt, M., Jost, K., Steinhauser, M., Falkenstein, M., Philipp, A.M., et al. (2010). Control and interference in task switching: a review. *Psychological Bulletin, 136*(5), 849–874.

Kim, J. S., & Choi-Kwon, S. (1996). Discriminative sensory dysfunction after unilateral stroke. *Stroke, 27*, 677–682.

Krupa, D. J., Ghazanfar, A. A., & Nicolelis, M. A. (1999). Immediate thalamic sensory plasticity depends on corticothalamic feedback. *Proceedings of the National Academy of Sciences USA, 96*(14), 8200–8205.

Kusoffsky, A., Wadell, I., & Nilsson, B. Y. (1982). The relationship between sensory impairment and motor recovery in patients with hemiplegia. *Scandinavian Journal of Rehabilitation Medicine, 14*, 27–32.

Lederman, S. J., & Klatzky, R. L. (1993). Extracting object properties through haptic exploration. *Acta Psychologica, 84*, 29–40.

Lewis, C. M., Baldassarre, A., Committeri, G., Romani, G. L., & Corbetta, M. (2009). Learning sculpts the spontaneous activity of the resting human brain. *Proceedings of the National Academy of Sciences USA, 106*(41), 17558–17563.

Loubinoux, I., Carel, C., Alary, F., Boulanouar, K., Viallard, G., Manelfe, C., et al. (2001). Within-session and between-session reproducibility of cerebral sensorimotor activation: a test-retest effect evidenced with functional magnetic resonance imaging. *Journal of Cerebral Blood Flow and Metabolism, 21*, 592–607.

Lynch, E. A., Hillier, S. L., Stiller, K., Campanella, R. R., & Fisher, P. H. (2007). Sensory retraining of the lower limb after acute stroke: a randomized controlled pilot trial. *Archives of Physical Medicine and Rehabilitation, 88*, 1101–1107.

Lyons, W. (2010). *Left of Tomorrow.* Glen Waverley: Sid Harta Publishers.

Macaluso, E., & Maravita, A. (2010). The representation of space near the body through touch and vision. *Neuropsychologia, 48*(3), 782–795.

Mastos, M., & Carey, L. (2010). *Occupation-based outcomes associated with sensory retraining post-stroke.* Paper presented at the 21st Annual Scientific Meeting of the Stroke Society of Australasia Melbourne, Australia.

Mesulam, M.-M. (1998). From sensation to cognition. *Brain, 121*, 1013–1052.

Molinari, M., Chiricozzi, F., Clausi, S., Tedesco, A., De Lisa, M., & Leggio, M. (2008). Cerebellum and detection of sequences, from perception to cognition. *Cerebellum, 7*(4), 611–615.

Molinari, M., Filippini, V., & Leggio, M. G. (2002). Neuronal plasticity of interrelated cerebellar and cortical networks. *Neuroscience, 111*(4), 863–870.

Moore, C. I., Stern, C. E., Corkin, S., Fischl, B., Gray, A. C., Rosen, B. R., et al. (2000). Segregation of somatosensory activation in the human rolandic cortex using fMRI. *Journal of Neurophysiology, 84*(1), 558–569.

Mountcastle, V. B. (1997). The columnar organization of the neocortex. *Brain, 120*, 701–722.

Murray, E. A., & Mishkin, M. (1984). Relative contribution of SII and area 5 to tactile discrimination in monkeys. *Behavioural Brain Research, 11*, 67–83.

Naito, E., Roland, P. E., Grefkes, C., Choi, H. J., Eickhoff, S., Geyer, S., et al. (2005). Dominance of the right hemisphere and role of area 2 in human kinesthesia. *Journal of Neurophysiology, 93*(2), 1020–1034.

Nicolelis, M. A. (2005). Computing with thalamocortical ensembles during different behavioural states. *Journal of Physiology, 566*(pt 1), 37–47.

Nowak, D., Hermsdörfer, J., & Topka, H. (2003). Deficits of predictive grip force control during object manipulation in acute stroke. *Journal of Neurology, 250*, 850–860.

O'Reilly, J. X., Beckmann, C. F., Tomassini, V., Ramnani, N., & Johansen-Berg, H. (2010). Distinct and overlapping functional zones in the cerebellum defined by resting state functional connectivity. *Cerebral Cortex, 20*(4), 953–965.

Olsson, C. J., Jonsson, B., & Nyberg, L. (2008). Learning by doing and learning by thinking: an fMRI study of combining motor and mental training. *Frontiers in Human Neuroscience, 2,* Article 5.

Op de Beeck, H. P., & Baker, C. I. (2010). The neural basis of visual object learning. *TRENDS in Cognitive Sciences, 14*(1), 22–30.

Patel, A. T., Duncan, P. W., Lai, S.-M., & Studenski, S. (2000). The relation between impairments and functional outcomes poststroke. *Archives of Physical Medicine and Rehabilitation, 81*, 1357–1363.

Peltier, S., Stilla, R., Mariola, E., LaConte, S., Hu, X., & Sathian, K. (2007). Activity and effective connectivity of parietal and occipital cortical regions during haptic shape perception. *Neuropsychologia, 45*(3), 476–483.

Puce, A., & Carey, L. (2010). Somatosensory function. In I. B. Weiner, W. E. Craighead & C. B. Nemeroff (Eds.), *The Corsini encyclopedia of psychology*. (4th ed. pp. 1678–1680.). New York: John Wiley & Sons, Inc.

Raos, V., & Bentivoglio, M. (1993). Crosstalk between the two sides of the thalamus through the reticular nucleus: a retrograde and anterograde tracing study in the rat. *Journal of Comparative Neurology, 332*(2), 145–154.

Reding, M. J., & Potes, E. (1988). Rehabilitation outcome following initial unilateral hemispheric stroke: life table analysis approach. *Stroke, 19*, 1354–1358.

Reed, C. (2007). Divisions within the posterior parietal cortex help touch meet vision. *Behavioral and Brain Sciences, 30*(2), 218.

Remy, P., Zilbovicius, M., Cesaro, P., Amarenco, P., Degos, J. D., & Samson, Y. (1999). Primary somatosensory cortex activation is not altered in patients with ventroposterior thalamic lesions: a PET study. *Stroke, 30*(12), 2651–2658.

Roberts, P. D., & Leen, T. K. (2010). Anti-Hebbian spike-timing-dependent plasticity and adaptive sensory processing. *Frontiers in Computational Neuroscience, 4*, Article 156.

Roland, P. E. (1981). Somatotopical tuning of postcentral gyrus during focal attention in man: a regional cerebral blood flow study. *Journal of Neurophysiology, 46*, 744–754.

Rossini, P. M., Altamura, C., Ferreri, F., Melgari, J.-M., Tecchio, F., Tombini, M., et al. (2007). Neuroimaging experimental studies on brain plasticity in recovery from stroke. *Eura Medicophys, 43*, 241–254.

Rossini, P. M., Tecchio, F., Pizzella, V., Lupoi, D., Cassetta, E., & Pasqualetti, P. (2001). Interhemispheric differences of sensory hand areas after monohemispheric stroke: MEG/MRI integrative study. *NeuroImage, 14*(2), 474–485.

Ruben, J., Schwiemann, J., Deuchert, M., Meyer, R., Krause, T., Curio, G., et al. (2001). Somatotopic organization of human secondary somatosensory cortex. *Cerebral Cortex, 11*(5), 463–473.

Sathian, K. (2005). Visual cortical activity during tactile perception in the sighted and the visually deprived. *Developmental Psychobiology, 46*(3), 279–286.

Sathian, K. (2006). Cross-modal plasticity in sensory systems. In M. E. Selzer, S. Clarke, L. G. Cohen, P. W. Duncan, & F. H. Gage (Eds.), *Textbook of neural repair and rehabilitation: Vol. 1. Neural repair and plasticity*. (Vol. I, pp. 180–193). Cambridge: Cambridge Uni Press.

Sathian, K., Zangaladze, A., Hoffman, J. M., & Grafton, S. T. (1997). Feeling with the mind's eye. *NeuroReport, 8*(18), 3877–3881.

Savini, N., Babiloni, C., Brunetti, M., Caulo, M., Del Gratta, C., Perrucci, M. G., et al. (2010). Passive tactile recognition of geometrical shape in humans: an fMRI study. *Brain Research Bulletin, 83*(5), 223–231.

Schabrun, S. M., Stinear, C. M., Byblow, W. D., & Ridding, M. C. (2009). Normalizing motor cortex representations in focal hand dystonia. *Cerebral Cortex, 19*(9), 1968–1977.

Schaechter, J. D., Moore, C. I., Connell, B. D., Rosen, B. R., & Dijkhuizen, R. M. (2006). Structural and functional plasticity in the somatosensory cortex of chronic stroke patients. *Brain, 129*(10), 2722–2733.

Seidler, R. D. (2010). Neural correlates of motor learning, transfer of learning, and learning to learn. *Exercise Sport Science Research, 38*(1), 3–9.

Selzer, M., Clarke, S., Cohen, L., Duncan, P., & Gage, F. (2006). *Textbook of neural repair and rehabilitation: Vol I. Neural repair and plasticity*. Cambridge: Cambridge University Press.

Sharma, N., Baron, J. C., & Rowe, J. B. (2009). Motor imagery after stroke: Relating outcome to motor network connectivity. *Annals of Neurology, 66*(5), 604–616.

Shoham, D., & Grinvald, A. (2001). The cortical representation of the hand in macaque and human area S-I: High resolution optical imaging. *Journal of Neuroscience, 21*(17), 6820–6835.

Smania, N., Montagnana, B., Faccioli, S., Fiaschi, A., Aglioti, S.M. (2003). Rehabilitation of somatic sensation and related deficit of motor control in patients with pure sensory stroke. *Archives of Physical Medicine and Rehabilitation, 84*, 1692–1702.

Sommerfeld, D. K., & von Arbin, M. H. (2004). The impact of somatosensory function on activity performance and length of hospital stay in geriatric patients with stroke. *Clinical Rehabilitation, 18*(2), 149–155.

Song, Y. Y., Hu, S. Y., Li, X. T., Li, W., & Liu, J. (2010). The role of top-down task context in learning to perceive objects. *Journal of Neuroscience, 30*(29), 9869–9876.

Staines, W. R., Black, S. E., Graham, S. J., & McIlroy, W. E. (2002). Somatosensory gating and recovery from stroke involving the thalamus. *Stroke, 33*(11), 2642–2651.

Staines, W. R., Graham, S. J., Black, S. E., & McIlroy, W. E. (2002). Task-relevant modulation of contralateral and ipsilateral primary somatosensory cortex and the role of prefrontal-cortical sensory gating systems. *NeuroImage, 15*(1), 190–199.

Sullivan, J. E., & Hedman, L. D. (2008). Sensory dysfunction following stroke: incidence, significance, examination, and intervention. *Topics in Stroke Rehabilitation, 15*(3), 200–217.

Tal, N., & Amedi, A. (2009). Multisensory visual-tactile object related network in humans: insights gained using a novel crossmodal adaptation approach. *Experimental Brain Research, 198*(2–3, Sp. Iss. SI), 165–182.

Talsma, D., Senkowski, D., Soto-Faraco, S., & Woldorff, M. G. (2010). The multifaceted interplay between attention and multisensory integration. *TRENDS in Cognitive Sciences, 14*(9), 400–410.

Taskin, B., Jungehulsing, G. J., Ruben, J., Brunecker, P., Krause, T., Blankenburg, F., et al. (2006). Preserved responsiveness of secondary somatosensory cortex in patients with thalamic stroke. *Cerebral Cortex, 16*(10), 1431–1439.

Tesche, C. D., & Karhu, J. J. T. (2000). Anticipatory cerebellar responses during somatosensory omission in man. *Human Brain Mapping, 9*(3), 119–142.

Thach, W. T. (1998). A role for the cerebellum in learning movement coordination. *Neurobiology of Learning and Memory, 70*(1–2), 177–188.

Tyson, S. F., Hanley, M., Chillala, J., Selley, A. B., & Tallis, R. C. (2008). Sensory loss in hospital-admitted people with stroke: characteristics, associated factors, and relationship with function. *Neurorehabilitation and Neural Repair, 22*(2), 166–172.

Van Deusen Fox, J. (1964). Cutaneous stimulation: effects on selected tests of perception. *American Journal of Occupational Therapy, 18*, 53–55.

Voller, B., Flöel, A., Werhahn, K. J., Ravindran, S., Wu, C. W., & Cohen, L. G. (2006). Contralateral hand anesthesia transiently improves poststroke sensory deficits. *Annals of Neurology, 59*(2), 385–388.

Weder, B., Knorr, U., Herzog, H., Nebeling, B., Kleinschmidt, A., Huang, Y., et al. (1994). Tactile exploration of shape after subcortical ischaemic infarction studied with PET. *Brain, 117*(3), 593–605.

Wing, A. M., Flanagan, J. R., & Richardson, J. (1997). Anticipatory postural adjustments in stance and grip. *Experimental Brain Research, 116*(1), 122–130.

Winward, C. E., Halligan, P. W., & Wade, D. T. (2002). The Rivermead Assessment of Somatosensory Performance (RASP): standardization and reliability data. *Clinical Rehabilitation, 16*(5), 523–533.

Wu, X., Nestrasil, I., Ashe, J., Tuite, P., & Bushara, K. (2010). Inferior olive response to passive tactile and visual stimulation with variable interstimulus intervals. *Cerebellum, 9*(4), 598–602.

Yekutiel, M. (2000). *Sensory re-education of the hand after stroke.* London: Whurr Publishers.

Yekutiel, M., & Guttman, E. (1993). A controlled trial of the retraining of the sensory function of the hand in stroke patients. *Journal of Neurology, Neurosurgery and Psychiatry, 56*, 241–244.

Zangaladze, A., Epstein, C. M., Grafton, S. T., & Sathian, K. (1999). Involvement of visual cortex in tactile discrimination of orientation. *Nature, 401*(6753), 587–590.

Zhang, D. Y., Snyder, A. Z., Fox, M.D., Sansbury, M. W., Shimony, J. S., & Raichle, M. E. (2008). Intrinsic functional relations between human cerebral cortex and thalamus. *Journal of Neurophysiology, 100*(4), 1740–1748.

Zhang, J. X., & Kourtzi, Z. (2010). Learning-dependent plasticity with and without training in the human brain. *Proceedings of the National Academy of Sciences of the United States of America, 107*(30), 13503–13508.

13 | VISION

AMY BRODTMANN

13.1 INTRODUCTION

The human visual system is an extraordinarily complex sensory system. Despite many decades of research, not all of its components are fully described or understood. Its widely distributed nature renders it vulnerable to insults along its long pathways. Visual deficits are particularly common after stroke. It has been estimated that in Europe and the United States, between 90,000 and 100,000 new cases of cerebral blindness occur each year (Sahraie, 2007). *Cerebral blindness* is a term used to describe visual field deficits following ischemic damage to the visual pathways.

In this chapter a summary of the complex pathways of the human visual system will be presented, using evidence from primate and other mammalian models where appropriate. This is to introduce the reader to the concepts potentially underlying recovery in the visual cortical system (see Table 13.1). The focus of the background discussion will be on the ventral and dorsal pathways—the "what" and "where" pathways. It will not be on the division of object vision versus action (the "what" and "how" pathways).

The introduction to the complex visual system will be followed by a discussion of current thinking about visual rehabilitation and visual restorative strategies. The clinical focus of this chapter would be the patient presenting with a visual field deficit, who may be asking: Will this recover? Is there anything I can do to improve my vision? The answer to these questions a decade ago would have been resoundingly negative, but there is now hope that new restorative therapies may assist some people in gaining cortical visual function.

13.2 ANATOMY OF VISUAL PATHWAYS

13.2.1 THE RETINOGENICULATE PATHWAY

Information processing in the visual pathway begins at the photoreceptors in the outer layer of the retina, the earliest visual part of the central nervous system. Light passes through the cornea overlying the pupil, with the image being inverted by the lens and inversely projected onto the retina. Two types of cells, the rods and cones, detect light: these are known as *photoreceptors*. Rods detect form and color, and bear most responsibility for day vision, while cones mediate night vision, when most stimuli are too weak to excite the cone system (Hecht, 1937; Young, 1970). A well-characterized chain of synaptic events from receptor cells to other neurons in the retina then follows. Photoreceptor impulses are transmitted to bipolar cells in the intermediate zone, which represent the primary afferent neurons of the visual system. Their short axons terminate on the retinal ganglion cells constituting the inner layer of the retina. These cells are structurally and functionally divided into several categories, known as X-, Y-, and W-cells in the cat (Stone, 1972; Stone & Fukuda, 1974). Analogous cells have been identified in monkey models, and the corresponding monkey retinal cells are the B-, A-, and C-cells (Leventhal, Rodieck, & Dreher, 1981). The subdivisions are important, as the three types of cells have different terminal targets. W-cells (C-cells in the monkey) constitute 10% of the total ganglion cells in the retina, and mostly project to the superior colliculus due to their involvement in head and neck movements (Hubel & Wiesel, 1963; Enroth-Cugell & Robson, 1966). The Y-cells (A-cells in the monkey; 10% of total) project exclusively to the magnocellular cells of the lateral geniculate body (layers 1 and 2, and see below), and respond to motion and

TABLE 13.1 Selected Visual Cortex Nomenclature Used in This Chapter.

ANATOMICAL DESCRIPTION	BRODMANN AREA	OLD FUNCTIONAL DESCRIPTION	REGIONAL NAME	FUNCTIONAL SPECIALIZATION EXAMPLE
Striate or calcarine cortex	Area 17	Primary visual cortex	V1	Edge detection
Pericalcarine cortex	Area 18	Visual association cortex	V2	Depth perception
Extrastriate cortex	Areas 18 and 19	Visual association cortex	V3 (V3$_{dorsal}$ and V3$_{ventral}$)	Orientation selective
		Visual association cortex	V3a (or V3$_{accessory}$)	Direction discrimination
Lateral aspect of collateral sulcus of fusiform gyrus		Visual association cortex	V4 (V4$_v$ and V4$_d$) or V8 or VO	Human color area
Lateral occipitotemporal junction	Areas 21/22?	Visual association cortex	V5 or MT or MT+	Motion sensitive areas
Fusiform gyrus	Area 20?	Visual association cortex	Fusiform face area (FFA)	Face selective
Parahippocampal gyrus		Visual association cortex	Parahippocampal place area (PPA)	Place/location specific
Lateral occipital gyri			Lateral occipital complex (LOC)	Object sensitive

NOTE: *Nomenclature is based on a table by Watson (Watson, 2000) modified after Tootell (Tootell, Tsao, & Vanduffel, 2003). Areas included are examples only, to introduce visual cognitive novices to the range of terms used.*

the gross features of the stimulus, such as contrast (Hubel & Wiesel, 1959, 1962). The X-cells (A-cells in the monkey; 80% of total) project mainly to the parvocellular layers (they have some projections to the magnocellular layers), and are concerned with fine visual detail (Perry & Cowey, 1981; Perry, Oehler, & Cowey, 1984). Retinal cellular position largely determines their functional pathway, with the population of Y-cells increasing with greater eccentricity in the retina (Hubel & Wiesel, 1959, 1962). Centrally (parafoveal), retinal cells feed selectively into the parvocellular system, responsible for excellent spatial resolution, while extrafoveal cells (placed further from the retinal center) link into the magnocellular system, which is a low–spatial resolution, highly motion sensitive pathway (Leventhal, 1979; Tootell, Hamilton, & Switkes, 1988). These two parallel information processing pathways are often referred to as the *X-parvocellular* and *Y-magnocellular pathways* (Stone, Dreher, & Leventhal, 1979).

The fovea-macular projection (papillomacular bundle) is the major ocular-cortical outflow, with the central 5° of retina subserved by 25% of the axons, and the central 20° by 90% of the axons (Nieuwenhuys, Voogd, & van Huijzen, 1988). The axons of the retinal ganglion cells converge to form the optic nerve, and acquire a myelin sheath once leaving the retina. The optic nerves pass to the optic chiasm and undergo a partial decussation (crossing), with fibers from the nasal halves of the retina (and therefore the temporal halves of the visual field) crossing to the opposite side, and the temporal fibers remaining uncrossed. See Figure 13.1 for a diagram of the major anatomical structures comprising the human retinogeniculostriate pathway.

The fibers then course retrochiasmically as two diverging optic tracts, which arch around the diencephalon to reach the lateral geniculate nucleus (LGN). Once the optic tract reaches the thalamus, it divides into two branches. The larger of the two terminates in

the LGN. In the monkey, about 90% of retinal ganglion cells (the A-cells and B-cells) terminate in the LGN—the remaining 10% (mainly C-cells) project to the superior colliculi, nuclei of the accessory optic system, and pretectal regions (and see extrageniculate pathways below; Perry et al., 1984; Perry, Silveira, & Cowey, 1990; Stone & Dreher, 1982). Some of these retinofugal fibers or collaterals leave the optic chiasm, enter the anterior hypothalamus, and terminate in the suprachiasmatic nucleus. It is via this retinohypothalamic projection that the visual system is believed to participate in the regulation of diurnal rhythms (Nieuwenhuys

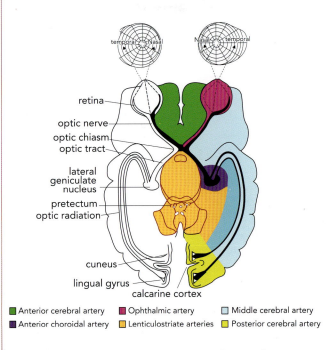

Figure 13.1 Diagram of the human striatogeniculate visual system depicting major anatomical structures and their blood supply—see legend at bottom.

et al., 1988). The monkey visual system is analogous to the human system and the preceding statements are believed to be relevant to human visual anatomy.

In the mid-1990s, it was observed that retrograde tracers labeled cells with different markers when injected into the superficial layers and deeper layers of V1, with different laminar patterns of projection (Hendry & Yoshioka, 1994). These observations triggered investigation of a third, koniocellular (K) pathway (Casagrande, 1994). Separate definitions of the K pathway have emerged at different levels in the visual pathway, and the precise nature of this pathway is still being characterized (Callaway, 2005; Nassi & Callaway, 2009).

13.2.2 THE GENICULOSTRIATE PATHWAY

Most of the fibers of the optic tract terminate in the lateral geniculate nucleus, a vital thalamic center for vision. The LGN has a distinctively laminar structure composed of six concentric layers, numbered 1–6, beginning ventromedially. Layers 1 and 2 are known as *magnocellular laminae*, as their cells are larger than the others, and the remainder are therefore termed *parvocellular* (Stone, Dreher, & Leventhal, 1979). The retinal fibers terminate in an exquisitely ordered fashion, with layers 2, 3, and 5 receiving fibers from the ipsilateral eye, layers 1, 4, and 6 receiving fibers from the contralateral eye. As mentioned above, in the monkey, A-cells project to the magnocellular (M-cell pathway) and B-cells to the parvocellular laminae (P-cell pathway; Stone & Dreher, 1982; Perry et al., 1984, 1990). The efferent fibers of the LGN form the optic radiation (or geniculocalcarine tract), and first course past the retrolenticular part of the internal capsule before arching around the lateral ventricle and then proceeding back toward the occipital cortex (see Figure 13.1).

The primary visual cortex is often referred to as the *striate cortex* (V1, striate cortex, or Brodmann's area 17), named by Gennari, who first described the macroscopically distinctive laminated or striated appearance, caused by a visible layer of myelinated fibers bisecting the internal granular layer. Those from the lateral part of the LGN sweep anteriorly into the temporal lobe before passing posteriorly to the striate cortex. Most of the fibers terminate in primary visual cortex, and there is a precise point-to-point (retinotopic) projection from the retina via the LGN to the striate cortex (Dobelle, Turkel, Henderson, & Evans, 1979; Chen, Zhu, Thulborn, & Ugurbil, 1999). In addition, the arching nature of the optic radiation projections mean that the lower retinal halves (superior quadrants) project to the striate cortex below the calcarine sulcus, while the upper retinal halves (inferior quadrants) project to the striate cortex above the sulcus (Holmes, 1918, 1945). The retinal areas concerned with central (macular) vision project to a relatively large area, which forms the posterior part of the striate cortex (Fox, Miezin, Allman,

Van Essen, & Raichle, 1987). The parts of the retina concerning more peripheral aspects of the visual field project to a smaller, intermediate part, while the nasal periphery of the retina (most temporal regions of the visual field, which are monocular) project to the extreme anterior portion of the striate region (Tootell, Switkes, Silverman, & Hamilton, 1988).

This understanding of the topographic organization of the striate cortex has only come about in the last two decades. The revised maps expand the area of striate cortex subserving central vision, with a proportional reduction in that used for peripheral vision (Horton & Hoyt, 1991; McFadzean, Brosnahan, Hadley, & Mutlukan, 1994). These revisions accord with clinical observations and explain why visual field defects confined to the monocular temporal crescent are rare, given the fact that the anterior striate cortex subserving this region constitutes less than 10% of the total striate area. In addition, it justifies the use of computerized testing strategies that test the central 24° to 30° of visual field, as this actually assesses 80%–83% of the striate cortex, making it unlikely to miss cortical occipital lesions (Currie, 1997). They also help to explain the phenomenon of macular sparing in homonymous hemianopia.

The occipital pole is supplied by both the middle cerebral artery (MCA) and posterior cerebral artery (PCA) in a minority of people. In the advent of PCA occlusion, the posterior half of the striate cortex will remain perfused. Because of the large distribution of the central visual field over the posterior half of the striate cortex, a variable amount of this cortex, subserving macular vision, will be spared. Thus the presence of a homonymous hemianopia with macular sparing is said to be pathognomonic of an occipital lesion. The disproportionately large cortical area devoted to macular vision has been confirmed in experimental animals and termed the *cortical magnification factor* (Daniel & Whitteridge, 1961). Its description represented a landmark in the conceptualization of the functional anatomy of the visual system.

13.2.3 EXTRAGENICULOSTRIATE PATHWAYS

Extrageniculostriate pathways, paralleling the retinogeniculocalcarine pathway, have been demonstrated in monkeys (Yukie & Iwai, 1981; Cowey, Stoerig, & Bannister, 1994) and similar pathways have been shown in humans (Weiskrantz, Barbur, & Sahraie, 1995; Ffytche, Howseman, Edwards, Sandeman, & Zeki, 2000). In the monkey these account for less than 10% of retinal ganglion cell projections (Stone & Dreher, 1982). There are three successive components: retinotectal fibers (Itaya, 1980; Hutchins & Weber, 1985; Itaya & Itaya, 1985), fibers that originate in the superior colliculus and terminate in the pulvinar (Holstege & Collewijn, 1982), and fibers that arise from the pulvinar and project to the striate and extrastriate

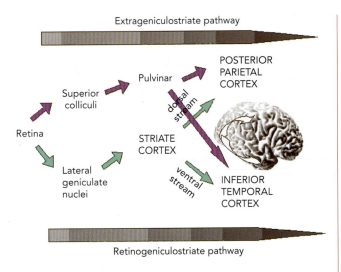

Figure 13.2 Cartoon summarizing the major visual information pathways. *Extrageniculostriate pathway* refers to the top group of arrows; *retinogeniculostriate pathway* refers to the bottom and central arrows.

areas (Berman, 1977). The first two form the accessory optic system, while this latter component of the extrageniculate pathway appears to be involved in orientation and attention (Perry & Cowey, 1984).

In the first, axons from the retinal ganglion cells continue in a mediocaudal direction and terminate directly in the superior colliculus, pulvinar, and terminal nuclei of the accessory visual system (nucleus terminalis medialis, lateralis, and dorsalis; Itaya, 1980; Holstege & Collewijn, 1982; Itaya & Itaya, 1985). Their fibers link the visual system with nuclei regulating the intrinsic and extrinsic musculature of the eye. In rodents, rabbits, and cats, these terminal nuclei are intimately involved in visual-vestibular interactions (Itaya, 1980; Holstege & Collewijn, 1982; Itaya & Itaya, 1985). The pretectal region consists of a group of five nuclei in most mammals, with a similar complex existing in and around the pulvinar in primates (Berman, 1977; Hutchins & Weber, 1985). These complexes have dense bilateral projections, and elements in this group also form a retinocerebellar relay to pontine nuclei and the inferior olivary nucleus (Terasawa, Ottani, & Yamada, 1979; Hutchins & Weber, 1985).

Efferents are also sent from the pulvinar and the superior colliculi to the striate and extrastriate cortices (Holstege & Collewijn, 1982). These are in addition to those efferents from these sites that synapse in the pulvinar before projecting to the visual cortical areas (Terasawa et al., 1979). It should be noted that these extrageniculate pathways lack the strict retinotopically ordered mapping of the geniculostriate pathways.

In 2004, Sincich et al. described a direct geniculate input to V1, using a retrograde tracing technique in the macaque monkey (Sincich, Park, Wohlgemuth, & Horton, 2004). They reported that the constituent neurons in this pathway sent almost no collateral axons to primary visual cortex, and constituted around 10% of the V1 population innervating MT. This finding further explains the phenomenon of blindsight, and suggests that residual perception after damage to primary visual cortex could arise from direct thalamic input to "secondary" or heteromodal cortical areas.

13.3 IPSILATERAL REPRESENTATION OF THE VISUAL HEMIFIELD

In primates and other mammals, it was accepted that visual input to each cerebral hemisphere comes solely or largely from the contralateral visual field. In macaque monkeys, input to V1 was believed to be only from the contralateral visual field (Dow, Snyder, Vautin, & Bauer, 1981; Tootell, Switkes, et al., 1988). Electrophysiological studies have demonstrated that as neurons are progressively further removed from striate cortex, their receptive fields become correspondingly larger, losing the strict retinotopy of V1 and V2 but receiving a larger visual field input from the ipsilateral side. In striate cortex, the ipsilateral input occurs mainly near the retinotopic representation of the vertical meridian, the "seam" along which the left and right hemifield representations are united. In extrastriate areas, receptive fields become so large and bilateral that retinotopy is rendered difficult to demonstrate. However, there is evidence that the same relationship of callosal terminations along a coarsely defined vertical meridian is preserved (Van Essen, Newsome, & Maunsell, 1984). Even in those extrastriate areas where retinotopy cannot be resolved, neurons vary in the extent of their ipsilateral input, with differences having been identified in the macaque MST area and immediately adjacent MT area (Albright, 1984; Ungerleider & Desimone, 1986). In addition, there are differences between the excitatory hemispheric overlap of the lateral intraparietal area in the macaque (LIP) and V4, which both show very little activity (Blatt, Andersen, & Stoner, 1990), and the inferotemporal cortex, which displays a great deal of ipsilateral activation (Desimone, Moran, Schein, & Mishkin, 1993). These electrophysiological variations are thought to reflect differences in the corresponding densities of callosal input within the same cortical regions (DeYoe, Felleman, Van Essen, & McClendon, 1994).

In the 1990s the ipsilateral representation of the visual field in the human striate cortex was also identified (Clarke & Miklossy, 1990; Tootell, Mendola, Hadjikhani, Liu, & Dale, 1998). The first fMRI maps of ipsilateral activation were published in 1998 by Tootell and colleagues, and they found a corresponding expansion of ipsilateral activity extending anteriorly, particularly into the temporal lobe when naturalistic stimuli were used (Tootell, Mendola, et al., 1998). The findings were consistent with the idea that color and form are processed in a more ventral stream,

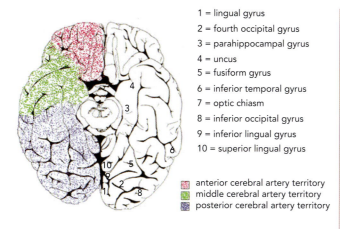

1 = lingual gyrus
2 = fourth occipital gyrus
3 = parahippocampal gyrus
4 = uncus
5 = fusiform gyrus
6 = inferior temporal gyrus
7 = optic chiasm
8 = inferior occipital gyrus
9 = inferior lingual gyrus
10 = superior lingual gyrus

anterior cerebral artery territory
middle cerebral artery territory
posterior cerebral artery territory

Figure 13.3 Cartoon of inferior (ventral) surface of the brain depicting cerebral blood supply of these areas.

with motion and spatial relations being processed more dorsally (and see below). They found that:

"Human visual information is processed first in the contralateral visual field, the processing gradually crosses the vertical meridian as receptive fields become larger and extend into the ipsilateral visual field. Visual information is represented even more bilaterally in correspondingly more anterior areas, with much larger receptive fields and without demonstrable retinotopy. Converging fMRI evidence suggests that human area MT and the lateral occipital region have such bilaterally responsive, large, poorly retinotopic receptive fields." (Tootell, Mendola, et al., 1998)

These findings were important because not only did they concord with theories of visual processing streams for objects versus movement, they also highlighted the importance of transcallosal inputs in visual processing, which may be important pathways in the recovery of visual function following lesions to striate cortex.

13.4 STRIATE–EXTRASTRIATE CONNECTIONS—THE "WHAT" AND "WHERE" PATHWAYS

The striate cortex projects an array of efferents into a number of different extrastriate areas (Felleman & Van Essen, 1991). Two broad streams of connections were identified in the macaque monkey in the early 1980s, further described by Felleman and Van Essen in their seminal paper in 1991 (Felleman & Van Essen, 1991). In monkeys, these are the ventral or "what" stream projecting into inferotemporal cortex, and the dorsal or "where" stream projecting into posterior parietal cortex (Ungerleider & Mishkin, 1982; Zeki, 1990, 1993; Felleman & Van Essen, 1991;

Ungerleider & Haxby, 1994). In addition, the extrageniculostriate projection connects the superior colliculi to the dorsal stream via the pulvinar (see Figure 13.2). These pathways were identified in humans in the 1990s with PET and fMRI (Haxby et al., 1991, 1994; Ungerleider & Haxby, 1994).

Ungerleider and Mishkin went on to argue that these two pathways separated and maintained their separation from early on, in extrastriate stratification (Desimone & Ungerleider, 1986; Ungerleider & Desimone, 1986). They argued that neurons in striate cortex projected simultaneously into extrastriate cortical sites, quickly separating the object and movement pathways (Ungerleider & Mishkin, 1982). Lesion-based case studies in humans initially provided compelling evidence of an identical system in the human brain, but some recent studies have proposed a more synergistic model. In particular, Goodale and Milner have hypothesized that both streams process information about object features and about their spatial location at the same time (Milner & Goodale, 2008). Most researchers now agree that there are separate processing pathways: "vision for perception" and "vision for action."

13.5 VENTRAL EXTRASTRIATE CORTEX: VISUAL OBJECT RECOGNITION AND PROCESSING

The ventral stream comprises the inferior part of the occipital pole, including parts of the lingual gyrus and the inferior and fourth occipital gyri, extending anteriorly into the inferotemporal cortex. It includes the fusiform gyrus and the parahippocampal gyrus, as well as the inferior temporal gyrus (see Figure 13.3). Various areas within this system have been identified as being specifically activated by differing stimuli. Some examples of specialized neural modules include the fusiform face area and the parahippocampal place area.

Researchers in the early 1990s used electrophysiological techniques to study the temporal cortex of monkeys and found regions that responded selectively to faces and not to other stimulus categories (Desimone, 1991; Harries & Perrett, 1991). Sergent and colleagues first described the functional specialization of areas of the ventral extrastriate cortex for faces in humans with PET in 1992 (Sergent, Ohta, & MacDonald, 1992; Sergent & Signoret, 1992), and their findings were later confirmed by Haxby et al. with a PET study comparing activation to faces and locations (Haxby et al., 1994). Whole faces appear disproportionately represented in the fusiform face area (FFA), but building blocks of faces are represented in occipitotemporal cortex (Summerfield, Egner, Mangels, & Hirsch, 2006; Steeves et al., 2009; Nichols, Betts, & Wilson, 2010).

Several authors have revealed activation to images of locations and images in the parahippocampal gyrus (Haxby et al., 1991; Epstein & Kanwisher, 1998). However, this region differs from the FFA in that it appears to be intimately involved in place encoding to memory, not just to location perception (Epstein, Harris, Stanley, & Kanwisher, 1999; Kanwisher, 2000). The evidence for the parahippocampal place area (PPA) appeared well supported by pathological case studies of patients with topographic disorientation associated with parahippocampal lesions, which is rarely described (Habib & Sirigu, 1987). Many scene-selective regions in human visual cortex are now recognized, such as the parahippocampal place area (PPA), transverse occipital sulcus, and retrosplenial cortex, each of which has been linked to higher-order functions such as navigation, scene perception and recognition, and contextual association (Nasr et al., 2011). A number of category-sensitive regions for the human body have also been identified, such as the OFA mentioned above, and body-sensitive cortex in the extrastriate body area (J. C. Taylor & Downing, 2011). These regions are particularly interesting, as they appear to be vital for human social cognition (Brefczynski-Lewis, Berrebi, McNeely, Prostko, & Puce, 2011).

Most of these studies used standard BOLD fMRI techniques to identify regions. The whole field of category-selective processing has been recently challenged by the concept of distributed processing, with authors such as Kriegeskorte arguing that perceptual and cognitive content is represented in the brain by patterns of activity across populations of neurons (Kriegeskorte, 2009). At the time of writing this chapter, researchers from Gallant's group demonstrated that quantitative modeling of human brain activity could provide insights about cortical representations, potentially forming the basis for brain decoding devices. They modeled brain activity elicited by static visual patterns using a new motion-energy encoding model (Nishimoto et al., 2011). The field remains dynamic.

13.6 COLOR AND MOVEMENT

The color perception regions, as well as dorsal extrastriate cortices, will not be discussed as these regions are not directly relevant to this chapter.

13.6.1 DORSAL EXTRASTRIATE CORTEX: VISUAL MOTION PERCEPTION

The dorsal stream projects superiorly and laterally from the calcarine cortex into the posterior parietal region. It comprises the intraparietal sulcus, the superior temporal sulcus, the middle temporal gyrus, and the lateral occipital sulcus. Area V5, the region believed to be essential for human motion perception, lies at the border of the occipital and temporal lobes in part of infero-middle temporal gyrus (Cardoso-Leite & Gorea, 2010; Frost, 2010).

The monkey area MT, also known as V5, had been identified as critical for motion processing and contains a large proportion of neurons that are selectively sensitive to stimulus direction, speed, orientation, and depth (Albright, 1984). While the presence of motion-selective areas in the monkey brain had been known for some time, it is only since the 1990s that analogous areas in the human brain have been identified. This is in part due to the rarity of a human model for failed motion perception, known as *cerebral akinetopsia*. Indeed, the term was first used in a review by Zeki in 1991 (Zeki, 1991). There are case studies of akinetopsia—most famously a patient known in the literature as L. M., who suffered bilateral posterior hemispheric damage secondary to presumed venous sinus thrombosis—but the nature of the causative injuries was often too diffuse to infer much about the location of motion perception in the human brain (Zihl, von Cramon, & Mai, 1983). However, several researchers did identify a number of occipitotemporoparietal and parieto-occipital areas involved in patients with abnormalities of motion perception (Vaina, Lemay, Bienfang, Choi, & Nakayama, 1990; Vaina, Cowey, & Kennedy, 1999).

Functional neuroimaging led to the identification of an MT equivalent area in humans, called V5, in 1991 (Zeki, 1991). Further studies with PET and fMRI confirmed its location in the temporo-occipital junction, and also revealed the orientation selectivity of cells in V3 (Watson et al., 1993; Shipp, de Jong, Zihl, Frackowiak, & Zeki, 1994; Sereno et al., 1995; Shipp, Watson, Frackowiak, & Zeki, 1995). In addition, a third motion stimuli responsive area was identified in the superior parietal lobe, just anterior to the parieto-occipital fissure (Shipp et al., 1994). These results have been replicated by a number of researchers, and disorders of motion perception temporarily induced by transcranial magnetic stimulation (Thakral & Slotnick, 2011). Subsequent scanning of the patient L. M. confirmed bilateral damage to areas V5 and V3 (Shipp et al., 1994).

Since these early studies, there have been great advances made in the field of human motion processing. In particular, Vaina's group have systematically analyzed motion-sensitive areas of the brain in normal controls and post-stroke patients, and have concluded that there are at least three motion mechanisms in the human visual system: a low-level first-order and second-order motion mechanism and a high-level attention or position-based mechanism (Vaina et al., 2010; Vaina & Dumoulin, 2011).

13.7 VISUAL SYNDROMES CAUSED BY STROKE

Stroke can affect any part of the visual pathway from the retina to the primary visual cortex—see Figure 13.4. The site of the stroke determines the type of visual deficit. These deficits can be broadly divided into simple visual field abnormalities alone, or those associated with disorders of higher visual cognition. Up to two-thirds of patients with acute hemispheric stroke will have some visual field deficit (Gray et al., 1989). Visuospatial dysfunction is also known to confer a worse prognosis, particularly when associated with neglect (Jehkonen et al., 2000).

13.7.1 VISUAL FIELD DEFICITS FOLLOWING STROKE

The prevalence of visual field deficits associated with stroke is believed to be between 0.5%–1% (Geddes et al., 1996; H. R. Taylor, Livingston, Stanislavsky, & McCarty, 1997). A population-based study looking at the incidence of homonymous visual field defects and stroke found that 8% of patients who reported having a stroke had an homonymous visual field defect, with the overall prevalence in an older population (aged >49 years) being 0.8% (Gilhotra, Mitchell, Healey, Cumming, & Currie, 2002). This value also appeared to rise with increasing age over 70 years.

13.7.1.1 MONOCULAR VISUAL DEFICITS
Rarely, monocular temporal crescentic field loss can occur with posterior optic radiation or anterior occipital lobe

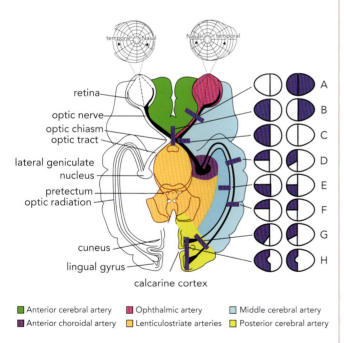

Figure 13.4 Diagram of the visual system depicting common visual field deficits (left), arterial supply (below), and their anatomical correlations. A = monocular full loss associated with retinal artery occlusion; B = bitemporal hemianopia; C = incongruous homonymous defect from anterior optic radiation involvement; D = asymmetrical congruous homonymous defect; E = inferior, and F = superior quadrantanopia from lesions in the E = parietal and F = temporal components of the optic radiation; G = incongruous partial homonymous hemianopia from anterior occipital infarction (non–macular sparing); H = classical macular sparing homonymous hemianopia from posterior calcarine infarction.

lesions that damage the projection of unpaired peripheral nasal fibers. However, these are uncommon, as monocular peripheral visual field defects arise from retinal lesions in the majority of cases. The reverse lesion can be seen in homonymous hemianopias caused by posterior occipital lobe lesions that may spare the anterior striate cortex, in essence causing a hemianopic defect with temporal crescent sparing.

13.7.2 HOMONYMOUS VISUAL DEFICITS

13.7.2.1 LATERAL GENICULATE NUCLEUS LESIONS
These are caused by lateral choroidal or anterior choroidal artery occlusion, and are rare. They are distinctive in that they break the visual field rule of respecting the horizontal meridian, and can manifest as a congruous wedge-shaped homonymous defect that straddles this horizontal watershed (McFadzean & Hadley, 1997; Jones, Waggoner, & Hoyt, 1999; Slotnick & Moo, 2003; see Figure 13.4).

13.7.2.2 QUADRANTANOPIC VISUAL FIELD DEFECTS
Quadrantanopic visual field defects can be caused by both striate and extrastriate cortical lesions (McFadzean & Hadley, 1997). Ventral extrastriate lesions tend to manifest with a superior quadrantanopia, as the fibers supplying the superior visual quadrant dip down near the ventral extrastriate cortex (Horton & Hoyt, 1991). Less commonly, lesions of the posterior parietal (dorsal extrastriate) cortex cause inferior quadrantanopia, as this is an area of the brain that is rarely infarcted with a solitary lesion. It is more likely to be included in a large MCA stroke, although small embolic strokes in this territory can occur (see Figure 13.4, D–F).

13.7.2.3 HEMIANOPIC VISUAL FIELD DEFECTS
Complete homonymous hemianopia in an individual patient has essentially no localizing value, as it can arise from a lesion in any retrochiasmal site. However, as a general principle the pattern of the defect in each eye becomes more congruous as the lesion approaches the occipital lobe. The optic radiations are often affected by middle cerebral artery (MCA) territory strokes, causing homonymous visual defects that are usually more incongruous than those caused by occipital lesions. Lesions of the striate cortex caused by posterior cerebral artery (PCA) territory strokes usually produce a complete homonymous hemianopia, with or without macular sparing, or exquisitely congruous homonymous scotomata that can be anatomically localized within the calcarine architecture (Horton

& Hoyt, 1991; R. McFadzean et al., 1994; Kitajima et al., 1998; see Figure 13.4, G–H).

In a series of 100 patients with homonymous hemianopia, 40% had occipital lobe, 33% parietal lobe, and 24% temporal lobe lesions (J. L. Smith, 1962). Optic tracts and lateral geniculate lesions were rare, and the majority (42%) were caused by stroke. Moreover, in another series of patients presenting with an isolated homonymous hemianopia, 89% were of vascular origin, 86% of which were due to PCA infarcts (Trobe, Lorber, & Schelzinger, 1973).

13.7.3 DISORDERS OF HIGHER VISUAL COGNITION COMMONLY CAUSED BY STROKE

Some of the classical neuropsychological syndromes that have helped shape concepts of human cognition have arisen from studies of stroke subjects. The description and anatomical localization of such conditions as Balint's syndrome, alexia without agraphia, prosopagnosia, blindsight, and neglect have been fundamental to the understanding of neuropsychological principles and cerebral anatomical organization. There are many visuospatial dysfunctions described in the neuropsychological literature, many of them not produced by stroke. In addition, the visual system, as in many of the distributed systems in the human brain, allows for a certain amount of redundancy and some visual syndromes are not seen until bilateral damage to visual cortex ensues.

13.8 MECHANISMS OF RECOVERY FOLLOWING STROKE

There are two major phases to recovery of function following stroke: an acute phase incorporating reperfusion with salvage of extant neurons in ischemic but not infarcted zones and resolution of edema; and a later, or chronic, phase including remodeling or reorganization of surviving cortex to resume or approximate impaired function—see Figure 13.5 and Chapter 6. Recovery predominantly occurs in the first few weeks, and plateaus by three months. However, ongoing improvements in a patient's function can occur over many years.

Recovery over the first few days is usually due to resolution of edema, thereby uncovering the extent of the deficit (Calautti & Baron, 2003). Reperfusion of the ischemic penumbra may also play a part, but it is not yet known to what extent this affects prognosis (Astrup, Siesjo, & Symon, 1981; Donnan & Davis, 2002). In addition, recovery of damaged or ischemic neural networks within the infarct may also contribute, particularly in areas of misery perfusion or chronic ischemia, but these latter two phenomena remain unproven in human studies (Cao, Vikingstad, George, Johnson, & Welch, 1999; Thulborn, Carpenter, & Just, 1999). Cellular level changes, such as

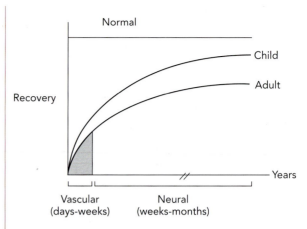

Figure 13.5 Graphical cartoon depicting stages of recovery from stroke. Children exhibit greater plasticity and hence their recovery at every stage is better. (Thanks to Geoffrey Donnan)

cortical reorganization via synaptic sprouting and the formation of new cortical connections, may also contribute to recovery (Darian-Smith & Gilbert, 1994). The majority of functional recovery is probably dependent on ongoing brain reorganization.

13.8.1 NEURAL PLASTICITY POST-STROKE

Neural plasticity has been defined as "short-term modulations of function and long-term structural changes" (Dobkin, 1996), but its mechanisms are poorly understood. It is now believed that sensory and motor cortical representations are dynamically maintained throughout life, in contrast to older theories alleging that while the human brain was enormously plastic during its development, its organization became "fixed" at a fairly early age. Localization concepts of brain function, enshrined by Broca, argued against the ability of the brain to utilize areas or networks that usually govern a different system.

Thankfully, work in primate and other mammalian models and in humans has shown this not to be the case (see also Chapter 3). It now appears clear that cerebral systems participate on both focal levels (as in calcarine cortex in the visual system; Horton & Hoyt, 1991) and distributed levels (widespread attentional networks, as discussed in the above section on neglect; Mesulam, 1981, 1990, 2000), and that functional localization remains a dynamic process even in the adult human brain (Dobkin, 1996; Chollet & Weiller, 2000).

Thus, the changes underlying plasticity seem to occur at both the cellular and systems level in the brain. Neuroimaging studies have built on previous pathophysiological data and suggest that the changes fall into three main groups: spontaneous metabolic reorganization (e.g., diaschisis), recruitment of remote areas via disinhibition or increased excitation, and extension of function into other specialized areas within the same network. Basal metabolic reorganization occurs in the lesioned brain within minutes to hours of infarct. These metabolic changes can be seen in the phenomenon of diaschisis and have been demonstrated by crossed cerebellar diaschisis (Baron, Bousser, Comar, & Castaigne, 1980; Feeney & Baron, 1986) and in multiple supratentorial areas (Lenzi, Frackowiak, & Jones, 1982; Martin & Raichle, 1983), as well as in visual cortex (Brodtmann, Puce, Darby, & Donnan, 2007).

The latter phenomenon includes expansion of cortical representation of the damaged area of the cortex into adjacent areas (peri-infarct), use of ipsilateral pathways in the intact hemisphere (contralesional recruitment), and activation of other cortical and subcortical regions distant to the lesion (vicariance; Chollet & Weiller, 2000; Nudo, 2007).

13.8.2 MECHANISMS OF RECOVERY FOLLOWING INJURY TO THE VISUAL SYSTEM

Natural history studies have generated different results in the estimation of visual field recovery after brain injury. Gray et al. (1989) estimated that less than 20% of completely hemianopic patients had full recovery of their visual fields after a month, while more than 70% of those with partial hemianopias recovered their vision fully in the same time frame. Zhang et al. found that spontaneous visual field defect recovery occurred in at least 50% of a group of 254 patients within 1 month of injury (Zhang, Kedar, Lynn, Newman, & Biousse, 2006a, 2006b).

How does this occur? Until recently, the human visual system had been thought to have an exquisitely contralateral representation and was thought to be one of least plastic parts of the brain (Tootell, Mendola, et al., 1998). Despite a blossoming of interest in mechanisms of cortical recovery following stroke affecting the somatosensory, motor, and language pathways, studies in which the visual cortex is examined are still in the minority. This may be a result of this widely held prior assumption that primary visual cortex, once damaged, was unable to recover because of its precise retinotopy and absence of ipsilateral visual field input. These assumptions have been heavily influenced by Hubel and Wiesel's seminal work on monocular deprivation (Hubel & Wiesel, 1963, 1970; Wiesel & Hubel, 1965) and strabismic rearing (Hubel & Wiesel, 1965). The findings from these early studies led to the concept of visual development being modified by visual experience during "critical periods" early in postnatal life, after which the cortical networks (ocular dominance columns, segregation of geniculocortical afferents) become "hard-wired" and were unable to be affected by further visual experience. However, as more knowledge emerged about the topographic organization of extrastriate visual areas (DeYoe et al., 1996; Baseler, Morland, & Wandell, 1999), retinotectal maps, and evidence of extrastriate cortical plasticity from studies of patients with blindsight and other visual syndromes (see below), it is becoming evident that the visual system, when studied broadly, retains plasticity into late adulthood.

13.8.3 CROSS-MODAL PLASTICITY IN THE VISUAL SYSTEM

Evidence for cross-modal plasticity emerged in the last decade, when functional neuroimaging researchers (using PET, TMS, and fMRI) revealed remarkable activation of the primary visual cortex during tactile tasks. These investigators demonstrated that both extrastriate and striate cortex could be utilized in a variety of tactile discrimination tasks, particularly Braille reading, and went some way in explaining the superior tactile perceptual abilities of subjects who were blind from an early age. However, the extrapolation of these studies was slow. Insights from case studies of patients with blindsight and the Riddoch syndrome suggested that non-striate areas, such as dorsal extrastriate cortex, direct subcortical projections, and even brainstem sites, could be recruited (Marshall & Halligan, 1988; Brogaard, 2011).

Indeed, regions in the visual system appear to be uniquely cross-modal. The cross-modal plasticity literature in the visual system is now extensive and at times revolutionary. There appear to be cross-modal interactions of auditory, visual, somatic and even olfactory inputs, with studies done on blind people demonstrating extraordinary levels of activation in occipital regions to auditory and tactile stimuli (Saenz, Lewis, Huth, Fine, & Koch, 2008; Collignon, Voss, Lassonde, & Lepore, 2009; Fiehler & Rosler, 2010; Lewis, Saenz, & Fine, 2010; Kupers et al., 2011; Striem-Amit, Dakwar, Reich, & Amedi, 2011; Wong, Gnanakumaran, & Goldreich, 2011). These findings represent some of the most exciting advances in cognitive neuroscience, as researchers explore the organizational principles that drive this cross-modal plasticity.

13.8.3.1 THE DORSAL EXTRASTRIATE PATHWAY—A POSSIBLE SITE FOR SURROGACY

It has been demonstrated in monkey models that dorsal extrastriate neurons (in MT) retain visual responsiveness in the presence of deactivated V1, whether this deactivation is via cooling or ablation (Cowey & Stoerig, 1989; Cowey, Stoerig, & Perry, 1989)—some neurons even retain directional tuning. Conversely, the ventral extrastriate regions seem more reliant on intact striate function (Girard, Salin, & Bullier, 1991; Girard, Lomber, & Bullier, 2002). Utilization of dorsal extrastriate sites may also be a reflection of the relative differences of the ventral and dorsal streams in their inherent modifiability. There is evidence of molecular differences between systems with varying levels of experience-dependent plasticity (Neville & Bavelier, 2002). The level of expression of immunoreactivity to the monoclonal antibody CAT 301 is positively correlated with systems with high levels of modifiability and experience-dependent plasticity (Sur, Frost, & Hockfield, 1988; Deyoe, Hockfield, Garren, & Van Essen, 1990). All levels of the dorsal pathway of the macaque monkey visual system display strong immunoreactivity for antibody CAT 301, while the ventral visual pathway displays very little labeling (Deyoe et al., 1990). There is also evidence that the expression of CAT 301 immunoreactivity may play a part in the guidance and stabilization of synaptic structure—important determinants of cortical plasticity (Sur et al., 1988). Another theory argues that the different levels of inherent modifiability are related to patterns of developmental plasticity and systems-based learning mechanisms (Neville & Bavelier, 2002). For example, systems that display experience-dependent change throughout life, such as the establishment of form, face, and object representations, may rely upon different developmental learning mechanisms than systems associated with mediating dynamically shifting relations and computations, such as motion and direction detection in the dorsal stream. Finally, the dorsal extrastriate cortex also has more abundant connections via the colliculo-pulvinar pathways compared to the ventral extrastriate cortex (Terasawa et al., 1979; Holstege & Collewijn, 1982).

13.9 VISUAL RECOVERY HYPOTHESES

There are a number of possible mechanisms for visual cortical plasticity. Some researchers argue that spared neurons within the banks of the calcarine and pericalcarine fissures remodel and assume activity for the extant retinogeniculate projections. The concept of "spared islands" of tissue had been most strongly presented by Fendrich and coworkers, who put forward evidence of residual neuronal activity based on high-resolution perimetry (Fendrich, Wessinger, & Gazzaniga, 1992). However, results from functional neuroimaging studies have not been able to support this hypothesis (Baseler et al., 1999; Schoenfeld et al., 2002).

Another hypothesis asserts that retinal information reaches extrastriate cortical locations directly via extrageniculostriate pathways, bypassing V1/striate cortex. Results from several fMRI experiments on patients with blindsight/Riddoch syndrome have demonstrated such ipsilesional extrastriate activation. However, the temporal hierarchy of these extrageniculostriate projections has not been fully clarified; namely, whether they project initially to lower-tier levels such as the cuneus and peristriate cortex (V2), to dorsal extrastriate cortex (V3), or to higher-tier levels, such as V5. Another contributing factor could be that recovery is occurring via recruitment

of transcallosal pathways and interhemispheric connections, which are known to cause the bilateral activation seen in unilateral presentation of visual images in normal subjects (Tootell et al., 1998; Tootell, Mendola, et al., 1998; Brandt, Stephan, Bense, Yousry, & Dieterich, 2000). As in studies of motor and sensory recovery, it could be that these pathways are "disinhibited" by the destruction of contralateral visual cortex, and the connectivity of these projections is enhanced (Liepert, Hamzei, & Weiller, 2000; Cicinelli et al., 2003). It has also been demonstrated that stroke-related injuries lead to the formation of new within-network intracortical connections via axonal reorganization (Dancause et al., 2005; Nudo, 2006, 2007, 2011). Benowitz and Carmichael (2010) have argued that this reorganization remains constrained by a number of factors, including extracellular growth inhibitors, limited trophic agents, and other factors that are intrinsic to neurons themselves.

Many researchers maintain that, as demonstrated in other brain areas, the "higher" the cortical visual area the less rigid the topographic mapping and the more bilaterality of representation, hence the greater ease of assumption of other visual roles to compensate in the event of injury. Data from fMRI studies in motor and sensory stroke support this, as do the findings from studies in stroke affecting visual pathways (Chollet et al., 1991; Chollet & Weiller, 2000; S.C. Cramer, Moore, Finklestein, & Rosen, 2000; Calautti, Leroy, Guincestre, & Baron, 2001, 2003; S. C. Cramer et al., 2001; Nelles et al., 2002; Calautti & Baron, 2003). In many of the more recent studies where researchers have focused on recovery and restorative therapies, the possible effects of these expanded receptive fields have been examined. There is good evidence that fMRI retinotopic maps do correlate with receptive fields. Smith et al. used fMRI to estimate the average receptive field sizes of neurons in several striate and extrastriate visual areas of the human cerebral cortex, and their results were consistent with neurophysiological data from macaque monkeys (A.T. Smith, Singh, Williams, & Greenlee, 2001).

13.9.1 EXPERIMENTS IN VISUAL RECOVERY FOLLOWING STROKE

13.9.1.1 PET STUDIES IN THE VISUAL SYSTEM FOLLOWING STROKE

Bosley and coworkers performed a series of PET studies in the mid to late1980s examining the effects of stroke, both PCA and MCA, on the visual system. They used serial 18-flouro-2-deoxyglucose PET to serially study five patients with strokes affecting the posterior afferent visual system causing homonymous hemianopia (Bosley et al., 1987). They demonstrated a reduction in size of the metabolic lesion and improvement in striate cortex metabolism in patients with visual recovery. These findings were not seen in patients with persistent visual field defects (Bosley et al., 1987). They also demonstrated evidence of diaschisis in the visual cortex when lesions were situated in the optic radiations. Three patients with damage limited to the optic radiation had decreased glucose metabolism in the portion of striate cortex appropriate for the visual field defect (Bosley et al., 1985). Changes in glucose metabolism were also noted to occur in undamaged ipsilateral thalamic and extrastriate cortical areas. In another cross-sectional study, where patients were examined 3–30 days following MCA stroke causing homonymous hemianopia, the investigators found diffuse hypometabolism throughout the ipsilesional cerebral hemisphere, including in areas that were not obviously ischemic on clinical examination or neuroimaging (Kiyosawa et al., 1990).

13.9.1.2 MRI STUDIES IN THE VISUAL SYSTEM FOLLOWING STROKE

13.9.1.2.1 Insights from Blindsight
A subset of patients with hemianopic loss retain the ability to detect the presence and direction of motion in the blind hemifield, without being able to assign other attributes (color, form) to the moving object. This phenomenon was called *Riddoch syndrome* by Zeki and Ffytche in 1998, after an army surgeon who originally described its occurrence in soldiers in 1917 (Zeki & Ffytche, 1998). It has been most extensively studied in G. Y., an English patient who was rendered hemianopic following a lesion affecting his primary visual cortex in his youth. It has now been retrospectively recognized following stroke (Zeki & Ffytche, 1998), although until the eponymous name was created, these individuals were probably described as having a form of blindsight (Stoerig, Kleinschmidt, & Frahm, 1998; Ptito, Fortin, & Ptito, 2001; Sahraie et al., 2003). Blindsight can also be induced with TMS, and this had allowed further understanding of this fascinating window into visual processing (Ro & Rafal, 2006).

Baseler and colleagues studied a G. Y. using fMRI with a retinotopic mapping paradigm (Baseler et al., 1999). When stimuli were confined to his blind hemifield, activation was seen mainly in dorsal extrastriate cortex, which exhibited abnormal retinotopic organization dependent on the stimulus condition (Baseler et al., 1999). Retinotopic mapping in the residual lesioned occipital cortex displayed a more conventional pattern. In a further case study on another subject who had suffered a left PCA hemorrhagic infarct 3 years previously, the investigators used MEG and fMRI (with a motion and color detection task) to study the spatial and temporal aspects of these connections (Schoenfeld et al., 2002). They found further evidence for subcortical mediation of spared visual capacities, and observed reorganization of visual inputs. The authors

suggested this was a function of increased connectivity between V5 and other extrastriate sites. However, the primary aim of these studies was to explain the phenomena of blindsight and the Riddoch syndrome, and researchers did not directly address the mechanisms of primary perceptual vision and visual field recovery following injury. Until the last decade, few investigators had attempted to correlate functional neuroimaging findings with visual field recovery post-stroke.

Baseler et al. performed fMRI retinotopic mapping on G. Y., in order to describe the extent that topographic maps in human extrastriate cortex reorganize after damage to the primary visual cortex. They sought to distinguish between the three possible consequences of a partial V1 lesion on extrastriate areas, these being no reorganization following injury, retention of normal topographic representation from extrageniculostriate or transcallosal (together subcortical) inputs, or the possibility that extrastriate cortex reorganizes and recruits inputs from spared regions or V1. Their findings supported the latter two theories, and particularly the presence of plasticity, colonization and reorganization in the surviving regions of occipital cortex (Baseler et al., 1999). Goebel et al. studied two patients (one of whom was G. Y.) with chronic traumatic brain injuries causing longstanding post-geniculate lesions of the left hemisphere (Goebel, Muckli, Zanella, Singer, & Stoerig, 2001). They used fMRI with two visual paradigms: a rotating spiral for dorsal extrastriate activation and colored images of natural objects for ventral stream activation. They were the first to demonstrate evidence of sustained ipsilesional ventral extrastriate activation to objects presented to the blind hemifield, but noted that despite pronounced cortical activity in both subjects, there was no accompanying awareness of the stimuli. This prompted the authors to conclude that this activation was not restorative, but more likely represented activity in stable resonant neuronal loops—circuits that have been proposed to be the neural correlates of conscious vision (Tononi & Edelman, 1998; Engel & Singer, 2001).

It had remained difficult to evaluate whether recovery involved the formation of new neural connections or whether functional change was due to recruitment of existing pathways. Bridge et al. used diffusion-weighted MRI to demonstrate an ipsilateral pathway in both controls and G. Y. between the LGN and MT+/V5, bypassing V1 (Bridge, Thomas, Jbabdi, & Cowey, 2008). G. Y. demonstrated two additional features absent in controls: a contralateral pathway from right LGN to left MT+/V5 and a substantial corticocortical connection between MT+/V5 regions bilaterally, with possible evidence for a pathway in G. Y. from the left LGN to the right MT+/V5. The authors concluded that these findings were evidence that utilizing alternative brain regions following childhood cortical damage might strengthen or establish specific connections.

13.9.1.2.2 Insights from Visual Field Deficits

Schoenfeld et al. (2002) were the first to examine the pathways that mediated preserved vision in a single patient with homonymous hemianopia and Riddoch syndrome following left striate cortical infarction 3 years previously. They used a combined fMRI and magnetoencephalographic (MEG) approach, in order to provide superior spatiotemporal resolution. Their findings suggested that retained motion perception in the blind hemifield (Riddoch syndrome) was mediated via subcortical pathways, bypassing V1, projecting first to extrastriate regions (V5 and V4/V8) before subsequently projecting back to peristriate regions (V2/V3). Their findings provided strong support to the hypothesis that input to (particularly dorsal) ipsilesional extrastriate regions arrives via subcortical colliculo-pulvinar connections, projecting mainly to V5/MT. They also demonstrated increased connectivity between V4/V8 and V5 in the lesioned hemisphere, suggested to be due to reorganization of the visual inputs to these areas following the striate lesion.

Nelles et al. (2002) then looked at a group of patients an average of 17 months following striate cortical infarction. Their aim was simply to investigate the patterns of brain activation in patients with post-stroke visual field defects after a single occipital stroke, using a hemifield stimulation paradigm to segregate brain activation during stimulation of the hemianopic versus normal side. They found pronounced ipsilateral (contralesional) activation of peristriate and extrastriate visual cortices, and absent striate cortical activation during stimulation of the blind hemifield. However, they were unable to distinguish whether this activation was via transcallosal pathways, deviations in central fixation, or disinhibition of the normal ipsilateral visual field representation. No comment was made on the presence of enhanced ipsilesional dorsal extrastriate activation, but it may be that this was not specifically the focus of the study.

Brodtmann and colleagues performed serial fMRI studies on patients with visual cortex infarction to evaluate early and late striate, ventral, and dorsal extrastriate cortical activation (Brodtmann, Puce, Darby, & Donnan, 2009). Patients were studied with fMRI within 10 days and at 6 months post-stroke, using a high-level visual activation task designed to activate ventral extrastriate cortex. These data were compared to those of age-appropriate healthy control subjects. Patients had infarcts involving striate and ventral extrastriate cortex. Patient activation patterns were markedly different to controls, demonstrating a reduction in bilateral striate and ventral extrastriate activation at both sessions, with preservation of dorsal extrastriate activated voxel counts. Conversely, mean percent magnetic resonance signal change increased in dorsal sites. We concluded that these results provided strong evidence of bilateral post-stroke functional depression of striate and ventral extrastriate cortices, and surrogate utilization or *vicariance* of the dorsal visual system following

stroke. In subsequent studies with fMRI as well as other advanced imaging techniques, such as diffusion tensor imaging, further evidence of visual cortical plasticity has been demonstrated after stroke and other brain injury (Nelles, de Greiff, Pscherer, Forsting, et al., 2007; Nelles, de Greiff, Pscherer, Stude et al., 2007; Polonara et al., 2011; Schmielau & Wong, 2007; Ho et al., 2009). Evidence for ipsilesional peri-infarct activation, changes in connectivity, and contralesional expansion of neural receptive fields has been demonstrated.

13.10 RESTORATIVE THERAPIES: REHABILITATING THE HUMAN VISUAL SYSTEM

In the late 1990s and early 2000s, a number of research groups postulated that deficits caused by acquired visual pathway injury in adulthood were potentially reversible through visual training strategies. In a special 2008 issue of *Restorative Neurology and Neuroscience* on the topic of "Visual System Restoration and Plasticity," Sabel stated that the "traditional view that visual system damage is permanent has given way to a more optimistic view" (Sabel, 2008). Researchers demonstrated evidence of visual field recovery in people with stable lesions, often with lesions that were many years old (Kasten et al., 1999; Poggel, Kasten, & Sabel, 2004; Kasten, Bunzenthal, & Sabel, 2006; Poggel, Kasten, Muller-Oehring, Bunzenthal, & Sabel, 2006; Chokron et al., 2008; Henriksson, Raninen, Nasanen, Hyvarinen, & Vanni, 2007; Jobke, Kasten, & Sabel, 2009; Kasten, Bunzenthal, Muller-Oehring, Mueller, & Sabel, 2007; Mueller, Gall, Kasten, & Sabel, 2008; Poggel, Mueller, Kasten, Bunzenthal, & Sabel, 2010; Raemaekers, Bergsma, van Wezel, van der Wildt, & van den Berg, 2011). The training usually consists of target detection during gaze fixation. During training, the subjects are asked to fix their gaze centrally while detecting stimuli in the border zone of the impaired and unimpaired visual fields, in other words on the edge of their visual field deficit, with attention measured. Results from these studies have demonstrated a gradual enlargement of their functional visual field, and concomitant reduction in their objective visual field deficit (Bergsma & van der Wildt, 2010).

However, these claims have not been without controversy. This is despite renewed interest in the possible benefits of newer forms of visual rehabilitation therapies that may improve outcome in some patients with chronic visual loss (Kasten, Wust, Behrens-Baumann, & Sabel, 1998; Poggel et al., 2004; Schreiber et al., 2006). It remains unclear whether such therapies are causing actual improvement of visual field deficits or whether they are adaptive, causing functional improvement by increased saccades into the affected hemifield (Reinhard et al., 2005; Glisson & Galetta, 2007). The introduction of kinetic stimuli into such newer computerized visual therapies is feasible (Spitzyna et al., 2007). When the early studies were first published, many researchers felt that the functional improvements demonstrated by the authors were due to better scanning and attention, rather than a true expansion of the visual field. In further studies, the field expansion was shown to be independent of eye movements (Kasten et al., 2006). Mueller, Mast, and Sabel performed a large clinical observational study of 302 patients before and after being treated with computer-based vision restoration therapy (VRT) for a period of 6 months at eight clinical centers. In around 70% of patients, VRT was associated with a 17% improvement in super-threshold stimuli detection in the blind hemifield. These detection gains were not significantly correlated with eye movements, and were validated by standard perimetry (Mueller, Mast, & Sabel, 2007).

These restorative studies have also allowed insights into the neuronal mechanisms underlying recovery. After intensive, prolonged (200 plus hours) training, Hendrikkson et al. (2007) found evidence of contralesional processing of visual information from both hemifields, suggesting that neurons in the intact hemisphere had massively expanded their receptive fields, or gained a second receptive field. However, Raemaekers et al. (2011) found no evidence for the emergence of a second representation in the contralesional cortex after training. Not surprisingly, training appears to be more beneficial in patients with extant ipsilesional cortex, and training effects are also influenced by spatial attention (Chokron et al., 2008).

There is still debate as to whether visual representation that is established via alternative routes, without parallel representation in the primary visual cortices, results in vision that is qualitatively comparable with normal vision. Sabel has argued that these residual structures have a "triple handicap to be fully functional" due to fewer neurons, inadequate and competing attentional resources, and temporally disturbed processing (Sabel, Henrich-Noack, Fedorov, & Gall, 2011). Extant pathways are rendered unable to make a meaningful contribution to everyday vision, and their coexisting and parallel "non-use" further impairs the capacity for developing functional improvements.

13.11 SUMMARY

The human visual system—despite or because of its complexity—now appears to be extraordinarily plastic. Neural plasticity can improve vision leading to visual recovery. There is now good evidence that this can occur many years after brain injury, at any age and in a range of visual pathway injuries. However, it appears in vision, as it is in all other areas of the brain, that the mantra of recovery is the same: practice, practice, practice.

REFERENCES

Albright, T. D. (1984). Direction and orientation selectivity of neurons in visual area MT of the macaque. *Journal of Neurophysiology, 52*, 1106–1130.

Astrup, J., Siesjo, B. K., & Symon, L. (1981). Thresholds in cerebral ischemia—the ischemic penumbra. *Stroke, 12*(6), 723–725.

Baron, J. C., Bousser, M. G., Comar, D., & Castaigne, P. (1980). "Crossed cerebellar diaschisis" in human supratentorial brain infarction. *Transactions of the American Neurological. Association, 105*, 459–461.

Baseler, H. A., Morland, A. B., & Wandell, B.A. (1999). Topographic organization of human visual areas in the absence of input from primary cortex. *Journal of Neuroscience, 19*(7), 2619–2627.

Benowitz, L. I., & Carmichael, S. T. (2010). Promoting axonal rewiring to improve outcome after stroke. *Neurobiological Disorders, 37*(2), 259–266.

Bergsma, D. P., & van der Wildt, G. (2010). Visual training of cerebral blindness patients gradually enlarges the visual field. *British Journal of Ophthalmology, 94*(1), 88–96.

Berman, N. (1977). Connections of the pretectum. *Journal of Computational Neurology, 174*, 227–254.

Blatt, G. J., Andersen, R. A., & Stoner, G. R. (1990). Visual receptive field organization and cortico-cortical connections of the lateral intraparietal area (area LIP) in the macaque. *Journal of Computational Neurology, 299*(4), 421–445.

Bosley, T. M., Dann, R., Silver, F. L., Alavi, A., Kushner, M., Chawluk, J. B., et al. (1987). Recovery of vision after ischemic lesions: positron emission tomography. *Annals of Neurology, 21*(5), 444–450.

Bosley, T. M., Rosenquist, A. C., Kushner, M., Burke, A., Stein, A., Dann, R., et al. (1985). Ischemic lesions of the occipital cortex and optic radiations: positron emission tomography. *Neurology, 35*(4), 470–484.

Brandt, T., Stephan, T., Bense, S., Yousry, T. A., & Dieterich, M. (2000). Hemifield visual motion stimulation: an example of interhemispheric crosstalk. *Neuroreport, 11*, 2803–2809.

Brefczynski-Lewis, J. A., Berrebi, M. E., McNeely, M. E., Prostko, A. L., & Puce, A. (2011). In the blink of an eye: neural responses elicited to viewing the eye blinks of another individual. *Frontiers in Human Neuroscience, 5*, 68.

Bridge, H., Thomas, O., Jbabdi, S., & Cowey, A. (2008). Changes in connectivity after visual cortical brain damage underlie altered visual function. *Brain, 131*(Pt 6), 1433–1444.

Brodtmann, A., Puce, A., Darby, D., & Donnan, G. (2007). fMRI demonstrates diaschisis in the extrastriate visual cortex. *Stroke, 38*(8), 2360–2363.

Brodtmann, A., Puce, A., Darby, D., & Donnan, G. (2009). Serial Functional Imaging Poststroke Reveals Visual Cortex Reorganization. *Neurorehabilitation and Neural Repair, 23*(2), 150–159.

Brogaard, B. (2011). Conscious vision for action versus unconscious vision for action? *Cognitive Science, 35*(6), 1076–1104.

Calautti, C., & Baron, J. C. (2003). Functional neuroimaging studies of motor recovery after stroke in adults: a review. *Stroke, 34*(6), 1553–1566.

Calautti, C., Leroy, F., Guincestre, J. Y., & Baron, J. C. (2001). Dynamics of motor network overactivation after striatocapsular stroke: a longitudinal PET study using a fixed-performance paradigm. *Stroke, 32*(11), 2534–2542.

Calautti, C., Leroy, F., Guincestre, J.Y., & Baron, J. C. (2003). Displacement of primary sensorimotor cortex activation after subcortical stroke: a longitudinal PET study with clinical correlation. *NeuroImage, 19*(4), 1650–1654.

Callaway, E. M. (2005). Neural substrates within primary visual cortex for interactions between parallel visual pathways. *Progress in Brain Research, 149*, 59–64.

Cao, Y., Vikingstad, B. S., George, K. P., Johnson, A. F., & Welch, K. M. A. (1999). Cortical language activation in stroke patients recovering from aphasia with functional MRI. *Stroke, 30*, 2331–2340.

Cardoso-Leite, P., & Gorea, A. (2010). On the perceptual/motor dissociation: a review of concepts, theory, experimental paradigms and data interpretations. *Seeing Perceiving, 23*(2), 89–151.

Chen, W., Zhu, X. H., Thulborn, K. R., & Ugurbil, K. (1999). Retinotopic mapping of lateral geniculate nucleus in humans using functional magnetic resonance imaging. *Proceedings of the National Academy of Science U S A, 96*(5), 2430–2434.

Chokron, S., Perez, C., Obadia, M., Gaudry, I., Laloum, L., & Gout, O. (2008). From blindsight to sight: cognitive rehabilitation of visual field defects. *Restorative Neurology and Neuroscience, 26*(4–5), 305–320.

Chollet, F., DiPiero, V., Wise, R. J., Brooks, D. J., Dolan, R. J., & Frackowiak, R. S. (1991). The functional anatomy of motor recovery after stroke in humans: a study with positron emission tomography. *Annals of Neurology, 29*(1), 63–71.

Chollet, F., & Weiller, C. (2000). Recovery of neurological function. In J. Mazziota, A. Toga, & R. S. Frackowiak (Eds.), *Brain mapping: The disorders* (pp. 587–597). San Diego: Academic Press.

Cicinelli, P., Pasqualetti, P., Zaccagnini, M., Traversa, R., Oliveri, M., & Rossini, P. M. (2003). Interhemispheric asymmetries of motor cortex excitability in the postacute stroke stage: a paired-pulse transcranial magnetic stimulation study. *Stroke, 34*(11), 2653–2658.

Clarke, S., & Miklossy, J. (1990). Occipital cortex in man: organization of callosal connections, related myelo- and cytoarchitecture, and putative boundaries of functional visual areas. *Journal of Computational Neurology, 298*(2), 188–214.

Collignon, O., Voss, P., Lassonde, M., & Lepore, F. (2009). Cross-modal plasticity for the spatial processing of sounds in visually deprived subjects. *Experimental Brain Research, 192*(3), 343–358.

Cowey, A., & Stoerig, P. (1989). Projection patterns of surviving neurons in the dorsal lateral geniculate nucleus following discrete lesions of striate cortex: implications for residual vision. *Experimental Brain Research, 75*(3), 691–705.

Cowey, A., Stoerig, P., & Bannister, M. (1994). Retinal ganglion cells labelled from the pulvinar nucleus in macaque monkeys. *Neuroscience, 1994*(61).

Cowey, A., Stoerig, P., & Perry, V.H. (1989). Transneuronal retrograde degeneration of retinal ganglion cells after damage to striate cortex in macaque monkeys: selective loss of P beta cells. *Neuroscience, 29*(1), 65–80.

Cramer, S. C., Moore, C. I., Finklestein, S. P., & Rosen, B. R. (2000). A pilot study of somatotopic mapping after cortical infarct. *Stroke, 31*, 668–671.

Cramer, S. C., Nelles, G., Schaechter, J. D., Kaplan, J. D., Finklestein, S. P., & Rosen, B. R. (2001). A functional MRI study of three motor tasks in the evaluation of stroke recovery. *Neurorehabilitation and Neural Repair, 15*(1), 1–8.

Currie, J. (1997). *Visual field abnormalities.*Unpublished manuscript, Sydney.

Dancause, N., Barbay, S., Frost, S. B., Plautz, E. J., Chen, D., Zoubina, E. V., et al. (2005). Extensive cortical rewiring after brain injury. *Journal of Neuroscience, 25*(44), 10167–10179.

Daniel, P. M., & Whitteridge, D. (1961). The representation of the visual field on the cerebral cortex in monkeys. *Journal of Physiology, 159*, 203–221.

Darian-Smith, C., & Gilbert, C. D. (1994). Axonal sprouting accompanies functional reorganization in adult cat striate cortex. *Nature, 368*, 737–740.

Desimone, R. (1991). Face-selective cells in the temporal cortex of monkeys. *Journal of Cognitive Neuroscience, 115*, 107–117.

Desimone, R., Moran, J., Schein, S. J., & Mishkin, M. (1993). A role for the corpus callosum in visual area V4 of the macaque. *Visual Neuroscience, 10*(1), 159–171.

Desimone, R., & Ungerleider, L. G. (1986). Multiple visual areas in the caudal superior temporal sulcus of the macaque. *Journal of Computational Neurology, 248*(2), 164–189.

DeYoe, E. A., Carman, G. J., Bandettini, P., Glickman, S., Wieser, J., Cox, R., et al. (1996). Mapping striate and extrastriate visual areas in human cerebral cortex. *Proceedings of the National Academy of Science U S A, 93*(6), 2382–2386.

DeYoe, E. A., Felleman, D. J., Van Essen, D. C., & McClendon, E. (1994). Multiple processing streams in occipitotemporal visual cortex. *Nature, 371*(6493), 151–154.

Deyoe, E. A., Hockfield, S., Garren, H., & Van Essen, D. C. (1990). Antibody labeling of functional subdivisions in visual cortex: Cat-301 immunoreactivity in striate and extrastriate cortex of the macaque monkey. *Visual Neuroscience, 5*(1), 67–81.

Dobelle, W. H., Turkel, J., Henderson, D. C., & Evans, J. R. (1979). Mapping the representation of the visual field by electrical stimulation of human visual cortex. *American Journal of Ophthalmology, 88*(4), 727–735.

Dobkin, D. H. (1996). Plasticity in motor and neural networks. In D. H. Dobkin (Ed.), *Neuroscientific foundations in rehabilitation* (pp. 4). Philadelphia: FA Davis Co.

Donnan, G. A., & Davis, S. M. (2002). Neuroimaging, the ischaemic penumbra, and selection of patients for acute stroke therapy. *Lancet Neurology, 1*(7), 417–425.

Dow, B. M., Snyder, A. Z., Vautin, R. G., & Bauer, R. (1981). Magnification factor and receptive field size in foveal striate cortex of the monkey. *Experimental Brain Research, 44*(2), 213–228.

Engel, A.K., & Singer, W. (2001). Temporal binding and the neural correlates of sensory awareness. *Trends in Cognitive Science, 5*, 16–25.

Enroth-Cugell, C., & Robson, J. G. (1966). The contrast sensitivity of retinal ganglion cells of the cat. *Journal of Physiology (Lond), 187*, 517–552.

Epstein, R., Harris, A., Stanley, D., & Kanwisher, N. (1999). The parahippocampal place area: recognition, navigation, or encoding? *Neuron, 23*(1), 115–125.

Epstein, R., & Kanwisher, N. (1998). A cortical representation of the local visual environment. *Nature, 392*(6676), 598–601.

Feeney, D. M., & Baron, J. C. (1986). Diaschisis. *Stroke, 17*, 817–830.

Felleman, D. J., & Van Essen, D. C. (1991). Distributed hierarchical processing in the primate cerebral cortex. *Cerebral Cortex, 1*(1), 1–47.

Fendrich, R., Wessinger, C. M., & Gazzaniga, M. S. (1992). Residual vision in a scotoma: implications for blindsight. *Science, 258*, 1489–1491.

Ffytche, D. H., Howseman, A., Edwards, R., Sandeman, D. R., & Zeki, S. (2000). Human area V5 and motion in the ipsilateral visual field. *European Journal of Neuroscience, 12*(8), 3015–3025.

Fiehler, K., & Rosler, F. (2010). Plasticity of multisensory dorsal stream functions: evidence from congenitally blind and sighted adults. *Restorative Neurology and Neuroscience, 28*(2), 193–205.

Fox, P. T., Miezin, F. M., Allman, J. M., Van Essen, D. C., & Raichle, M. E. (1987). Retinotopic organization of human visual cortex mapped with positron-emission tomography. *Journal of Neuroscience, 7*(3), 913–922.

Frost, B. J. (2010). A taxonomy of different forms of visual motion detection and their underlying neural mechanisms. *Brain Behavior Evolution, 75*(3), 218–235.

Geddes, J. M., Fear, J., Tennant, A., Pickering, A., Hillman, M., & Chamberlain, M. A. (1996). Prevalence of self-reported stroke in a population in northern England. *J Epidemiol Commun Health, 50*, 140–143.

Gilhotra, J. S., Mitchell, P., Healey, P. R., Cumming, R. G., & Currie, J. (2002). Homonymous visual field defects and stroke in an older population. *Stroke, 33*, 2417–2420.

Girard, P., Lomber, S. G., & Bullier, J. (2002). Shape discrimination deficits during reversible deactivation of area V4 in the macaque monkey. *Cerebral Cortex, 12*(11), 1146–1156.

Girard, P., Salin, P. A., & Bullier, J. (1991). Visual activity in macaque area V4 depends on area 17 input. *Neuroreport, 2*(2), 81–84.

Glisson, C. C., & Galetta, S. L. (2007). Visual rehabilitation: now you see it; now you don't. *Neurology, 68*(22), 1881–1882.

Goebel, R., Muckli, L., Zanella, F. E., Singer, W., & Stoerig, P. (2001). Sustained extrastriate cortical activation without visual awareness revealed by fMRI studies of hemianopic patients. *Vision Research, 41*(10–11), 1459–1474.

Gray, C. S., French, J. M., Bates, D., Cartlidge, N. E., Venables, G. S., & James, O. F. (1989). Recovery of visual fields in acute stroke: homonymous hemianopia associated with adverse prognosis. *Age and Ageing, 18*(6), 419–421.

Habib, M., & Sirigu, A. (1987). Pure topographical disorientation: a definition and anatomical basis. *Cortex, 23*, 73–85.

Harries, M. H., & Perrett, D. I. (1991). Visual processing of faces in temporal cortex: Physiological evidence for a modular organization and possible anatomical correlates. *Journal of Cognitive Neuroscience, 3*, 9–24.

Haxby, J., Grady, C., Horwitz, B., Ungerleider, L.G., Mishkin, M., Carson, R. E., et al. (1991). Dissociation of object and spatial visual processing pathways in the human extrastriate cortex. *Proceedings of the National Academy of Science USA, 88*, 1621–1625.

Haxby, J. V., Grady, C. L., Horwitz, B., Ungerleider, L. G., Mishkin, M., Carson, R. E., et al. (1991). Dissociation of object and spatial visual processing pathways in human extrastriate cortex. *Proceedings of the National Academy of Science U S A, 88*(5), 1621–1625.

Haxby, J. V., Horwitz, B., Ungerleider, L. G., Maisog, J. M., Pietrini, P., & Grady, C. L. (1994). The functional organization of human extrastriate cortex: a PET-rCBF study of selective attention to faces and locations. *Journal of Neuroscience, 14*(11 Pt 1), 6336–6353.

Hecht, S. (1937). Rods, cones, and the chemical basis of vision. *Physiology Reviews, 17*, 239–290.

Hendry, S. H. C., and Yoshioka, T. (1994). A neurochemically distinct third channel in macaque dorsal lateral geniculate nucleus. *Science 264:* 575–577.

Henriksson, L., Raninen, A., Nasanen, R., Hyvarinen, L., & Vanni, S. (2007). Training-induced cortical representation of a hemianopic hemifield. *Journal of Neurology, Neurosurgery and Psychiatry, 78*(1), 74–81.

Ho, Y. C., Cheze, A., Sitoh, Y. Y., Petersen, E. T., Goh, K. Y., Gjedde, A., et al. (2009). Residual neurovascular function and retinotopy in a case of hemianopia. *Annals of the Academy of Medicine Singapore, 38*(9), 827–831.

Holmes, G. (1918). Disturbances of vision by cerebral lesions. *British Journal of Ophthalmology, 2*, 353–384.

Holmes, G. (1945). The Ferrier Lecture: the organisation of the visual cortex in man. *Proceedings of the Royal Society (London), 132*, 348–361.

Holstege, G., & Collewijn, H. (1982). The efferent connections of the nucleus of the optic tract and the superior colliculus in the rabbit. *Journal of Computational Neurology, 209*, 139–175.

Horton, J. C., & Hoyt, W. F. (1991). Quadrantic visual field defects. A hallmark of lesions in extrastriate (V2/V3) cortex. *Brain, 114*, 1703–1718.

Horton, J. C., & Hoyt, W. F. (1991). The representation of the visual field in human striate cortex. A revision of the classic Holmes map. *Archives of Ophthalmology, 109*, 816–824.

Hubel, D. H., & Wiesel, T. N. (1959). Receptive fields of single neurons in the cat's striate cortex. *Journal of Physiology, 148*, 574–591.

Hubel, D. H., & Wiesel, T. N. (1962). Receptive fields, binocular interaction and functional architecture in the cat's visual cortex. *Journal of Physiology, 160*, 106–154.

Hubel, D. H., & Wiesel, T. N. (1963). Receptive fields of cells in striate cortex in very young, visually inexperienced kittens. *Journal of Neurophysiology, 26*, 994–1002.

Hubel, D. H., & Wiesel, T. N. (1965). Binocular interaction in striate cortex of kittens raised with artificial squint. *Journal of Neurophysiology, 28*, 1041–1059.

Hubel, D. H., & Wiesel, T. N. (1970). The period of susceptability to the physiological effects of unilateral eye closure in kittens. *Journal Physiology, 206*, 419–436.

Hutchins, B., & Weber, J. T. (1985). The pretectal complex of the monkey: a reinvestigation of the morphology and retinal terminations. *Journal of Computational Neurology, 232*, 425–442.

Itaya, S. K. (1980). Retinal efferents from the pretectal area in the rat. *Brain Research, 201*, 436–441.

Itaya, S. K., & Itaya, P. W. (1985). Centrifugal fibers to the rat retina from the periacqueductal grey matter. *Brain Research, 326*, 362–365.

Jehkonen, M., Ahonen, J. P., Dastidar, P., Koivisto, A. M., Laippala, P., Vilkki, J., et al. (2000). Visual neglect as a predictor of functional outcome one year after stroke. *Acta Neurologica Scandinavia, 101*(3), 195–201.

Jobke, S., Kasten, E., & Sabel, B. A. (2009). Vision restoration through extrastriate stimulation in patients with visual field defects: a double-blind and randomized experimental study. *Neurorehabilitation and Neural Repair, 23*(3), 246–255.

Jones, M. R., Waggoner, R., & Hoyt, W. F. (1999). Cerebral polyopia with extrastriate quadrantanopia: report of a case with magnetic resonance documentation of V2/V3 cortical infarction. *Journal of Neuroophthalmology, 19*(1), 1–6.

Kanwisher, N. (2000). Domain specificity in face perception. *Nature Neuroscience, 3*(8), 759–763.

Kasten, E., Bunzenthal, U., Muller-Oehring, E. M., Mueller, I., & Sabel, B. A. (2007). Vision restoration therapy does not benefit from costimulation: A pilot study. *Journal of Clinical and Experimental Neuropsychology, 29*(6), 569–584.

Kasten, E., Bunzenthal, U., & Sabel, B. A. (2006). Visual field recovery after vision restoration therapy (VRT) is independent of eye movements: an eye tracker study. *Behavioral Brain Research, 175*(1), 18–26.

Kasten, E., Poggel, D. A., Muller-Oehring, E., Gothe, J., Schulte, T., & Sabel, B. A. (1999). Restoration of vision II: residual functions and training-induced visual field enlargement in brain-damaged patients. *Restorative Neurology and Neuroscience, 15*(2–3), 273–287.

Kasten, E., Wust, S., Behrens-Baumann, W., & Sabel, B. A. (1998). Computer-based training for the treatment of partial blindness. *Nature Medicine, 4*(9), 1083–1087.

Kitajima, M., Korogi, Y., Kido, T., Ikeda, O., Morishita, S., & Takahashi, M. (1998). MRI in occipital lobe infarcts: classification by involvement of the striate cortex. *Neuroradiology, 40*(11), 710–715.

Kiyosawa, M., Bosley, T.M., Kushner, M., Jamieson, D., Alavi, A., & Reivich, M. (1990). Middle cerebral artery strokes causing homonymous hemianopia: positron emission tomography. *Annals Neurology, 28*(2), 180–183.

Kriegeskorte, N. (2009). Relating population-code representations between man, monkey, and computational models. *Frontiers Neuroscience, 3*(3), 363–373.

Kupers, R., Beaulieu-Lefebvre, M., Schneider, F.C., Kassuba, T., Paulson, O. B., Siebner, H.R., et al. (2011). Neural correlates of olfactory processing in congenital blindness. *Neuropsychologia, 49*(7), 2037–2044.

Lenzi, G., Frackowiak, R. S., & Jones, T. (1982). Cerebral oxygen metabolism and blood flow in human cerebral ischemic infarction. *Journal of Cerebral Blood Flow and Metabolism, 2*, 321–335.

Leventhal, A., Rodieck, R. W., & Dreher, B. (1981). Retinal ganglion cells in old-world monkey morphology and central projections. *Science, 213*, 1139–1142.

Leventhal, A. G. (1979). Evidence that the different classes of relay cells of the cat's lateral geniculate nucleus terminate in different layers of the striate cortex. *Experimental Brain Research, 37*(2), 349–372.

Lewis, L. B., Saenz, M., & Fine, I. (2010). Mechanisms of cross-modal plasticity in early-blind subjects. *Journal of Neurophysiology, 104*(6), 2995–3008.

Liepert, J., Hamzei, F., & Weiller, C. (2000). Motor cortex disinhibition of the unaffected hemisphere after acute stroke. *Muscle Nerve, 23*(11), 1761–1763.

Marshall, J. C., & Halligan, P. W. (1988). Blindsight and insight in visuo-spatial neglect. *Nature, 336*(6201), 766–767.

Martin, W., & Raichle, M. E. (1983). Cerebellar blood flow and metabolism in cerebral hemisphere infarction. *Annals of Neurology, 14*, 168–176.

McFadzean, R., Brosnahan, D., Hadley, D., & Mutlukan, E. (1994). Representation of the visual field in the occipital striate cortex. *British Journal Ophthalmology, 78*(3), 185–190.

McFadzean, R. M., & Hadley, D. M. (1997). Homonymous quadrantanopia respecting the horizontal meridian. A feature of striate and extrastriate cortical disease. *Neurology, 49*(6), 1741–1746.

Mesulam, M. M. (1981). A cortical network for directed attention and unilateral neglect. *Annals of Neurology, 10*, 309–325.

Mesulam, M. M. (1990). Large-scale neurocognitive networks and distribution processing for attention, language and memory. *Annals of Neurology, 28*, 597–603.

Mesulam, M. M. (2000). Attentional networks, confusional states and neglect syndromes. In M. M. Mesulam (Ed.), *Principles of behavioral and cognitive neurology* (pp. 194). New York: Oxford University Press.

Milner, A. D., & Goodale, M. A. (2008). Two visual systems re-viewed. *Neuropsychologia, 46*(3), 774–785.

Mueller, I., Gall, C., Kasten, E., & Sabel, B. A. (2008). Long-term learning of visual functions in patients after brain damage. *Behavioral Brain Research, 191*(1), 32–42.

Mueller, I., Mast, H., & Sabel, B. A. (2007). Recovery of visual field defects: a large clinical observational study using vision restoration therapy. *Restorative Neurology and Neuroscience, 25*(5–6), 563–572.

Nasr, S., Liu, N., Devaney, K. J., Yue, X., Rajimehr, R., Ungerleider, L. G., et al. (2011). Scene-selective cortical regions in human and nonhuman primates. *Journal of Neuroscience, 31*(39), 13771–13785.

Nassi, J. J., & Callaway, E. M. (2009). Parallel processing strategies of the primate visual system. *Nature Reviews Neuroscience, 10*(5), 360–372.

Nelles, G., de Greiff, A., Pscherer, A., Forsting, M., Gerhard, H., Esser, J., et al. (2007). Cortical activation in hemianopia after stroke. *Neuroscience Letters, 426*(1), 34–38.

Nelles, G., de Greiff, A., Pscherer, A., Stude, P., Forsting, M., Hufnagel, A., et al. (2007). Saccade induced cortical activation in patients with post-stroke visual field defects. *Journal of Neurology, 254*(9), 1244–1252.

Nelles, G., Widman, G., de Greiff, A., Meistrowitz, A., Dimitrova, A., Weber, J., et al. (2002). Brain representation of hemifield stimulation in poststroke visual field defects. *Stroke, 33*(5), 1286–1293.

Neville, H., & Bavelier, D. (2002). Human brain plasticity: evidence from sensory deprivation and altered language experience. *Progress in Brain Research, 138*, 177–188.

Nichols, D. F., Betts, L.R., & Wilson, H. R. (2010). Decoding of faces and face components in face-sensitive human visual cortex. *Frontiers in Psychology, 1*, 28.

Nieuwenhuys, R., Voogd, J., & van Huijzen, C. (1988). *The human central nervous system. A synopsis and atlas.* Berlin: Springer-Verlag.

Nishimoto, S., Vu, A. T., Naselaris, T., Benjami, Y., Yu, B., & Gallant, J. L. (2011). Reconstructing visual experiences from brain activity evoked by natural movies. *Current Biology, 21*(in press), 1–6.

Nudo, R. J. (2006). Plasticity. *NeuroRx, 3*(4), 420–427.

Nudo, R. J. (2007). Postinfarct cortical plasticity and behavioral recovery. *Stroke, 38*(2 Suppl), 840–845.

Nudo, R. J. (2011). Neural bases of recovery after brain injury. *Journal of Communication Disorders*, 2011 Sep–Oct; 44(5):515–20. Epub 2011 Apr 30. Review.

Perry, V. H., & Cowey, A. (1981). The morphological correlates of X- and Y-like retinal ganglion cells in the retina of monkeys. *Experimental Brain Research, 43*(2), 226–228.

Perry, V. H., & Cowey, A. (1984). Retinal ganglion cells that project to the superior colliculus and pretectum in the macaque monkey. *Neuroscience, 12*, 1125–1137.

Perry, V. H., Oehler, R., & Cowey, A. (1984). Retinal ganglion cells that project to the dorsal lateral geniculate nucleus in the macaque monkey. *Neuroscience, 12*(4), 1101–1123.

Perry, V. H., Silveira, L. C., & Cowey, A. (1990). Pathways mediating resolution in the primate retina. *Ciba Foundation Symposium, 155*, 5–14; discussion 14–21.

Poggel, D. A., Kasten, E., Muller-Oehring, E. M., Bunzenthal, U., & Sabel, B. A. (2006). Improving residual vision by attentional cueing in patients with brain lesions. *Brain Research, 1097*(1), 142–148.

Poggel, D. A., Kasten, E., & Sabel, B. A. (2004). Attentional cueing improves vision restoration therapy in patients with visual field defects. *Neurology, 63*(11), 2069–2076.

Poggel, D. A., Mueller, I., Kasten, E., Bunzenthal, U., & Sabel, B. A. (2010). Subjective and objective outcome measures of computer-based vision restoration training. *NeuroRehabilitation, 27*(2), 173–187.

Polonara, G., Salvolini, S., Fabri, M., Mascioli, G., Cavola, G. L., Neri, P., et al. (2011). Unilateral visual loss due to ischaemic injury in the right calcarine region: a functional magnetic resonance imaging and diffusion tension imaging follow-up study. *International Ophthalmology, 31*(2), 129–134.

Ptito, A., Fortin, A., & Ptito, M. (2001). "Seeing" in the blind hemifield following hemispherectomy. *Progress in Brain Research, 134*, 367–378.

Raemaekers, M., Bergsma, D. P., van Wezel, R. J., van der Wildt, G. J., & van den Berg, A. V. (2011). Effects of vision restoration training on early visual cortex in patients with cerebral blindness investigated with functional magnetic resonance imaging. *Journal of Neurophysiology, 105*(2), 872–882.

Reinhard, J., Schreiber, A., Schiefer, U., Kasten, E., Sabel, B. A., Kenkel, S., et al. (2005). Does visual restitution training change absolute homonymous visual field defects? A fundus controlled study. *British Journal of Ophthalmology, 89*(1), 30–35.

Ro, T., & Rafal, R. (2006). Visual restoration in cortical blindness: insights from natural and TMS-induced blindsight. *Neuropsychology Rehabilitation, 16*(4), 377–396.

Sabel, B. A. (2008). Plasticity and restoration of vision after visual system damage: an update. *Restorative Neurology and Neuroscience, 26*(4–5), 243–247.

Sabel, B. A., Henrich-Noack, P., Fedorov, A., & Gall, C. (2011). Vision restoration after brain and retina damage: the "residual vision activation theory." *Progress in Brain Research, 192*, 199–262.

Saenz, M., Lewis, L. B., Huth, A. G., Fine, I., & Koch, C. (2008). Visual motion area MT+/V5 responds to auditory motion in human sight-recovery subjects. *Journal of Neuroscience, 28*(20), 5141–5148.

Sahraie, A. (2007). Induced visual sensitivity changes in chronic hemianopia. *Current Opinions in Neurology, 20*(6), 661–666.

Sahraie, A., Trevethan, C.T., Weiskrantz, L., Olson, J., MacLeod, M. J., Murray, A. D., et al. (2003). Spatial channels of visual processing in cortical blindness. *European Journal of Neuroscience, 18*(5), 1189–1196.

Schmielau, F., & Wong, E. K., Jr. (2007). Recovery of visual fields in brain-lesioned patients by reaction perimetry treatment. *Journal of Neuroengineering and Rehabilitation, 4*, 31.

Schoenfeld, M. A., Noesselt, T., Poggel, D., Tempelmann, C., Hopf, J. M., Woldorff, M. G., et al. (2002). Analysis of pathways mediating preserved vision after striate cortex lesions. *Annals of Neurology, 52*(6), 814–824.

Schreiber, A., Vonthein, R., Reinhard, J., Trauzettel-Klosinski, S., Connert, C., & Schiefer, U. (2006). Effect of visual restitution training on absolute homonymous scotomas. *Neurology, 67*(1), 143–145.

Sereno, M. I., Dale, A. M., Reppas, J. B., Kwong, K. K., Belliveau, J. W., Brady, T. J., et al. (1995). Borders of multiple visual areas in humans revealed by functional magnetic resonance imaging. *Science, 268*(5212), 889–893.

Sergent, J., Ohta, S., & MacDonald, B. (1992). Functional neuroanatomy of face and object processing. A positron emission tomography study. *Brain, 115 Pt 1*, 15–36.

Sergent, J., & Signoret, J. L. (1992). Functional and anatomical decomposition of face processing: evidence from prosopagnosia and PET study of normal subjects. *Philosophical Transactions of the Royal Society London B: Biological Science, 335*(1273), 55–61.

Shipp, S., de Jong, B. M., Zihl, J., Frackowiak, R. S., & Zeki, S. (1994). The brain activity related to residual motion vision in a patient with bilateral lesions of V5. *Brain, 117 (Pt 5)*, 1023–1038.

Shipp, S., Watson, J. D., Frackowiak, R. S., & Zeki, S. (1995). Retinotopic maps in human prestriate visual cortex: the demarcation of areas V2 and V3. *NeuroImage, 2*(2), 125–132.

Sincich, L. C., Park, K. F., Wohlgemuth, M. J., & Horton, J. C. (2004). Bypassing V1: a direct geniculate input to area MT. *Nature Neuroscience, 7*(10), 1123–1128.

Slotnick, S. D., & Moo, L. R. (2003). Retinotopic mapping reveals extrastriate cortical basis of homonymous quadrantanopia. *Neuroreport, 14*(9), 1209–1213.

Smith, A. T., Singh, K. D., Williams, A. L., & Greenlee, M. W. (2001). Estimating receptive field size from fMRI data in human striate and extrastriate visual cortex. *Cerebral Cortex, 11*(12), 1182–1190.

Smith, J. L. (1962). Homonymous hemianopia: A review of a hundred cases. *American Journal of Ophthalmology, 54*, 616–622.

Spitzyna, G. A., Wise, R.J., McDonald, S.A., Plant, G.T., Kidd, D., Crewes, H., et al. (2007). Optokinetic therapy improves text reading in patients with hemianopic alexia: a controlled trial. *Neurology, 68*(22), 1922–1930.

Steeves, J., Dricot, L., Goltz, H. C., Sorger, B., Peters, J., Milner, A. D., et al. (2009). Abnormal face identity coding in the middle fusiform gyrus of two brain-damaged prosopagnosic patients. *Neuropsychologia, 47*(12), 2584–2592.

Stoerig, P., Kleinschmidt, A., & Frahm, J. (1998). No visual responses in denervated V1: high-resolution functional magnetic resonance imaging of a blindsight patient. *Neuroreport, 9*(1), 21–25.

Stone, J. (1972). Morphology and physiology of the geniculocortical synapse in the cat: the question of parallel input to the striate cortex. *Investigative Ophthalmology, 11*(5), 338–346.

Stone, J., & Dreher, B. (1982). Parallel processing of information in the visual pathways. A general principle of sensory coding? *Trends in Neuroscience, 5*, 441–446.

Stone, J., Dreher, B., & Leventhal, A. (1979). Hierarchical and parallel mechanisms in the organization of visual cortex. *Brain Research, 180*(3), 345–394.

Stone, J., Dreher, B., & Leventhal, A. G. (1979). Hierarchical and parallel mechanisms in the organization of visual cortex. *Brain Research Reviews, 1*, 345–394.

Stone, J., & Fukuda, Y. (1974). Properties of cat retinal ganglion cells: a comparison of W-cells with X- and Y-cells. *Journal of Neurophysiology, 37*(4), 722–748.

Striem-Amit, E., Dakwar, O., Reich, L., & Amedi, A. (2011). The large-scale organization of "visual" streams emerges without visual experience. *Cerebral Cortex*. epub 2011 September 21.

Summerfield, C., Egner, T., Mangels, J., & Hirsch, J. (2006). Mistaking a house for a face: neural correlates of misperception in healthy humans. *Cerebral Cortex, 16*(4), 500–508.

Sur, M., Frost, D. O., & Hockfield, S. (1988). Expression of a surface-associated antigen on Y-cells in the cat lateral geniculate nucleus is regulated by visual experience. *Journal of Neuroscience, 8*(3), 874–882.

Taylor, H. R., Livingston, P. M., Stanislavsky, Y. L., & McCarty, C. A. (1997). Visual impairment in Australia: distance visual acuity, near vision, and visual field findings of the Melbourne Visual Impairment Project. *American Journal of Ophthalmology, 123*, 328–337.

Taylor, J. C., & Downing, P. E. (2011). Division of labor between lateral and ventral extrastriate representations of faces, bodies, and objects. *Journal of Cognitive Neuroscience*. 2011 Dec;23(12):4122–37. Epub 2011 Jul 7.

Terasawa, K., Ottani, K., & Yamada, J. (1979). Descending pathways of the nucleus of the optic tract in the rat. *Brain Research, 173*, 405–417.

Thakral, P. P., & Slotnick, S. D. (2011). Disruption of MT impairs motion processing. *Neuroscience Letters, 490*(3), 226–230.

Thulborn, K. R., Carpenter, P. A., & Just, M. A. (1999). Plasticity of language-related brain function during recovery from stroke. *Stroke, 30*(4), 749–754.

Tononi, G., & Edelman, G. M. (1998). Consciousness and complexity. *Science, 282*, 1846–1851.

Tootell, R. B., Hadjikhani, N. K., Vanduffel, W., Liu, A. K., Mendola, J. D., Sereno, M. I., et al. (1998). Functional analysis of primary visual cortex (V1) in humans. *Proceedings of the National Academy of Science U S A, 95*(3), 811–817.

Tootell, R. B., Hamilton, S. L., & Switkes, E. (1988). Functional anatomy of macaque striate cortex. IV. Contrast and magno-parvo streams. *Journal of Neuroscience, 8*(5), 1594–1609.

Tootell, R. B., Mendola, J. D., Hadjikhani, N. K., Liu, A. K., & Dale, A. M. (1998). The representation of the ipsilateral visual field in human cerebral cortex. *Proceedings of the National Academy of Science U S A, 95*(3), 818–824.

Tootell, R. B., Switkes, E., Silverman, M. S., & Hamilton, S. L. (1988). Functional anatomy of macaque striate cortex. II. Retinotopic organization. *J Neurosci, 8*(5), 1531–1568.

Tootell R. B., Tsao D., Vanduffel W. J Neurosci. Neuroimaging weighs in: humans meet macaques in "primate" visual cortex J Neurosci. 2003 May 15;23(10):3981–3989.

Trobe, J. D., Lorber, M. L., & Schelzinger, N. S. (1973). Isolated homonymous hemianopsia. *Archives of Ophthalmology, 89*, 377–381.

Ungerleider, L. G., & Desimone, R. (1986). Cortical connections of visual area MT in the macaque. *Journal of Computational Neurology, 248*(2), 190–222.

Ungerleider, L. G., & Haxby, J. V. (1994). "What" and "where" in the human brain. *Current Opinions in Neurobiology, 4*(2), 157–165.

Ungerleider, L. G., & Mishkin, M. (1982). Two cortical visual systems. In D. J. Ingle, M. A. Goodale & R. J .W. Mansfield (Eds.), *Analysis of visual behavior* (pp. 549–586). Cambridge, Massachusetts: MIT Press.

Vaina, L. M., Cowey, A., & Kennedy, D. N. (1999). Perception of first- and second-order motion: Separable neurological mechanisms? *Human Brain Mapping, 7*, 67–77.

Vaina, L. M., & Dumoulin, S. O. (2011). Neuropsychological evidence for three distinct motion mechanisms. *Neuroscience Letters, 495*(2), 102–106.

Vaina, L. M., Lemay, M., Bienfang, C. D., Choi, A. Y., & Nakayama, K. (1990). Intact "biological motion" and "structure from motion" perception in a patient with impaired motion mechanisms. *Visual Neuroscience, 5*, 353–369.

Vaina, L. M., Sikoglu, E. M., Soloviev, S., LeMay, M., Squatrito, S., Pandiani, G., et al. (2010). Functional and anatomical profile of visual motion impairments in stroke patients correlate with fMRI in normal subjects. *Journal of Neuropsychology, 4*(Pt 2), 121–145.

Van Essen, D. C., Newsome, W. T., & Maunsell, J. H. (1984). The visual field representation in striate cortex of the macaque monkey: asymmetries, anisotropies, and individual variability. *Vision Research, 24*(5), 429–448.

Watson, J. "The Human Visual System" in Brain Mapping: The Systems edited by A. W. Toga and J. C. Mazziotta, (Academic Press, San Diego) 2000: pp. 263–289.

Watson, J. D., Myers, R., Frackowiak, R. S., Hajnal, J. V., Woods, R. P., & Mazziota, J. (1993). Area V5 of the human brain: Evidence from a combined study using positron emission tomography and magnetic resonance imaging. *Cerebral Cortex, 3*, 79–94.

Weiskrantz, L., Barbur, J. L., & Sahraie, A. (1995). Parameters affecting conscious versus unconscious visual discrimination with damage to the visual cortex (V1). *Proceedings of the National Academy of Science USA, 92*, 6122–6126.

Wiesel, T. N., & Hubel, D. H. (1965). Extent of recovery from the effects of visual deprivation in kittens. *Journal of Neurophysiology, 28*, 1060–1072.

Wong, M., Gnanakumaran, V., & Goldreich, D. (2011). Tactile spatial acuity enhancement in blindness: evidence for experience-dependent mechanisms. *Journal of Neuroscience, 31*(19), 7028–7037.

Young, R. W. (1970). Visual cells. *Scientific American, 223*(4), 80–91.

14 | GOAL-DRIVEN ATTENTION AND WORKING MEMORY

SHEILA GILLARD CREWTHER, NAHAL GOHARPEY, LOUISE C. BANNISTER, and GEMMA LAMP

14.1 INTRODUCTION

Stroke is a leading cause of disability (Mathers, Vos, & Stevenson, 1999; Thrift, Dewey, Macdonell, McNeil, & Donnan, 2000; Paul et al., 2005; Lloyd-Jones et al., 2009), with an estimated 62 million stroke survivors worldwide (Strong, Mathers, & Bonita, 2007). With advances in treatment and medication, the proportion of disabled stroke survivors is increasing (Carandang et al., 2006) with up to 20% continuing to experience very poor health-related quality of life (HRQoL) for at least 5 years after the event (Paul et al., 2005). Furthermore, at least 50% of long-term stroke survivors regard their recovery from stroke as incomplete (Bonita, Solomon, & Broad, 1997). Even patients with what is classified as a "mild" stroke (score of ≤5 on the National Institutes of Health Stroke Scale [NIHSS]) report residual stroke-related changes, such as depression and cognitive changes (Edwards, Hahn, Baum, & Dromerick, 2006). Such ongoing disabilities have serious implications for quality of life for the patient and for their families and friends (Mathers et al., 1999; Abegunde, Mathers, Adam, Ortegon, & Strong, 2007) and also induce significant social and financial cost (Thrift et al., 2000).

This chapter will argue that brain damage, whether it is a mild concussion or a severe stroke, almost guarantees that impaired attention, working memory, cognition, and ability to relearn will be the norm and not the exception in survivors. This can be attributed to lesion-induced cell death and consequential neuroinflammation, which is closely associated with "sickness behavior," fatigue, and depression post-stroke. *Sickness behavior* is a term coined to describe the archetypical adaptive behaviors (whether animal or human) that are induced by the immune system to cope effectively with infection and commonly referred to as "flu-like" symptoms; namely, fever, lethargy, depression, anxiety, lack of energy, lack of appetite, sleepiness, and hyperanalgesia (Hart, 1988). For new learning to occur in the rehabilitation process, motor behavior and basic perceptual mechanisms need to be retrained and reestablished.

14.1.1 FACTORS AFFECTING STROKE REHABILITATION

At least a third of stroke patients demonstrate cognitive impairment (Tatemichi et al., 1994; Nys et al., 2005), as identified using brief cognitive screens (Tatemichi et al., 1994) or neuropsychological evaluation (Nys et al., 2005). In particular, attention, including divided attention, sustained attention, selective attention, and speed of information processing are affected post-stroke (Tatemichi et al., 1994; Hochstenbach, Mulder, van Limbeel, Donders, & Schoonderwaldt, 1998; Stapleton, Ashburn, & Stack, 2001; Fisk, Owsley, & Mennemeier, 2002; Ballard et al., 2003) and can persist for a long time, even after supposedly good clinical recovery (Mori, Sadoshima, Ibayashi, Lino, & Fujishima, 1994; Edwards et al., 2006). Furthermore, mood disorders such as depression are becoming increasingly recognized as a common consequence of stroke, with clinically diagnosed post-stroke depression estimated to affect one-third to two-thirds of stroke patients at some point (Eslinger, Parkinson, & Shamay, 2002; Robinson & Starkstein, 2002; Hackett & Anderson, 2005; Linden, Blomstrand & Skoog, 2007), typically within the first two years following stroke (Linden et al., 2007). Depression and anxiety are clinically characterized by attention and concentration difficulties (Kauhanen et al., 1999; Lezak, Howieson, & Loring, 2004; Barker-Collo, 2007), as well as poor motivation (Mialet, Pope, & Yurgelun-Todd, 1996;

Austin, Mitchell, & Goodwin, 2001; Brose, Schmiedek, Lövdén, & Lindenberger, 2011). These difficulties are likely to further exacerbate cognitive dysfunction and may also impact the ability of individuals to benefit from rehabilitation. Stroke rehabilitation is broadly defined here as any aspect of stroke care (generally nonsurgical and nonpharmaceutical) that aims to reduce disability and handicap and promote activity and independent participation in everyday activities (Langhorne & Legg, 2003; National Stroke Foundation, 2005; Dewey, Sherry, & Collier, 2007; The Consensus Panel on the Stroke Rehabilitation System, 2007). Thus, rehabilitation may be operationally considered to be about learning how to achieve old skills in new ways.

The process of rehabilitation is likely affected by psychological and physiological stress and inflammatory changes associated with the ischemic areas following stroke (Pascoe, Crewther, Carey, & Crewther, 2011). The initial effects of stroke are due to the sudden interruption of blood supply to the brain (ischemia) by occlusion of the blood vessels, or hemorrhage following rupture of blood vessels (World Health Organization, 1992; Ropper & Brown, 2005). Hypoxia and hypoglycemia in the area supplied by the occluded artery lead to cell death and disintegration of cell membranes, release of toxic amounts of excitatory neurotransmitters, edema (Ropper & Brown, 2005; Liberato & Krakauer, 2007) and, most importantly, disruption to the blood-brain barrier (Kolb & Whishaw, 1998). Temporary hypoxia and glucose restriction in the minutes following stroke lead to impaired cell energy sources, disruption of ion dispersion within the neurons and extravascular space, and cellular volume changes, and induce an inflammatory response characterized by the release of key inflammatory mediators (cytokines, chemokines, and inflammatory cells) from nearby astroglia (Tedgui & Mallat, 2006; McColl, Allan, & Rothwell, 2007; Chapman et al., 2009; Denes, Thornton, Rothwell, & Allan, 2010) that disrupt blood brain permeability and lead to further invasion of the area by peripherally derived immune reagents. Over time, these ischemic damage-induced inflammatory responses come to be characterized by a constellation of nonspecific symptoms such as weakness, increased somnolence, inability to concentrate, lethargy, and depression, collectively termed sickness behavior (Hart, 1988; Dantzer, 2004). These inflammatory mediators have also been shown to modulate learning and memory processes (Dantzer, 2004), and are associated with clinically defined depressive symptoms (Anisman, Merali, & Hayley, 2008; Dantzer, O'Connor, Freund, & Kelley, 2008). What has not been established is for how long the presence of physiologically derived neuroinflammatory factors continue to limit relearning and rehabilitation. Thus, impairment in cognitive abilities such as attention and mood need to be considered as inherent early components of any model of stroke rehabilitation and recovery.

14.1.2 GOAL-DIRECTED ACTION AND THE VISUAL SYSTEM

Goal-directed action is predominately guided by vision, though visual attention for top-down manipulation of visual and sensory information receives constant supplementation and confirmation with information from the other senses (Corbetta & Shulman, 2002). Visual information predominates in terms of attention because accurate spatial and temporal information regarding potential threats can be collected from far and near, such as when driving a car or walking around a crowded room. Audition, on the other hand, often assumes greater importance to attention at near distances, due to its social relevance and role in language and social communication (Centelles, Assaiante, Nazarian, Anton, & Schmitz, 2011). However, it is interesting to note that even in social communication situations, auditory information is usually supplemented by rapid visual attention to the speaker and their "body language." Thus, vision and visual attention are likely to become even more important to the many stroke patients suffering from language and motor disabilities, particularly as they seek means to behaviorally compensate for residual disabilities that affect their ability to navigate their environment.

14.2 WHAT IS ATTENTION?

In 1890 William James defined attention as "the taking possession by the mind, in clear and vivid form, of one out of what seem several simultaneously possible objects or trains of thought … It implies withdrawal from some things in order to deal effectively with others" (James, 1890, pp. 403–404). Over a century later, the accepted definition of attention has changed very little, with a recent paper describing it as "a set of mechanisms that determine how particular sensory input, perceptual objects, trains of thought, or courses of action are selected for further processing from an array of concurrent possible stimuli, objects, thoughts and action" (Talsma, Senkowski, Soto-Faraco, & Woldorff, 2010, p. 400). The simplicity of these definitions belies the fact that attention is a complex and multifaceted cognitive construct that is manifest at the levels of behavior, brain systems, and single-neuron responses, but is always related back to the visually driven selective attention system (Wannig, Stanisor, & Roelfsema, 2011). Indeed, attention is essential and fundamental to any perceptual, cognitive, or behavioral process and is predominantly visual in origin in normal healthy humans (de Schotten et al., 2011).

As alluded to above, vision may be considered by far the most important sensory input for higher animals, especially humans and other primates and birds of prey. Not surprisingly, then, the human and primate visual systems

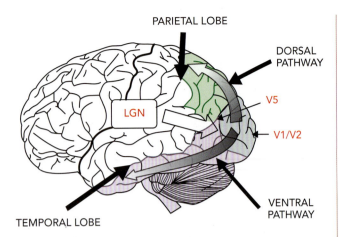

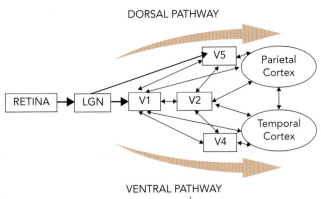

Figure 14.1 The Conscious Human Visual System—A Functional Model. The magnocellular (large retinal ganglion cell) projection of visual information arrives in V1 20–25 msc (Klistorner, Crewther, & Crewther, 1997) before the slower projection from the smaller parvocellular ganglion cells, and thence project dorsally to V5 to both alert the parietofrontal lobes attention systems, and simultaneously allow a first foreground/background segregation of visual information before feedback into V1/V2 (Bullier, 2001). This early M type information then joins with the slower incoming parvocellular input, to project ventrally to inferotemporal cortex to object recognition areas. Modified from Laycock and Crewther (2008) by Felicity Della Nogare, Honors Thesis, 2011, School of Psychological Science, La Trobe University.

Figure 14.2 The Magnocellular Advantage Model of Feedforward/Feedback Visual Processing. The magnocellular (large retinal ganglion cell) projection of visual information arrives in V1 20–25 msc (Klistorner, Crewther, & Crewther, 1997) before the slower projection from the smaller parvocellular ganglion cells, and thence projects dorsally to V5 to both alert the parietal and frontal lobes alert attention systems and allow a first foreground/background segregation of visual information before feedback into V1/V2 (Bullier, 2001) to meet the incoming parvocellular input, prior to together processing ventrally to inferotemporal cortex for object recognition. Note the presence of a projection from the visual thalamus, the lateral geniculate nucleus (LGN) direct to V5 (Nassi & Callaway, 2009). This figure was modified from Felicity Della Nogare, Honors Thesis, 2011, School of Psychological Science, La Trobe University.

comprise more than one third of the cortical mantle (Van Essen & Drury, 1997; Van Essen, Drury, Joshi, & Miller, 1998), sending and receiving inputs from most areas and, as such, guiding and directing selective attention. This complex anatomy is comparatively well understood and has been well mapped out since the work of Allman and Kaas (1971a, 1971b) and Van Essen and colleagues in the 1970s and 1980s. Information beyond primary visual cortex (V1) is conceptualized to be processed in a feed-forward feed-back manner (Bullier, 2001; Laycock, Crewther, & Crewther, 2007) via two initially segregated visual pathways. The two major visual streams comprise a more dorsal "where" pathway, projecting to the parietal cortex and then to the frontal areas, and a more ventral "what" pathway projecting to the temporal cortex (see also Chapter 13).

The "where" pathway (V5, V7) responds preferentially to motion and fast movement and requires less spatial information, and so in projecting to the parietal cortex is involved in driving the localized attention pathways for both overt and covert spatial attention, connecting with regions that control eye and hand movements. Not surprisingly, parietal pathways play a central role in guiding attention, and hence behaviors, to spatial locations (Lewis & Van Essen, 2000); thus their integrity and involvement is particularly important post-stroke. In contrast, the ventral "what" pathway (lateral occipital complex, V4, V8) projects to the temporal cortex and is involved in the recognition, identification, and categorization of visual objects (e.g., the lateral occipital complex

responds to entire objects). While there is specialization within the dorsal and ventral visual pathways, there is also much communication between areas and other sensory systems, as well as feedback loops within visual areas (Bullier, 2001; Laycock et al., 2007). Indeed, speech areas involved in aphasia are also located adjacent and superior to ventral visual areas and receive mutual projections. See Figures 14.1 and 14.2 that illustrate the visual projections.

14.2.1 NEUROANATOMICAL INTERACTION BETWEEN THE ATTENTION AND VISUAL SYSTEMS

According to Corbetta and Shulman (2002), attention in the human brain is carried out by at least two extensive interconnected neural networks that have their derivation in the visual sensory system. At a functional level there is a top-down system dorsal network (driven by our goals, expectations, and knowledge) and a bottom-up system ventral network (driven by our incoming sensory environment) that interact with one another in order to determine where visual attention and actions will be directed at any one time (Corbetta & Shulman, 2002). The first system is the more dorsal frontoparietal attention network that is primarily involved in higher-order "top down," goal-driven attention. It includes the primary visual regions, intraparietal sulcus (IPS), superior parietal lobule, frontal eye fields, and superior frontal cortex (Corbetta & Shulman, 2002; Yantis & Serences, 2003; Woldorff et al., 2004; Corbetta,

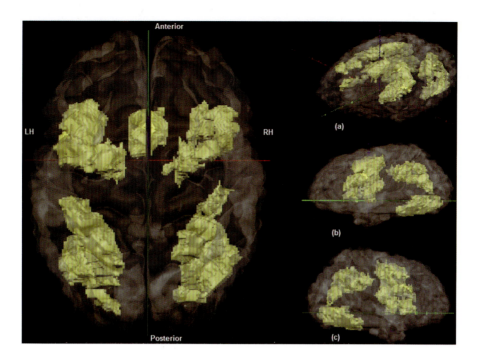

Figure 14.3 Visual Attention Related To Difficulty in N-back Working Memory Tasks. This figure is adapted from the study by Crewther, Lamp, Sanchez-Rockliffe, and Crewther (2010), and demonstrates common patterns of bilateral activation of the frontoparietal networks for both attention and working memory. The brain on the left shows the planes of dissection for the smaller figures on the right and the bilateral activation in middle frontal gyri, premotor cortex (BA 6), occipital lobes, anterior cingulate cortex (BA 24), and parietal lobes, particularly superior parietal (BA 7), and frontal eye fields. Figure 14.3 (a) shows almost complete activation of both the more dorsal and more ventral attention networks for left hemisphere; (b) medial networks, including much of anterior and posterior cingulate cortex, parieto-occipital areas, and parahippocampal and fusiform areas; (c) shows similar right hemisphere activations of extrastriate visual areas, including ventral areas of lateral occipital up to both the ventral attention stream around temporal parietal junction and the more dorsal intraparietal sulcus.

Patel, & Shulman, 2008). The second system is the ventral attention network (VAN), which is primarily involved in the detection of behaviorally relevant "bottom up" stimuli (Corbetta & Shulman, 2002; Moore, Armstrong, & Fallah, 2003; Yantis & Serences, 2003; Woldorff et al., 2004; Corbetta et al., 2008). The VAN system includes the temporoparietal junction (TPJ), the supramarginal gyrus, and middle and inferior prefrontal cortex, and is largely lateralized to the right hemisphere. Stimulus-driven attention seems to operate in concert with rapid subcortical networks that include the superior colliculi that subserve eye movements via frontal eye fields and project onto the frontal cortex (Kim et al., 1999; Corbetta & Shulman, 2002). Furthermore, both the lateral intraparietal cortex (LIP) and the frontal eye fields have been found to play roles in attention, memory and eye movements; in other words, LIP and front eye fields control all the processes that underlie overt shifts in attention (Bruce & Goldberg, 1985; Gnadt & Andersen, 1988; Colby, Duhamel, & Goldberg, 1996), explaining the severe problems with the rapid shifting of attention needed for social interactions that occur post-stroke.

Visual attention is a balance between the control regions of the dorsal frontoparietal cortex, which generates and maintains expectations, and the more occipital regions that are primarily involved in sensory analysis. The ventral attentional network is hypothesized to act as a "circuit breaker" for the dorsal system, directing attention to salient events (where relative salience is a measure of importance or relevance of particular pieces of information to the goal-directed actions of an individual) when they are outside the focus of processing (Corbetta & Shulman, 2002). This "circuit breaking" function is hypothesized to lie in the interaction between TPJ and the IPS, whereby the IPS informs the TPJ of the behavioral relevance of the stimuli either directly or indirectly through top-down modulation of the visual cortex (Corbetta & Shulman, 2002).

New learning (such as social information and planning for meals, etc.) is constantly being sought and acquired by everyone, including stroke survivors. Thus, new approaches to rehabilitation post-stroke need to consider how best to utilize both ventral and dorsal attention systems. It is known that lesions to the ventral prefrontal cortex result in deficits in the ability to adapt to novel situations or stimuli (Clark, Cools, & Robbins, 2004), and so it has been suggested that the ventral attention system may be responsible for the evaluation of new stimuli. Furthermore, in order for humans to be able to adapt to a constantly changing environment, new stimulus–response associations (or mappings) are constantly and often very rapidly required.

It has been suggested that such new stimulus–response associations are laid down in the dorsal posterior parietal cortex, which lies alongside the intraparietal sulcus and contains Brodmann's areas 5, 7, 40, and 39, particularly in the left hemisphere (Kimberg, Aguirre, & D'Esposito, 2000; Sohn, Ursu, Anderson, Stenger, & Carter, 2000; Shulman, d'Avossa, Tansy, & Corbetta, 2002). Indeed, the dorsal attentional system is proposed to link sensory representations to motor responses in areas of the frontoparietal network (Corbetta & Shulman, 2002) and facilitate decision making, implying that lesion damage to this network will severely incapacitate normal purposeful behavior.

The attentional system is believed to have a supramodal function (Driver & Spence, 1998; Macaluso, Frith, & Driver, 2002). For example, the ventral attentional system has been associated with the detection of salient stimuli in the auditory and tactile domains, as well as in the visual domain (Downar, Crawley, Mikulis, & Davis, 2000). Similar dorsal and ventral parietal and frontal regions are modulated by reorienting to invalid targets in other modalities (Arrington, Carr, Mayer, & Rao, 2001; Macaluso et al., 2002; Mayer, Harrington, Adair, & Lee, 2006; Vossel, Thiel, & Fink, 2006). Indeed, it is well recognized that attention is coded as raised arousal levels in all visual areas from thalamus through cortex (McAlonan, Cavanaugh, & Wurtz, 2008). Such enhanced electrical activity leads to permanent morphological changes in neurons (Mueller, Brehmer, von Oertzen, Li, & Lindenberger, 2008; Van der Lubbe, Buitenweg, Boschker, Gerdes, & Jongsma, 2011) and encoding of functional memories. In the absence of such attention-driven enhancement of electrical processes, as often occurs in many fatigued and/or depressed stroke patients, effective new learning is less likely to occur.

14.2.2 ATTENTION AND MULTISENSORY INTEGRATION

Multisensory integration (MSI) refers to the integration of information from different senses into a unified percept (Shimojo & Shams, 2001; Sathian, 2006) that ensures faster response times (Todd, 1912; Miller, 1982). Thus, in the case of stroke survivors MSI is even more likely to be necessary for adequate performance by any of the impaired sensorimotor systems. MSI would be expected to facilitate the additive attentional effects of several sensory streams needed to enable compensatory motor or language responses and to maintain and adequately drive goal-directed behaviors. Multisensory integration is a critical stage of sensory perception, and occurs in a bottom-up fashion when there is low competition between stimuli and through top-down modulation during high competition between stimuli (Talsma et al., 2010). During multisensory integration, pieces of information arriving from the individual sensory modalities (e.g., vision, audition, and touch) interact, influence processing in other sensory modalities,

and combine together to produce a unified experience of multisensory events (Talsma et al., 2010). Regions can be defined as *multisensory* if they receive afferent connections from more than one sensory cortical area (E. G. Jones & Powell, 1970; Cappe & Barone, 2005), or if neural activation in the area is enhanced when cross-modal stimuli are presented (Calvert, 2001). Such areas are necessary if one is to identify and find a ringing telephone or switch off a boiling kettle, for example.

At a neural level, temporally and spatially aligned sensory inputs across different modalities have a higher chance of capturing an individual's attention and undergoing further processing than do nonaligned stimuli—indicating that attention tends to orient more easily toward multisensory inputs (Talsma et al., 2010). As well as having a role in multisensory integration, it has been proposed that the posterior parietal cortex acts as a cross-modal focus for attention and as an organizer of top-down inputs (Buchel et al., 1998), capable of mediating attention to simple streams from several modalities relevant to salient behavior (Andersen, 1997).

Multisensory processing involves extensive networks of cortical and subcortical regions at early and late stages of processing, as has been shown using neurophysiology, neuroimaging, and neuroanatomical techniques, including event-related potentials (ERPs), fMRI, positron emission tomography (PET), single-cell recordings, lesion studies, and retrograde tracing (McIntosh, Cabeza, & Lobaugh, 1998). Key subcortical regions implicated in multisensory integration include the thalamus (Crick, 1984; Cappe, Morel, Barone, & Rouiller, 2009) and superior colliculus (May, 2006). The superior colliculus has also been shown to contain multisensory neurons in animals (Gordon, 1973; Stein & Meredith, 1993; Wallace, Wilkinson, & Stein, 1996), and is involved in reflexive orienting of attention toward salient stimuli (Talsma et al., 2010). The superior colliculus is the only multilayered structure in the brain receiving visual, auditory, and motor signals from different discrete layers that connect to motor regions adjacent, allowing the 10ms sensory input information to drive attention to actions (Wallace, 2004).

At a cortical level, complex integration of information from different senses, particularly vision, has been shown to take place in the posterior parietal cortex (Burton et al., 1999; Johansen-Berg & Lloyd, 2000; Eimer & Forster, 2003; Bear, Connors, & Paradiso, 2007; Puce & Carey, 2010). The intraparietal sulcus (IPS) has also been implicated in the attentional aspects of multisensory integration (Calvert, 2001; Schroeder et al., 2003). Superior temporal sulcus and gyrus have also been implicated, because neurons here are responsive to auditory, visual, and somatosensory input (Hikosaka, Iwai, Saito, & Tanaka, 1988; Schroeder et al., 2003). In addition, the temporoparietal junction (TPJ) has been proposed as a site of multisensory integration of visuospatial, vestibular, and body-related signals—the alignment of these signals generates and helps maintain an individual's sense of bodily self (Blanke & Arzy, 2005). Multisensory learning also involves the prefrontal cortex (Fuster, Bodner, & Kroger, 2000).

Multisensory processing is not simply hierarchical, but can show early influences in primary sensory areas (Driver & Noesselt, 2008). For example, combined ERP and fMRI studies have demonstrated multisensory integration between the tactile, visual (Amedi, Jacobson, Hendler, Malach, & Zohary, 2002), somatosensory, and auditory domains (Foxe et al., 2000) at early processing times. Secondary processing areas within other modalities involve multisensory integration; for example, neurons in macaque secondary auditory cortex have also been shown to be responsive to somatosensory stimulation (Fu et al., 2003).

14.3 LEARNING NEEDS ATTENTION, WORKING MEMORY, AND MOTIVATION

14.3.1 NEURAL PLASTICITY: LEARNING IN THE BRAIN

Humans and animals are consistently being required to adapt their behavior to ensure effective responses to a constantly changing environment. These behavioral changes are associated with permanent structural changes in the brain (Mateer & Kerns, 2000; Gazzaniga, 2004; Kolb, Teskey, & Gibb, 2010), referred to as *evidence of neuroplasticity*. Neuroplasticity refers to the ability of the nervous system to change its structure, function, and connections in response to experience or the environment (Held, 1965; Hubel & Wiesel, 1968; Kolb, 1996; Merzenich et al., 2002; Ward, 2005; Greenwood & Parasuraman, 2010; Cramer et al., 2011). More broadly, the term *plasticity* may be used to refer to any changes at different levels of the nervous system, ranging from molecular events, to cellular events such as growth of new neurons (neurogenesis) and synapses (synaptogenesis), to behavior (Shaw & McEachern, 2001; Cramer et al., 2011). Neural plasticity is also the mechanism underlying conscious learning. Attention modulates neural plasticity and is necessarily involved in new learning and the laying down of new memory traces (Sathian & Burton, 1991; Ahissar, Abeles, Ahissar, Haidarliu, & Vaadia, 1998; Goldstone, 1998; Noppeney, Waberski, Gobbele, & Buchner, 1999; Ngezahayo, Schachner, & Artola, 2000; Jagadeesh, 2006; Polley, Steinberg, & Merzenich, 2006; Mukai et al., 2007). For example, in one study, Stefan, Wycislo, and Classen (2004) demonstrated that the use of paired associative stimulation and transcranial magnetic stimulation (TMS) on a region of the motor cortex (on subject's hand) resulted in neural plasticity *only* when the subject's attention was on the treated hand. Neural plasticity did not occur when the subject did not attend to the treated hand during the procedure.

Although there are critical periods early in life when neural networks are more receptive to synaptic change and development (Daw, 2005), changes associated with neural reorganization continue throughout the lifespan (Steward, 2006; Nudo, 2007), as evident in the ability of humans to continue to learn new information throughout life. Attention to unpleasant or fearful stimuli or events (negative attention) leads to the laying down of the most intense memories, such as in post-trauma syndrome, whereas positive valence attention (motivation) is suggested to be a key modulator of neural plasticity by promoting attention on task. For example, Castro-Alamancos and Borrell (1995) found that rats would more readily engage in reaching rehabilitation tasks if they received food treats (reward) as a result. Additionally, stimulation of the ventral tegmental area (a reward circuit in the brain) was associated with an increased performance on the reaching rehabilitation tasks in the rats tested, which further highlights the role of motivation in the learning process.

14.3.2 ATTENTION AND WORKING MEMORY

Attention and working memory share similar fMRI activation areas in the brain and are both fundamentally important for the most basic learning processes (Owen, McMillan, Laird, & Bullmore, 2005). Working memory is the ability to maintain and manipulate the interaction between new information and older memories online in the presence of other information or distractions. According to the commonly acknowledged Baddeley and Hitch (2000) working memory model, working memory is commonly considered to comprise four subsystems that each serve a different function. These subtypes include the *central executive*, which controls and coordinates incoming information; the *visual-spatial sketchpad*, which is responsible for manipulating visual information; the *phonological loop*, which rehearses verbal information; and the *episodic buffer*, which is primarily responsible for temporal storage of information. It has been suggested that working memory subsystems are differentiated functionally but not anatomically, as the prefrontal cortex has been shown to be activated by all the subcomponents. Müller and Knight (2006) report in a review paper that according to evidence found from lesion studies, the visual-spatial sketchpad of working memory can be further divided into the conscious ventral stream and the dorsal stream. The ventral stream is derived from the occipital visual cortex area V1 and projects to temporal cortex, where it is involved in object recognition, whereas the dorsal stream facilitates object recognition by connecting the occipital and parietal cortex and frontoparietal attention networks.

Working memory and selective attention also share overlapping areas in the parietal cortex, as shown by common activation of the posterior parietal cortex during both working memory and attention type tasks (Rawley

& Constantinidis, 2009). The posterior parietal cortex receives its major input from the visual system via the dorsal stream. It also has numerous connections to other sensory modalities, frontal regions, limbic structures, superior colliculus, and basal ganglia (Rawley & Constantinidis, 2009) and receives projections from auditory and somatosensory areas (primary [SI] and secondary [SII] somatosensory cortices; Friedman, Murray, O'Neill, & Mishkin, 1986; Pons & Kaas, 1986; Disbrow, Litinas, Recanzone, Padberg, & Krubitzer, 2003) and thalamic nuclei (Friedman & Murray, 1986). The posterior parietal cortex, in turn, projects back to SII, premotor cortex, the limbic cortex, and the superior temporal sulcus (Kaas, 2004). In addition, part of SII (parietal operculum, OP 1) has also been suggested to subserve tactile working memory (Romo, Hernandez, Zainos, Lemus, & Brody, 2002; Pleger et al., 2003; Burton, Sinclair, & McLaren, 2008; Burton, Sinclair, Wingert, & Dierker, 2008).

This similarity in the brain regions for activation of attention and working memory has led to speculation as to whether attention and working memory are necessarily different processes (Awh & Jonides, 2001). We suggest that what makes attention and working memory processes separate or different are their temporal characteristics. That is, attention precedes working memory and selects stimuli that are to be maintained and processed in working memory, while directing access to different aspects of working memory. Indeed, a recent study demonstrated that while working memory needs attention, attention does not need working memory (Buehner, Krumm, & Pick, 2005). This is conceptually logical, given that it is critical to selectively attend to information while maintaining other information online, but one may attend to only one bit of new information at a time, and thus not require reference to long-term memory or the online working memory component of information processing. Not surprisingly, when the posterior parietal cortex of the brain is damaged due to brain lesions (e.g., a stroke), the result is grave impairment in attention, working memory, and learning.

14.3.3 SELECTIVE ATTENTION IS ALSO GUIDED BY EMOTIVE AND MOTIVATIONAL EVALUATION OF THE TARGET STIMULI

The brain has a limited capacity to process information; thus, it is important to prioritize the selection of items of information to be attended and processed in working memory first, in order to achieve immediate and long-term goals (Raymond, 2009). As has been shown in many studies utilizing visual attention type paradigms, such as spatial cueing, one's emotional evaluation of stimuli (positive or negative) influences the rate of change of attention allocation and speed of object recognition (Raymond, 2009). For example, studies have shown that adults attend longer

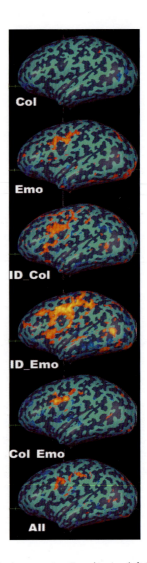

Figure 14.4 FMRI brain reconstruction showing left hemisphere sites of activation for one subject correctly performing a working memory task known as an *n-back* task, and demonstrating overlapping nature of attention and working memory networks and lack of activation recorded when tasks are consciously "too difficult." N-back tasks require identification of similar stimuli that appear *n* places apart in a rapid serial presentation task. In this case we used a 1-back task utilizing familiar cartoon faces. The criteria requiring identification by button presses here were (i) same faces (ID) though in different colors (Col); (ii) different identities but same color (Col); (iii) same emotions (Emo) on any faces; and then combinations of (iv) ID and Col but any emotion; (v) ID Emo but any color; (vi) Col and Emo but any face; and (vii) all 3 features have to be present. Note the similarity of activations to that normally seen when imaging attention. Note also that the single conditions were relatively easy, though judging emotion was reportedly the most difficult of these three conditions as indicated by personal report and the extent of activation in the upper three brains. The combined ID-Emo condition induced greatest activation despite being reported as less difficult than the last two conditions, where this participant reported "giving up." Photo—Crewther, D. P., Panioutyis A., & Crewther, S. G., original unpublished data.

to emotive stimuli (e.g., an angry face) than to either neutral or novel stimuli (Lipp, Price, & Tellegen, 2009).

This prioritization of information selection is also influenced by the predictive value of the stimuli and determines how much of one's finite attentional resources will be committed to the fastest processing of the stimuli most relevant to one's immediate goal (Raymond, 2009). Such attentional resources would be expected to be even more limited in any brain-damaged patient suffering fatigue and possibly clinical depression associated with inflammation. The actual mechanisms underlying prioritization of the incoming stimuli are necessarily based on prior learning of the reward or punishment value associated with the stimuli and, obviously, stored in long-term memory (Raymond, 2009). In common parlance, this prioritization is referred to as the degree of *motivation* of the individual and is recognized by clinicians and health practitioners as being an extraordinarily important aspect of prognosis of stroke recovery.

A distributed network of cortical and subcortical regions have been said to be involved in the emotional evaluation processes (LeDoux, 1996; Heller, 2004). In particular, the amygdala that is the site of cortisol action, and an important component of the hypothalamic-pituitary-adrenal axis, is also believed to be involved in processing physical responses to emotional stimuli (Damasio, 1996) and hence potentially plays an important role in monitoring, updating, and integrating sensory signals (Schaefer et al., 2006; Schaefer & Gray, 2007). In particular, the amygdala has been shown to receive emotionally salient sensory information from unisensory and multisensory nuclei in the thalamus (Smiley & Falchier, 2009), suggesting that it could be an important nucleus in integrating the emotional and motivational factors that are carried in sensory signals (e.g., the emotional understanding that grows out of attending to body language). Thus, the amygdala must play an important role in overall perception (Raymond, 2009) and possibly be responsible for the reputedly more local or self-centered view of the world associated with all types of "sickness behavior" (Dantzer, 2004), including stroke.

Indeed, the anterior cingulate cortex (ACC), amygdala, and orbitofrontal cortex have been proposed as key regions linking attention, emotion, and motivation (Raymond, 2009). The ACC has also been suggested to play an important role in the regulation of bodily states of arousal and to meet concurrent behavioral demands (Iacovella & Hasson, 2011). It appears to be one of the most important brain mediators between peripherally generated sympathetic information and brain activity (Iacovella & Hasson, 2011). The insula (lateral to ACC) has been linked to subjective awareness and affective processing of bodily signals (Craig, 2002) and has been found to show correlated activity with variation in heart rate, suggesting that it could also be involved in the representation of afferent information from the autonomic nervous system toward the cortex. The insula has been suggested to be a critical node for the relay of visual, auditory, and somatosensory information from the parietal cortex to the amygdala and hippocampus (Smiley & Falchier, 2009). Thus, it seems that these key regions—the amygdala, ACC, orbitofrontal cortex, and insula—are likely to play a key role in assigning emotional value to sensory information in order to guide behavior (Damasio, 1996; LeDoux, 1996; Raymond, 2009).

In conclusion, emotional and motivational evaluation of stimuli appears to improve sensory perception and enhance the perceptual benefits of attention (Mesulam, 1998; Phelps, Ling, & Carrasco, 2006; Pessoa, 2008; Raymond, 2009). Such a concept has previously not been sufficiently addressed in the context of recovery and rehabilitation post-stroke, but certainly needs to be, particularly given that mood disorders are common post-stroke (Robinson & Starkstein, 2002; Linden et al., 2007; Pascoe et al., 2011; see also Chapter 8).

14.3.4 THE CASE OF DEPRESSION

As referred to earlier, patients with post-stroke depression regularly report severe fatigue and reduced motivation that would be expected to affect their ability to attend, remember, or hold information in working memory, and which must impede their ability to relearn. Depression has also long been known to be associated with higher psychological and physiological stress, increased neurodegeneration, and reduced neurogenesis leading to impaired attention, motivation, and working memory (Mialet et al., 1996; Austin et al., 2001; Brose et al., 2011). Thus, it is not surprising that neural plasticity has also been found to be low in depressed individuals (Hayley, Poulter, Merali, & Anisman, 2005; Pittenger & Duman, 2007). Indeed, it has been suggested in the literature that neural cell death and physiologically reduced neural plasticity may be an underlying cause of behavioral depression (Dantzer, 2004). Increased levels of neurotoxic peptides (such as cortisol, cortisol releasing hormone, and gamma-aminobutyric acid) are often found in patients with chronic stress or depression and result in neural cell death, particularly in the hippocampus, which is on average relatively smaller in depressed individuals (Hayley et al., 2005; Pascoe et al., 2011). Cell death and low neuroplasticity have also found to result in low levels of neurotransmitters such as serotonin, which may explain the low serotonin levels often reported in depression (Hayley et al., 2005). With the high incidence of depression post-stroke it is important to both assess and treat depression (Pascoe et al., 2011) properly before attempting intensive rehabilitation. Otherwise, rehabilitation may not be particularly effective in producing the neural changes and long-term plasticity needed for better cognition and quality of life and behavioral performance in post-stroke patients.

14.4 THE EFFECT OF BRAIN LESIONS ON ATTENTION

Brain damage—whether it is a mild traumatic brain injury (mTBI; i.e., transient alteration to consciousness;

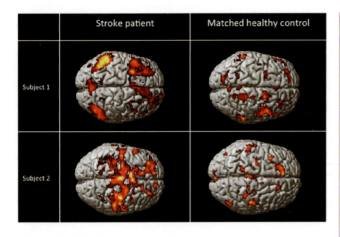

	Stroke patient	Matched healthy control
Subject 1		
Subject 2		

Figure 14.5 Functional connectivity networks for two patients at 1 month post-stroke and for matched healthy controls.

Functional connectivity analysis of low frequency resting-state functional magnetic resonance imaging data (fcMRI) is a method that can be used to study brain networks during undirected behavior. Correlations between low frequency fluctuations of the blood oxygen level dependent (BOLD) signal have been identified between a region of interest in the somatosensory area of the ventroposterior thalamus, and the regions illustrated above in Figure 14.5. In both stroke patients, stronger functional correlations between the thalamus and bilateral frontoparietal regions can be seen relative to matched healthy control individuals. The need for greater attentional demands on stroke patients during planning and execution of sensorimotor tasks is likely to be reflected in strengthened functional connections between thalamus and frontoparietal attention regions. These regions (see above) are present even in the absence of explicit task performance. Adapted from Bannister, Crewther, Gavrilescu, & Carey (2010).

Halterman et al., 2006) such as a concussion, or more severe injury such as a stroke—results in neural atrophy in affected regions and changes in the brain's connectivity. Such damage to the brain negatively affects the attention network and the process of learning (Kleim & Jones, 2008).

Halterman and colleagues (2006) compared individuals with mTBI to healthy control individuals (matched on gender, age, height, weight, and activity level) in terms of alerting, orienting, and executive components of visual attention. They showed that those with mTBI sustained impairment in executive component of attention up to 1 month post-injury, suggesting that attentional mechanisms are particularly vulnerable even to mild brain damage, and for prolonged times after. More severe damage to the brain, such as a stroke, commonly results in lesions to the parietal cortex, thus even more drastically limiting the vascular supply to this important area of sensory integration. This results in even more severe impairment in the attention and/or working memory systems.

Unilateral spatial neglect is a common neurological deficit caused by a stroke, characterized by an inability to attend to objects in the opposite side of the lesion despite showing normal vision or somatosensory input. It is estimated to affect between 25%–30% of patients, which is estimated to be approximately 250,000 patients in the United States per year (Corbetta & Shulman, 2011). Spatial neglect can occur following lesions to either hemisphere of the brain, but is more obvious when it affects the right hemisphere. Affected individuals also present with reduced speed of information processing and arousal, lack of awareness of their illness, and lack of ownership of their own body. Corbetta and Shulman (2011) have proposed that spatial neglect is due to impairment in the attentional networks of the brain. More specifically, they suggest that the bias in spatial attention to objects and locations on the side of the lesion seen in patients with neglect is a result of impairment to the *more dorsal* frontoparietal network that controls attention, while nonspatial deficits of neglect, such as reduced arousal, can be attributed to damage to the *more ventral* attentional stream.

One of the more severe effects of a parietal lesion is Balint's syndrome, which is the inability to direct vision away from the fovea or to scan the visual world and coordinate one's hand movements toward objects, as well as the inability to perceive more than one object at any one time (Corbetta & Shulman, 2011). Visual neglect caused by parietal lesions (right or bilateral) can also be accompanied by impairments in spatial working memory for both the object and its location. Another potential impairment for patients with neglect is the inability to attend to more than one memory at a time (i.e., memory simultanagnosia). This could also be more generally seen as evidence of impaired working memory capacity and efficiency.

14.5 REHABILITATION POST-STROKE

Rehabilitation approaches that are founded on the potential for and evidence of neuroplastic changes in the brain (Kolb & Whishaw, 1998; Azari & Seitz, 2000; Mateer & Kerns, 2000; Nudo, 2003; McEwen, 2004; Selzer, Clarke, Cohen, Duncan, & Gage, 2006), have been shown to be behaviorally beneficial for many stroke survivors (Outpatient Service Trialists, 2003; Dobkin, 2004; Barnes, Dobkin, & Bogousslavsky, 2005; Hodics, Cohen, & Cramer, 2006; Legg, Drummond, & Langhorne, 2006). Some degree of spontaneous behavioral improvement also occurs post-stroke via multiple cellular and molecular events (Barone & Feuerstein, 1999). In the hours after stroke, functional improvement may be mediated by restoration of blood flow (Rossini, Caluatti, Pauri, & Baron, 2003; Lezak et al., 2004; Seitz, Butefisch, Kleiser, & Homberg, 2004; Ropper & Brown, 2005). From 3 days to around 4 weeks after stroke, clinical improvement, usually measured in terms of motor function, is largely due to the spontaneous regression of brain edema (Wei, Erinjeri, Rovainen, & Woolsey, 2001; Katsman, Zheng, Spinelli, & Carmichael, 2003; Seitz et al., 2004). Slower, more sustained functional improvement in outcomes such as motor performance continues in the following months (Wade, Wood, & Langton Hewer, 1985; Binkofski et al., 2001; Kwakkel, Kollen, van der Grond, & Prevo, 2003; Carey & Seitz, 2007), though it is both associated with and limited by excessive fatigue and prolonged neuroinflammatory-induced "sickness behavior" (Dantzer, 2004).

On the other hand, later improvements in behavior are likely to be underpinned by the reduction in neuroinflammation and the long-term neuroanatomical and neurophysiological changes that occur during any learning and behavioral change (Kolb & Whishaw, 1998; Rossini et al., 2003; Seitz et al., 2004; Selzer et al., 2006; Carey & Seitz, 2007). Post-stroke molecular and cellular processes of neural plasticity have been demonstrated in animal models to take place in both perilesional and remote brain regions (Schallert, Leasure, & Kolb, 2000; Carmichael, 2003; Kolb, 2003; Dancause et al., 2005). For example, increased expression of developmental proteins such as vascular endothelial growth factor (VEGF) has been shown in animal models in the hours and days after stroke, both in the infarct and peri-infarct regions and in more remote cortical areas (Carmichael et al., 2005; Stowe et al., 2007). These proteins are involved in neuronal growth, apoptosis, angiogenesis, and cellular differentiation (Carmichael et al., 2005; Stowe et al., 2007). Structural changes, such as increased dendritic branching (T. A. Jones & Schallert, 1992) and synaptogenesis—increases in the number of synapses per neuron and the volume and membrane surface area of dendritic processes per neuron (T. A. Jones, Kleim, & Greenough, 1996)—have been found to occur in contralateral motor cortex of adult rats several weeks after experimentally induced stroke. There is evidence of increased hyperexcitability in perilesional and contralateral cortex after focal lesions in the sensory area in rats (Buchkremer-Ratzmann, August, Hagemann, & Witte, 1996).

Importantly, these neuroplastic changes can be modified by behavioral experiences such as skill training (Nudo, 2007; T. A. Jones et al., 2009;). For example, environmental enrichment (Johansson & Belichenko, 2002; Komitova, Perfilieva, Mattsson, Eriksson, & Johansson, 2002; Dahlqvist et al., 2003) and social interaction (Dahlqvist et al., 2003) have been shown to produce improved behavioral outcomes and measurable neuroanatomical changes in rat models of stroke. Examples of such changes include increased dendritic spine density in pyramidal neurons contralateral to a cortical infarct (Johansson & Belichenko, 2002) and increased ipsilateral production of astrocytes (Komitova et al., 2002), following post-ischemic exposure to an enriched environment. Task-specific rehabilitative therapy, in the form of daily skilled-reach training, has been shown in a rat model of stroke to result in behavioral improvement as well as enhanced dendritic complexity and length in the undamaged motor cortex, in rats who underwent training compared to those who received standard intervention (Biernaskie & Corbett, 2001). However, animal models of stroke recovery have typically been carried out on healthy young animals with few of the vascular risk factors, such as high cholesterol, high blood pressure, and diabetes, that are common in older stroke victims, thus limiting their applicability to humans and leading to problems in translation of findings from the lab to the clinic (Kolb et al., 2010).

In humans, a growing body of evidence from functional imaging studies indicates that behavioral manipulations in the form of attention-based rehabilitation protocols can lead to changes in the brain after stroke that are associated with improved outcomes (Hodics et al., 2006; Carey & Seitz, 2007; Richards, Stewart, Woodbury, Senesac, & Cauraugh, 2008; Stinear, Barber, Coxon, Fleming, & Byblow, 2008). Preliminary evidence using structural imaging in long-term stroke survivors has shown increased cortical thickness in the same areas that showed functional plasticity (Schaechter, Moore, Connell, Rosen, & Dijkhuizen, 2006; Gauthier et al., 2008). Further work is needed to better characterize the exact mechanisms underlying this relationship, and these results need to be more widely replicated in larger samples. Nonetheless, they provide early evidence of changes in the human brain that might underlie behavioral improvement after brain injury.

14.5.1 TRAINING ATTENTION POST-STROKE

It is not surprising that attention skills have been shown to predict outcome after stroke, given that they are critical for new learning and memory (Goldstone, 1998; Polley et al., 2006; Mukai et al., 2007), and that attention networks and greater blood flow may need to be recruited to compensate for reduced function in specific brain areas (Ferdon & Murphy, 2003; Madden, Whiting, Provenzale, & Huettel, 2004; Minati, Grisoli, & Bruzzone, 2007). Specifically, retained attentional abilities, such as sustained concentration (Robertson, Ridgeway, Greenfield, & Parr, 1997), ability to shift attention between several salient stimuli (McDowd, Filion, Pohl, Richards, & Stiers, 2003), and working memory capacity (Malouin, Belleville, Richards, Desrosiers, & Doyon, 2004) strongly predict patients' potential to benefit from rehabilitation and their long-term functional improvement on physical and social outcomes (Robertson et al., 1997; McDowd et al., 2003; Nys et al., 2005). Conversely, executive deficits have been found to predict poor functional outcome a year after stroke (Lesniak, Bak, Czepiel, Seniow, & Czlonkowska, 2008; see Chapter 15).

At a neural level, attention selectively enhances the single-cell responses conveying information about relevant sensory attributes (Burton & Sinclair, 2000) through enhanced neuronal responses to relevant stimuli

(Mountcastle, Andersen, & Motter, 1981; Lamme, 2000), suppressed responses to distracting stimuli (Burton & Sinclair, 2000), and enhanced synchronization of activity (Alonso, Usrey, & Reid, 1996; Larkum, Zhu, & Sakmann, 1999; Azouz & Gray, 2000; Usrey, Alonso, & Reid, 2000; Fries, Reynolds, Rorie, & Desimone, 2001; Wannig et al., 2011). The reticular nucleus of the thalamus receives inhibitory inputs from novelty-activated, ascending cholinergic brainstem pathways, and it has been suggested that during periods of arousal, the suppression of the reticular nucleus would enhance cortical plasticity (Kaas & Ebner, 1998; Kaas, 1999). Attention is also associated with the activation of modulatory neurotransmitters such as acetylcholine (Bear & Singer, 1986). Overall, the changes in brain activity associated with arousal and attention create an environment in which permanent learning can best occur.

The brain's attention systems are also vital in compensating for the impairment of function-specific brain areas due to aging or injury (Ferdon & Murphy, 2003; Madden et al., 2004; Maruishi, Miyatani, Nakao, & Muranaka, 2007; Minati et al., 2007). In a study of patients with diffuse axonal injury, Maruishi et al. (2007) reported that patients showed greater activation of the right prefrontal area when carrying out a working memory task at similar performance levels to controls, presumably because more attentional resources were required to maintain the same standard of performance. In stroke patients, it is well established that increased attention is required for previously simple tasks such as walking (Jueptner et al., 1997; Haggard, Cockburn, Cock, Fordham, & Wade, 2000; Bowen et al., 2001; Rowe, Friston, Frackowiak, & Passingham, 2002).

Interestingly, subtle attentional deficits in patients considered clinically "recovered" have been shown to be associated with poor social functioning. In a study by McDowd, Filion, Pohl, Richards, and Stiers (2003) 6 months post-stroke, patients living independently with a Mini-Mental State Exam (MMSE; Folstein, Folstein, & McHugh, 1975) of at least 18, still showed impaired sustained and divided attention on a series of computer-based attentional tasks compared to healthy older adults. The extent of these attention deficits were also found to be negatively associated with the degree of social participation of the recovered patients, highlighting the fact that ability to disengage and reengage attention is likely to be associated with the ability to carry on a conversation and switch from one topic to another rapidly, as happens in normal everyday life. Findings of this study suggested that new, more sensitive assessment measures are required in order to effectively characterize patients' cognitive deficits post-stroke and that these tests should be applied even for patients who appear cognitively intact.

In regard to rehabilitation practices, attention training has been suggested by Ponsford and Willmott (2004) as one means of improving attention post-stoke. Attention training typically involves exercises designed to remediate attention impairments using stimulus–response paradigms that require subjects to identify and select among relevant auditory and visual stimuli, often using speeded stimulus presentations (Cicerone et al., 2000). There is now substantial evidence to support attention interventions after TBI, such as strategy training for post-acute attention deficits (Cicerone et al., 2005, 2011). In their meta-analysis of 30 studies of attention rehabilitation after acquired brain injury (ABI; predominantly TBI, mean age 29.5) or stroke (mean age 54.3), Park and Ingles (2001) found that performance improved significantly after attention training in young patients with ABI.

In contrast to the many studies with TBI populations, few studies have specifically evaluated the efficacy of training nonspatial attention post-stroke. One study by McDowd et al. (2003) has shown that patients with stroke show improvements on attention type tasks if they have been practicing tasks that require those attention mechanisms (McDowd et al., 2003), but that the training is unlikely to generalize to other types of tasks requiring attention. One Cochrane review has been published that included two randomized controlled trials (Lincoln, Majid, & Weyman, 2000). Attention training was shown to improve alertness and sustained attention; however, neither study measured the effect of training on secondary measures such as of activities of daily living. Thus, the effect of post-stroke attention training on everyday functional abilities remains unknown.

Learning in stroke patients has also been shown to be facilitated by delivering instructions accounting for their attention deficits. For example, Carey and Matyas (2005) have suggested that a patient may be more successful in rehabilitation if cues are used to help the patient allocate his/her attention appropriately, as well as the use of clear explicit instructions and pausing before switching from one activity or instruction to another, to provide the patient with sufficient time to reallocate attention (Sohlberg & Mateer, 2001; Carey & Matyas, 2005). Research is still needed to determine whether such approaches will facilitate rehabilitation training but they do highlight the importance of ensuring attention is activated if learning is to occur. Importantly, the quality of the therapist/patient interaction beyond the specific training tasks has been shown to impact the effectiveness of treatment, such as through the use of feedback, reinforcement, and confidence-building (Ponsford & Kinsella, 1988; Wilson & Robertson, 1992; Cicerone, 2002). Thus, attention and motivation and goals are critical components of stroke rehabilitation training programs (Yekutiel, 2000; Carey, 2006; Shaughnessy & Resnick, 2009), and need to be further explored in future studies.

14.6 SUMMARY AND CONCLUSION

Stroke continues to be a cause of prolonged disability worldwide. Thus, rehabilitation training post-stroke must provide an opportunity for relearning and progress toward greater independence. Such rehabilitation and post-stroke recovery is theoretically likely to be mediated by attention-facilitated learning and neural reorganization. Evidence of the role of attention in recovery after stroke (Robertson et al., 1997; McDowd et al., 2003; Nys et al., 2005), as well as learning (Polley et al., 2006) and plasticity (Noppeney et al., 1999), allows us to make predictions regarding the neural networks involved in facilitating recovery of attentional function after stroke (Corbetta & Shulman, 2011; de Schotten et al., 2011). Potentially, the integrity of attentional networks, as well as multisensory pathways and interactions with circuits involved in motivation and emotion, are likely to predict an individual's level of impairment, suggesting that the promotion of goal-driven attention, working memory, and motivation in rehabilitation should facilitate relearning and post-stroke recovery. Thus, in the context of recovery post-stroke, training neural systems related to attention, working memory, learning, and motivation are presumably fundamental to any improvement in behavior and the prospect of greater independence.

REFERENCES

Abegunde, D. O., Mathers, C. D., Adam, T., Ortegon, M., & Strong, K. (2007). The burden and costs of chronic diseases in low-income and middle-income countries. *The Lancet, 370*(9603), 1929–1938.

Ahissar, E., Abeles, M., Ahissar, M., Haidarliu, S., & Vaadia, E. (1998). Hebbian-like functional plasticity in the auditory cortex of the behaving monkey. *Neuropharmacology, 37*, 633–655.

Allman, J. M., & Kaas, J. H. (1971a). Representation of the visual field in striate and adjoining cortex of the owl monkey (Aotus trivirgatus). *Brain research, 35*(1), 89–106.

Allman, J. M., & Kaas, J. H. (1971b). A representation of the visual field in the caudal third of the middle temporal gyrus of the owl monkey (Aotus trivirgatus). *Brain research, 31*(1), 85–105.

Alonso, J.-M., Usrey, W. M., & Reid, R. C. (1996). Precisely correlated firing in cells of the lateral geniculate nucleus. *Nature, 383*, 815–819.

Amedi, A., Jacobson, G., Hendler, T., Malach, R., & Zohary, E. (2002). Convergence of visual and tactile shape processing in the human lateral occipital complex. *Cerebral Cortex, 12*, 1202–1212.

Andersen, R. A. (1997). Multimodal integration for the representation of space in the posterior parietal cortex. *Philosophical Transactions of the Royal Society of London, Series B: Biological Sciences, 352*, 1421–1428.

Anisman, H., Merali, Z., & Hayley, S. (2008). Neurotransmitter, peptide and cytokine processes in relation to depressive disorder: Comorbidity between depression and neurodegenerative disorders. *Progress in Neurobiology, 85*, 1–74.

Arrington, C. M., Carr, T. H., Mayer, A. R., & Rao, S. M. (2001). Neural mechanisms of visual attention: Object-based selection of a region in space. *Journal of Cognitive Neuroscience, 12*(SUPPL. 2), 106–117.

Austin, M. P., Mitchell, P., & Goodwin, G. M. (2001). Cognitive deficits in depression: possible implications for functional neuropathology. *The British Journal of Psychiatry, 178*(3), 200–206.

Awh, E., & Jonides, J. (2001). Overlapping mechanisms of attention and spatial working memory. *Trends in cognitive sciences, 5*(3), 119–126.

Azari, N. P., & Seitz, R. J. (2000). Brain plasticity and recovery from stroke. *American Scientist, 88*, 426–451.

Azouz, R., & Gray, C. M. (2000). Dynamic spike threshold reveals a mechanism for synaptic coincidence detection in cortical neurons in vivo. *Proceedings of the National Academy of Sciences of the United States of America, 97*, 8110–8115.

Baddeley, A. D., & Hitch, G. J. (2000). Development of working memory: Should the Pascual-Leone and the Baddeley and Hitch models be merged?. *Journal of Experimental Child Psychology, 77*(2), 128–137.

Ballard, C., Stephens, S., Kenny, R., Kalaria, R., Tovee, M., & O'Brien, J. (2003). Profile of neuropsychological deficits in older stroke survivors without dementia. *Dementia and Geriatric Cognitive Disorders, 16*, 52–56.

Bannister, L. C., Crewther, S. C., Gavrilescu, M. Carey, L. M., (2010). Somatosensory networks in stroke survivors with somatosensory impairment: new insights from resting state functional connectivity. *European Stroke Conference 2010*. Barcelona.

Barker-Collo, S. L. (2007). Depression and anxiety 3 months post stroke: Prevalence and correlates. *Archives of Clinical Neuropsychology, 22*, 519–531.

Barker-Collo, S. L., Feigin, V., Lawes, C., Senior, H., & Parag, V. (2010). Natural History of Attention Deficits and Their Influence on Functional Recovery from Acute Stages to 6 Months after Stroke. *Neuroepidemiology, 35*(4), 255–262.

Barnes, M. P., Dobkin, B. H., & Bogousslavsky, J. (2005). *Recovery after stroke*. New York: Cambridge University Press.

Barone, F. C., & Feuerstein, G. Z. (1999). Inflammatory mediators and stroke: New opportunities for novel therapeutics. *Journal of Cerebral Blood Flow and Metabolism, 19*, 819–834.

Bear, M. F., Connors, B. W., & Paradiso, M. A. (2007). *Neuroscience: Exploring the brain* (3rd ed.). Baltimore, MD: Lippincott Williams & Wilkins.

Bear, M. F., & Singer, W. (1986). Modulation of visual cortical plasticity by acetylcholine and noradrenaline. *Nature, 320*, 172–176.

Biernaskie, J., & Corbett, D. (2001). Enriched rehabilitative training promotes improved forelimb motor function and enhanced dendritic growth after focal ischemic injury. *Journal of Neuroscience, 21*, 5272–5280.

Binkofski, F., Seitz, R. J., Hackländer, T., Pawelec, D., Mau, J., & Freund, H.-J. (2001). Recovery of motor functions following hemiparetic stroke: A clinical and magnetic resonance-morphometric study. *Cerebrovascular Diseases, 11*, 273–281.

Blanke, O., & Arzy, S. (2005). The out-of-body experience: Disturbed self-processing at the temporo-parietal junction. *Neuroscientist, 11*, 16–24.

Bonita, R., Solomon, N., & Broad, J. B. (1997). Prevalence of stroke and stroke-related disability. *Stroke, 28*, 1898–1902.

Bowen, A., Wenman, R., Mickelborough, J., Foster, J., Hill, E., & Tallis, R. (2001). Dual-task effects of talking while walking on velocity and balance following a stroke. *Age and Ageing, 30*, 319–323.

Brose, A., Schmiedek, F., Lövdén, M., & Lindenberger, U. (2011). Daily variability in working memory is coupled with negative affect: The role of attention and motivation. *Emotion*, July 25, DOI: 10.1037/a0024436

Bruce, C. J., & Goldberg, M. E. (1985). Primate frontal eye fields. I. Single neurons discharging before saccades. *Journal of Neurophysiology, 53*, 603–635.

Buchel, C., Josephs, O., Rees, G., Turner, R., Frith, C. D., & Friston, K. J. (1998). The functional anatomy of attention to visual motion: A functional MRI study. *Brain, 121*, 1281–1294.

Buchkremer-Ratzmann, I., August, M., Hagemann, G., & Witte, O. W. (1996). Electrophysiological transcortical diaschisis after cortical photothrombosis in rat brain. *Stroke, 27*, 1105–1109.

Buehner, M., Krumm, S., & Pick, M. (2005). Reasoning=working memory [not equal to] attention. *Intelligence, 33*(3), 251–272.

Bullier, J. (2001). Integrated model of visual processing. *Brain Research Reviews, 36*, 96–107.

Burton, H., Abend, N. S., MacLeod, A. M., Sinclair, R. J., Snyder, R. J., & Raichle, M. E. (1999). Tactile attention tasks enhance activation in somatosensory regions of parietal cortex: A positron emission tomography study. *Cerebral Cortex, 9*, 662–674.

Burton, H., & Sinclair, R. J. (2000). Attending to and remembering tactile stimuli: A review of brain imaging data and single-neuron responses. *Journal of Clinical Neurophysiology, 17*, 575–591.

Burton, H., Sinclair, R. J., & McLaren, D. G. (2008). Cortical network for vibrotactile attention: A fMRI study. *Human Brain Mapping, 29*, 207–221.

Burton, H., Sinclair, R. J., Wingert, J. R., & Dierker, D. L. (2008). Multiple parietal operculum subdivisions in humans: Tactile activation maps. *Somatosensory and Motor Research, 25*, 149–162.

Calvert, G. A. (2001). Crossmodal processing in the human brain: Insights from functional neuroimaging studies. *Cerebral Cortex, 11*, 1110–1123.

Cappe, C., & Barone, P. (2005). Heteromodal connections supporting multisensory integration at low levels of cortical processing in the monkey. *European Journal of Neuroscience, 22*, 2886–2902.

Cappe, C., Morel, A., Barone, P., & Rouiller, E. M. (2009). The thalamocortical projection systems in primate: An anatomical support for multisensory and sensorimotor interplay. *Cerebral Cortex, 19*, 2025–2037.

Carandang, R., Seshadri, S., Beiser, A., Kelly-Hayes, M., Kase, C. S., Kannel, W. B., & Wolf, P. A. (2006). Trends in incidence, lifetime risk, severity, and 30-day mortality of stroke over the past 50 years. *Journal of the American Medical Association, 296*(24), 2939.

Carey, L. M. (2006). Loss of somatic sensation. In M. Selzer, S. Clarke, L. Cohen, P. Duncan, & F. Gage (Eds.), *Textbook of neural repair and rehabilitation* (Vol. 2, pp. 231–247). Cambridge: Cambridge University Press.

Carey, L. M., & Matyas, T. A. (2005). Training of somatosensory discrimination after stroke: Facilitation of stimulus generalization. *American Journal of Physical Medicine and Rehabilitation, 74*, 428–442.

Carey, L. M., & Seitz, R. J. (2007). Functional neuroimaging in stroke recovery and neurorehabilitation: Conceptual issues and perspectives. *International Journal of Stroke, 2*, 245–264.

Carmichael, S. T. (2003). Plasticity of cortical projections after stroke. *The Neuroscientist, 9*, 64–75.

Carmichael, S. T., Archibeque, I., Luke, L., Nolan, T., Momiy, J., & Li, S. (2005). Growth-associated gene expression after stroke: Evidence for a growth-promoting region in the peri-infarct cortex. *Experimental Neurology, 193*, 291–311.

Castro-Alamancos, M., & Borrell, J. (1995). Functional recovery of forelimb response capacity after forelimb primary motor cortex damage in the rat is due to the reorganization of adjacent areas of cortex. *Neuroscience, 68*(3), 793–805.

Centelles, L., Assaiante, C., Nazarian, B., Anton, J.-L., & Schmitz, C. (2011). Recruitment of both the mirror and the mentalizing networks when observing social interactions depicted by point-lights: A neuroimaging study. *Public Library of Science ONE, 6*, e15749.

Chapman, K. Z., Dale, V. Q., Denes, A., Bennett, G., Rothwell, N. J., Allan, S. M., & McColl, B. W. (2009). A rapid and transient peripheral inflammatory response precedes brain inflammation after experimental stroke. *Journal of Cerebral Blood Flow and Metabolism, 29*, 1764–1768.

Cicerone, K. D. (2002). Remediation of "working attention" in mild traumatic brain injury. *Brain Injury, 16*, 185–195.

Cicerone, K. D., Dahlberg, C., Kalmar, K., Langenbahn, D. M., Malec, J. F., Bergquist, T. F., t al. (2000). Evidence-based cognitive rehabilitation: Recommendations for clinical practice. *Archives of Physical Medicine and Rehabilitation, 81*, 1596–1615.

Cicerone, K. D., Dahlberg, C., Malec, J. F., Langenbahn, D. M., Felicetti, T., Kneipp, S., et al. (2005). Evidence-based cognitive rehabilitation: Updated review of the literature from 1998 through 2002. *Archives of Physical Medicine and Rehabilitation, 86*, 1681–1692.

Cicerone, K. D., Langenbahn, D. M., Braden, C., Malec, J. F., Kalmar, K., Fraas, M., et al. (2011). Evidence-based cognitive rehabilitation: Updated review of the literature from 2003 through 2008. *Archives of Physical Medicine and Rehabilitation, 92*, 519–530.

Clark, L., Cools, R., & Robbins, T. W. (2004). The neuropsychology of ventral prefrontal cortex: Decision-making and reversal learning. *Brain and Cognition, 55*(1), 41–53.

Colby, C. L., Duhamel, J. R., & Goldberg, M. E. (1996). Visual, presaccadic, and cognitive activation of single neurons in monkey lateral intraparietal area. *Journal of Neurophysiology, 76*, 2841–2852.

Corbetta, M., Patel, G., & Shulman, G. L. (2008). The reorienting system of the human brain: From environment to theory of mind. *Neuron, 58*, 306–324.

Corbetta, M., & Shulman, G. (2011). Spatial neglect and attention networks. *Annual Review of Neuroscience, 34*, 569–599.

Corbetta, M., & Shulman, G.L. (2002). Control of goal-directed and stimulus-driven attention in the brain. *Nature Reviews. Neuroscience, 3*, 201–215.

Craig, A. D. (2002). How do you feel? Interoception: The sense of the physiological condition of the body. *Nature Reviews. Neuroscience, 3*, 655–666.

Cramer, S. C., Sur, M., Dobkin, B. H., O'Brien, C., Sanger, T. D., Trojanowski, J. Q., et al. (2011). Harnessing neuroplasticity for clinical applications. *Brain, 134*, 1591–1609.

Crewther, S., Lamp, G., Sanchez-Rockliffe, A., & Crewther, D. (2010). Visual attention related to difficulty in n-back tasks. *Journal of Vision, 10*(7), 221.

Crick, F. (1984). Function of the thalamic reticular complex: The search-light hypothesis. *Proceedings of the National Academy of Sciences of the United States of America, 81*, 4586–4590.

Dahlqvist, P., Ronnback, A., Risedal, A., Nergardh, R., Johansson, I. M., Seckl, J. R., et al. (2003). Effects of postischemic environment on transcription factor and serotonin receptor expression after permanent focal cortical ischemia in rats. *Neuroscience, 119*, 643–652.

Damasio, A. R. (1996). The somatic marker hypothesis and the possible functions of the prefrontal cortex. *Philosophical Transactions of the Royal Society of London, Series B: Biological Sciences, 351*, 1413–1420.

Dancause, N., Barbay, S., Frost, S. B., Plautz, E. J., Chen, D., Zoubina, E. V., et al. (2005). Extensive cortical rewiring after brain injury. *Journal of Neuroscience, 25*, 10167–10179.

Dantzer, R. (2004). Cytokine-induced sickness behaviour: A neuroimmune response to activation of innate immunity. *European Journal of Pharmacology, 500*, 399–411.

Dantzer, R., O'Connor, J. C., Freund, G. G., & Kelley, K. W. (2008). From inflammation to sickness and depression: When the immune system subjugates the brain. *Nature Reviews. Neuroscience, 9*, 46–57.

Daw, N. W. (2005). *Visual development* (2nd ed.). New Haven, Connecticut: Springer.

de Schotten, M. T., Dell'acqua, F., Forkel, S. J., Simmons, A., Vergani, F., Murphy, D. G., & Catani, M. (2011). A lateralized brain network for visuospatial attention. *Nature Neuroscience, 14*, 1245–1246.

Denes, A., Thornton, P., Rothwell, N. J., & Allan, S. M. (2010). Inflammation and brain injury: Acute cerebral ischaemia, peripheral and central inflammation. *Brain, Behavior, and Immunity, 24*, 708–723.

Dewey, H. M., Sherry, L. J., & Collier, J. M. (2007). Stroke rehabilitation 2007: What should it be? *International Journal of Stroke, 2,* 191–200.

Disbrow, E., Litinas, E., Recanzone, G. H., Padberg, J., & Krubitzer, L. (2003). Cortical connections of the second somatosensory area and the parietal ventral area in macaque monkeys. *Journal of Comparative Neurology, 462,* 382–399.

Dobkin, B. (2004). Strategies for stroke rehabilitation. *Lancet Neurology, 3,* 528–536.

Downar, J., Crawley, A. P., Mikulis, D. J., & Davis, K. D. (2000). A multimodal cortical network for the detection of changes in the sensory environment. *Nature Neuroscience, 3*(3), 277–283.

Driver, J., & Noesselt, T. (2008). Multisensory interplay reveals crossmodal influences on "sensory-specific" brain regions, neural responses, and judgments. *Neuron, 57,* 11–23.

Driver, J., & Spence, C. (1998). Cross-modal links in spatial attention. *Philosophical Transactions of the Royal Society B: Biological Sciences, 353*(1373), 1319–1331.

Edwards, D. F., Hahn, M. G., Baum, C. M., & Dromerick, A. W. (2006). The impact of mild stroke on meaningful activity and life satisfaction. *Journal of Stroke and Cerebrovascular Diseases, 15,* 151–157.

Eimer, M., & Forster, B. (2003). Modulations of early somatosensory ERP components by transient and sustained spatial attention. *Experimental Brain Research, 151,* 24–31.

Eslinger, P. J., Parkinson, K., & Shamay, S. G. (2002). Empathy and social-emotional factors in recovery from stroke. *Current Opinion in Neurology, 15,* 91–97.

Ferdon, S., & Murphy, C. (2003). The cerebellum and olfaction in the aging brain: A functional magnetic resonance imaging study. *Neuroimage, 20,* 12–21.

Fisk, G. D., Owsley, C., & Mennemeier, M. (2002). Vision, attention, and self-reported driving behaviors in community-dwelling stroke survivors. *Archives of Physical Medicine and Rehabilitation, 83,* 469–477.

Folstein, M. F., Folstein, S. E., & McHugh, P. R. (1975). "Mini-mental state." A practical method for grading the cognitive state of patients for the clinician. *Journal of Psychiatric Research, 12,* 189–198.

Foxe, J. J., Morocz, I. A., Murray, M. M., Higgins, B. A., Javitt, D. C., & Schroeder, C. E. (2000). Multisensory auditory-somatosensory interactions in early cortical processing revealed by high-density electrical mapping. *Cognitive Brain Research, 10,* 77–83.

Friedman, D. P., & Murray, E. A. (1986). Thalamic connectivity of the second somatosensory area and neighboring somatosensory fields of the lateral sulcus of the macaque. *Journal of Comparative Neurology, 252,* 348–373.

Friedman, D. P., Murray, E. A., O'Neill, J. B., & Mishkin, M. (1986). Cortical connections of the somatosensory fields of the lateral sulcus of macaques: Evidence for a corticolimbic pathway for touch. *Journal of Comparative Neurology, 252,* 323–347.

Fries, P., Reynolds, J. H., Rorie, A. E., & Desimone, R. (2001). Modulation of oscillatory neuronal synchronization by selective visual attention. *Science, 291,* 1560–1563.

Fu, K .M., Johnston, T. A., Shah, A. S., Arnold, L., Smiley, J., Hackett, T. A., et al. (2003). Auditory cortical neurons respond to somatosensory stimulation. *Journal of Neuroscience, 23,* 7510–7515.

Fuster, J. M., Bodner, M., & Kroger, J. K. (2000). Cross-modal and cross-temporal association in neurons of frontal cortex. *Nature, 405,* 347–351.

Gauthier, L. V., Taub, E., Perkins, C., Ortmann, M., Mark, V. W., & Uswatte, G. (2008). Remodeling the brain: Plastic structural brain changes produced by different motor therapies after stroke. *Stroke, 39,* 1520–1525.

Gazzaniga, M. S. (Ed.). (2004). *The cognitive neurosciences* (3rd ed.). Cambridge, MA: MIT Press.

Gnadt, J. W., & Andersen, R. A. (1988). Memory related motor planning activity in posterior parietal cortex of macaque. *Experimental Brain Research, 70,* 216–220.

Goldstone, R. L. (1998). Perceptual learning. *Annual Review of Psychology, 49,* 585–612.

Gordon, B. (1973). Receptive fields in deep layers of cat superior colliculus. *Journal of Neurophysiology, 36,* 157–178.

Greenwood, P. M., & Parasuraman, R. (2010). Neuronal and cognitive plasticity: A neurocognitive framework for ameliorating cognitive aging. *Frontiers in Aging Neuroscience, 2*(150), 1–14.

Hackett, M. L., & Anderson, C. S. (2005). Predictors of depression after stroke: A systematic review of observational studies. *Stroke, 36,* 2296–2301.

Haggard, P., Cockburn, J., Cock, J., Fordham, C., & Wade, D. (2000). Interference between gait and cognitive tasks in a rehabilitating neurological population. *Journal of Neurology, Neurosurgery and Psychiatry, 69,* 479–486.

Halterman, C. I., Langan, J., Drew, A., Rodriguez, E., Osternig, L. R., Chou, L. S., & Donkelaar, P. (2006). Tracking the recovery of visuospatial attention deficits in mild traumatic brain injury. *Brain, 129*(3), 747–753.

Hart, B. L. (1988). Biological basis of the behavior of sick animals. *Neuroscience and Biobehavioral Reviews, 12,* 123–137.

Hayley, S., Poulter, M., Merali, Z., & Anisman, H. (2005). The pathogenesis of clinical depression: stressor-and cytokine-induced alterations of neuroplasticity. *Neuroscience, 135*(3), 659–678.

Held, R. (1965). Plasticity in sensory-motor systems. *Scientific American, 213,* 84–94.

Heller, W. (2004). Emotion. In M. T. Banich (Ed.), *Cognitive neuroscience and neuropsychology* (pp. 393–428). Boston: Houghton Mifflin Company.

Hikosaka, K., Iwai, E., Saito, H., & Tanaka, K. (1988). Polysensory properties of neurons in the anterior bank of the caudal superior temporal sulcus of the macaque monkey. *Journal of Neurophysiology, 60,* 1615–1637.

Hochstenbach, J., Mulder, T., van Limbeel, J., Donders, R., & Schoonderwaldt, H. (1998). Cognitive decline following stroke: A comprehensive study of cognitive decline following stroke. *Journal of Clinical and Experimental Neuropsychology, 20,* 503–517.

Hodics, T., Cohen, L. G., & Cramer, S. C. (2006). Functional imaging of intervention effects in stroke motor rehabilitation. *Archives of Physical Medicine and Rehabilitation, 87,* S36–S42.

Hubel, D. H., & Wiesel, T. N. (1968). Receptive fields and functional architecture of monkey striate cortex. *Journal of Physiology, 195,* 215–243.

Iacovella, V., & Hasson, U. (2011). The relationship between BOLD signal and autonomic nervous system functions: Implications for processing of "physiological noise." *Magnetic Resonance Imaging, 29*(10), 1338–1345.

Jagadeesh, B. (2006). Attentional modulation of cortical plasticity. In M. Selzer, S. Clarke, L. Cohen, P. Duncan & F. Gage (Eds.), *Textbook of neural repair and rehabilitation* (Vol. 1, pp. 194–206). Cambridge: Cambridge University Press.

James, W. (1890). *The principles of psychology.* New York: Dover.

Johansen-Berg, H., & Lloyd, D. (2000). The physiology and psychology of selective attention to touch. *Frontiers in Bioscience, 5,* 894–904.

Johansson, B. B., & Belichenko, P. V. (2002). Neuronal plasticity and dendritic spines: Effect of environmental enrichment on intact and postischemic rat brain. *Journal of Cerebral Blood Flow and Metabolism, 22,* 89–96.

Jones, E. G., & Powell, T. P. (1970). An anatomical study of converging sensory pathways within the cerebral cortex of the monkey. *Brain, 93,* 793–820.

Jones, T. A., Allred, R. P., Adkins, D. L., Hsu, J. E., O'Bryant, A., & Maldonado, M. A. (2009). Remodeling the brain with behavioral experience after stroke. *Stroke, 40,* S136–S138.

Jones, T. A., Kleim, J. A., & Greenough, W. T. (1996). Synaptogenesis and dendritic growth in the cortex opposite unilateral sensorimotor cortex damage in adult rats: A quantitative electron microscopic examination. *Brain Research, 733,* 142–148.

Jones, T. A., & Schallert, T. (1992). Overgrowth and pruning of dendrites in adult rats recovering from neocortical damage. *Brain Research, 581,* 156–160.

Jueptner, M., Stephan, K. M., Frith, C. D., Brooks, D. J., Frackowiak, R. S. J., & Passingham, R. E. (1997). Anatomy of motor learning. I. Frontal cortex and attention to action. *Journal of Neurophysiology, 77,* 1313–1324.

Kaas, J., & Ebner, F. (1998). Intrathalamic connections: A new way to modulate cortical plasticity? *Nature Neuroscience, 1,* 341–342.

Kaas, J. H. (1999). Is most of neural plasticity in the thalamus cortical? *Proceedings of the National Academy of Sciences, 96,* 7622–7623.

Kaas, J. H. (2004). Somatosensory system. In G. Paxinos & J.K. Mai (Eds.), *The human nervous system* (pp. 1059–1092). New York: Elsevier Academic Press.

Katsman, D., Zheng, J., Spinelli, K., & Carmichael, S. T. (2003). Tissue microenvironments wihtin functional cortical subdivisions adjacent to focal stroke. *Journal of Cerebral Blood Flow and Metabolism, 23,* 997–1009.

Kauhanen, M., Korpelainen, J. T., Hiltunen, P., Brusin, E., Mononen, H., Maatta, R., et al. (1999). Poststroke depression correlates with cognitive impairment and neurological deficits. *Stroke, 30,* 1875–1880.

Kim, Y. H., Gitelman, D. R., Nobre, A. C., Parrish, T. B., LaBar, K. S., & Mesulam, M. M. (1999). The large-scale neural network for spatial attention displays multifunctional overlap but differential asymmetry. *Neuroimage, 9,* 269–277.

Kimberg, D. Y., Aguirre, G. K., & D'Esposito, M. (2000). Modulation of task-related neural activity in task-switching: An fMRI study. *Cognitive Brain Research, 10*(1–2), 189–196.

Kleim, J. A., & Jones, T. A. (2008). Principles of experience-dependent neural plasticity: Implications for rehabilitation after brain damage. *Journal of Speech, Language, and Hearing Research, 51,* S225–S239.

Klistorner, A., Crewther, D. P., & Crewther, S. G. (1997). Separate magnocellular and parvocellular contributions from temporal analysis of the multifocal VEP. *Vision Research, 37*(15), 2161–2169.

Kolb, B. (1996). *Brain plasticity and behavior.* Hillsdale: Erlbaum.

Kolb, B. (2003). Overview of cortical plasticity and recovery from brain injury. *Physical Medicine and Rehabilitation Clinics of North America, 14*(1, Supplement), 7–25.

Kolb, B., Teskey, G. C., & Gibb, R. (2010). Factors influencing cerebral plasticity in the normal and injured brain. *Frontiers in Human Neuroscience, 4*(204), 1–12.

Kolb, B., & Whishaw, I. Q. (1998). Brain plasticity and behavior. *Annual Review of Psychology, 49,* 43–64.

Komitova, M., Perfilieva, E., Mattsson, B., Eriksson, P. S., & Johansson, B. B. (2002). Effects of cortical ischemia and postischemic environmental enrichment on hippocampal cell genesis and differentiation in the adult rat. *Journal of Cerebral Blood Flow and Metabolism, 22,* 852–860.

Kwakkel, G., Kollen, B. J., van der Grond, J., & Prevo, A. J. H. (2003). Probability of regaining dexterity in the flaccid upper limb: Impact of severity of paresis and time since onset in acute stroke. *Stroke, 34,* 2181–2186.

Lamme, V. A. F. (2000). Neural mechanisms of visual awareness: A linking proposition. *Brain and Mind, 1,* 385–406.

Langhorne, P., & Legg, L. (2003). Evidence behind stroke rehabilitation. *Journal of Neurology, Neurosurgery and Psychiatry, 74*(Suppl IV), 18–21.

Larkum, M. E., Zhu, J. J., & Sakmann, B. (1999). A new cellular mechanism for coupling inputs arriving at different cortical layers. *Nature, 398,* 338–341.

Laycock, R., & Crewther, S. G. (2008). Towards an understanding of the role of the "magnocellular advantage" in fluent reading. *Neuroscience and Biobehavioral Reviews, 32,* 1494–1506.

Laycock, R., & Crewther, S. G. (2008). Towards an understanding of the role of the "magnocellular advantage" in fluent reading. *Neuroscience & Biobehavioral Reviews, 32*(8), 1494–1506.

Laycock, R., Crewther, S. G., & Crewther, D. P. (2007). A role for the "magnocellular advantage" in visual impairments in neurodevelopmental and psychiatric disorders. *Neuroscience and Biobehavioral Reviews, 31,* 363–376.

LeDoux, J. (1996). *The emotional brain.* New York: Simon & Schuster.

Legg, L., Drummond, A., & Langhorne, P. (2006). Occupational therapy for patients with problems in activities of daily living after stroke. *Cochrane Database of Systematic Reviews, 4.* CD003585.

Lesniak, M., Bak, T., Czepiel, W., Seniow, J., & Czlonkowska, A. (2008). Frequency and prognostic value of cognitive disorders in stroke patients. *Dementia and Geriatric Cognitive Disorders, 26,* 356–363.

Lewis, J. W., & Van Essen, D. C. (2000). Corticocortical connections of visual, sensorimotor, and multimodal processing areas in the parietal lobe of the macaque monkey. *The Journal of comparative neurology, 428*(1), 112–137.

Lezak, M. D., Howieson, D. B., & Loring, D. W. (2004). *Neuropsychological assessment* (4th ed.). New York: Oxford University Press.

Liberato, B., & Krakauer, J. W. (2007). *Ischemic stroke: Mechanisms, evaluation, and treatment.* Philadelphia: Elsevier.

Lincoln, N. B., Majid, M.J., & Weyman, N. (2000). Cognitive rehabilitation for attentional deficits following stroke. *Cochrane Database of Systematic Reviews, Issue 4,* Art. No.: CD002842.

Linden, T., Blomstrand, C., & Skoog, I. (2007). Depressive disorders after 20 months in elderly stroke patients: A case-control study. *Stroke, 38,* 1860–1863.

Lipp, O. V., Price, S. M., & Tellegen, C. L. (2009). Emotional faces in neutral crowds: Detecting displays of anger, happiness, and sadness on schematic and photographic images of faces. *Motivation and Emotion, 33*(3), 249–260.

Lloyd-Jones, D., Adams, R., Carnethon, M., De Simone, G., Ferguson, T. B., Flegal, K., et al. (2009). Heart Disease and Stroke Statistics—2009 Update. *Circulation, 119*(3), 480–486.

Macaluso, E., Frith, C. D., & Driver, J. (2002). Supramodal effects of covert spatial orienting triggered by visual or tactile events. *Journal of Cognitive Neuroscience, 14*(3), 389–401.

Madden, D. J., Whiting, W. L., Provenzale, J. M., & Huettel, S. A. (2004). Age-related changes in neural activity during visual target detection measured by fMRI. *Cerebral Cortex, 14,* 143–155.

Malouin, F., Belleville, S., Richards, C. L., Desrosiers, J., & Doyon, J. (2004). Working memory and mental practice outcomes after stroke. *Archives of Physical Medicine and Rehabilitation, 85,* 177–183.

Maruishi, M., Miyatani, M., Nakao, T., & Muranaka, H. (2007). Compensatory cortical activation during performance of an attention task by patients with diffuse axonal injury: A functional magnetic resonance imaging study. *Journal of Neurology, Neurosurgery and Psychiatry, 78,* 168–173.

Mateer, C. A., & Kerns, K. A. (2000). Capitilizing on neuroplasticity. *Brain and Cognition, 42,* 106–109.

Mathers, C., Vos, T., & Stevenson, C. (1999). *The burden of disease and injury in australia.* Canberra: Australian Institute of Health and Welfare.

May, P. J. (2006). The mammalian superior colliculus: Laminar structure and connections. *Progress in Brain Research, 151,* 321–378.

Mayer, A. R., Harrington, D., Adair, J. C., & Lee, R. (2006). The neural networks underlying endogenous auditory covert orienting and reorienting. *NeuroImage, 30*(3), 938–949.

McAlonan, K., Cavanaugh, J., & Wurtz, R. H. (2008). Guarding the gateway to cortex with attention in visual thalamus. *Nature, 456,* 391–394.

McColl, B. W., Allan, S. M., & Rothwell, N. J. (2007). Systemic inflammation and stroke: Aetiology, pathology and targets for therapy. *Biochemical Society Transactions, 35,* 1163–1165.

McDowd, J. M., Filion, D. L., Pohl, P. S., Richards, L. G., & Stiers, W. (2003). Attentional abilities and functional outcomes following stroke. *Journal of Gerontology, 58B*, 45–53.

McEwen, B. S. (2004). How sex and stress hormones regulate the structural and functional plasticity of the hippocampus. In M. S. Gazzaniga (Ed.), *The cognitive neurosciences* (3rd ed.). Cambridge, MA: MIT Press.

McIntosh, A. R., Cabeza, R. E., & Lobaugh, N. J. (1998). Analysis of neural interactions explains the activation of occipital cortex by an auditory stimulus. *Journal of Neurophysiology, 80*, 2790–2796.

Merzenich, M. M., Wright, B. A., Jenkins, W., Xerri, C., Byl, N., Miller, S., & Tallal, P. (Eds.). (2002). *Cortical plasticity underlying perceptual, motor, and cognitive skill development: Implications for neurorehabilitation*. Malden, MA: Blackwell Publishing.

Mesulam, M. M. (1998). From sensation to cognition. *Brain, 121*, 1013–1052.

Mialet, J., Pope, H., & Yurgelun-Todd, D. (1996). Impaired attention in depressive states: a non-specific deficit? *Psychological Medicine, 26*(5), 1009–1020.

Miller, J. (1982). Divided attention: Evidence for coactivation with redundant signals. *Cognitive Psychology, 14*(2), 247–279.

Minati, L., Grisoli, M., & Bruzzone, M. G. (2007). MR spectroscopy, functional MRI, and diffusion-tensor imaging in the aging brain: A conceptual review. *Journal of Geriatric Psychiatry and Neurology, 20*, 3–21.

Moore, T., Armstrong, K. M., & Fallah, M. (2003). Visuomotor origins of covert spatial attention. *Neuron, 40*, 671–683.

Mori, S., Sadoshima, S., Ibayashi, S., Lino, K., & Fujishima, M. (1994). Relation of cerebral blood flow to motor and cognitive functions in chronic stroke patients. *Stroke, 25*, 309–317.

Mountcastle, V. B., Andersen, R. A., & Motter, B. C. (1981). The influence of attentive fixation upon the excitability of the light-sensitive neurons of the posterior parietal cortex. *Journal of Neuroscience, 1*, 1218–1225.

Mueller, V., Brehmer, Y., von Oertzen, T., Li, S. C., & Lindenberger, U. (2008). Electrophysiological correlates of selective attention: A lifespan comparison. *BMC Neuroscience, 9*, 18.

Mukai, I., Kim, D., Fukunaga, M., Japee, S., Marrett, S., & Ungerleider, L. G. (2007). Activations in visual and attention-related areas predict and correlate with the degree of perceptual learning. *Journal of Neuroscience, 27*, 11401–11411.

Müller, N., & Knight, R. (2006). The functional neuroanatomy of working memory: contributions of human brain lesion studies. *Neuroscience, 139*(1), 51–58.

Nassi, J. J., & Callaway, E. M. (2009). Parallel processing strategies of the primate visual system. *Nature Reviews. Neuroscience, 10*, 360–372.

National Stroke Foundation. (2005). *Clinical guidelines for stroke rehabilitation and recovery*. Melbourne: National Stroke Foundation.

Ngezahayo, A., Schachner, M., & Artola, A. (2000). Synaptic activity modulates the induction of bidirectional synaptic changes in adult mouse hippocampus. *Journal of Neuroscience, 20*, 2451–2458.

Noppeney, U., Waberski, T. D., Gobbele, R., & Buchner, H. (1999). Spatial attention modulates the cortical somatosensory representation of the digits in humans. *Neuroreport, 10*, 3137–3141.

Nudo, R. J. (2003). Adaptive plasticity in motor cortex: Implications for rehabilitation after brain injury. *Journal of Rehabilitation Medicine, 41*, 7–10.

Nudo, R. J. (2007). Postinfarct cortical plasticity and behavioural recovery. *Stroke, 38*, 840–845.

Nys, G. M., van Zandvoort, M. J., de Kort, P. L., van der Worp, H. B., Jansen, B. P., Algra, A., et al. (2005). The prognostic value of domain-specific cognitive abilities in acute first-ever stroke. *Neurology, 64*, 821–827.

Outpatient Service Trialists. (2003). Therapy-based rehabilitation services for stroke patients at home. *Cochrane Database of Systematic Reviews, 1*. CD002925

Owen, A. M., McMillan, K. M., Laird, A. R., & Bullmore, E. (2005). N-back working memory paradigm: a meta-analysis of normative functional neuroimaging studies. *Human brain mapping, 25*(1), 46–59.

Park, N. W., & Ingles, J. L. (2001). Effectiveness of attention rehabilitation after an acquired brain injury: A meta-analysis. *Neuropsychology, 15*, 199–210.

Pascoe, M. C., Crewther, S. G., Carey, L. M., & Crewther, D. P. (2011). Inflammation and depression: Why poststroke depression may be the norm and not the exception. *International Journal of Stroke, 6*, 128–135.

Paul, S. L., Sturm, J. W., Dewey, H. M., Donnan, G. A., Macdonell, R. A., & Thrift, A. G. (2005). Long-term outcome in the north east melbourne stroke incidence study: Predictors of quality of life at 5 years after stroke. *Stroke, 36*, 2082–2086.

Pessoa, L. (2008). On the relationship between emotion and cognition. *Nature Reviews. Neuroscience, 9*, 148–158.

Phelps, E. A., Ling, S., & Carrasco, M. (2006). Emotion facilitates perception and potentiates the perceptual benefits of attention. *Psychological Science, 17*, 292–299.

Pittenger, C., & Duman, R. S. (2007). Stress, depression, and neuroplasticity: a convergence of mechanisms. *Neuropsychopharmacology, 33*(1), 88–109.

Pleger, B., Foerster, A. F., Ragert, P., Dinse, H. R., Schwenkreis, P., Malin, J. P., et al. (2003). Functional imaging of perceptual learning in human primary and secondary somatosensory cortex. *Neuron, 40*, 643–653.

Polley, D. B., Steinberg, E. E., & Merzenich, M. M. (2006). Perceptual learning directs auditory cortical map reorganization through top-down influences. *Journal of Neuroscience, 26*, 4970–4982.

Pons, T. P., & Kaas, J. H. (1986). Corticocortical connections of area 2 of somatosensory cortex in macaque monkeys: A correlative anatomical and electrophysiological study. *Journal of Comparative Neurology, 248*, 313–335.

Ponsford, J., & Willmott, C. (2004). Rehabilitation of nonspatial attention. In J. Ponsford (Ed.), *Cognitive and behavioral rehabilitation* (pp. 59–99). New York: The Guilford Press.

Ponsford, J. L., & Kinsella, G. (1988). Evaluation of a remedial programme for attentional deficits following closed-head injury. *Journal of Clinical and Experimental Neuropsychology, 10*, 693–708.

Puce, A., & Carey, L. M. (2010). Somatosensory function. In I.B. Weiner, W.E. Craighead & C. B. Nemeroff (Eds.), *The Corsini encyclopedia of psychology* (4th ed., pp. 929–931). New York: John Wiley & Sons.

Rawley, J. B., & Constantinidis, C. (2009). Neural correlates of learning and working memory in the primate posterior parietal cortex. *Neurobiology of learning and memory, 91*(2), 129–138.

Raymond, J. (2009). Interactions of attention, emotion and motivation. *Progress in Brain Research, 176*, 293–308.

Richards, L. G., Stewart, K. C., Woodbury, M. L., Senesac, C., & Cauraugh, J. H. (2008). Movement-dependent stroke recovery: A systematic review and meta-analysis of TMS and fMRI evidence. *Neuropsychologia, 46*, 3–11.

Robertson, I. H., Ridgeway, V., Greenfield, E., & Parr, A. (1997). Motor recovery after stroke depends on intact sustained attention: A 2-year follow-up study. *Neuropsychology, 11*, 290–295.

Robinson, R. G., & Starkstein, S. E. (2002). Neuropsychiatric aspects of cerebrovascular disorders. In S.C. Yudofsky & R.E. Hales (Eds.), *Essentials of Neuropsychiatry and Behavioural Neurosciences* (2nd ed., pp.299–322). Washington, D.C.: American Psychiatric Press.

Romo, R., Hernandez, A., Zainos, A., Lemus, L., & Brody, C. D. (2002). Neuronal correlates of decision-making in secondary somatosensory cortex. *Nature Neuroscience, 5*, 1217–1225.

Ropper, A. H., & Brown, R. H. (Eds.). (2005). *Adams and Victor's principles of neurology*. New York: McGraw-Hill Medical Pub. Division.

Rossini, P. M., Caluatti, C., Pauri, F., & Baron, J. C. (2003). Poststroke plastic reorganisation in the adult brain. *Lancet Neurology, 2*, 493–502.

Rowe, J., Friston, K. J., Frackowiak, R. S. J., & Passingham, R. E. (2002). Attention to action: Specific modulation of corticocortical interactions in humans. *Neuroimage, 17*, 988–998.

Sathian, K. (2006). Cross-modal plasticity in sensory systems. In M. Selzer, S. Clarke, L. Cohen, P. Duncan & F. Gage (Eds.), *Textbook of neural repair and rehabilitation* (Vol. 1, pp. 180–193). Cambridge: Cambridge University Press.

Sathian, K., & Burton, H. (1991). The role of spatially selective attention in the tactile perception of texture. *Perception and Psychophysics, 50*, 237–248.

Schaechter, J. D., Moore, C. I., Connell, B. D., Rosen, B. R., & Dijkhuizen, R. M. (2006). Structural and functional plasticity in the somatosensory cortex of chronic stroke patients. *Brain, 129*, 2722–2733.

Schaefer, A., Braver, T. S., Reynolds, J. R., Burgess, G. C., Yarkoni, T., & Gray, J. R. (2006). Individual differences in amygdala activity predict response speed during working memory. *Journal of Neuroscience, 26*, 10120–10128.

Schaefer, A., & Gray, J. R. (2007). A role for the human amygdala in higher cognition. *Reviews in the Neurosciences, 18*, 355–363.

Schallert, T., Leasure, J. L., & Kolb, B. (2000). Experience-associated structural events, subependymal cellular proliferative activity, and functional recovery after injury to the central nervous system. *Journal of Cerebral Blood Flow and Metabolism, 20*, 1513–1528.

Schroeder, C. E., Smiley, J., Fu, K. G., McGinnis, T., O'Connell, M. N., & Hackett, T. A. (2003). Anatomical mechanisms and functional implications of multisensory convergence in early cortical processing. *International Journal of Psychophysiology, 50*, 5–17.

Seitz, R. J., Butefisch, C. M., Kleiser, R., & Homberg, V. (2004). Reorganisation of cerebral circuits in human ischemic brain disease. *Restorative Neurology and Neuroscience, 22*, 207–229.

Selzer, M., Clarke, S., Cohen, L., Duncan, P., & Gage, F. (2006). *Textbook of neural repair and rehabilitation.* Cambridge: Cambridge University Press.

Shaughnessy, M., & Resnick, B. M. (2009). Using theory to develop an exercise intervention for patients post stroke. *Topics in Stroke Rehabilitation, 16*, 140–146.

Shaw, C. A., & McEachern, J. C. (Eds.). (2001). *Toward a theory of neuroplasticity.* Philadelphia, PA: Psychology Press.

Shimojo, S., & Shams, L. (2001). Sensory modalities are not separate modalities: Plasticity and interactions. *Current Opinion in Neurobiology, 11*, 505–509.

Shulman, G. L., d'Avossa, G., Tansy, A. P., & Corbetta, M. (2002). Two attentional processes in the parietal lobe. *Cerebral Cortex, 12*(11), 1124–1131.

Smiley, J. F., & Falchier, A. (2009). Multisensory connections of monkey auditory cerebral cortex. *Hearing Research, 258*, 37–46.

Sohlberg, M. M., & Mateer, C. A. (2001). *Cognitive rehabilitation: An integrative neuropsychological approach.* New York: The Guilford Press.

Sohn, M. H., Ursu, S., Anderson, J. R., Stenger, V. A., & Carter, C. S. (2000). The role of prefrontal cortex and posterior parietal cortex in task switching. *Proceedings of the National Academy of Sciences of the United States of America, 97*(24), 13448–13453.

Stapleton, T., Ashburn, A., & Stack, E. (2001). A pilot study of attention deficits, balance control and falls in the subacute stage following stroke. *Clinical Rehabilitation, 15*, 437–444.

Stefan, K., Wycislo, M., & Classen, J. (2004). Modulation of associative human motor cortical plasticity by attention. *Journal of Neurophysiology, 92*(1), 66.

Stein, B. E., & Meredith, M. A. (1993). *The merging of the senses.* Cambridge, MA: MIT Press.

Steward, O. (2006). Anatomical and biochemical plasticity of neurons: Regenerative growth of axons, sprouting, pruning and denervation supersensitivity. In M. Selzer, S. Clarke, L. Cohen, P. Duncan & F. Gage (Eds.), *Textbook of neural repair and rehabilitation:* Vol I. Neural repair and plasticity. (pp. 5–25). Cambridge, UK: Cambridge University Press.

Stinear, C. M., Barber, P. A., Coxon, J. P., Fleming, M. K., & Byblow, W. D. (2008). Priming the motor system enhances the effects of upper limb therapy in chronic stroke. *Brain, 131*, 1381–1390.

Stowe, A. M., Plautz, E. J., Eisner-Janowicz, I., Frost, S. B., Barbay, S., Zoubina, E. V., et al. (2007). VEGF protein associates to neurons in remote regions following cortical infarct. *Journal of Cerebral Blood Flow and Metabolism, 27*, 76–85.

Strong, K., Mathers, C., & Bonita, R. (2007). Preventing stroke: saving lives around the world. *The Lancet Neurology, 6*(2), 182–187.

Talsma, D., Senkowski, D., Soto-Faraco, S., & Woldorff, M. G. (2010). The multifaceted interplay between attention and multisensory integration. *Trends in Cognitive Sciences, 14*, 400–410.

Tatemichi, T. K., Desmond, D. W., Stern, Y., Paik, M., Sano, M., & Bagiella, E. (1994). Cognitive impairment after stroke: Frequency, patterns, and relationship to functional abilities. *Journal of Neurology, Neurosurgery and Psychiatry, 57*, 202–207.

Tedgui, A., & Mallat, Z. (2006). Cytokines in atherosclerosis: Pathogenic and regulatory pathways. *Physiological Reviews, 86*, 515–581.

The Consensus Panel on the Stroke Rehabilitation System. (2007). *Consensus panel on the stroke rehabilitation system: "Time is function." A report from the consensus panel on the stroke rehabilitation system to the Ministry of Health and Long-Term Care.* Ontario: Heart and Stroke Foundation of Ontario.

Thrift, A. G., Dewey, H. M., Macdonell, R. A. L., McNeil, J. J., & Donnan, G. A. (2000). Stroke incidence on the east coast of Australia: the north east Melbourne stroke incidence study (NEMESIS). *Stroke, 31*(9), 2087–2092.

Todd, J. W. (1912). Reaction to multiple stimuli. In R. S. Woodworth (Ed.), *Archives of psychology, No. 25. Columbia contributions to philosophy and psychology.* New York: The Science Press.

Usrey, W. M., Alonso, J.-M., & Reid, R. C. (2000). Synaptic interactions between thalamic inputs to simple cells in cat visual cortex. *Journal of Neuroscience, 19*, 7591–7602.

Van der Lubbe, R. H., Buitenweg, J. R., Boschker, M., Gerdes, B., & Jongsma, M. L. (2011). The influence of transient spatial attention on the processing of intracutaneous electrical stimuli examined with ERPs. *Clinical Neurophysiology, In Press.* DOI: http://dx.doi.org/10.1016/j.clinph.2011.08.034

Van Essen, D. C., & Drury, H. A. (1997). Structural and functional analyses of human cerebral cortex using a surface-based atlas. *The Journal of neuroscience, 17*(18), 7079–7102.

Van Essen, D. C., Drury, H. A., Joshi, S., & Miller, M. I. (1998). Functional and structural mapping of human cerebral cortex: solutions are in the surfaces. *Proceedings of the National Academy of Sciences,* U. S. A. *95*(3), 788–795.

Vossel, S., Thiel, C. M., & Fink, G.R. (2006). Cue validity modulates the neural correlates of covert endogenous orienting of attention in parietal and frontal cortex. *NeuroImage, 32*(3), 1257–1264.

Wade, D. T., Wood, V. A., & Langton Hewer, R. (1985). Recovery after stroke: The first 3 months. *Journal of Neurology, Neurosurgery and Psychiatry, 48*, 7–13.

Wallace, M. T. (2004). The development of multisensory processes. *Cognitive Processing, 5*, 69–83.

Wallace, M. T., Wilkinson, L. K., & Stein, B. E. (1996). Representation and integration of multiple sensory inputs in primate superior colliculus. *Journal of Neurophysiology, 76*, 1246–1266.

Wannig, A., Stanisor, L., & Roelfsema, P. R. (2011). Automatic spread of attentional response modulation along Gestalt criteria in primary visual cortex. *Nature Neuroscience, 14*, 1243–1244.

Ward, N. S. (2005). Mechanisms underlying recovery of motor function after stroke. *Postgraduate Medical Journal, 81*, 510–514.

Wei, L., Erinjeri, J., Rovainen, C., & Woolsey, T. (2001). Collateral growth and angiogenesis around cortical stroke. *Stroke, 32,* 2179–2184.

Wilson, C., & Robertson, I. H. (1992). A home-based intervention for attentional slips during reading following head injury: A single case study. *Neuropsychological Rehabilitation, 2,* 193–205.

Woldorff, M. G., Hazlett, C. J., Fichtenholtz, H. M., Weissman, D. H., Dale, A. M., & Song, A. W. (2004). Functional parcellation of attentional control regions of the brain. *Journal of Cognitive Neuroscience, 16,* 149–165.

World Health Organization. (1992). *The ICD-10 classification of mental and behavioural disorders: Clinical descriptions and diagnostic guidelines.* Geneva: World Health Organization.

Yantis, S., & Serences, J. T. (2003). Cortical mechanisms of space-based and object-based attentional control. *Current Opinion in Neurobiology, 13,* 187–193.

Yekutiel, M. (2000). *Sensory re-education of the hand after stroke.* London: Whurr Publishers.

15 | EXECUTIVE FUNCTIONS

SUSAN M. FITZPATRICK and CAROLYN M. BAUM

15.1 STROKE REHABILITATION: THE ROLE OF EXECUTIVE FUNCTIONS

Rehabilitation for people recovering from stroke focuses on restoring the ability to perform the activities required for living independently. For the most part, clinical neurorehabilitation concentrates on interventions designed to treat motor and language impairments. The difficulties an individual may experience from impairments of high-level cognitive functions, typically labeled *executive functions,* are not always apparent in clinical settings and are often not the focus of therapy. Part of the reason executive functions may be somewhat overlooked in clinical care is that executive functions have been defined in a number of contexts ranging from experimental cognitive studies to neuropsychological assessments. There is no commonly agreed set of cognitive abilities or neural structures uniquely identified as supporting executive functions. Rebecca Elliot (2003) provides a good summary of why the term *executive functions* is not a unitary concept. In this chapter, we will attempt to integrate across the behavioral, cognitive, and neural descriptions of executive functions in an effort to identify gaps in our knowledge that, if filled, could be helpful in translating research findings into clinical practice.

In general, cognitive psychologists describe executive functions as (i) the ability to exhibit flexible adaptive behavior, (ii) the use of appropriate problem-solving strategies as required for maintaining and updating goals, (iii) the capacity to monitor the consequences of actions, and (iv) the ability to use prior knowledge to correctly interpret future events (Miyake & Shah, 1999). Cognitively, the term *executive functions* also derives in part from the idea of top-down control by a central executive, as proposed in models of working memory (Baddeley, 2001) or of attentional control (Posner & Petersen, 1990). From a performance-based perspective, executive functions are called on when individuals make plans, initiate actions, and modify activities as problems are experienced or information from the environment changes. A performance-based approach to executive functions starts with an examination of how well a person is able to run errands, multitask at work, or quickly alter a route because of road congestion, and then attempt to identify the underlying cognitive and neural substrates.

Chen et al. (2006) suggest that the brain networks supporting executive functions are central to learning, and thus executive functions are important to the relearning and retraining necessary for successful rehabilitation as measured by real-world performance. Clinicians are encouraged to exercise care during client evaluations. Individuals with executive dysfunction can often perform adequately on standard neuropsychological evaluations because they are administered in a structured and supportive environment (Lezak, 1982, 2000; Prigatano, 1999; Dosenbach et al., 2008). Their difficulties may not become apparent until they attempt to resume unstructured activities at home, work, or in social situations. Chan et al. (2008) provide a comprehensive review of the various cognitive neuroscience models proposed for executive functioning and discuss some of the difficulties with assessing cognitive contributions to complex behaviors in the laboratory, in clinical settings, and in everyday life.

Brain injury as a result of stroke is a leading cause of individuals becoming unable to carry out the activities central to their daily life (Cardol et al., 2002). Considering the impact of stroke on everyday functioning, it is surprising that 85% of people who survive a stroke return home (Reutter-Bernays & Rentsch, 1993). Stroke can result in a wide range of deficits, including executive function deficits. When not identified and managed, these functional deficits lead to restrictions in home, work, and community activities, even if by clinical assessment the deficits are considered "mild" (Pohjasvaara et al., 2002; Rochette et al., 2007). The cognitive deficits associated with stroke vary in type and severity from individual to individual, based on site and lesion(s) location, but Zinn, Bosworth, Hoenig, and Swartzwelder (2007) found that nearly 50% of individuals show deficits in executive function. We suspect this number underestimates the true incidence of high-level cognitive difficulties.

The Cognitive Rehabilitation Research Group (CRRG) at Washington University in St. Louis maintains a large database of information regarding stroke patients admitted to Barnes-Jewish Hospital. As of December 2009, the CRRG research team had classified 9000 patients hospitalized for stroke. Although stroke is often associated with elderly populations, nearly half of the patients (46%) were younger than age 65. About 4500 patients (50%), were classified as having mild stroke (National Institute of Health Stroke Scale score = 0 to 5). In a subsample of 110 patients, 65% were found to have executive dysfunction as measured on behavior and performance tests (Baum, 2009; Wolf et al., 2009). The demographics of stroke evidenced in the Washington University database—younger and with milder disease—presents an eye-opening challenge for rehabilitation professionals. Younger stroke survivors had higher expectations of returning to work and to the myriad demands of active family and social life. Unlike older stroke survivors, whose lives may be more structured and thus more readily routinized, younger individuals were engaged in precisely the kind of activities most reliant on the flexibility provided by intact executive functioning (Wolf et al., 2009; O'Brien & Wolf, 2010). To meet the needs and expectations of younger stroke patients, neurorehabilitation must be prepared to address deficits in executive functions.

In this chapter, our performance-based definition of *executive functions* and *executive dysfunction* overlaps with but is not synonymous with *frontal lobe functions* or *frontal syndrome*, respectively. These have been described most notably by Stuss and colleagues (for review see Levine, Turner, & Stuss, 2008). Individual performance on some behavioral measures provides strong support that executive function shares characteristics with, but need not be identical to, neuropsychological tasks primarily reliant on working memory (Frank, Loughy, & OReilly, 2001) or with "top-down" control mechanisms (Dosenbach, 2008). Due to the complex nature of the tasks dependent upon executive functions it is likely that executive functions are supported by networks of brain region comprised of cortical, subcortical, and cerebellar regions (Chen et al., 2006; Dosenbach, 2008; Pessoa, 2008).

The ability of individuals to carry out the behavioral tasks associated with intact or disrupted executive functions is an active area of research in a number of distinct but overlapping disciplines, including neurorehabilitation, cognitive psychology, and cognitive neuroscience (Elliot, 2003). Rather than exhaustively review the decades of research pertinent to executive functions, including the large bodies of research carried out on working memory and attention, we decided to use this chapter as an opportunity to explore how the concept "executive function" is used by different disciplines, in what ways the uses of the concept are similar or different, and the opportunities and challenges to be met when integrating findings from across the disciplines to yield a coherent understanding at the neural, cognitive, and behavioral/performance levels, so that research findings can be used to inform clinical practice aimed at ameliorating executive dysfunction. It is our goal to identify the language and knowledge gaps that could be hindering the successful translation of experimental knowledge into practical applications for individuals recovering from stroke. It is not possible to overemphasize how difficult such integrative work can be. For the past several years, the James S. McDonnell Foundation has been encouraging working groups composed of basic cognitive neuroscientists and academic clinicians to develop consensus reviews for diagnosis and treatment based on a cognitive neuroscience model called CAP (computation-anatomy-psychology; Corbetta & Fitzpatrick, 2011). The first series of papers, on action rehabilitation, recently appeared as a special supplement to *Neurorehabilitation and Repair* (Frey et al., 2011; Pomeroy et al., 2011; Sathian et al., 2011) and serves as one model for developing mutually agreed-upon language and concepts.

In this chapter, we review the measures used to identify executive dysfunction and the interventions targeted to executive dysfunction at the neural, behavior, and performance levels. For the purposes of this chapter, only key findings from the cited papers pertinent to the chapter's goals are provided; readers are encouraged to consult the original papers for more complete details. The approach we've selected begins with examining the current understanding of executive function at the multiple levels of analysis we call *Brain* (including neural and cognitive systems), *Behavior*, and *Performance*. Figure 15.1 provides a

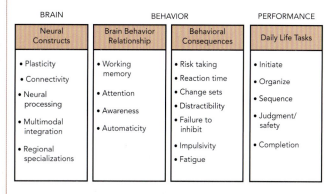

Figure 15.1 The Language of Executive Function At Multiple Levels

summary of some of the language commonly used at each of the levels.

What is readily observable is that there is very little overlap in terminology across the levels. A major barrier, in our view, of cross-disciplinary research and attempts to translate research into practice is the lack of a shared, mutually understood language. Recognizing that at present there are few effective, theory-driven, experimentally tested interventions for executive dysfunction, our purpose is to review the groundwork and suggest the research agenda needed if the field of neurorehabilitation is to use cognitive neuroscience findings to inform the development of therapeutic approaches. For cognitive neuroscientists, it is also critically important that theories and explanations concerning brain function be tested and refined as needed in the context of real world behaviors. Well-structured neurological and cognitive theories concerning information processing and performance should have some informative and predictive power for post-stroke rehabilitation. The practice of rehabilitation is often built on asking the patient to participate in relearning or retraining. This may create an ongoing tension between the natural need for neural systems to be both resilient (stable following perturbations) and plastic (able to alter with experience). It is imperative that we understand how injury and therapeutic interventions interact with, and can be helped or hindered by, the resilient and plastic aspects of neural systems. Figures 15.2 and 15.3 will serve as a reference for the measures and interventions that will be discussed in this paper.

15.2 OVERVIEW OF A MULTI-LEVEL UNDERSTANDING OF EXECUTIVE FUNCTIONS

Executive functions are needed to perform complex tasks. Complex tasks require goals to be formulated, and performance requires a particular sequence of actions. In carrying out complex tasks, the task rules or contexts can

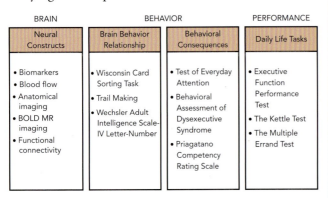

Figure 15.2 Measures of Executive Function at Multiple Levels. Note: *This list is not exhaustive but is meant to introduce measures at different levels.*

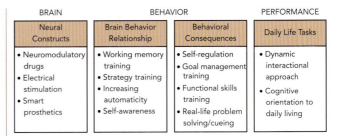

Figure 15.3 Interventions for Executive Function at Multiple Levels. Note: *This list is not exhaustive but is meant to introduce interventions at different levels.*

change, and there is often competing stimuli that must be ignored to accomplish the task (Burgess & Shallice, 1996; Kaplan & Berman, 2010). When considering performance, at least five cognitive constructs have empirical support as major components of executive functioning: (i) inhibition, (ii) working memory, (iii) strategic processing, (iv) set shifting, and (v) emotional regulation (Norman & Shallice, 1986; Shallice, Levin, Eisenberg, & Benton, 1991; Baddeley, 1996; Goldman-Rakic, 1996; Smith & Jonides, 1999; Jonides & Smith, 1997; Miyake et al., 2000; Braver, Cohen, & Barch, 2002; Diamond, 2002). In essence, executive functions make it possible for humans to successfully encounter novelty. Executive functions allow humans to synthesize information coming from the external environment, as well as from memory stores in the brain, to generate, implement, and correctly implement strategies necessary to accomplish tasks (Goldberg, 2001; Manchester, Priestley, & Jackson, 2004). These abilities are among the most complex functions of the human brain and are central to being able to perform activities at home, work, and in community life.

Both experimental and clinical findings indicate that frontal lobes of the human brain are a primary center of executive functions. It is also clear that executive functions rely on connections to other areas throughout the brain. For years the healthcare community attributed executive dysfunction only to frontal lobe injury; however, we now are aware that individuals can experience executive dysfunction even in absence of frontal lobe injury (Tranel, Anderson, & Benton, 1994; Manchester et al., 2004). In fact, there has been some evidence to support the theory that executive dysfunction is more likely attributed to diffuse lesions in the brain (Stuss & Levine, 2002; Pessoa, 2008). Almost any brain injury disrupting the networks supporting executive function can be expected to lead to cognitive, behavioral, and performance problems to a greater or lesser extent. Being able to identify patterns of neural injury predictive of the nature and extent of executive dysfunction is central to creating a feasible post-stroke treatment plan. If, as we discuss above, the concept of "executive functions" does not neatly map onto identifiable cognitive operations, it is even more difficult to map the disruptions of executive functions suspected of supporting complex human behaviors onto discrete neural structures. In part, the difficulty derives from the observation that executive functions are behaviorally context-dependent, and are characterized as the dynamic deployment of cognitive resources. Although published more than 2 decades ago, a review by Posner and Petersen (1990) provides a cogent discussion of the challenges inherent in the attempts to map processes described at the cognitive level of analysis onto neural substrates. Posner and Petersen's concerns remain relevant today and should guide practical interpretation of research findings.

Neurorehabilitation researchers and clinicians should be cautious of overgeneralizing from brain models of executive functions proposed by cognitive neuroscientists, particularly if based primarily on functional imaging studies, because imaging results are dependent on the task performed during data acquisition and on the experimental context. The current use of task-free resting state functional connectivity imaging does not completely mitigate the challenges of translating findings from research to practice, particularly in the context of the altered physiological context of the human brain post-stroke. Cognitive neuroscience studies of attention, working memory, or set-shifting with experimental tasks designed to probe specific cognitive processes (e.g., Stroop task, N-back test, or Wisconsin card sorting task) should not be taken as complete proxies for more complex behaviors (see discussion in Chan et al., 2008).

Translating from cognitive neuroscience to neurorehabilitation (and vice versa) also requires contending with a suite of challenges posed by the multi-scale nature of brain function. The neural elements implicated in performance-dependent executive functions span temporal scales ranging from milliseconds to years, and spatial scales ranging from the molecular to whole organisms interacting with environments. The scale an investigator chooses for monitoring function, for measuring the loss of function, and for determining recovery has far-reaching implications for the validity of the conclusions and generalizations that can be made at other scales.

It is not possible for this chapter to review the extensive functional brain imaging literature relating to executive functions that has been amassed in the past two decades. Rather, we describe a limited number of recently proposed working models derived from cognitive neuroscience research that have sufficient detail to make predictions about the neural underpinnings of executive functions and the risk for dysfunction as a result of injury or disease that can and should be tested in both clinical and real-world environments. We do not mean to imply that information should flow in only one direction—from cognitive neuroscience toward rehabilitation. Rather, we believe it is imperative that researchers and clinicians work together to generate knowledge and to validate findings. Testing predictions in the real-world settings of neurorehabilitation yields information needed to refine or correct neural and cognitive models.

15.3 NEURAL SUBSTRATES OF EXECUTIVE FUNCTIONS

Much of what is known about the neural systems supporting executive functions has been derived from neuropsychological studies with patients with brain lesions, mostly resulting from trauma (reviewed in Zoccolotti et al., 2011). Increasingly, the availability of noninvasive imaging methodologies has allowed cognitive neuroscientists to study the neural basis of cognitive functions in intact subjects, in neurological patients with well-characterized structural lesions, and in psychiatric populations. In general, however, experimental constraints make it impossible for cognitive neuroscientists to study complex, real-world behaviors and, as a result, most functional imaging studies focus on dissociable components of executive functions as previously defined in this chapter (e.g., working memory, inhibition, set-shifting).

One component of executive functions extensively studied is top-down control (or voluntary control) over automatic processes (see Cohen, Dunbar, & McClelland, 1990; and Robbins & Arnsten, 2009 for review). It is commonly agreed that top-down control involves areas of the prefrontal cortex, specifically the dorsal lateral prefrontal cortex, and the dorsal anterior cingulate cortex/medial superior frontal cortex (Miller & Cohen, 2001). However, new experimental data from imaging studies indicate that top-down control is likely to involve a larger number of interacting brain regions organized into two distinct networks operating at different temporal scales (Seeley et al, 2007; Dosenbach et al., 2008). The evidence supports one network, described by Dosenbach and colleagues as "fronto-parietal" and a second as "cingulo-opercular" (2008). The frontoparietal network responds with fast dynamics to cues signifying task onset and, in the experimental laboratory setting, plays a role in initiating and adjusting control of performance on a trial-by-trial basis. The frontoparietal network responds differentially depending on whether participants perform correctly or incorrectly on individual trials, indicating the network's activity is sensitive to feedback. The cingulo-opercular network, which includes the thalamus, operates at a slower temporal scale and is involved with maintaining set (the ability to be prepared to respond in a particular way) over many trials (Dosenbach et al., 2006) during what might be considered the entire task epoch. The cingulo-opercular network also monitors response choices in light of task goals. A set of interacting cerebellar regions, functionally connected to both the frontoparietal and cingulo-opercular networks and ascribed with processing error-related activity contributing to improvement of task performance, were also found during the experiments summarized by Dosenbach et al. (2008) and are included in the rather comprehensive and updated model they provide for the neural systems responsible for human top-down control.

In an interesting *Nature Reviews Neuroscience* opinion article, Luiz Pessoa (2008) proposes an expanded model of interacting brain regions contributing to executive functions. Pessoa's model describes integrated cognitive-emotional networks supporting complex, flexible behaviors, and adds the amygdala and nucleus accumbens to the frontal executive network. A particularly intriguing aspect of Pessoa's model is the conceptual proposal he puts forward: that particular brain areas could be characterized along a gradient of connectivity. Highly connected brain areas serve as hubs regulating the flow and integration of information (for details see Figure 4 in Pessoa, 2008). It is tempting to speculate that focal disruption of a highly connected hub would result in global dysfunction, while a lesion localized to sparsely connected regions would yield a specific behavioral impairment. Considering that areas implicated as integrative hubs are also the brain regions affected in the most common clinical strokes resulting from vascular accidents involving the middle cerebral artery and anterior cerebral artery, it should be anticipated that stroke patients will experience some degree of executive dysfunction (Levine, Turner, & Stuss, 2008). Chen et al. (2006) have also put forward a conceptual rubric for considering structure/function relations in the human brain that suggest that there are regions in the brain that carry out specific cognitive functions, while other cognitive processes require interactions among a network of brain regions. Damage to brain areas as a result of stroke should be expected to yield both specific impairments and impairments of a more generalized nature, such as executive dysfunction.

It is important to keep in mind that the characterization of these networks derive from data obtained in experimental contexts. The operations of task-dependent, experimentally determined functional networks in real-world, everyday tasks (e.g., packing for a trip) remains to be determined. It is also important to keep in mind that functional models based on brain imaging tools must be interpreted in light of the numerous assumptions built into the protocols for acquiring, processing, and interpreting functional imaging data (Fitzpatrick and Rothman, 2002). The assumptions made regarding the requisite hemodynamics and brain tissue properties may or may not generalize to patients after brain injury. A final caveat for consideration is that most basic science functional imaging studies report findings obtained from data averaged across subjects. To be useful in clinical rehabilitation research, it will be necessary to be able to extrapolate group findings or general principles to an individual.

Evidence is accumulating on how neuromodulatory neurotransmitters influence activity in cortical-striatal circuits responsible for performance of complex cognitive tasks, such as those known to rely on working memory, a key component of executive functions (for reviews see Cools & D'Esposito, 2009; Robbins & Arnsten, 2009). In particular, converging evidence from cognitive neuroscience studies carried out with rodent, nonhuman primates, and human subjects underscore the importance of dopamine neuromodulation on performance of working memory dependent tasks.

Although most of the functional imaging studies reporting results on the role of neurotransmitters and neuromodulators during performance of cognitive tasks are typically carried out with healthy participants without neurological deficits, a few studies have also been carried out with patient populations. People with Parkinson's disease are, not surprisingly, important for studies looking at the effects of dopamine on cognitive function. The results of such studies taken together with theoretical models describing how different brain regions interact to accomplish complex tasks are intriguing enough to encourage further experimental studies and are of potential interest to rehabilitation. Before pharmacological interventions can be used effectively, much remains to be learned from studies with defined patient populations with an eye toward delineating how pharmacological approaches may or may not be helpful with individuals with compromised neurological function and difficulties performing complex working-memory dependent tasks.

The current understanding is that neurons in the prefrontal cortex, an area known to be important in the performance of working memory–dependent tasks, receive modulatory input from ascending fibers from dopamine-releasing midbrain (i.e., the striatum) neurons (for review see Cools & D'Esposito, 2009). Communication between the prefrontal cortex (PFC) and the striatum is important for optimal working memory performance. In theory, the role of these ascending fibers is to stabilize task-relevant working memory representations or, in other words, to decrease an individual's susceptibility to distractions during task performance.

It can be tempting in light of the experimental evidence to consider the possibility that neurological patients suffering from working memory deficits could be helped by the administration of dopamine agonists, either alone or in conjunction with rehabilitation. However, a series of publications from Mark D'Esposito's laboratory, reviewed below, provide a case study underscoring the care that must be taken when rehabilitation practitioners look to translate experimental results. Attempting to modulate cognitive performance by tinkering with the complex, dynamic, and adaptive nature of chemical neurotransmission requires detailed understanding of mechanisms.

Wallace et al. (2011) evaluated the influence of dopaminergic modulation on measures of prefrontal cortex-striatal functional connectivity by reanalyzing data from a study with healthy human subjects (Gibbs & D'Esposito, 2005) that monitored the effects of the dopamine D2 receptor agonist bromocriptine in conjunction with a functional neuroimaging study during performance on verbal delayed recognition tasks. The principle finding was that bromocriptine appeared to modulate the putative PFC-dependent retrieval rate, but not the encoding or retention stages of the task.

Following up the previous findings, Wallace et al. (2011) reanalyzed the neuroimaging data obtained from subjects in the Gibbs and D'Esposito 2005 study in an effort to tease out the effects of bromocriptine on the functional connectivity of the prefrontal cortex and the striatum during working memory tasks. Before exploring the neuroimaging results, it is critical to note the behavioral observation that dopamine augmentation yields an inverted U-shaped curve with respect to task performance. Too little or too much dopamine appears to negatively influence behavior (see discussion in Gjedde et al., 2010). Behaviorally, individuals can be characterized as belonging to either a high-span working memory group or a low-span working memory group. Interestingly, bromocriptine administration improved task-related speed and accuracy only in low working memory span individuals. High working memory span individuals trended toward a decrement in performance. Importantly, the effects are not explained by changes in either motor speed or vigilance. The findings raise important implications for use of dopamine augmentation in rehabilitation, as discussed below.

When Wallace et al. (2011) analyzed the imaging data to obtain a measure of frontal-striatal connectivity, the principal finding was that bromocriptine administration increased the measured connectivity in low working memory span individuals and was positively correlated with the improved behavioral performance on the experimental task. Similarly, bromocriptine exerted a negative effect on frontal-striatal connectivity in the high working memory span individuals, again correlating with the behavioral data, although both the imaging and the performance data failed to reach statistical significance, possibly due to the small sample size.

The findings, albeit obtained from healthy young participants in a carefully controlled experimental setting, still offer some intriguing implications for additional research, particularly with individuals recovering from mild or moderate stroke demonstrating deficits in working memory–dependent function. Additional research is needed that can specifically address the needs of clinical populations with neurological insults affecting large neural networks and

multiple neurotransmitter systems. Some of the questions that will need to be answered include the following:

- Could dopamine augmentation help individuals demonstrating post-stroke deficits dependent on working memory functions?

- Are there diagnostic measurements that could reliably ascertain which patients are likely to benefit?

- Knowing that undertreatment or overtreatment could result in negative effects, how will the optimal dose be determined for individual patients?

- How could dopamine augmentation be optimally paired with behavioral interventions?

- Will pharmacological resistance develop over time as part of an adaptive response?

- What are the unwanted effects?

- Will dopamine augmentation yield behaviorally meaningful improvement?

Answering these questions, and the myriad others expected to arise in the clinical setting, suggests some general translational research principles regarding what needs to be determined prior to adoption of neurochemical adjuvants to behavioral rehabilitation interventions. This will be the case whether the neuromodulation is obtained via pharmacological treatments or by the application of electrical stimulation (for further discussion see Bütefisch, 2004, and Chapter 10). Carrying out such research will require the infrastructure and resources needed to support multidisciplinary teams with expertise in neuroscience, computational modeling, imaging, cognitive psychology, neurology, and rehabilitation.

15.3.1 NEURAL MEASURES AND INTERVENTIONS

It is important that stroke patients be assessed with structural neural imaging methods to determine the full extent of their injuries. Refer to Figure 15.2 and 15.3. It is useful to have anatomical imaging (CT or MRI) to make a determination of the structural integrity of the brain, and diffusion tensor or diffusion weight imaging to assess white matter integrity. Ramirez, Gao, and Black (2008) provide a detailed overview of clinical brain imaging methods and how these tools can contribute to a neuroanatomical/neurophysiological context for neurorehabilitation (see also Chapter 4). Increasingly, resting state functional connectivity blood oxygenation level dependent (BOLD) magnetic resonance imaging (fcMRI) is being called upon to identify functional neural networks in both intact and patient populations (for a historical review of this measurement see Lowe, 2010). Other approaches for assessing functional connectivity have been proposed, most notably the use of perfusion MR imaging, which monitors changes in cerebral blood flow (CBF), rather than the BOLD signal, which is dependent on changes in blood oxygenation, CBF. and cerebral blood volume (CBV; Chuang et al., 2008). Despite more than a decade of research, it remains to be seen how useful resting state functional connectivity measurements will be when they are used in neurorehabilitation, particularly in the context of the altered cerebrovascular milieu characteristic of patients post-stroke.

Urgently needed to advance the science of neurorehabilitation is the development of methods amenable to the clinical rehabilitation and outpatient settings that allow temporally dynamic measurements of the neural changes accompanying behavioral change. We think it would also be beneficial to have long-term studies of individuals post-stroke. The ability to capture the neural changes occurring at different grain sizes that continue to shape the brain years after injury will be especially useful with the younger populations of patients, many of whom can expect to live decades after a stroke.

Very few rehabilitative interventions for executive dysfunction are directed at the neural level. It is most likely that interventions directed at the neural level will be pharmacological or based on the use of electrical stimulation. Not surprisingly, a recent review summarizing the usefulness of pharmacological interventions or cortical stimulation protocols to aid recovery in patients following stroke (Floel & Cohen, 2010) primarily focused on motor and language impairment, areas of rehabilitative need where the authors could identify experimental findings and small-scale trials data. We agree with the general conclusions drawn by authors of this review that there remain many open questions that require answers before the neurorehabilitation community can implement such adjuvant therapy to traditional practice. In particular, research is needed on determining optimal dosing, timing, and duration of treatment. Considering the heterogeneity of stroke patients, determining the correct pairings of drugs and behavioral interventions will require careful titration for each patient in the context of the neural and cognitive sequelae of stroke, and individual goals for rehabilitation. This was essentially the conclusion reached in a review on the use of amphetamines for improving recovery after stroke (Martinsson, Hardemark, & Eksborg, 2007).

There is some evidence that antidepressant therapy can have a positive effect on executive functioning post-stroke (Narushima et al., 2007). The authors propose that the effect could be mediated via a monoaminergic modulation of frontal-striatal networks. Robbins and Arnsten (2009) have published an authoritative and comprehensive review of experimental and clinical evidence for the role of monoaminergic modulation of executive functions in the context of mental disorders that is recommended

for all researchers and clinicians interested in considering how neuropharmacology could influence the mechanism of post-stroke dysfunction or recovery. Narushima and colleagues also suggest that antidepressant therapy may aid recovery of executive functions by upregulating neurotropins and thereby enhancing neuroplasticity (Narushima et al., 2007). A similar mechanism of action has been suggested, based on experimental studies with murine brain slices, as contributing to the action of cortical stimulation techniques (Fritsch et al., 2010).

We admit that it is appealing to consider the use of pharmacological agents to alter plasticity and network reorganization to make the state of the system more responsive to rehabilitation. However, a reading of the cautionary "case study" provided in Box 1 exposes the knowledge gaps that must be bridged if the field of neurorehabilitation is to translate experimental findings into clinical applications. The challenge for any intervention directed at the neural level is demonstrating that the resulting changes are not confined to the neural level but can yield or enable changes and meaningful improvements at higher levels of analysis. If an intervention is to be useful in rehabilitation, it is not enough to demonstrate that a pharmacological agent may increase, for example, long-term potentiation (LTP) as a proxy for synaptic plasticity unless there is also evidence that alterations in synaptic plasticity allows for meaningful, beneficial gains in behavior and performance.

Chen and colleagues (2006) have also proposed a theoretical framework for executive dysfunction interventions based on cognitive neuroscience/functional neuroimaging findings (Chen et al., 2006). The level of the interventions they propose and the predictions they make for determining outcome, however, are at the cognitive-behavioral level and not the neural level. It remains to be seen whether multi-level combinations of pharmacology, targeted cognitive retraining, and behavioral interventions will not only improve performance on targeted tasks but also improve patients' performance on everyday tasks. Restoring or augmenting cognitive processes may very well turn out to be necessary but not sufficient to meet patient-centered rehabilitation goals (Swartz, 1997).

15.4 BEHAVIORAL MEASURES AND INTERVENTIONS

Persons with executive dysfunction have difficulty planning, lack insight, are distractible, make poor decisions, and have little concern for social rules (Burgess & Simons, 2005). Executive functions are needed to fulfill roles in family, work, and community life, and post-stroke deficits should be identified and addressed as a part of rehabilitation services. In this section of the chapter we focus less on what has been learned from cognitive neuroscience research and more on what can be learned from neuropsychology, a subspecialty of the field of psychology that focuses on the relationship between brain functioning and behavior. Lezak's (1982) work describes the characteristics of the person with brain injury and challenges neuropsychologists to develop tools to better characterize these behaviors. Two levels of neuropsychological tests describe both the brain function and the behavioral consequences of executive function. Several instruments in each category will be described. Figure 15.2 lists the measures that will be discussed.

15.4.1 MEASURES TO IDENTIFY BRAIN-RELATED BEHAVIORS

The **Wisconsin Card Sorting Test** (WCST; Grant & Berg, 1948; Heaton, Cheelune, Talley, Kay & Curtiss, 1993) is a test of set-shifting. It measures the person's ability to display flexibility as he is presented with changing schedules of reinforcement. In a sample of 112 persons with stroke, the WCST-64 resulted in a three dimensional model: (i) inflexibility, (ii) ineffective hypothesis-testing strategy, and (iii) set maintenance (Su Lin, Kwan, & Guo, 2008).

The **Trail Making Test** (Reitan & Wolfson, 1995) provides information regarding attention, visual scanning, and executive function. Part A requires the participant to draw lines to connect 25 numbers scattered on a page. Part B requires the connection of numbers and letters (a trail) in order, alternating between letters and numbers without lifting the pencil from the paper. The time it takes for the person to connect the trail is reported. If the person makes an error, the administrator points out the error so she can correct it. The two scores reflect the total time in seconds required to complete each task.

The **Wechsler Adult Intelligence Scale-IV (WAIS-IV) Working Memory Index.** The WAIS was created in 1955 (Wechsler, 1955) and revised in 2008 (WAIS_IV) after being standardized on 2,200 persons in the United States and 688 in Canada (http://cps.nova.edu/~cpphelp/WAIS-R.html). The Working Memory Index has three tests: **Digit Span,** which measures working memory/attention, concentration, and mental control; **Arithmetic,** which measures concentration while the subject manipulates mental mathematical problems; and **Letter-Number Sequencing** (a supplemental task), which measures attention and working memory. The test can be used with people with brain injury to identify the area of the brain that has been affected, and specific subtests identify the extent of the damage.

15.4.2 MEASURES TO IDENTIFY THE BEHAVIORAL CONSEQUENCES OF STROKE

The tests discussed in this section were designed to respond to the concerns that neuropsychological tests were failing to generalize to performance in naturalistic settings. In response to the criticisms, new neuropsychological tests were developed that do not rely on the performance of single tasks delivered in a controlled environment but rather provide more complex tasks closer to the demands made in "real life" situations (Wilson et al., 1996). However, it is an important caveat that these are still administered in testing rooms under controlled conditions and therefore do not fully mimic the rich complexity of real life situations. It is not always necessary that tests be carried out in fully naturalized settings to be valid for assessing performance. However, to be useful in rehabilitative practice, we believe it is necessary that an individual's performance on such tests (i) be highly correlated with performance in everyday life, (ii) reveal in a meaningful way the underlying neural or cognitive deficits that are contributing to poor performance, and (iii) guide therapy.

The **Test of Everyday Attention** (TEA; Robertson, Ward, Ridgeway & Nimmo-Smith, 1994) uses a range of attentional tasks that are necessary in everyday life (searching maps, using a telephone directory, listening to lottery number broadcasts). The factors of sustained attention, selective attention, attentional switching, and auditory-verbal working memory match the current evidence for functionally independent attentional circuits in the brain (Posner & Petersen, 1990). The data from the TEA reveal problems with attention that will require rehabilitation professionals to engage with the patient, caregivers, and prospective employers in devising a care plan. Strategies may include training on subtasks that are made routine, thereby increasing automaticity and allowing working memory and attentional resources to be deployed to more "on-line" task demands.

Behavioral Assessment of the Dysexecutive Syndrome (BADS; Wilson, Alderman, Burgess, Emslie, & Evans, 1996). The BADS is a battery of six tests and two questionnaires that requires the person to plan, initiate, monitor, and adjust behavior in response to the explicit and implicit demands of a series of tasks. The tasks include a "rule shift" to demonstrate shifting between two rules in a card task; an "action program" requiring a solution to a practical problem of getting a cork out of a narrow tube using rules; "key search," which identifies the ability to solve a problem; "temporal judgment," requiring estimating times for everyday events; "zoo map," which requires the ability to follow a route through a map that does not break rules; and "modified six elements," which assess time management with the person dividing the available time between a number of tasks while not breaking rules. The assessment also includes the Dysexecutive Questionaire (DEX), a behavioral questionnaire to identify the occurrence of behaviors. It can be used as a measure of awareness, as one version is for the respondent and the second for a family member to rate the respondent.

The **Patient Competency Rating Scale** (Prigatano, 1986) is a measure of self-awareness or the ability to appraise one's strengths and weaknesses in activities of daily living, behavioral and emotional function, and cognitive and physical function following brain injury. The respondent's responses are compared to a relative's or therapist's observations. Awareness is a serious problem when a person experiences executive dysfunction, since the first step in learning new strategies to manage an executive function deficit is to know that you have a problem that needs new strategies.

15.4.3 PERFORMANCE-BASED TESTS

Neuropsychological tests are designed to document the relationship between brain function and behavior. The intent of neuropsychological assessment is to provide an accurate depiction of an individual's specific cognitive impairments (e.g., working memory deficit), as well as assessing how well component cognitive processes work together to accomplish a task. However, these tasks tend to ignore the person–environment interaction. The natural and built environment can both support and hinder performance in ways that might not be obvious in the absence of a complete understanding of what cognitive resources are actually required. Clarity in the task demands and the available affordances are critical in planning interventions and working with patients and their families to help them learn to manage the consequences of executive dysfunction. Performance tests, primarily developed by occupational therapists, take a different approach from what we have described for neuropsychological tests and seek to answer a different question about brain function: "How does the brain and cognition support the everyday performance of tasks necessary to live independently, be safe, to manage daily affairs?" Using a performance approach, executive function is examined as a person performs an entire task, an actual task that is necessary in everyday life. Clearly, linking performance to the underlying neural structures supporting performance requires intermediate cognitive models. A discussion of this point in the context of education carries important lessons for rehabilitation (Bruer, 1997).

It should not be assumed that impairment in a cognitive process will result in impairments in overall functional capacity, because activities can be accomplished by employing different strategies and by different levels of motivation, interest, and different environments. For example, there are many ways individuals can navigate a grocery store even if the end goal, buying all the items on a list as quickly as possible, is identical. By conceptualizing the task differently, different cognitive resources and brain networks are brought to the goal. It is, however, important to learn how it is that a person plans and executes a task, responds to errors, and how much external support is needed in order to be successful. Assessing the level of support required is key, because support is the variable most likely to determine if someone can remain at home or

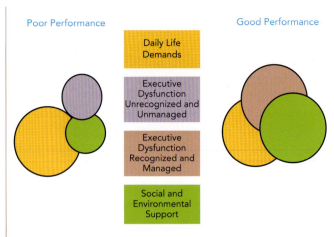

Figure 15.4 Factors Contributing to Resuming Participation Post-Stroke. This figure depicts how rehabilitation directed at executive dysfunction, including environmental and social support systems can result in vastly different outcomes for individuals with similar post stroke clinical profiles.

return to work (see Figure 15.4 for a summary). Support is also the variable that is most dependent on social, cultural, and political norms.

In our view, it is unwise to base an intervention strategy solely on the results of functional imaging studies or the results from a neuropsychological battery. At this time there are still gaps in our ability to interpret brain and cognitive measures in terms of what is or is not sufficient for determining an individual's overall ability to function. The results of neuropsychological assessments should be supplemented with performance-based assessments (Burgess et al., 2006) in the hope that more insightful measurements can be created with a combination of these two assessment strategies.

The Executive Function Performance Test (EFPT) was developed by Baum et al. (2003) in an effort to address some of the challenges raised above. The EFPT provides a record of executive functions serving in the performance of a task. It has been validated in studies with the elderly, with individuals with stroke, and with clients with schizophrenia (Katz, Tadmor, Felzen, & Hartman-Maeir, 2007; Baum, Connor, Morrison, Hahn, Dromerick, & Edwards, 2008; Wolf, Stith, Connor, & Baum, 2010). The EFPT includes 4 standardized instrumental activities of daily living (IADL) tasks (cooking, telephone use, medication management, and bill paying) that the client has to perform to live independently at home. The clinician provides a series of graded cues: (1) a verbal prompt, (2) a gestural prompt, (3) direct verbal instruction, (4) physical assistance, and (5) cessation of the task because the person is not capable of completing it. A total score is determined based on the individual's ability to initiate the task, execute the task (including organization, sequencing, judgment, and safety), and complete the task. Importantly, the EFPT does not simply determine successful or unsuccessful task completion; rather, it identifies what an individual can do and how much assistance is needed for him or her to carry out a task. Via the cueing system, a wider range of abilities, previously thought to be untestable, are captured in persons. This cueing system is standardized and is associated with the degree of cognitive impairment. Because the EFPT can be used in both the clinic and the home, it is a bridge linking the data obtained in controlled research studies with the rehabilitation goal of assessing an individual's ability to perform in everyday life.

The Kettle Test (Hartman-Maier et al., 2009) is designed to indicate one's ability to perform daily tasks. The patient's task is to prepare two hot drinks, one for the clinician and one for the patient. The clinician and patient make the decisions about the details of the task to be completed from some options of coffee, tea, hot chocolate; and the clinician observes while the patient completes the task. The performance is scored for each element of the task, including assembling the kettle, obtaining the water and ingredients, putting the ingredient into the cup, and serving the beverage (a 12-step task). Each of the steps is scored based upon the speed, receipt of cues, incomplete performance, and necessity of assistance. Following completion of the task performance, the therapist engages the client in a debriefing that focuses on the client's evaluation of the performance.

The Multiple Errand Test by Shallice and Burgess (1991), which was adapted and studied in clients with traumatic brain injury (Knight et al., 2002; Alderman et al., 2003) and following stroke (Dawson et al., 2009), is a multiple sub-goal task performed in a shopping district or a health facility. It was developed to elucidate cognitive problems persons have in managing the challenges of everyday life. The person being tested must accomplish 6 tasks: buy 3 items (using only a specific amount of money), make a phone call, mail something, and meet the investigator 10 minutes after starting the assessment. They also must collect information about opening and closing times, identify the cost of an item, and say when they are finished. They are scored in terms of errors (omissions, partially completed tasks, inefficiencies, and the strategies used). By observing the task failures, rehabilitation professionals may find it helpful to identify strategies they can use to help individuals either learn new strategies or learn compensation strategies to help them function after an injury that results in executive dysfunction (Alderman et al., 2003).

15.5 BEHAVIORAL AND PERFORMANCE INTERVENTIONS

Throughout this chapter we have made the point that *executive functions* serves as an "umbrella term" for a constellation of cognitive processes supporting complex behaviors

(Elliot, 2003). It should not come as a surprise that, as a result of this complexity, individuals with executive function are somewhat resistant to rehabilitative efforts. There are some promising strategies addressing the rehabilitation of executive functions that deserve further study. Of course, rehabilitation interventions for executive functions share many of the problems encountered in rehabilitation more generally, including lack of well-designed intervention trials with outcome measures linked to the stated outcome goals. Four promising intervention strategies will be presented, two at the behavioral level and two at the performance level. Refer to Figure 15.3.

15.5.1 INTERVENTIONS AT THE BEHAVIORAL LEVEL

Goal Management Training (GMT) is a neuropsychological intervention developed to teach patients with brain injury a strategy to improve their ability to plan activities and to structure their intentions. It is based on Duncan's theory of goal neglect. The theory states that any activity requires the person to establish goals and/or task requirements to create the structure to guide the actions that can lead to the goals being achieved. While performing a task, the current state of affairs and the goal state are compared, and actions or mental operations are selected to address the mismatch. This process continues until there is no mismatch between the current state and the goal state. Because there can be many actions associated with a task, it is important to inhibit irrelevant actions that will not contribute to a particular goal. The GMT contains several stages that are based on this notion: (i) Stop! Alerts and orients the person to the task; (ii) the person defines the main tasks, (iii) lists the main steps, (iv) learns the steps, and (v) checks or monitors the process. In the final stage, "checking," the outcome of the selected actions is compared with the goals to be achieved (Levine, Robertson, Clare, Carter, Hong, Wilson, et al., 2000). It is likely that these operations map onto the frontoparietal and cingulo-opercular networks discussed earlier in this chapter, and are likely to be disrupted by the damage caused by strokes to anterior regions of the brain (Dosenbach et al., 2008).

The Neurofunctional Retraining Approach, an occupational therapy intervention, recognizes the impairments faced by persons with brain injury and trains them to develop habits and routines for real-world skills with the goal of developing behavioral automaticity and a greater reliance on the environment, including cueing (Giles, 2005). Such an approach is used to train clients in behavioral routines when there is little expectation of generalized application of strategies to novel circumstances encountered in the real world. For example, to train in a specific morning routine, therapy would involve repeating the sequence and activities over many days until the process becomes automatic. Another example of therapy for a circumstance encountered in everyday life would be training a person to walk to the same restaurant on the same route with specific instructions of where to turn, how to look before crossing a street, how to obey street lights, etc. Training would also cover what the individual should do upon arrival to the restaurant, how to become familiar with the staff and the menu, and how to use the menu and order a dish. The aim is to maintain a schedule that can become routine, doing the same activities in the same sequence each day (Baum & Katz, 2009).

Neurofunctional retraining considers the person's learning capacity in the design and implementation of programs. The specific cognitive capacities are not the target of the interventions; however, the person's capacities—particularly memory, attention, and executive function—must be considered in the design of functional skills training. One problem associated with cognitive impairments is when the person fails to recognize limitations, a lack of awareness called *anosognosia*. Therapy enables the individual to integrate awareness of deficits of memory, attention, and executive control in order to allow the individual to have a new view of self after brain injury. There may be a distinction between a motivated lack of awareness (embarrassment) and an organic lack of awareness (McGlynn & Schacter, 1989). This lack of awareness hinders the individual from engaging in everyday life; thus, integration of awareness into interventions is critical.

15.5.2 INTERVENTIONS AT THE PERFORMANCE LEVEL

Toglia (1993, 2005), an occupational therapist, proposes **a strategy learning and awareness approach** that encourages the clinician to discover the cognitive capacities and processing strategies that can influence the person's performance. Treatment focuses on helping the person develop strategies and become aware of how deficits require modification of activity demands and the environment (Toglia, 1991, 2005; Toglia & Kirk, 2000). This strategy conceptualizes cognition as the dynamic interaction among the person, activity, and environment, and operates on the premise that cognition is modifiable under certain conditions. Although there is a fixed or structural limit in the individual's capacity to process information, there are differences in the way that capacity can be used. The same activity can require different amounts of processing capacity depending on how and where it is performed; thus, efficiency in the performance is critical. The efficient allocation of limited processing resources is central to learning and cognition (Flavell, Miller, & Miller, 1993). This approach focuses on changing the activity demands, the environment, and the person's use of strategies and level of awareness, with the goal of the person being trained to learn strategies that can be used in different activities and conditions. This approach requires the clinician to pres-

ent opportunities for the individual to experience different environments, different levels of demands of the activity, and bring to consciousness a new level of awareness (Baum & Katz, 2009).

Cognitive Orientation to Daily Occupational Performance (CO-OP), also developed by occupational therapists, is a client-centered, performance-based, problem-solving approach that enables the person to acquire skills through a process of strategy use and guided discovery (Polatajko & Mandich, 2004, 2005; see also Chapter 2). CO-OP fosters skill acquisition, cognitive strategy use, generalization, and transfer of learning. The foundational theories are drawn from behavioral and cognitive psychology, movement science, and occupational therapy. Behavioral theories focus on the relationship between stimulus, response, and consequence. Learning is viewed as a permanent change in the form, duration, or frequency of a behavior. Reinforcement is seen as an integral component of learning. CO-OP uses reinforcement, modeling, shaping, prompting, fading, and chaining techniques to support skill acquisition (Polatajko & Mandich, 2004). CO-OP requires the mental organization of knowledge (problem solving, reasoning, and thinking) in the acquisition and performance of skills (Schunk, 2000). The problem-solving strategy used in CO-OP is "GOAL, PLAN, DO, CHECK." It was adopted from Meichenbaum (1977, 1994) as a framework for guiding the discovery of self-generated domain-specific strategies that support skill acquisition.

The Fitts and Posner (1967) model of motor learning provides theoretical support for CO-OP. Their three-stage model of motor learning guides the process. The *cognitive stage* guides the individual as he or she seeks to understand the task and how to perform it; the *associative stage* is where the individual focuses attention and performs with greater speed and precision; and the *autonomous stage* is where the skill is performed consistently and in a coordinated pattern. CO-OP is based on a learning paradigm that acknowledges that new skills emerge from an interaction with the environment. The clinician creates the learning environment to support optimal learning. In this approach, cognition acts as the mediator between the individual's ability and the performance that is the goal of the individual; as such, a certain level of cognitive abilities is required in order to develop the new desirable skills. CO-OP creates a learning paradigm that helps individuals develop skills to support their daily life activities (Baum & Katz, 2009).

15.6 CONCLUSIONS

The executive dysfunction difficulties faced by individuals who have had a stroke requires the continued work and communication of cognitive and rehabilitation scientists.

The following reflect the gaps we identified that can be addressed:

- Cognitive and rehabilitation scientists need to develop a shared language that will allow cross-level validation of interventions and outcome measures. Specifically, there needs to be better definitions and assessment of executive functions at all levels. For example, to understand the effectiveness of behavioral interventions, a good starting point would be to use outcome measures at both the behavioral and performance levels. This approach could lead to a greater understanding of the neural and cognitive contributions to behavioral performance.

- Questions that need to be addressed about the performance of tasks include: What cognitive resources are needed to accomplish everyday tasks? What is automated? What requires attentional resources? How is task set maintained over an entire task epoch? How many independent ways are there to complete a task? At the cognitive and neural levels, are different strategies truly independent?

- We need to develop and maintain shared databases of patients that include comprehensive clinical evaluations, results from neuropsychological tests, performance-based tests, and self and caregiver reports. These databases must be maintained over time to begin to understand the consequences of aging with a brain injury. Such information is necessary to guide interventions and anticipate outcomes.

- Patient-centered outcomes will always rely on the interactions among the nature of the injury, the recovery processes, patients' expectations, their life demands, and their environments. Each will make contributions to actual and perceived outcomes. This is the complexity of neurorehabilitation and the challenges to those who study executive function. In Figure 15.4 we have made an attempt to capture the complexity of these interactions and demonstrate the importance of social and environmental support.

REFERENCES

Alderman, N., Burgess, P. W., Knight, C., & Henman, C. (2003). Ecological validity of a simplified version of the multiple errands shopping test. *Journal of the International Neuropsychological Society, 9*(1), 31–44.

Baddeley, A. (1996). Exploring the central executive. *The Quarterly Journal of Experimental Psychology A, 49*(1), 5–28.

Baddeley, A. D. (2001). Is working memory still working? *American Psychologist, 56*, 849–864.

Baum, C. (2009, May) Linking neuroscience to everyday life [Data summary and slide presentation]. Symposium *Stroke Rehabilitation: Focus on Symptom Management*, New York-Presbyterian Department of Rehabilitation Science, the University Hospital of Columbia and Cornell, Weill Cornell Medical College, New York.

Baum, C., & Katz, N. (2009). Occupational therapy approach to assessing the relationship between cognition and function. In T. D. Marcotte & I. Grant (Eds.), *Neuropsychology of everyday functioning* (pp. 62–91). New York: Guilford Press.

Baum, C., Morrison, T., Hahn, M., & Edwards, D. (2003). *Executive Function Performance Test: Test protocol booklet*. St. Louis, MO: Program in Occupational Therapy, Washington University School of Medicine.

Baum, C. M., Connor, L. T., Morrison, T., Hahn, M., Dromerick, A. W., & Edwards, D. F. (2008). Reliability, validity, and clinical utility of the Executive Function Performance Test: A measure of executive function in a sample of people with stroke. *American Journal of Occupational Therapy, 62*(4), 446–455.

Braver, T. S., Cohen, J. D., & Barch, D. M. (2002). The role of the prefrontal cortex in normal and disordered cognitive control: A cognitive neuroscience perspective. In D. T. Stuss & R. T. Knight (Eds.), *Principles of frontal lobe function* (pp. 428–448). Oxford: Oxford University Press.

Bruer, J. B. (1997). Education and the brain: A bridge too far. *Educational Researcher, 26*(8), 4–16.

Burgess, P. W., & Shallice, T. (1996). Response suppression, initiation and strategy use following frontal lobe lesions. *Neuropsychologia, 34*(4), 263–273.

Burgess, P. W., Alderman, N., Forbes, C., Costello, A., Coates, L. M-A., Dawson, D. R., et al.(2006). The case for the development and use of "ecologically valid" measures of executive function in experimental and clinical neuropsychology. *Journal of International Neuropsychological Society, 12*(2), 194–209.

Burgess, P. W., & Simons, J. S. (2005). Theories of frontal lobe executive function: Clinical applications. In P. W. Halligan & D. T. Wade (Eds.), *Effectiveness of rehabilitation for cognitive deficits* (pp. 211–231). Oxford: Oxford University Press.

Bütefisch, C. M. (2004). Plasticity in the human cerebral cortex: Lessons from the normal brain and from stroke. *Neuroscientist, 10*(2): 163–173.

Cardol, M., Beelen, A., van den Bos, G. A., den Jong, B. A., de Groot, I. J., & de Haan, R. J. (2002). Responsiveness of the impact on participation and autonomy questionnaire. *Archives of Physical Medicine and Rehabilitation, 83*(11), 1524–1529.

Chan, R. C. K., Shum, D., Toulopoulou, T., Chen, E. Y. H. (2008). Assessment of executive functions: Review of instruments and identification of critical issues. *Archives of Clinical Neuropsychology, 23*(2), 201–216.

Chen, A. J. W., Abrams, G. M., & D'Esposito, M. (2006). Functional reintegration of prefrontal neural networks for enhancing recovery after brain injury. *Journal of Head Trauma Rehabilitation, 21*(2), 107–118.

Chuang, K.-H., van Gelderen, P., Merkle, H., Bodurka, J., Ikonomidou, V. N., Koretsky A. P., et al. (2008). Mapping resting-state functional connectivity using perfusion MRI. *NeuroImage, 40*(4): 1595–1605.

Cohen, J. D., Dunbar, K., & McClelland, J. L. (1990). On the control of automatic processes: A parallel-distributed processing account of the Stroop Effect. *Psychological Review, 97*(3), 332–361.

Cools, R., & D'Esposito, M. (2009). Dopaminergic modulation of flexible control in humans. In A. Bjorkland, S. B. Dunnett, L. L. Iversen, & S. D. Iversen (Eds.), *Dopamine handbook* (pp. 249–261). Oxford: Oxford University Press.

Corbetta, M., & Fitzpatrick, S. M. (2011). Neural rehabilitation: action and manipulation. *Neurorehabilitation and Neural Repair, 25*(5 Suppl), 3S–5S.

Dawson, D. R., Anderson, N. D., Burgess, P., Cooper, E., Krpan, K. M., Stuss, D.T. (2009). Further development of the Multiple Errands Test: Standardized scoring, reliability, and ecological validity for the Baycrest version. *Archives of Physical Medicine and Rehabilitation, 90*(11 Suppl), S41–S51.

Diamond, A. (2002). Normal development of prefrontal cortex from birth to young adulthood: Cognitive functions, anatomy, and biochemistry. In D. T. Stuss & R. T. Knight (Eds.), *Principles of frontal lobe function* (pp. 466–503). Oxford: Oxford University Press.

Dosenbach, N. U. F., Visscher, K. M., Palmer, E. D., Miezin, F. M., Wenger, K. K., Kang, H. C., et al. (2006). A core system for the implementation of task sets. *Neuron, 50*(5), 799–812.

Dosenbach, N. U. F., Fair, D. A., Cohen, A. L., Schlaggar, B. L., & Petersen, S. E. (2008). A dual-networks architecture of top-down control. *Trends in Cognitive Science, 12*(3), 99–105.

Elliot, R. (2003). Executive functions and their disorders. *British Medical Bulletin, 65*(1), 49–59.

Fitts, P. M., & Posner, M. I. (1967). *Learning and skilled performance in human performance*. Belmont CA: Brock-Cole.

Fitzpatrick, S. M., & Rothman, D. L. (2002). Meeting report: Choosing the right MR tools for the job. *Journal of Cognitive Neuroscience, 14*(5), 806–815.

Flavell, J. H., Miller, P. H., & Miller, S. A. (1993). *Cognitive development* (3rd ed.). Englewood Cliffs, NJ: Prentice-Hall.

Floel, A., & Cohen, L. G. (2010). Recovery of function in humans: Cortical stimulation and pharmacological treatments after stroke. *Neurobiology of Disease, 37*(2), 243–251.

Frank, M. J., Loughry, B., & O'Reilly, R.C. (2001). Interactions between frontal cortex and basal ganglia in working memory: A computational model. *Cognitive, Affective, & Behavioral Neuroscience, 1*(2) 137–160.

Frey, S. H., Fogassi, L., Grafton, S., Picard, N., Rothwell, J. C., Schweighofer, N., Fitzpatrick, S. M. (2011). Neurological principles and rehabilitation of action disorders: Computation, anatomy, and physiology (CAP) model. *Neurorehabilitation and Neural Repair, 25*(5 Suppl), 6S–20S.

Fritsch, B., Reis, J., Martinowich, K., Schambra, H. M., Yuanyuan, J., Cohen, L. G., and Lu, B. (2010). Direct current stimulation promotes BDNF-dependent synaptic plasticity: Potential implications for motor learning. *Neuron, 66*(2) 198–204.

Gibbs, S. E., & D'Esposito, M. (2005). Individual capacity differences predict working memory performance and prefrontal activity following dopamine receptor stimulation. *Cognitive, Affective & Behavioral Neuroscience, 5*(2), 212–221.

Giles, G. M. (2005). A neurofunctional approach to rehabilitation following severe brain injury. In N. Katz (Ed.), *Cognition and occupation across the life span: Models for intervention in occupational therapy* (pp. 139–165). Bethesda, MD: AOTA Press.

Gjedde, A., Kumakura, Y., Cumming, P., Linnet, J., Møller, A. (2010). Inverted-U-shaped correlation between dopamine receptor availability in striatum and sensation-seeking. *Proceedings of the National Academy of Sciences, 107*(8), 3870–3875. Retrieved from: http://www.pnas.org/cgi/doi/10.1073/pnas.0912319107.

Goldberg, E. (2001). *The executive brain*. New York: Oxford University Press.

Goldman-Rakic, P. S. (1996). The prefrontal landscape: Implications of functional architecture for understanding human mentation and the central executive. In A. C. Roberts, T. W. Robbins & L. Weiskrantz (Eds.), *The prefrontal cortex: Executive and cognitive functions* (pp. 87–103). Oxford: Oxford University Press.

Grant, D. A., & Berg, E. A. (1948). A behavioral analysis of degree of reinforcement and ease of shifting to new responses in a Weigl-type card-sorting problem. *Journal of Experimental Psychology, 38*(4), 404–411.

Hartman-Maeir, A., Harel, H., & Katz, N. (2009). Kettle Test—A brief measure of cognitive functional performance: Reliability and validity in stroke rehabilitation. *American Journal of Occupational Therapy, 63*(5), 592–599.

Heaton, R. K., Chelune, G. J., Talley, J. L., Kay, G. G., & Curtiss, G. (1993). Wisconsin Card Sorting Test manual: Revised and expanded. Odessa, FL: Psychological Assessment Resources.

Jonides, J., & Smith, E. E. (1997). The architecture of working memory. In M. D. Rugg (Ed.), *Cognitive neuroscience* (pp. 243–276). Cambridge, MA: MIT Press.

Kaplan, S., & Berman, M. G. (2010). Directed attention as a common resource for executive functioning and self-regulation. *Perspectives on Psychological Science, 5*(1), 43–57.

Katz, N., Tadmor, I., Felzen, B., & Hartman-Maeir, A. (2007). Validity of the Executive Function Performance Test in individuals with schizophrenia. *Occupational Therapy Journal of Research, 27*(2), 44–51.

Knight, C., Alderman, N., & Burgess, P. (2002). Development of a simplified version of the multiple errands test for use in hospital settings. *Neuropsychological Rehabilitation, 12*(3), 231–255.

Levine, B., Robertson, I. H., Clare, L., Carter, G., Hong, J., Wilson, B. A., Stuss, D. T. (2000). Rehabilitation of executive functioning: An experimental–clinical validation of goal management training. *Journal of International Neuropsychological Society, 6*(3), 299–312.

Levine, B., Turner, G. R., & Stuss, D. T. (2008). Rehabilitation of frontal lobe functions. In D. T. Stuss, G. Winocur, & I. H. Robinson (Eds.), *Cognitive neurorehabilitation: Evidence and application* (pp. 464–486). Cambridge: Cambridge University Press.

Lezak, M. D. (1982). The problem of assessing executive functions. *International Journal of Psychology, 17*(1), 281–297.

Lezak, M. D. (2000). Nature, applications and limitations of neuropsychological assessment following traumatic brain injury. In A. Christensen & B. P. Uzzell (Eds.), *International handbook of neuropsychological rehabilitation* (pp. 67–80). New York: Kluwer Academic/Plenum.

Lowe, M. J. (2010). A historical perspective on the evolution of resting-state functional connectivity with MRI. *Magnetic Resonance Materials in Physics, Biology and Medicine, 23*(5–6), 279–288.

Manchester, D., Priestley, N., & Jackson, H. (2004). The assessment of executive functions: Coming out of the office. *Brain Injury, 18*(11), 1067–1081.

Martinsson, L., Hårdemark, H., & Eksborg, S. (2007). Amphetamines for improving recovery after stroke. *Cochrane Database of Systematic Reviews,* (1), Article CD002090.

McGlynn, S. M., & Schacter, D. L. (1989). Unawareness of deficits in neuropsychological syndromes. *Journal of Clinical and Experimental Neuropsychology, 11*(2), 143–205.

Meichenbaum, D. (1977). Cognitive behavioral modification: An integrative approach. New York: Plenum Press.

Meichenbaum, D. (1994). A clinical handbook/practical therapist manual for assessing and treating adults with post traumatic stress disorder. Waterloo, Ontario: Institute Press.

Miller, E. K., & Cohen, J. D. (2001). An integrative theory of prefrontal cortex function. *Annual Review of Neuroscience, 24*(1), 167–202.

Miyake, A., & Shah, P. (1999). Toward unified theories of working memory: Emerging general consensus, unresolved theoretical issues and future directions. In A. Miyake & P. Shah (Eds.), *Models of working memory: Mechanisms of active maintenance and executive control* (pp. 28–61). Cambridge, England: Cambridge University Press.

Miyake, A., Friedman, N. P., Emerson, M. J., Witzki, A. H., Howerter, A., & Wager, T. D. (2000). The unity and diversity of executive functions and their contributions to complex "frontal lobe" tasks: A latent variable analysis. *Cognitive Psychology, 41*(1), 49–100.

Narushima, K., Paradiso, S., Moser, D. J., Jorge, R., Robinson, R. G. (2007). Effect of antidepressant therapy on executive function after stroke. *The British Journal of Psychiatry, 190,* 260–265.

Norman, D. A., & Shallice, T. (1986). Attention to action: Willed and automatic control of behavior. In R. J. Davidson, G. E. Schwartz, & D. Shapiro (Eds.), *Consciousness and self-regulation* (Vol. 4, pp. 1–18). New York: Plenum Press.

O'Brien, A. N., & Wolf, T. J. (2010). Determining work outcomes in mild to moderate stroke survivors. *Work, 36*(4), 441–447.

Pessoa, L. (2008). On the relationship between emotion and cognition. *Nature Reviews Neuroscience, 9*(2), 148–158.

Pohjasvaara T., Vataja, R., Leppävuori, A., Kaste, M., & Erkinjuntti, T. (2002). Cognitive functions and depression as predictors of poor outcome 15 months after stroke. *Cerebrovascular Diseases, 14*(3–4), 228–233.

Polatajko, H. & Mandich, A. (2004). *Enabling occupation in children: The cognitive orientation to daily occupational performance (CO-OP) approach.* Ottawa, ON: CAOT Publications ACE.

Polatajko, H. J., & Mandich, A. (2005). Cognitive orientation to daily occupational performance with children with developmental coordination disorders. In Katz, N. (Ed.), *Cognition and occupation across the life span: Models for intervention in occupational therapy* (pp. 237–259). Bethesda, MD: American Occupational Therapy Association.

Pomeroy, V., Aglioti, S.M., Mark, V. W., McFarland, D., Stinear, C., Wolf, S.L., et al. (2011). Neurological principles and rehabilitation of action disorders: Rehabilitation interventions. *Neurorehabilitation and Neural Repair, 25*(5 Suppl), 33S–43S.

Posner, M. I., & Petersen, S. E. (1990). The attention system of the human brain. *Annual Review of Neuroscience, 13*(1), 25–42.

Prigatano, G. P. (1986). Personality and psychosocial consequences of brain injury. In G. P. Prigatano, D. J. Fordyce, H. K. Zeiner, J. R. Roueche, M. Pepping, & B. C. Wood (Eds.), *Neuropsychological rehabilitation after brain injury* (pp. 29–50). Baltimore: Johns Hopkins University Press.

Prigatano, G. P. (1990). *Principals of Neuropsychological Rehabilitation.* New York: Oxford University Press.

Ramirez, J., Gao, F., & Black, S. E. (2008). Structural neuroimaging: Defining the cerebral context for cognitive rehabilitation. In I. H. Robertson, G. Winocur, & D. T. Stuss (Eds.), *Cognitive neurorehabilitation: Evidence and applications* (pp. 124–148). Cambridge: Cambridge University Press.

Reitan, R. M., & Wolfson, D. (1995). Category test and trail making test as measures of frontal lobe functions. *Clinical Neuropsychologist, 9*(1), 50–56.

Reutter-Bernays, D., & Rentsch, H. P. (1993). Rehabilitation of the elderly patient with stroke: An analysis of short-term and long-term results. *Disability and Rehabilitation, 15*(2), 90–95.

Robbins, T. W., & Arnsten, A. F. T. (2009). The neuropsychopharmacology of fronto-executive function: Monoaminergic modulation. *Annual Review of Neuroscience, 32*(1), 267–287.

Robertson, I. H., Ward, T., Ridgeway, V., & Nimmo-Smith, I. (1994). *The test of everyday attention manual.* Flempton: Thames Valley Test Company.

Rochette, A., Desrosiers, J., Bravo, G., St-Cyr-Tribble, D., & Bourget, A. (2007). Changes in participation after a mild stroke: Quantitative and qualitative perspectives. *Topics in Stroke Rehabilitation, 14*(3), 59–68.

Sathian, K., Buxbaum, L. J., Cohen, L. G., Krakauer, J. W., Lang, C. E., Corbetta, M., et al. (2011). Neurological principles and rehabilitation of action disorders: Common clinical deficits. *Neurorehabilitation and Neural Repair, 25*(5 Suppl), 21S–32S.

Schunk, D. H. (2000). *Learning theories: an educational perspective* (3rd ed.). Upper Saddle River, NJ: Merrill/Prentice-Hall.

Seeley, W. W., Menon, V. Schatzberg, A. F., Keller, J. Glover, G. H., Kenna, H., Reiss, A. L., and Greicius, M. D. (2007). Dissociable Intrinsic Connectivity Networks for Salience Processing and Executive Control. *Journal of Neuroscience, 27*(9), 2349–2346.

Shallice, T., & Burgess, P. W. (1991). Deficits in strategy application following frontal lobe damage in man. *Brain,* 114(2), 727–741.

Shallice, T., Levin, H. S., Eisenberg, H. M., & Benton, A. L. (Eds.). (1991). *Frontal lobe function and dysfunction.* Oxford: Oxford University Press.

Smith, E. E., & Jonides, J. (1999). Storage and executive processes in the frontal lobes. *Science,* 283(5408), 1657–1661.

Stuss, D. T., & Levine, B. (2002). Adult clinical neuropsychology: Lessons from studies of the frontal lobes. *Annual Review of Psychology, 53*(1), 401–433.

Su, C. Y., Lin, Y. H., Kwan, A. L., & Guo, N. W. (2008). Construct validity of the Wisconsin Card Sorting Test-64 in patients with stroke. *Clinical Neuropsychology,* 22 (2), 273–287.

Swartz, N. (1997). *The concept of necessary conditions and sufficient conditions.* Retrieved from http://www.sfu.ca/~swartz/conditions1.htm.

Toglia, J., & Kirk, U. (2000). Understanding awareness deficits following brain injury. *NeuroRehabilitation,* 15(1), 57–70.

Toglia, J. P. (1991). Generalization of treatment: a multicontextual approach to cognitive perceptual impairment in the brain-injured adult. *American Journal of Occupational Therapy,* 45(6), 505–516.

Toglia, J. P. (1993). *Contextual Memory Test.* San Antonio, TX: The Psychological Corporation.

Toglia J. P. (2005). A dynamic interactional approach to cognitive rehabilitation. In N. Katz (Ed.), *Cognition and occupation across the life span: Models for intervention in occupational therapy* (pp. 29–72). Bethesda MD: American Occupational Therapy Association.

Tranel, D., Anderson, S. W., & Benton, A. L. (1994). Development of the concept of "executive function" and its relationship to the frontal lobes. In F. Boller & J. Grafman (Eds.), *Handbook of Neuropsychology* (Vol. 9, pp. 125–148). Amsterdam: Elsevier.

Wallace, D. L., Vytlacil, J. J., Nomura, E. M., Gibbs, S. E. B., D'Esposito, M. (2011). The dopamine agonist bromocriptine differentially affects fronto-striatal functional connectivity during working memory. *Frontiers in Human Neuroscience,* 5(32) 1–6.

Wechsler, D. (1955). Wechsler Adult Intelligence Scale: Manual. New York: The Psychological Corporation.

Wilson, B. A., Alderman, N., Burgess, P. W., Emslie, H., & Evans, J. J. (1996). Behavioural assessment of dysexecutive syndrome. St. Edmunds, UK: Thames Valley Test Company.

Wolf, T. J., Baum, C., & Connor, L. T. (2009). Changing face of stroke: implications for occupational therapy practice. *American Journal of Occupational Therapy,* 63(5), 621–625.

Wolf, T., Stift, S., Connor, L., & Baum, C. (2010). Feasibility of the EFPT at the acute stage of stroke to detect executive function deficits that impact return to work. *Work,* 36(4), 405–412.

Zinn, S., Bosworth, H. B., Hoenig, H. M., Swartzwelder, H. S. (2007). Executive function deficits in acute stroke. *Archives of Physical Medicine and Rehabilitation,* 88(2), 173–180.

Zoccolotti, P., Cantagallo, A., De Luca, M., Guariglia, C., Serino, A., & Trojano, I. (2011). Selective and integrated rehabilitation programs for disturbances of visual/spatial attention and executive function after brain damage: A neuropsychological evidence-based review. *European Journal of Physical Rehabilitation Medicine,* 47(1), 123–147.

16 | LANGUAGE

LISA TABOR CONNOR

16.1 NEUROSCIENCE OF LANGUAGE: NEUROPSYCHOLOGICAL AND LESION-SYMPTOM MAPPING EVIDENCE

Until the advent of modern-day functional neuroimaging techniques in the 1980s, the neuroscientific understanding of language had largely been based on 150 years of lesion-symptom mapping. The first widely publicized cerebral localization data came from Paul Broca's 1861 paper delivered to the Societé d'Anatomie in Paris describing the case of Monsieur Leborgne. Leborgne's case provided the first evidence that a lesion of the third frontal convolution of the left hemisphere produced a deficit of "articulate speech." Carl Wernicke followed in 1874 with a more nuanced model of language representation in the brain that included a center in the posterior aspect of the left superior temporal lobe that when lesioned, produced a deficit in the ability to comprehend speech (Finger, 1994). Wernicke proposed, moreover, that the articulation center and the comprehension center were somehow connected and that lesions of the connection between the regions would produce conduction aphasia (characterized by "misapplied" words and the inability to read, but with good comprehension and fluent expression), whereas lesions of both regions simultaneously would produce "total aphasia." This model of how language is represented in the brain has been elaborated upon and refined over the intervening years by neurolinguistics researchers, but has stood as a general framework.

More recently, several investigators have utilized modern-day imaging techniques to extend the lesion-symptom mapping approach. Bates, Wilson, Saygin, Dick, Sereno, Knight, et al. (2003) demonstrated with voxel-based lesion-symptom mapping that Broca's region may not be the most critical in disorders of fluency, but instead the anterior insula may be the region primarily associated with fluency deficits in people with aphasia, apraxia of speech, or both. Likewise, although Wernicke's region in the superior temporal gyrus was found to be associated with comprehension deficits using this approach, the primary region lesioned in those with comprehension deficits was the middle temporal gyrus. These regions, crucial for production and comprehension of language, have also been implicated in functional neuroimaging studies of language.

Another, more dynamic approach to the question of how language is represented in the brain is the perfusion-symptom mapping approach utilized by Hillis and colleagues (e.g., Hillis, Kane, Tuffiash, Ulatowski, Barker, Beauchamp, et al., 2001; Hillis, Barker, Wityk, Aldrich, Restrepo, Breese, et al., 2004; Hillis, Kleinman, Newhart, Heidler-Gary, Gottesman, Barker, et al., 2006). Hillis and colleagues have used perfusion-weighted magnetic resonance imaging coupled with a detailed lexical function test battery to examine regions of hypoperfusion in the brain shortly after stroke that correlate with aspects of lexical deficit. For instance, a patient with a deficit in lexical semantics was found to have hypoperfusion of Wernicke's area. A pharmacologic intervention that raised mean blood pressure, thereby reperfusing Wernicke's area, resulted in restoration of lexical semantic function in this patient (Hillis, et al., 2001). Similar studies have been done to examine associations of brain regions with picture naming (Hillis, et al., 2006) and the role of basal ganglia regions in aphasia (Hillis, et al., 2004). The allure of this technique for lesion-symptom mapping is that it is done within hours of stroke and thus, the results obtained using this technique are less likely to be contaminated by reorganization of language "centers" in the chronic stage of aphasia recovery.

16.2 FUNCTIONAL NEUROIMAGING OF LANGUAGE AND RECOVERY

Functional neuroimaging techniques, such as positron emission tomography (PET), functional magnetic resonance imaging (fMRI), and magnetoencephalography (MEG), have figured significantly in the development of understanding how language is represented in the brain. Because brain lesions are not precise and language theories are unable to be tested in animal models, functional neuroimaging techniques have been utilized in healthy adults to uncover regions of the brain involved in aspects of the production and comprehension of language, including reading and writing. The literature on verbal production and auditory comprehension of language in healthy adults has exploded to such an extent that Price (2010) published a review of 100 fMRI studies focused on this topic in 2009 alone. In her review, Price indicated that the convergence of primarily single word production and comprehension studies establishes a comprehension network that includes prelexical speech perception involving bilateral superior temporal gyri, comprehension of meaningful words in middle and inferior temporal cortices (converging with the meta-analysis conducted by Binder, Desai, Graves and Conant, 2009), retrieval of semantic knowledge involving left angular gyrus and pars orbitalis, with sentence comprehension involving bilateral superior temporal sulci. Verbal production studies revealed activation of the comprehension network; in addition, word retrieval activated left middle frontal cortex, articulatory planning involved left anterior insula, and initiation of speech production involved left putamen, pre-supplementary motor area (SMA), SMA, and motor cortex. Activation studies and meta-analyses (Binder, et al., 2009; Vigneau, Beaucousin, Herve, Duffau, Crivello, Houde et al. 2006) have begun to converge on the "nodes" in the language network, but further work will be needed to reveal anatomical and functional connections among these nodes.

Neuroimaging techniques have also been utilized to examine brain regions associated with recovery from aphasia and with aphasia treatment. One of the early studies that examined changes in brain activity over a recovery period was a PET study conducted by Musso and colleagues (1999). They examined people with aphasia before and after a short training session of comprehension treatment that was administered between PET scans. Changes in activity that were most strongly associated with changes in Token Test performance were increases in the posterior portion of right superior temporal gyrus and left precuneus, arguing that regions of the brain not normally participating in comprehension were now active in people with aphasia and responsible for their improvements in performance. Shortly thereafter, Rosen, Petersen, Linenweber, Snyder, White, Chapman, et al. (2000) provided data suggesting that verbal production performance in chronic patients with good outcomes was largely due to perilesional left hemisphere activity; those people with chronic aphasia and poorer performance had brain activity localized to the right hemisphere homolog of Broca's area.

More recently Saur and colleagues (2006) conducted an fMRI study over 3 sessions in the first year post-stroke: at 2 days, 2 weeks, and 10 months. They concluded that the brain activity pattern observed is highly dependent upon when imaging was conducted during the first year. Their data suggest that brain reorganization during language recovery happens in phases. First, activation in the expected left hemisphere is severely reduced in the acute phase. Second, regions homologous to the traditional language regions in right hemisphere are recruited that correlate with language improvement. Finally, a normalization of activation is observed with shifts in activity back to the left hemisphere, possibly reflecting consolidation in the language system due to recovery or treatment.

Several imaging studies have been conducted pretreatment and posttreatment to document brain-related changed due to rehabilitation. One of the first of these studies (Belin, Van Eeckhout, Zilbovicius, Remy, Francois, Guillaume, et al., 1996) found that after Melodic Intonation Therapy, reactivation of left prefrontal cortex and suppression of initially activated right hemisphere homologs resulted in the best performance changes in their seven chronic patients. This finding supported Rosen et al.'s and Saur et al.'s contention that right frontal activity may not be optimal for recovery. More recent treatment studies, one utilizing MEG and two utilizing transcranial magnetic stimulation (TMS), further add to the evidence that good aphasia recovery and treatment outcome are associated with return of left hemisphere perilesional regions and suppression of right hemisphere homologs. Cornelissen, Laine, Tarkiainen, Jarvensivu, Martin, and Salmelin (2003) performed MEG pretreatment and posttreatment for anomia. They reported that left inferior parietal lobe changes were associated with improvements in naming performance on treated items. Naeser and colleagues have conducted several studies using TMS to improve picture naming (e.g., Naeser, Martin, Nicholas, Baker, Seekins, Kobayashi, et al., 2005; Naeser, Martin, Theoret, Kobayashi, Fregni, Nicholas, et al., 2011). In participants with aphasia, suppression of right pars triangularis led to improvements in pictures naming coupled with decreases in response latency. Suppression of right pars opercularis, however, produced longer response latencies for picture naming but did not change the number of pictures named. Most compelling, healthy controls showed the same pattern of performance after right hemisphere TMS as did participants with aphasia, suggesting that the right hemisphere may have heretofore unrecognized contributions to verbal production that can be unmasked after aphasia.

16.2.1 WHITE MATTER TRACTOGRAPHY

Further elaboration of a model of the neural bases of language has been made possible using white matter imaging, also known as diffusion tensor or diffusion-weighted imaging with tractography (see Johansen-Berg & Rushworth, 2009; Jbabdi & Johansen-Berg, 2011; see Chapter 4). Diffusion imaging is based upon the physical properties of water diffusing directionally along a tube, in this case along bundles of myelinated axons. Regions of interest may be specified in a tractography model and tracts that connect these regions can be mathematically reconstructed. For example, Broca's and Wernicke's regions can be specified and the arcuate and longitudinal fasciculi can be constructed for individual subjects. The diffusion in these tracts can be compared between healthy individuals and those with lesions of white matter after stroke. Catani and colleagues (2005) applied the region-based tractography approach to peri-Sylvian language regions and found that the superior longitudinal fasciculus and arcuate fasciculus both traversed from Broca's to Wernicke's regions. A direct connection between these key regions exists via the arcuate. Many fibers from the superior longitudinal fasciculus terminate, however, in an intermediate region in the inferior parietal lobe in the left hemisphere, a region that has been implicated in functional imaging studies of language (e.g., Price, 2000; Wise, Scott, Blank, Mummery, Murphy, & Warburton, 2001; Cornelissen, et al., 2003). This parietal region Catani and colleagues called *Geschwind's territory*, with further tracts found to be connecting Geschwind's territory with Wernicke's area. DTI has thus uncovered an indirect pathway from Broca's to Wernicke's regions, helping to explain some of the anatomical variability in the lesions of people with conduction aphasia.

16.2.2 FUNCTIONAL CONNECTIVITY MRI

At rest, and even during sleep, the brain has slow (<0.01 Hz) synchronized activity that co-varies over time across spatially distinct regions. Recent work has examined these spontaneous fluctuations of blood oxygen level dependent (BOLD) signals using fMRI at rest, now termed resting-state functional MRI (rs-fMRI: e.g., Biswal, Yetkin, Haughton, & Hyde, 1995; Fox, Snyder, Vincent, Corbetta, Van Essen, & Raichle, 2005; Biswal, Mennes, Zuo, Guohel, Kelly, Smith, et al., 2010; Friston, 2011). The temporal correlation of these fluctuations between regions defines functional connectivity networks. The networks examined thus far are quite similar to the networks defined by task-evoked fMRI. That is, regions activated while a participant is performing an attention task in the scanner (Corbetta, Kincade, Lewis, Snyder, & Sapir, 2005) are the same regions whose resting state BOLD signal fluctuations co-vary temporally (He, Snyder, Vincent, Epstein, Shulman, & Corbetta, 2007).

There is a small, but growing, number of studies attempting to define the language system via resting state fMRI (Hampson, Peterson, Skudlarski, Gatenby, & Gore, 2002; Hampson, Tokoglu, Sun, Schafer, Skudlarski, & Gore, et al., 2006; Saur, Schelter, Schnell, Kratochvil, Kupper, Kellmeyer, et al., 2010; Xiang, Fonteijn, Norris, & Hagoort, 2010; Koyama, Di Martino, Zuo, Kelly, Mennes, Jutagir, et al., 2011; Perani, Saccuman, Scifo, Anwander, Spada, Baldoli, et al., 2011). The starting point of rs-fMRI is seed regions established through task-evoked fMRI studies. These early functional connectivity studies of language have extracted seed regions from data acquired during single word reading, single word verbal output, sentence reading, and sentence comprehension tasks. Once seed regions are selected, the whole brain is interrogated for temporal correlations with these seed regions. Relatively few language regions have been recovered thus far, but the temporal fluctuations in activity in Broca's and Wernicke's regions have consistently been found to correlate in the left hemisphere across studies. Broca's and Wernicke's areas have also been found in an effective connectivity study (Eickhoff, Heim, Zilles, & Amunts, 2009) to correlate with regions outside of the language network per se that would be involved in language-production tasks. These correlated regions included the anterior insula, basal ganglia, cerebellum, premotor cortex, and primary motor cortex. Koyama and colleagues (2011) have examined connectivity networks underlying reading competence that are common and divergent in adults and children. Broca's and Wernicke's areas were part of the common reading network for adults and children, with greater connectivity strength corresponding to better reading. In adults only, however, better reading also corresponded with stronger correlations between the fusiform gyrus, a region implicated in visual word form processing, and Broca's area.

Xiang et al. (2010) recently conducted an rs-fMRI study in healthy adults to refine and expand information about the functional connectivity of sub-regions in Broca's "complex" to other regions throughout peri-Sylvian cortex and their putative roles in language processing. Instead of examining the correlation of Broca's area with other language regions in the brain using a single seed region, the authors seeded a broader swath of Broca's "complex" with three contiguous seeds in regions reported in the literature to be active in different aspects of language processing in task-evoked fMRI studies: pars opercularis (BA 44), pars triangularis (BA 45), and pars orbitalis (BA 47). These three sub-regions have been associated with phonological (BA 44), syntactic (BA 44/45), and semantic (BA 47/45) processing. Additionally, the authors compared connectivity networks developed using left versus right hemisphere seed regions to measure the hemispheric specialization of the uncovered networks. The three seed regions in Broca's complex displayed three separable networks in the left hemisphere that involved distinct regions in prefrontal, inferior parietal, and temporal cortices, with some cross-correlations among regions suggesting a mechanism to integrate language information across networks, whereas the right hemisphere seeds did not produce distinct networks.

Only a few rs-fMRI studies have examined changes in networks due to training (Lewis, Baldassarre, Committeri, Romani, & Corbetta, 2009), stroke recovery (He, et al., 2007; Warren, Crinion, Lambon Ralph, & Wise, 2009; Carter, Astafiev, Lang, Connor, Rengachary, Strube, et al., 2010), or development (e.g., Fair, Cohen, Power, Dosenbach, Church, Miezen, et al., 2009; Friederici, Brauer & Lohmann, 2011; Perani, et al., 2011). A single study, by Warren and colleagues (2009), reports on the relationship between functional connectivity in the language network and functional outcomes in persons with aphasia. Individuals with better preserved intertemporal connectivity had better receptive language abilities. Clearly, more research in this area is needed to understand at the systems level changes in functional connectivity due to aphasia, its recovery, and the effects of treatment.

16.3 CURRENT MODELS OF LANGUAGE REHABILITATION

For modern-day speech/language pathologists there are several guiding frameworks for aphasia rehabilitation from which to choose. Although one of the possible frameworks takes a psychosocial/functional approach to rehabilitation, we will focus here on the traditional treatment approaches based on stimulation, neuropsychological, and neurolinguistic theories as they most directly dovetail with the neuroscience of language (see Chapey, 2008 for coverage of each of these approaches).

The most influential thinker of her time in aphasia rehabilitation, Hildred Schuell, articulated the stimulation framework for aphasia treatment after years of observing language deficits and attempting to ameliorate them in soldiers returning from World War II (Coelho, Sinotte, & Duffy, 2008). Schuell and colleagues, including Wepman (e.g., 1951), conceived of aphasia as "a general language deficit that crosses all language modalities and may or may not be complicated by other sequelae of brain damage" (Schuell, Jenkins, & Jiménez-Pabón, 1964). This definition, as a multimodal entity affecting speaking, auditory comprehension, reading, and writing, guided the development of assessment tools, observation, and data collection approaches, as well as treatment for persons with aphasia. Further assumptions of this approach are that (i) aphasia is not a *loss* of language, but a disruption to the already learned language system; and (ii) that the primary means to reorganize the language system is through inputs via the auditory modality. The cornerstone of stimulation treatment is to provide carefully controlled, strong stimulation to the auditory system of the person with aphasia in order to reorganize the disrupted language system. Although the stimulation approach wasn't based explicitly on neuroscientific principles, it does have two essential components that have been shown by neuroscience research to aid in rehabilitation—stimulation that is sufficient to register with the sensory system, and the need for many repetitions to reorganize the damaged language system.

A second commonly used treatment approach is based on cognitive neuropsychological models of language processing (see Hillis, 1993; Rapp, 2005; Hillis & Newhart, 2008). These types of models posit that the brain possesses a series of information processing modules with connections among them. Each processing module represents and decodes different aspects of language; once processing is done for that type of information, the products of that step are passed on in the network to another stage of processing. For instance, naming a line drawing of a tree involves accessing visual object representations in order to recognize the object as a tree, then accessing semantic features of the tree category to decide if the object is simply a generic tree or a specific type of tree, such as an elm. The semantic information about the tree must then be connected up with the phonological representation of the sounds comprising the word "tree." These phonological representations are then transferred to the motor planning module to articulate the word "tree." These types of models may be represented visually with box-and-arrow diagrams or may be instantiated in a connectionist network.

Primarily, these models are used to understand the nature of the language deficit manifest by a specific pattern of behavioral errors on language tasks given to the person with aphasia. Based on the pattern of errors, the nature of the language deficit is pinpointed in the system. The value of this detailed knowledge is that the therapist may determine whether a course of therapy will be targeted at the point of the deficit itself to remediate the problem, or will entail compensatory strategies designed to sidestep the "broken" neuropsychological process. Remediation therapies based on the cognitive neuropsychological framework have been quite successful (e.g., Beeson, Rewega, Vail, & Rapcsak, 2000; Friedman, Sample, & Lott, 2000; DeLeon, Gottesman, Kleinman, Neunart, Davis, Lee, et al., 2007) and many treatments based on this framework have been developed (e.g., Raymer, Thompson, Jacobs, & LeGrand, 1993; see also Raymer & Gonzalez Rothi, 2008). What these models are unable to do, however, is either to prescribe whether a remedial or compensatory treatment will be more effective, or to guide the therapist in the manner in which the treatment ought to be given. The strength of the cognitive neuropsychological approach is that models of the language system that form its basis were developed from the accumulation of knowledge and research regarding lesion–behavior relationships. Thus, patients can be grouped by the language deficits that they exhibit; treatment programs targeted at that level of representation can be assumed to be effective for all patients that share this particular pattern of errors, especially if they also share a lesion location in the brain.

Clearly, the assumptions of the cognitive neuropsychological framework differ dramatically from the stimulation framework. The cognitive neuropsychological framework insists that aphasia is not a multimodal deficit of language affecting reading, writing, speaking, and comprehending (unless the lesion extent covers multiple regions in the language zone); rather, the nature of aphasia in an individual depends on precisely where in the language network a lesion is located. Moreover, a remedial approach to aphasia using this framework dictates that treatment should not be general, but targeted at the specific processes affected by that lesion.

A final framework for treatment is a variation, or fine-tuning, of the cognitive neuropsychological approach. The cognitive neurolinguistic approach uses an information processing framework, but the important addition is its reliance on linguistic theory to propose specific methods for rehabilitation and a means to generate linguistic theory-based hypotheses about the generalization of trained materials (see Thompson, 2008). Treatment for aphasia begins, as in the cognitive neuropsychological approach, with a detailed assessment of language abilities that are intact and impaired, including grammatical structures. Patients demonstrating a deficit in grammatical structures may exhibit a pattern of verbal production whereby primarily content words are produced, with fewer verbs than nouns. In addition, the production of subject-verb-object sentences may be disordered, with missing arguments or agents, and mismatched verb agreement. Based on this pattern of errors, treatments are prescribed focused on the underlying grammatical processes that are impaired. Several treatments for agrammatism have been developed based on this cognitive linguistic framework (Loverso, Prescott, & Selinger 1986; Schwartz, Saffran, Fink, Myers, & Martin, 1994; Rochon, Laird, Bose, & Scofield, 2005). Thompson and colleagues, however, argue that most of these approaches do not produce generalization to untrained forms because they are not targeting underlying grammatical structure directly. Treatment of Underlying Forms (TUF: Thompson & Shapiro, 2005) not only improves the trained sentence types, but produces generalization to sentences that are linguistically related to those trained (e.g., Thompson, Ballard, & Shapiro, 1998; Ballard & Thompson, 1999); these treatment effects also extend to changes in spontaneous discourse production (Ballard & Thompson, 1999). The cognitive linguistic approach has provided principles from linguistic theory to guide the rehabilitation of persons with agrammatic aphasia, demonstrating that generalization can be built into treatment in a systematic manner. Neuroimaging studies, however, have not provided a narrow set of brain regions that subserve syntactic processing, even though the clinical manifestation of agrammatism is mainly associated with lesions of the left frontal lobe (Vanier & Caplan, 1990; Thompson, 2008).

16.4 TREATMENT PRINCIPLES/ STRATEGIES ARISING FROM NEUROSCIENCE AND COGNITIVE NEUROSCIENCE

A neuroscientifically guided approach to language treatment needs to not merely rely upon knowledge of the regions involved in language processing and their anatomical and functional connectivities. A neuroscientifically guided approach to language treatment must also include knowledge about learning principles that apply to the rehabilitation process itself (see Chapter 2 for more information about the Rehab-Learn model). Both behavioral studies of humans and lesion studies with animals on recovery from stroke have indicated that the largest relearning effects require that the treatment program be delivered with sufficient intensity. Hinckley and Craig (1998), Bhogal, Teasell, and Speechley (2003), and Cherney, Patterson, Raymer, Frymark, and Schooling (2008) have all provided evidence that aphasia treatment must be delivered on an intense schedule to maximize improvement in language functions.

Unfortunately, these reviews point out that the intensity of practice that is given in traditional rehabilitation settings, especially outpatient therapy, is delivered in a format that is suboptimal. One hour of therapy, delivered 2 or 3 times per week in the outpatient setting, is not sufficient to produce the maximum amount of change. Animal studies of motor recovery indicate that hundreds, if not thousands, of repetitions of a motor activity are required to produce changes in cortical mapping post-stroke (Nudo, Wise, SiFuentes, & Milliken, 1996; Kleim, Barbay, & Nudo, 1998). Lang and colleagues (2009) counted the number of repetitions in typical physical and occupational therapy sessions across seven rehabilitation facilities in North America. The average number of repetitions of upper extremity treatment in a session was 32 as compared to the 400–600 in animal upper extremity studies; the average number of gait steps in a treatment session was 357 as compared to the 1000–2000 steps in animal lower extremity studies. Although the number of repetitions was quite low in the observed treatment sessions, the number of responses made by a patient in a typical speech therapy session is likely to be similar.

To combat this lack of intensity in language treatment and to incorporate principles gleaned from the animal learning literature, several investigators have implemented treatment in a more intense format, akin to constraint-induced movement therapy (CIMT: see Wolf, Winstein, Miller, Taub, Uswatte, Morris, et al., 2006). Constraint-induced aphasia treatment (CIAT) is typically delivered in 2–3 hour sessions on 5 consecutive days over a 2-week interval (Pulvermüller, Neininger, Elbert, Mohr, Rockstroh, Koebbel, et al., 2001; Maher, Kendall, Swearengin, Rodriguez, Leon, Pingel, et al., 2006; Meinzer, Elbert, Djundja, Taub, & Rockstroh, 2007). The constraint in CIAT is twofold. Patients are only able to respond with verbal language; no attempt to communicate with gestures or writing is reinforced. Patients are constrained to produce the type of verbal response that is considered to be correct for a given set of trials. In addition to constrained massed practice, the treatment includes a shaping component (Taub, Crago, Burgio, Groomes, Cook III, DeLuca, et al., 1994). Patients are progressively given more and more demanding constraints for the format of their verbal output to more closely approximate language production in healthy speakers. Results of CIAT for people with chronic aphasia have been promising. Verbal production improves by the end of treatment using the CIAT format and gains may be maintained over time (e.g., Meinzer, et al., 2005), though retention has not generally been studied in all studies of CIAT.

16.5 TOWARD A NEUROSCIENTIFICALLY BASED MODEL OF APHASIA REHABILITATION

On the whole, how does this information gained from neuroscience inform the recovery and treatment of aphasia? What have we learned and where are we going? What still needs to be done? Three components of the neuroscientific approach to aphasia rehabilitation are now well established and two components are in development. Well established and well supported by the literature are the clinical rehabilitation frameworks of the stimulation approach, the cognitive neuropsychological approach, and the cognitive neurolinguistic approach, although it is not always obvious which approach is best for which patients. Knowledge gained from white matter tractography and functional resting-state connectivity studies may aid in determining which approach may yield better outcomes. For instance, a person with aphasia who has damage throughout the language system of the left hemisphere may not respond well to cognitive neuropsychological or cognitive neurolinguistic treatments, due to the lack of remaining plasticity in the neural system for language. Similarly, the cognitive neurolinguistic approach of targeting underlying syntactic forms may be most successful when imaging reveals that critical constituents of the syntactic subnetwork of the left hemisphere are still intact.

A second component, recently bolstered by an explosion of neuroimaging studies of language, is general agreement regarding regions that comprise the language system. Many task-evoked fMRI studies (literally hundreds) have converged on critical regions involved in phonological, semantic, and syntactic production and comprehension,

though single word production and comprehension studies predominate. Sentence production and comprehension studies (if not discourse studies) are needed, as it is clear that single word processing represents only a sliver of the full complement of language processing.

A third well-established neuroscientific contribution is that stimulation that can change the brain must be strong so that it registers, and treatment regimens must be intense, though sadly this information is underutilized in the current clinical environment. Massed practice is currently the primary means to move a brain from its current state to a new, more functional state in rehabilitation, but other interventions that serve as neuromodulators, such as drug therapies (see Berthier, Pulvermüller, Davila, Casares, & Guitierrez, 2011 for review), transcranial magnetic stimulation (Naeser, et al., 2005; Winhuisen, Thiel, Schumacher, Kessler, Rudolf, Haupt, et al., 2005), or direct current stimulation (Baker, Rorden, & Fridriksson, 2010) coupled with directed aphasia therapies can also provide a means to reorganize language functions after brain injury.

Two areas in need of further development to contribute to a stronger neuroscientific foundation of rehabilitation, especially in aphasia rehabilitation, are diffusion tractography and resting-state functional connectivity. These techniques are now being widely used to understand neural systems supporting cognition, but are only beginning to be utilized to understand recovery after brain injury and dynamic reorganization due to training. Functional connectivity studies of treatment will, no doubt, be forthcoming. It will likely take some time and concerted effort to make sense of those findings in order to benefit the rehabilitation programs for individual patients in the future.

The work that remains to be done is considerable, although there is a base of older literature to draw upon and some promising new studies that have begun to combine several of these techniques to a positive end. One of the relatively neglected areas of research in rehabilitation that will serve as a bridge from neuroscientific principles to rehabilitation techniques is the application of cognitive principles of learning. As mentioned above, massed practice is now a cornerstone of rehabilitative therapies, although the cognitive learning and memory literature has long supported the effectiveness of spaced retrieval to produce robust retention of memory and motor skills (e.g., Glenberg, 1979). Fridriksson, Holland, Beeson, and Morrow (2005) successfully applied the principle of spaced retrieval to an anomia treatment and found it to produce gains equivalent to or better than an alternative treatment approach that relied upon cuing hierarchies, with superior long-term retention. No studies to date have examined the benefits of massed versus spaced practice schedules on aphasia treatment and long-term retention. Further, seminal work on the development of automaticity by Shiffrin and Schneider (1977; Schneider & Shiffrin, 1977) ought to be applied to aphasia rehabilitation to maximize the

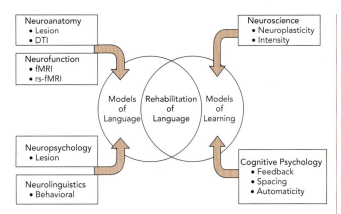

Figure 16.1 Influences on language rehabilitation. DTI = Diffusion tensor imaging; fMRI = functional magnetic resonance imaging; rs-fMRI = resting state functional magnetic resonance imaging.

fluidity of language production and comprehension skills developed in therapy. Finally, principles developed in the motor learning literature on the role of feedback, namely that less is more (e.g., Winstein & Schmidt, 1990), should also be examined as it applies to aphasia treatment. Cognitive learning principles can be utilized to develop the best techniques for treatment delivery.

In a similar vein, principles learned from cognitive neurolinguistics should not be forgotten when coupling neuroscience with treatment of aphasia. A notable development in the treatment literature is the Complexity Account of Treatment Efficacy (Kiran & Thompson, 2003; Thompson, Shapiro, Kiran, & Sobecks, 2003). Both in training syntactic forms and in training retrieval of lexical items, training is more effective if more complex structures or items are trained first; transfer then occurs without training simpler structures. Kiran and Thompson (2003) demonstrated this principle in a treatment study of naming. Participants were either trained on typical exemplars from the bird category, such as robin, or on more atypical exemplars, such as penguin. Those who received training on retrieval of atypical exemplars were also able to retrieve typical exemplars without additional training; the converse was not true. These types of studies help therapists design treatment materials to optimize rehabilitation services.

A complete neuroscientifically based model of aphasia rehabilitation, then, should encompass the structure of the language system, its anatomical and functional connectivity, principles of neuroplasticity that enable the brain to reorganize after aphasia-producing injury, effective therapeutic frameworks, cognitive principles of learning and retention, and principles of neurolinguistics in order to optimize language recovery in persons with aphasia (see Figure 16.1). Using neuroscientific principles, coupled with the psychosocial components that contribute to living with aphasia, we will be able to better understand how to foster participation in the activities and roles that people with aphasia need and want to do when they leave rehabilitation to resume community living.

REFERENCES

Baker, J., Rorden, C., & Fridriksson, J. (2010). Using transcranial direct current stimulation (tDCS) to treat stroke patients with aphasia. *Stroke, 41,* 1229–1236.

Ballard, K. J., & Thompson, C. K. (1999). Treatment and generalization of complex sentence production in agrammatism. *Journal of Speech, Language, and Hearing Research, 42,* 690–707.

Bates, E., Wilson, S. M., Saygin, A. P., Dick, F., Sereno, M. I., Knight, R. T., & Dronkers, N. F. (2003). Voxel-based lesion-symptom mapping, *Nature Neuroscience, 6,* 448–450.

Belin, P., Van Eeckhout, P., Zilbovicius, M., Remy, P., Francois, C., Guillaume, S., et al. (1996). Recovery from nonfluent aphasia after melodic intonation therapy: A PET study. *Neurology, 47,* 1504–1511.

Beeson, P. M., Rewega, M., Vail, S., & Rapcsak, S. Z. (2000). Problem-solving approach to agraphia treatment: Interactive use of lexical and sublexical spelling routes. *Aphasiology, 14,* 551–565.

Berthier, M. L., Pulvermüller, F., Davila, G., Casares N. G., & Guitierrez, A. (2011). Drug therapy of post-stroke aphasia: A review of current evidence. Neuropsychology Review, 21, 302–317.

Bhogal, S. K., Teasell, R., & Speechley, M. (2003). Intensity of aphasia therapy, impact on recovery. *Stroke, 34*(4), 987–993.

Binder, J. R., Desai, R. H., Graves, W. W., & Conant, L. L. (2009). Where is the semantic system? A critical review and meta-analysis of 120 functional neuroimaging studies. *Cerebral Cortex, 19,* 2767–2796.

Biswal, B. B., Mennes, M., Zuo, X. N., Gohel, S., Kelly, C., & Smith, S. M., et al. (2010). Toward discovery science of human brain function. *Proceedings of the National Academy of Sciences USA, 107,* 4734–4739.

Biswal, B., Yetkin, F. Z., Haughton, V. M., & Hyde, J. S. (1995). Functional connectivity in the motor cortex of resting human brain using echo-planar MRI. *Magnetic Resonance in Medicine, 34,* 537–541.

Broca, P. (1861). Remarques sur le siege de la faculte du langage articule; suivies d'une observation d'aphemie (perte del la parole). Bulletins de la Societe Anatomique (Paris), 6, 330–357, 398–407. In G. von Bonin, Some papers on the cerebral cortex. Translated as, "Remarks on the seat of the faculty of articulate language, followed by an observation of aphemia." Springfield, IL: Charles C. Thomas, 1960, pp. 49–72.

Carter, A. R., Astafiev, S. V., Lang, C. E., Connor, L. T., Rengachary, J., Strube, M. J., et al. (2010). Resting interhemispheric functional magnetic resonance imaging connectivity predicts performance after stroke. *Annals of Neurology, 67,* 365–375.

Catani, M., Jones, D., & Ffytche, D. (2005). Perisylvian language networks of the human brain. *Annals of Neurology, 57,* 8–16.

Chapey, R. (Ed.). (2008). *Language intervention strategies in aphasia and related Neurogenic communication disorders,* 5th Edition. Philadelphia: Wolters Kluwer Health.

Cherney, L. R., Patterson, J. P., Raymer, A., Frymark, T., & Schooling, T. (2008). Evidence-based systematic review: Effects of intensity of treatment and constraint-induced language therapy for individuals with stroke-induced aphasia. *Journal of Speech, Language, and Hearing Research, 51*(5), 1282–1299.

Coelho, C. A., Sinotte, M. P., & Duffy, J. R. (2008). Schuell's stimulation approach to rehabilitation. In R. Chapey (Ed.) *Language intervention strategies in aphasia and related Neurogenic communication disorders,* 5th Edition (pp. 403–449). Philadelphia: Wolters Kluwer Health.

Corbetta, M., Kincade, M. J., Lewis, C., Snyder, A. Z., & Sapir, A. (2005). Neural basis and recovery of spatial attention deficits in spatial neglect. *Nature Neuroscience, 8,* 1603–1610.

Cornelissen, K., Laine, M., Tarkiainen, A., Järvensivu, T., Martin, N., & Salmelin, R. (2003). Adult brain plasticity elicited by anomia treatment. *Journal of Cognitive Neuroscience, 15,* 444–461.

DeLeon, J., Gottesman, R. F., Kleinman, J. T., Neunart, M., Davis, C., Lee, A., et al. (2007). Neural regions essential for distinct cognitive processes underlying picture naming. *Brain, 130*, 1408–1422.

Eickhoff, S. B., Heim, S., Zilles, K., & Amunts, K. (2009). A systems perspective on the effective connectivity of overt speech production. *Philosophical Transactions, Series A. Mathematical, Physical and Engineering Sciences, 367*, 2399–2421.

Fair, D. A., Cohen, A. L., Power, J. D., Dosenbach, N.U., Church, J. A., Miezen, F. M., et al. (2009). Functional brain networks develop from a "local to distributed" organization. *Public Library of Science Computational Biology,5*, e1000381.

Finger, S. (1994). *Origins of neuroscience: A history of explorations into brain function.* New York: Oxford University Press.

Fox, M. D., Snyder, A. Z., Vincent, J. L., Corbetta, M., Van Essen, D. C., & Raichle, M. E. (2005). The human brain is intrinsically organized into dynamic, anticorrelated functional networks. *Proceedings of the National Academy of Sciences USA, 102*, 9673–9678.

Fridriksson, J., Holland, A. L., Beeson, P., & Morrow, L. (2005). Spaced retrieval treatment of anomia. *Aphasiology, 19*, 99–109.

Friederici, A. D., Brauer, J., & Lohmann, G. (2011). Maturation of the language network: From inter- to intrahemispheric connectivities. *Public Library of Science One, 6*, e20726.

Friedman, R. B., Sample, D. M., & Lott, S. N. (2000). The role of level of representation in the use of paired associate learning for rehabilitation of alexia. *Neuropsychologia, 40*, 223–234.

Friston, K. J. (2011). Functional and effective connectivity: A review. *Brain Connectivity, 1*, 13–36.

Glenberg, A.M. (1979). Component-level theory of the effects of spacing on repetitions on recall and recognition. *Memory & Cognition, 7*, 95–112.

Hampson, M., Peterson, B. S., Skudlarski, P., Gatenby, J. C. & Gore, J. C. (2002). Detection of functional connectivity using temporal correlations in MR images. *Human Brain Mapping, 15*, 247–262.

Hampson, M., Tokoglu, F., Sun, Z., Schafer, R. J., Skudlarski, P., Gore, J. C., et al. (2006). Connectivity-behavior analysis reveals that functional connectivity between left BA39 and Broca's area varies with reading ability. *NeuroImage, 31*, 513–519.

He, B. J., Snyder, A. Z., Vincent, J. L., Epstein, A., Shulman, G. L., & Corbetta, M. (2007) Breakdown of intrinsic brain synchrony in spatial neglect: A novel mechanism to explain brain-behavior relationships after stroke. *Neuron, 53*, 905–918.

Hillis, A. E. (1993). The role of models of language processing in rehabilitation of language impairments. *Aphasiology, 7*, 5–26.

Hillis, A. E., Barker, P. B., Wityk, R. J., Aldrich, E. M., Restrepo, L., Breese, E. L., et al. (2004). Variability in subcortical aphasia is due to variable sites of cortical hypoperfusion. *Brain and Language, 89*, 524–530.

Hillis, A. E., Kane, A., Tuffiash, E., Ulatowski, J. A., Barker, P. B., Beauchamp, N. J., et al. (2001). Reperfusion of specific brain regions by raising blood pressure restores selective language functions in subacute stroke. *Brain and Language, 79*, 495–510.

Hillis, A. E., Kleinman, J. T., Newhart, M., Heidler-Gary, J., Gottesman, R., Barker, P. B., et al. (2006). Restoring cerebral blood flow reveals neural regions critical for naming. *The Journal of Neuroscience, 26*(31), 8069–8073.

Hillis, A. E., & Newhart, M. (2008). Cognitive neuropsychological approaches to treatment of language disorders: Introduction. In R. Chapey (Ed.), *Language intervention strategies in aphasia and related Neurogenic communication disorders,* 5th Edition (pp. 595–604). Philadelphia: Wolters Kluwer Health.

Hinckley, J. J., & Craig, H. K. (1998). Influence of rate of treatment on the naming abilities of adults with chronic aphasia. *Aphasiology, 12*, 989–1006.

Jbabdi, S., & Johansen-Berg, H. (2011). Tractography: Where do we go from here? *Brain Connectivity, 1*(3), 169–183.

Johansen-Berg, H., & Rushworth, M. F. (2009). Using diffusion imaging to study human connectional anatomy. *Annual Review of Neuroscience, 32*, 75–94.

Kiran, S., & Thompson, C. K. (2003). The role of semantic complexity in treatment of naming deficits: Training semantic categories in

fluent aphasia by controlling exemplar typicality. *Journal of Speech Language and Hearing Research, 46*, 608–622.

Kleim, J. A., Barbay, S., & Nudo, R. J. (1998). Functional reorganization of the rat motor cortex following motor skill learning. *Journal of Neurophysiology, 80*, 3321–3325.

Koyama, M. S., Di Martino, A., Zuo, X.-N., Kelly, C., Mennes, M., Jutagir, D. R., et al. (2011). Resting-state functional connectivity indexes reading competence in children and adults. *Journal of Neuroscience, 31*, 8617–8624.

Lang, C. E., Macdonald, J. R., Reisman, D. S., Boyd, L., Jacobson, K. T., Schindler-Ivens, S. M., et al. (2009). Observation of amounts of movement practice provided during stroke rehabilitation. *Archives of Physical Medicine and Rehabilitation, 90*(10), 1692–1698.

Lewis, C. M., Baldassarre, A., Committeri, G., Romani, G. L., & Corbetta, M. (2009). Learning sculpts the spontaneous activity of the resting human brain. *Proceedings of the National Academy of Sciences USA, 106*, 17558–17568.

Loverso, F. L., Prescott, T. E., & Selinger, M. (1986). Cueing verbs: A treatment strategy for aphasic adults. *Journal of Rehabilitation Research, 25*, 47–60.

Maher, L. M., Kendall, D., Swearengin, J. A., Rodriguez, A., Leon, S. A., Pingel, K., et al. (2006). A pilot study of use-dependent learning in the context of constraint induced language therapy. *Journal of the International Neuropsychological Society, 12*(6), 843–852.

Meinzer, M., Djundja, D., Barthel, G., Elbert, T., & Rockstroh, B. (2005). Long-term stability of improved language functions in chronic aphasia after constraint-induced aphasia therapy. *Stroke, 36*, 1462–1466.

Meinzer, M., Elbert, T., Djundja, D., Taub, E., & Rockstroh, B. (2007). Extending the constraint-induced movement therapy (CIMT) approach to cognitive functions: Constraint-induced aphasia therapy (CIAT) of chronic aphasia. *NeuroRehabilitation, 22*, 311–318.

Musso, M., Weiller, C., Kiebel, S., Müller, S. P., Bülau, P., & Rijntjes, M. (1999). Training-induced brain plasticity in aphasia. *Brain, 122*, 1781–1790.

Naeser, M. A., Martin, P. I., Nicholas, M., Baker, E. H., Seekins, H., Kobayashi, M., et al. (2005). Improved picture naming in chronic aphasia after TMS to part of right Broca's area: An open-protocol study. *Brain and Language, 93*, 95–105.

Naeser, M. A., Martin, P. I., Theoret, H., Kobayashi, M., Fregni, F., Nicholas, M., et al. (2011). TMS suppression of right pars triangularis, but not pars opercularis, improves naming in aphasia. *Brain and Language, 119*, 206–213.

Nudo, R. J., Wise, B. M., SiFuentes, F., & Milliken, G. W. (1996). Neural substrates for the effects of rehabilitative training on motor recovery after ischemic infarct. *Science, 272*, 1791–1794.

Perani, D., Saccuman, M. C., Scifo, P., Anwander, A., Spada, D., Baldoli, C., et al. (2011). Neural language networks at birth. *Proceedings of the National Academy of Sciences USA, 108*, 16056–16061.

Price, C. J. (2000). The anatomy of language: Contributions from functional neuroimaging. *Journal of Anatomy, 197*, 335–359.

Price, C. J. (2010). The anatomy of language: A Review of 100 fMRI studies published in 2009. *Annals of the New York Academy of Sciences, 1191*(1), 62–88.

Pulvermüller, F., Neininger, B., Elbert, T., Mohr, B., Rockstroh, B., Koebbel, P., et al. (2001). Constraint-induced therapy of chronic aphasia after stroke. *Stroke, 32*(7), 1621–1626.

Rapp, B. (2005). The relationship between treatment outcomes and the underlying cognitive deficit: Evidence from the remediation of acquired dysgraphia. *Aphasiology, 19*, 994–1008.

Raymer, A. M., & Gonzalez Rothi, L. J. (2008). Impairments of word comprehension and production. In R. Chapey (Ed.), *Language intervention strategies in aphasia and related Neurogenic communication disorders*, 5th Edition (pp. 607–631). Philadelphia: Wolters Kluwer Health.

Raymer, A. M., Thompson, C. K., Jacobs, B., & LeGrand, H. R. (1993). Phonological treatment of naming deficits in aphasia: Model-based generalization analysis. *Aphasiology, 7*, 27–53.

Rochon, E., Laird, L., Bose, A., & Scofield, J. (2005). Mapping Therapy for sentence production impairments in non-fluent aphasia. *Neuropsychological Rehabilitation, 15*, 1–36.

Rosen, H. J., Petersen, S. E., Linenweber, M. R., Snyder, A. Z., White, D. A., Chapman, L., et al. (2000). Neural correlates of recovery from aphasia after damage to left inferior frontal cortex. *Neurology, 55*, 1883–1894.

Saur, D., Lange, R., Baumgaertner, A., Schraknepper, V., Willmes, K., Rijntjes, M., et al. (2006). Dynamics of language reorganization after stroke. *Brain, 129(Pt 6)*, 1371–1384.

Saur, D., Schelter, B., Schnell, S., Kratochvil, D., Küpper, H., Kellmeyer, P., et al., (2010). Combining functional and anatomical connectivity reveals brain networks for auditory language comprehension. *NeuroImage, 49*, 3187–3197.

Schuell, H., Jenkins, J. J., & Jiménez-Pabón, E. (1964). *Aphasia in adults.* New York: Harper & Row.

Schwartz, M. F., Saffran, E. M., Fink, R. B., Myers, J. L., & Martin, N. (1994). Mapping Therapy: A treatment programme for agrammatism. *Aphasiology, 8*, 19–54.

Shiffrin, R. M., & Schneider, W. (1977). Controlled and automatic human information processing: II. Perceptual learning, automatic attending, and a general theory. *Psychological Review, 84*, 127–190.

Schneider, W., & Shiffrin, R. M. (1977). Controlled and automatic human information processing: I. Detection, search, and attention. *Psychological Review, 84*, 1–66.

Taub, E., Crago, J. E., Burgio, L. D., Groomes, T. E., Cook E. W. III, DeLuca, S. C., et al. (1994). An operant approach to rehabilitation medicine: Overcoming learned nonuse by shaping. *Journal of Experimental Analysis of Behavior, 61*, 281–293.

Thompson, C. K. (2008). Treatment of syntactic and morphologic deficits in agrammatic aphasia: Treatment of underlying forms. In R. Chapey (Ed.), *Language intervention strategies in aphasia and related Neurogenic communication disorders*, 5th Edition (pp. 735–753). Philadelphia: Wolters Kluwer Health.

Thompson, C. K., Ballard, K. J., & Shapiro, L. P. (1998). The role of syntactic complexity in training wh-movement structures in agrammatic aphasia: Optimal order for promoting generalization. *Journal of the International Neuropsychological Society, 4*, 661–674.

Thompson, C. K., & Shapiro, L. P. (2005). Treating agrammatic aphasia within a linguistic framework: Treatment of Underlying Forms. *Aphasiology, 19*, 1021–1036.

Thompson, C. K., Shapiro, L. P., Kiran, S., & Sobecks, J. (2003). The role of syntactic complexity in treatment of sentence deficits in agrammatic aphasia: The complexity account of treatment efficacy (CATE*). Journal of Speech, Language, and Hearing Research, 46*, 591–607.

Vanier, M., & Caplan, D. (1990). CT-scan correlates of agrammatism. In L. Menn & L. Obler (Eds.), *Agrammatic aphasia: A cross-language narrative sourcebook* (pp. 37–114). Philadelphia: John Benjamins.

Vigneau, M., Beaucousin, V., Hervé, P. Y., Duffau, H., Crivello, F., Houdé, O., et al. (2006). Meta-analyzing left hemisphere language areas: Phonology, semantics, and sentence processing. *NeuroImage, 30*, 1414–1432.

Warren, J. E., Crinion, J. T., Lambon Ralph, M. A., & Wise, R. J. (2009). Anterior temporal lobe connectivity correlates with functional outcome after aphasic stroke. *Brain, 132*, 3428–3442.

Wepman, J. M. (1951). *Recovery from aphasia.* New York: Ronald Press.

Winhuisen, L., Thiel, A., Schumacher, B., Kessler, J., Rudolf, J., Haupt, W. F., et al. (2005). Role of the contralateral inferior frontal gyrus in recovery of language function in poststroke aphasia: A combined repetitive transcranial magnetic stimulation and Positron Emission Tomography study. *Stroke, 36*, 1759–1763.

Winstein, C. J., & Schmidt, R. A. (1990). Reduced frequency of knowledge of results enhances motor skill learning. *Journal of Experimental Psychology: Learning, Memory, and Cognition, 16*, 677–691.

Wise, R. J. S., Scott, S. K., Blank, S. C., Mummery, C. J., Murphy, K., & Warburton, E. A. (2001). Separate neural subsystems within "Wernicke's area." *Brain, 124*, 83–95.

Wolf, S. L., Winstein, C. J., Miller, J. P., Taub, E., Uswatte, G., Morris, D., et al. (2006). Effect of constraint-induced movement therapy on upper extremity function 3 to 9 months after stroke: The EXCITE randomized clinical trial. *Journal of the American Medical Association, 296*(17), 2095–2104.

Xiang, H.-D., Fonteijn, H. M., Norris, D. G., & Hagoort, P. (2010). Topographical functional connectivity pattern in the peri-Sylvian language networks. *Cerebral Cortex, 20*, 549–560.

PART E | NEW PERSPECTIVES AND DIRECTIONS FOR STROKE REHABILITATION RESEARCH

17 | TARGETING VIABLE BRAIN NETWORKS TO IMPROVE OUTCOMES AFTER STROKE

CATHY STINEAR and WINSTON BYBLOW

17.1 INTRODUCTION

Neuroscience is helping us to understand how the brain recovers after stroke, and how we might shape this process through rehabilitation therapy. New therapeutic approaches and adjunct techniques are being developed, based on the principles of neural plasticity. These techniques need to be targeted to selected patients, rather than applied in a one-size-fits-all way. As the number of rehabilitation "tools in the toolbox" increases, the selection of an appropriate combination of techniques for each patient will become increasingly challenging for therapists and clinicians. Neuroscience can inform this process in a number of ways. For example, neurophysiological and neuroimaging tools can be used to predict whether there is enough residual capacity in the ipsilesional neural network to support recovery, and to what extent the contralesional network is likely to support compensation. Knowing this will help clinicians to select therapies and adjunct techniques that will promote reorganization in residual networks.

This chapter describes emerging approaches to predicting and promoting neural plasticity and recovery after stroke. Most of the research in this area has focused on the motor system, though the principles are likely to hold for other functional domains. Recent developments indicate that rehabilitation planning and delivery is likely to become more tailored and optimized for individual patients based on measures of the remaining connectivity in the neural networks affected by stroke.

17.2 MEASURING CONNECTIVITY TO PREDICT MOTOR OUTCOMES

Predicting recovery after stroke for individual patients is difficult. Generally, prognosis is less favorable when more functional domains are initially impaired. For example, Patel et al. (2000) documented motor, sensory, and visual impairments in 360 patients 14 days after stroke. They found that the extent of dependence in activities of daily living 3, 6, and 12 months later was predicted by the number of domains initially impaired. Motor impairment was the strongest predictor of subsequent dependence, while additional sensory and/or visual impairment predicted greater dependence at all three follow-up time points. However, the recovery of independence varied greatly between patients, even those with the same initial impairments. Assessing how many functions are initially impaired doesn't allow accurate predictions of recovery to be made for individual patients.

Within the motor domain, greater initial impairment is related to less subsequent recovery of function (Kwakkel & Kollen, 2007; S.Y. Chen & Winstein, 2009). For example, greater impairment in shoulder flexion and finger extension predicts less recovery of upper limb function (Smania et al., 2007; Beebe & Lang, 2009). Similarly, greater impairment in leg motor power predicts less recovery of gait (Wandel, Jorgensen, Nakayama, Raaschou, & Olsen, 2000). While the relationship between initial motor impairment and subsequent motor function is fairly clear when data are pooled from a group of patients, it's highly variable from patient to patient. Two patients may be similarly impaired and experience quite different recovery trajectories. This means that making an accurate prediction of recovery on the basis of clinical scores for an individual patient is very difficult.

Information is needed about how the stroke has affected the patient's brain structures and pathways, in order to predict how they might recover and/or benefit from specific therapies. Some work has been done on this approach in the motor system, where TMS and MRI have been used to determine the extent of damage to key motor pathways. Most of the research to date has focused on the recovery of upper limb function, described below.

17.2.1 FUNCTIONAL INTEGRITY OF MOTOR PATHWAYS

17.2.1.1 CROSSED CORTICOSPINAL TRACT

The extent to which an individual patient will achieve good recovery of upper limb motor function depends on the integrity of the descending motor pathways, and in particular the lateral corticospinal tract (CST; Stinear et al., 2007). The lateral CST is predominantly a crossed pathway, which is why damage leads to a contralateral paresis and, in some cases, paralysis. Most patients are unable to carry out fine motor activities with the affected hand after complete injury of the lateral CST (Davidoff, 1990). But how much damage is too much? How much remaining connectivity in the CST is required to support an ipsilesional pattern of reorganization that would lead to good recovery of motor function? And how can this be measured? Here, we describe emerging approaches to measuring descending motor pathway integrity for the purposes of predicting an individual patient's recovery profile and tailoring rehabilitation prescription accordingly.

The functional integrity of the CST can be assessed by using single-pulse transcranial magnetic stimulation (TMS) of the ipsilesional primary motor cortex to elicit motor evoked potentials (MEPs) in paretic limb muscles (Heald, Bates, Cartlidge, French, & Miller, 1993; Catano, Houa, Caroyer, Ducarne, & Noel, 1996; Trompetto, Assini, Buccolieri, Marchese, & Abbruzzese, 2000; see also Chapter 5). Damage is usually indicated by prolonged latency of the MEP on the paretic side relative to the healthy side, or diminished size of the MEP for an equivalent strength of stimulation compared to the healthy side (Talelli, Greenwood, & Rothwell, 2006). The presence of MEPs is indicative of residual functional integrity of the CST and is usually associated with better motor outcomes (Stinear et al., 2007; Stinear, 2010). TMS may be a particularly useful prognostic tool in patients who initially demonstrate severe upper limb impairment (Hendricks, Pasman, van Limbeek, & Zwarts, 2003; Pizzi et al., 2009). Those with initially severe impairment who still demonstrate MEPs in response to TMS of the affected M1 have residual capacity for recovery that might otherwise go unrecognized (Stinear, 2010).

Information about the functional integrity of the CST can also inform the clinician about the expected pattern of reorganization in the cortical motor network (Swayne, Rothwell, Ward, & Greenwood, 2008). Patients with residual connectivity in the ipsilesional CST are more likely to recover function through plastic reorganization in the ipsilesional motor network (Ward et al., 2006). Primary motor, pre-motor and supplementary motor areas all project to the spinal cord. Spared pathways may regain some control over paretic muscles through neural plasticity in response to rehabilitation therapies. Patients without residual connectivity in the ipsilesional CST are likely to have sustained damage to corticomotor pathways from a range of motor areas. Under these circumstances, reorganization in the ipsilesional motor network is likely to be of limited benefit if the connectivity between the cortical network and spinal cord has been lost.

Beyond the simple presence or absence of MEPs, it is not yet clear whether the pattern of recovery also relates to the input–output properties of the affected CST (how the size of MEPs vary with stimulation strength). This will continue to be the subject of future research, with contemporary studies exploring whether the slope of the input–output curve is a marker CST functional integrity after stroke (Ward et al., 2006; Ward et al., 2007).

17.2.1.2 UNCROSSED CORTICOSPINAL TRACT

The primary motor cortex has direct uncrossed connections to alpha motoneurons innervating ipsilateral muscles, particularly the proximal muscles (MacKinnon, Quartarone, & Rothwell, 2004). Uncrossed connections to the alpha motoneurons innervating distal hand muscles are sparse, and their functional importance in adults is not well understood. It has been suggested that sprouting of new synapses between the uncrossed CST and ipsilateral alpha motoneurons could allow some control of the paretic upper limb after injury to the crossed CST (Dum & Strick, 1996; Jankowska & Edgley, 2006). For patients without viable ipsilesional descending motor pathways, increased activation and plastic reorganization in contralesional motor areas could therefore support some improvements in paretic limb function, though full recovery is highly unlikely. However, there is good reason to suspect that increasing input from the contralesional uncrossed CST to the spinal cord may be maladaptive when ipsilesional pathways remain intact. This is because the descending commands from the contralesional motor cortex may interfere at the level of the spinal cord with descending commands from the ipsilesional motor cortex, particularly for proximal upper limb musculature. Indirect evidence for this is supplied by studies showing that chronic stroke patients in whom TMS of the contralesional M1 produces a MEP in the affected pectoralis major muscle have greater upper limb impairment (Schwerin et al., 2008). This indicates that greater functional connectivity between contralesional M1 and muscles of the affected upper limb can be a disadvantage.

One interesting possibility is that repetitive magnetic or direct current brain stimulation protocols that suppress contralesional motor cortical areas might reduce interference of commands originating in the contralesional hemisphere, either within the motor cortex or at the level of the spinal cord. This novel idea has been demonstrated recently in healthy adults (Bradnam, Stinear, & Byblow, 2011; McCambridge, Bradnam, Stinear, & Byblow, 2011). After stroke, suppressing the activity of contralesional M1 may be beneficial or deleterious, depending on the extent of damage to ipsilesional corticomotor pathways. This is discussed in a subsequent section, and highlights the potential value of individualized therapy.

17.2.1.3 INTERHEMISPHERIC PATHWAYS

As noted in previous chapters (e.g., Chapters 5 and 10), impaired output from the stroke hemisphere can result in an increase in contralesional hemisphere activation and M1 excitability. After stroke, an increase in excitability of the contralesional M1 and reduced excitability of the ipsilesional M1 are commonly observed together and likely share a common mechanism, namely reduced inhibition from the ipsilesional motor cortex to the contralesional motor cortex via transcallosal pathways (Traversa, Cicinelli, Pasqualetti, Filippi, & Rossini, 1998; Murase, Duque, Mazzocchio, & Cohen, 2004; Duque et al., 2005; Nowak, Grefkes, Ameli, & Fink, 2009; see Chapter 5). TMS can be used to assess the interaction between the ipsilesional and contralesional hemisphere by measuring interhemispheric inhibition (IHI) with single-pulse or dual-pulse (dual coil) techniques (R. Chen et al., 2008). Using TMS to determine the presence or absence of abnormalities in IHI early after stroke may provide useful prognostic information in future neurophysiological or clinical rehabilitation studies.

Reduced IHI may lead to disinhibition and extensive contralesional reorganization. This might only be desirable in certain cases. In patients with a severely impaired upper limb, the excitability of contralesional M1 gradually increases with motor recovery, indicating that reorganization within the contralesional hemisphere may be an adaptive response in these patients (Gerloff et al., 2006; see Figure 17.1). However, in less impaired patients facilitated contralesional excitability may lead to maladaptive plasticity, such as increased prevalence and size of ipsilateral MEPs and greater upper limb impairment as described above. To date, there have been very few attempts to measure interhemispheric inhibition directly over the course of recovery from stroke, although many studies of patients at the chronic stage attribute changes in excitability across both hemispheres to altered IHI (Mansur et al., 2005; Nowak et al., 2008, 2009). Future studies will need to more closely examine how the functional connectivity between the hemispheres evolves with recovery after stroke.

17.2.2 STRUCTURAL IMAGING OF MOTOR PATHWAYS

Whereas TMS can be used to assess the functional integrity of the motor pathways, the structural integrity of the CST can be assessed with diffusion-weighted MRI (DW-MRI). As described in Chapter 4, this imaging technique detects the diffusion of water molecules throughout the brain, indicating where bundles of myelinated axons are present. CST integrity can be quantified by measuring fractional anisotropy (FA) within a particular brain region or pathway of interest, as FA is sensitive to white matter disruption. A low FA value in a particular brain region compared to the equivalent region in the healthy hemisphere is indicative of damage along the pathway and compromised integrity. To determine integrity of the CST and secondary descending motor pathways, the average FA is typically calculated within the posterior limb of the internal capsules (Zarei et al., 2007). The absolute value of FA is a fraction (a number between 0 and 1) and is variable between individuals and MRI scanners. Therefore, an asymmetry index of FA is used to compare the motor pathways in the ipsilesional hemisphere to those in the contralesional hemisphere. The asymmetry index ranges between -1 and +1, with zero indicating perfect symmetry, and appears to be a sensitive normalization technique for prognosis (Stinear et al., 2007).

To understand how FA adds prognostic value beyond knowledge of functional integrity of the CST, consider a patient with limited upper limb function, moderate to severe impairment, and no evoked responses to TMS before rehabilitation. The absence of MEPs may not be able to predict whether or not secondary ipsilesional motor pathways have sufficient connectivity to support ipsilesional reorganization and some reduction of impairment. A measure of structural integrity, such as FA asymmetry, may provide important information in this regard. Combining neurophysiological and imaging techniques for prognosis is described in the following section.

17.2.3 COMBINED APPROACHES

TMS and DW-MRI techniques are complementary, in that measures made with both relate to upper limb impairment (Stinear et al., 2007; Ward et al., 2007; Jang, 2009; Schaechter et al., 2009). Recently these techniques were combined to determine their prognostic value for predicting response to upper limb therapy at the chronic stage after stroke (Stinear et al., 2007). Functional integrity of the CST was indicated by the presence of MEPs in the affected wrist extensor muscles. Structural integrity of the CST was indicated by FA asymmetry, measured in the posterior limbs of the internal capsules. Both of these measures were strongly related to upper limb impairment at baseline, before patients completed a 30-day program of motor practice with their affected upper limb. The reduction in upper limb impairment after the motor practice program was predicted by the presence of MEPs in the affected upper limb. Upper limb impairment also decreased in patients without MEPs, provided FA asymmetry did not exceed a "point of no return." Stinear and colleagues estimated that chronic patients with an FA asymmetry >0.25 have very limited or no potential for further upper limb recovery. Interestingly, factors like baseline clinical scores, side of stroke, and size of lesion did not predict the potential for recovery.

Information about the residual connectivity in key motor pathways can, therefore, predict an individual's potential for recovery of motor function. This information could inform rehabilitation goal-setting and planning at the subacute stage. Algorithms for predicting the potential for motor recovery are in development and are described in the following section.

17.2.4 ALGORITHM FOR PREDICTING UPPER LIMB MOTOR OUTCOMES

Clinical, neurophysiological, and neuroimaging measures of CST integrity can be made in a step-wise manner to predict recovery of upper limb function at the subacute stage (Stinear, 2010). Algorithms for setting rehabilitation goals on the basis of an individual's residual motor network connectivity are in the early stages of development and require validation. The example algorithm in Figure 17.1 is designed to predict whether the patient has the capacity for recovery of upper limb function, or rehabilitation should be aimed at compensation or substitution strategies. These terms are defined below, based on work by Levin and colleagues (Levin, Kleim, & Wolf, 2009), and see also Chapter 2.

Recovery: Motor tasks are performed with the same effectors and movement patterns as before the stroke. For example, the patient recovers the ability to feed himself or herself by bringing a fork to the mouth using the paretic upper limb with a normal pattern of shoulder, elbow, wrist, and hand movements.

Compensation: Motor tasks are performed with the same effectors as before the stroke, but with new patterns of movement. For example, the patient may compensate for upper limb impairment during feeding by flexing the trunk and elevating the shoulder.

Substitution: Motor tasks are performed with new effectors or devices. For example, the patient may learn to use his/her nonparetic upper limb for feeding, or a motorized wheelchair for mobility.

Clearly, the best possible motor outcome after stroke is recovery of all affected motor functions. However, recovery is limited by the extent of damage to essential elements of the motor system, particularly the primary motor cortex and corticospinal tracts (Davidoff, 1990; Stinear et al., 2007). When damage to these essential elements exceeds a certain level, recovery is no longer possible and voluntary movement will remain impaired to some extent. Under these circumstances, compensation and substitution are more realistic rehabilitation goals.

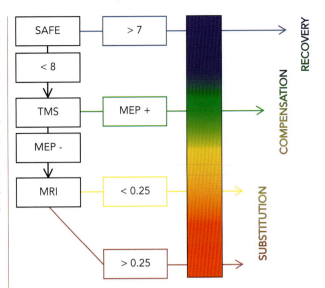

Figure 17.1 Proposed algorithm for predicting recovery of upper limb function at the acute stage of stroke. SAFE=Shoulder Abduction Finger Extension (SAFE) score, which is the sum of the Medical Research Council strength grades (0–5) for each movement. If the SAFE score 72 h after stroke is >7, the patient is expected to make a complete recovery of upper limb function by 12 weeks after stroke. If the SAFE score 72 h after stroke is <8, TMS is then used to evaluate the functional integrity of the corticomotor pathway to the wrist extensors of the affected upper limb. If MEPs are present in the affected wrist extensors (MEP +), upper limb function is expected to improve via a combination of recovery and compensation. If MEPs are absent (MEP -), MRI is used to acquire diffusion-weighted images and evaluate the structural integrity of the posterior limbs of the internal capsules. An asymmetry index is calculated and, when <0.25, limited improvement in upper limb function via compensation is expected and substitution will be needed for many activities. When the asymmetry index is >0.25, no meaningful improvement in upper limb function can be expected and the patient will need to use substitution strategies. Patients with a SAFE score >7, and/or MEPs in the affected wrist extensor muscles, may benefit from priming techniques designed to facilitate ipsilesional cortical excitability or suppress contralesional cortical excitability. These approaches may promote recovery and compensation by enhancing neural plasticity within the ipsilesional motor network. In contrast, patients without MEPs may benefit from priming techniques designed to facilitate contralesional cortical excitability, in order to promote proximal compensation and substitution via neural plasticity within the contralesional motor network. (Adapted from Stinear, 2010).

17.2.5 THE LOWER LIMB

Most studies have focused on the upper limb as a model for motor recovery, and stressed the critical importance of the ipsilesional CST in determining prognosis and extent of brain reorganization within and across hemispheres. To date, there is no algorithm for predicting recovery of lower limb function, but current evidence suggests both TMS and FA will have some prognostic value. However, there is currently no strong consensus regarding the importance of the lateral CST in recovery of walking after stroke.

A neuroimaging study found that some patients with complete lesions of the lateral CST regained walking ability within six months of stroke (Ahn, Ahn, Kim, Hong, & Jang, 2006) but it's not clear whether the CST or other secondary motor pathways were responsible for the recovery of gait. A neurophysiological study found that patients with no recordable MEPs in tibialis anterior 1 month post-stroke never regained walking ability, whereas patients with MEPs regained independent gait at discharge (Piron, Piccione, Tonin, & Dam, 2005). These findings illustrate the importance of CST functional integrity for recovery of lower limb function. Further work is needed to determine the minimal level of functional connectivity required in the motor system to support recovery of walking after stroke.

17.2.6 CONCLUSIONS

Neuroscience is improving our understanding of the key nodes and pathways within various neural networks that support recovery after stroke. For motor function, the crossed corticospinal tract is an essential pathway, connecting the cortical motor network to the spinal cord. Recovery of motor function depends in large part on the extent of damage to this pathway and the pattern of reorganization in the cortical motor network. In general, ipsilesional reorganization that utilizes a functionally intact crossed CST will lead to the best motor outcomes. When this is precluded by damage to the ipsilesional CST, bilateral reorganization may allow the contralesional motor network and uncrossed contralesional CST to provide some compensation. The general observation that recovery of ipsilesional neural activity is linked to better outcomes also holds true for other functions, such as somatosensation, language, and visuospatial attention. In the future, therapy teams may be able to tailor rehabilitation plans and goals for individual patients on the basis of a detailed understanding of the residual functional and structural connectivity within the neural networks affected by stroke. This understanding may also allow therapists to select appropriate adjunct techniques for promoting plasticity and reorganization within key components of neural networks, as described in the following section.

17.3 PRIMING APPROACHES

A question being addressed in current neurorehabilitation research is whether or not the brain can be made more responsive to physical therapy. A commonly studied approach is noninvasive brain stimulation, which is a potential adjunct to therapy described in Chapter 10. The main modalities are repetitive TMS (rTMS) and transcranial direct current stimulation (tDCS). These are commonly used because they can either increase or decrease neuronal excitability in a target area, depending on the protocol. The use of these techniques in stroke rehabilitation research has been summarized in many recent reviews (Hummel & Cohen, 2006; Hummel et al., 2008; Nowak

et al., 2009; Ackerley & Stinear, 2010), and in Chapter 10. The focus of this section is how to select a particular protocol given the characteristics of an individual patient.

A key decision is whether to make recovery, compensation, or substitution the goal for a given function. In order to achieve this, one might rely on algorithms such as that for the upper limb described above. Using this algorithm as an example, we can see how priming techniques might be used to promote recovery of upper limb function. When recovery or compensation are the goals, the aim of priming is to promote plasticity within ipsilesional nodes of the network to make these areas more responsive to therapy. This strategy is viable because the descending motor pathways remain intact. Priming may be achieved by using noninvasive brain stimulation protocols designed to promote disinhibition and create enduring increases in ipsilesional motor cortex excitability. At the same time, it may also be advantageous to apply techniques that dampen the output from contralesional motor cortex with the aim of reducing interference arising from contralesional nodes. This can be achieved by using low-frequency rTMS of the contralesional M1 (Grefkes et al., 2008) or contralesional cathodal direct current stimulation (Bradnam, Stinear, Barber, & Byblow, 2011), for example.

When damage to ipsilesional motor pathways is more severe and full recovery unlikely, then compensation or substitution are the only viable options. Now the aim of priming is to promote contributions from the wider neural network in both hemispheres, in the case of compensation, or strictly in contralesional nodes in the case of substitution. For example, facilitatory noninvasive brain stimulation of ipsilesional sensorimotor cortex may be appropriate if the descending pathways are not damaged beyond a critical point, and there remains viable ipsilesional connectivity to brainstem or spinal cord. As mentioned previously, this can only be determined by using combined approaches of TMS and DW-MRI to assess integrity of the descending pathways. When ipsilesional networks are no longer viable, priming approaches that incorporate and upregulate the contralesional hemisphere may be required. Facilitation of contralesional M1 may make use of uncrossed pathways that project predominantly to proximal upper limb muscles. Bimanual training approaches such as bilateral isokinetic therapy (Mudie & Matyas, 2000), and active–passive bilateral training (Stinear & Byblow 2004; Stinear et al., 2008) may facilitate compensation by specifically engaging both hemispheres to promote disinhibition and enhance subsequent use-dependent plasticity. Priming strategies for compensation or substitution need to avoid suppressing contralesional nodes, as these may have an important role to play. Small-scale studies have shown that more severely affected patients experience transient functional decrements in response to suppression of contralesional motor areas (Johansen-Berg et al., 2002; Bradnam et al., 2011). However, there is currently no evidence that priming to upregulate contralesional hemisphere activity confers a functional advantage in more severely affected patients. Furthermore, while the examples above are relevant to selecting rehabilitation goals and optimizing upper limb recovery, determining the balance of ipsilesional and contralesional priming for lower limb recovery remains an ongoing challenge (Jayaram & Stinear, 2009; Madhavan, Rogers, & Stinear, 2010; Madhavan & Stinear, 2010).

Future research might also consider genotype when selecting a priming technique for an individual patient. Neural plasticity is affected by the release of brain derived neurotrophic factor (BDNF; Murphy & Corbett, 2009). The gene that encodes BDNF has a common variation, called the *Val66Met* polymorphism. Most Caucasian adults have two copies of the *Valine* allele, while about a third have one or two copies of the *Methionine* allele. Adults with this variation of the BDNF gene have a blunted response to some noninvasive brain stimulation techniques (Cheeran et al., 2008; Antal et al., 2010) and may not benefit from certain priming techniques. Further research is needed to determine the clinical importance of common genetic variations, in terms of their impact on neural plasticity and recovery after stroke.

17.4 CONCLUSIONS

Neuroscience research is deepening our understanding of the mechanisms underlying recovery after stroke. Neural plasticity and reorganization within remaining networks is required to support recovery and compensation, and the aim of rehabilitation is to facilitate this process. Prognosis and priming techniques are being trialed with the aim of predicting and maximizing individual patients' recovery based on the residual anatomical and functional connectivity within affected neural networks. Future developments are likely to include the selection of rehabilitation goals, priming adjuncts, and therapy techniques for individual patients based on a more detailed understanding of their remaining capacity for neural reorganization. Factors affecting neural plasticity, such as genotype, may be included in future rehabilitation decision making. Cognitive and affective impairments will also need to be considered, as these may limit the patient's engagement in rehabilitation and their recovery of other functions, such as movement and communication.

REFERENCES

Ackerley, S. J. & Stinear, C. M. Stimulating stimulation: Can we improve motor recovery following stroke using repetitive transcranial magnetic stimulation?. *Physical Therapy Reviews* 15, 302–308 (2010).

Ackerley, S. J., & Stinear, C. M. (2010). Stimulating stimulation: can we improve motor recovery following stroke using repetitive transcranial magnetic stimulation? *Physical Therapy Reviews, 15*(4), 302–308.

Ahn, Y. H., Ahn, S. H., Kim, H., Hong, J. H., & Jang, S. H. (2006). Can stroke patients walk after complete lateral corticospinal tract injury of the affected hemisphere? *Neuroreport, 17*(10), 987–990.

Antal, A., Chaieb, L., Moliadze, V., Monte-Silva, K., Poreisz, C., Thirugnanasambandam, N., et al. (2010). Brain-derived neurotrophic factor (BDNF) gene polymorphisms shape cortical plasticity in humans. *Brain Stimulation, 3*(4), 230–237.

Beebe, J. A., & Lang, C. E. (2009). Active range of motion predicts upper extremity function 3 months after stroke. *Stroke, 40*(5), 1772–1779.

Bradnam, L. V., Stinear, C. M., Barber, P. A., & Byblow, W. D. (2011). Contralesional hemisphere control of the proximal paretic upper limb following stroke. *Cerebral Cortex,* DOI: 10.1093/cercor/bhr344.

Bradnam, L. V., Stinear, C. M., & Byblow, W. D. (2011). Cathodal transcranial direct current stimulation suppresses ipsilateral projections to presumed propriospinal neurons of the proximal upper limb. *Journal of Neurophysiology, 105*(5), 2582–2589

Catano, A., Houa, M., Caroyer, J. M., Ducarne, H., & Noel, P. (1996). Magnetic transcranial stimulation in acute stroke: early excitation threshold and functional prognosis. *Electroencephalography and Clinical Neurophysiology, 101*(3), 233–239.

Cheeran, B., Talelli, P., Mori, F., Koch, G., Suppa, A., Edwards, M., et al. (2008). A common polymorphism in the brain derived neurotrophic factor gene (BDNF) modulates human cortical plasticity and the response to rTMS. *Journal of Physiology, 586* (23), 5717–5725.

Chen, R., Cros, D., Curra, A., Di Lazzaro, V., Lefaucheur, J. P., Magistris, M. R., et al. (2008). The clinical diagnostic utility of transcranial magnetic stimulation: report of an IFCN committee. *Clinical Neurophysiology, 119*(3), 504–532.

Chen, S. Y., & Winstein, C. J. (2009). A systematic review of voluntary arm recovery in hemiparetic stroke: critical predictors for meaningful outcomes using the international classification of functioning, disability, and health. *Journal of Neurology and Physical Therapy, 33*(1), 2–13.

Davidoff, R. A. (1990). The pyramidal tract. *Neurology, 40*(2), 332–339.

Dum, R. P., & Strick, P. L. (1996). Spinal cord terminations of the medial wall motor areas in macaque monkeys. *Journal of Neuroscience, 16*(20), 6513–6525.

Duque, J., Hummel, F., Celnik, P., Murase, N., Mazzocchio, R., & Cohen, L. G. (2005). Transcallosal inhibition in chronic subcortical stroke. *NeuroImage, 28*(4), 940–946.

Gerloff, C., Bushara, K., Sailer, A., Wassermann, E. M., Chen, R., Matsuoka, T., et al. (2006). Multimodal imaging of brain reorganization in motor areas of the contralesional hemisphere of well recovered patients after capsular stroke. *Brain, 129*(Pt 3), 791–808.

Grefkes, C., Nowak, D. A., Eickhoff, S. B., Dafotakis, M., Kust, J., Karbe, H., et al. (2008). Cortical connectivity after subcortical stroke assessed with functional magnetic resonance imaging. *Annals of Neurology, 63*(2), 236–246.

Heald, A., Bates, D., Cartlidge, N. E., French, J. M., & Miller, S. (1993). Longitudinal study of central motor conduction time following stroke. 2. Central motor conduction measured within 72 h after stroke as a predictor of functional outcome at 12 months. *Brain, 116 (Pt 6)*, 1371–1385.

Hendricks, H. T., Pasman, J. W., van Limbeek, J., & Zwarts, M. J. (2003). Motor evoked potentials in predicting recovery from upper extremity paralysis after acute stroke. *Cerebrovascular Disease, 16*(3), 265–271.

Hummel, F. C., Celnik, P., Pascual-Leone, A., Fregni, F., Byblow, W. D., Buetefisch, C. M., et al. (2008). Controversy: Noninvasive and invasive cortical stimulation show efficacy in treating stroke patients. *Brain Stimulation, Oct 1*(4), 370–382.

Hummel, F. C., & Cohen, L. G. (2006). Non-invasive brain stimulation: a new strategy to improve neurorehabilitation after stroke? *The Lancet Neurology, 5*, 708–712.

Jang, S. H. (2009). The role of the corticospinal tract in motor recovery in patients with a stroke: a review. *NeuroRehabilitation, 24*(3), 285–290.

Jankowska, E., & Edgley, S. A. (2006). How can corticospinal tract neurons contribute to ipsilateral movements? A question with implications for recovery of motor functions. *Neuroscientist, 12*(1), 67–79.

Jayaram, G., & Stinear, J. W. (2009). The effects of transcranial stimulation on paretic lower limb motor excitability during walking. *Journal of Clinical Neurophysiology, 26*(4), 272–279.

Johansen-Berg, H., Rushworth, M. F., Bogdanovic, M. D., Kischka, U., Wimalaratna, S., & Matthews, P. M. (2002). The role of ipsilateral premotor cortex in hand movement after stroke. *Proceedings of the National Academy of Science U S A, 99*(22), 14518–14523.

Kwakkel, G., & Kollen, B. (2007). Predicting improvement in the upper paretic limb after stroke: a longitudinal prospective study. *Restorative Neurology and Neuroscience, 25*(5–6), 453–460.

Levin, M. F., Kleim, J. A., & Wolf, S. L. (2009). What do motor "recovery" and "compensation" mean in patients following stroke? *Neurorehabilitation and Neural Repair, 23*(4), 313–319.

MacKinnon, C. D., Quartarone, A., & Rothwell, J. C. (2004). Interhemispheric asymmetry of ipsilateral corticofugal projections to proximal muscles in humans. *Experimental Brain Research, 157*(2), 225–233.

Madhavan, S., Rogers, L. M., & Stinear, J. W. (2010). A paradox: after stroke, the non-lesioned lower limb motor cortex may be maladaptive. *European Journal of Neuroscience, 32*(6), 1032–1039.

Madhavan, S., & Stinear, J. W. (2010). Focal and bi-directional modulation of lower limb motor cortex using anodal transcranial direct current stimulation. *Brain Stimulation, 3*(1), 42.

Mansur, C. G., Fregni, F., Boggio, P. S., Riberto, M., Gallucci-Neto, J., Santos, C. M., et al. (2005). A sham stimulation-controlled trial of rTMS of the unaffected hemisphere in stroke patients. *Neurology, 64*(10), 1802–1804.

McCambridge, A. B., Bradnam, L. V., Stinear, C. M., & Byblow, W. D. (2011). Cathodal transcranial direct current stimulation of the primary motor cortex improves selective muscle activation in the ipsilateral arm. *Journal of Neurophysiology, 105*(6), 2937–2942.

Mudie, M. H. & Matyas, T. A. Can simultaneous bilateral movement involve the undamaged hemisphere in reconstruction of neural networks damaged by stroke? *Disability and Rehabilitation 22*, 23–37 (2000).

Murase, N., Duque, J., Mazzocchio, R., & Cohen, L. G. (2004). Influence of interhemispheric interactions on motor function in chronic stroke. *Annals of Neurology, 55*(3), 400–409.

Murphy, T. H., & Corbett, D. (2009). Plasticity during stroke recovery: from synapse to behaviour. *Nature Reviews Neuroscience, 10*(12), 861–872.

Nowak, D. A., Grefkes, C., Ameli, M., & Fink, G. R. (2009). Interhemispheric competition after stroke: brain stimulation to enhance recovery of function of the affected hand. *Neurorehabilitation and Neural Repair, 23*(7), 641–656.

Nowak, D. A., Grefkes, C., Dafotakis, M., Eickhoff, S., Kust, J., Karbe, H., et al. (2008). Effects of low-frequency repetitive transcranial magnetic stimulation of the contralesional primary motor cortex on movement kinematics and neural activity in subcortical stroke. *Archives of Neurology, 65*(6), 741–747.

Patel, A. T., Duncan, P. W., Lai, S. M., & Studenski, S. (2000). The relation between impairments and functional outcomes poststroke. *Archives of Physical Medicine and Rehabilitation, 81*(10), 1357–1363.

Piron, L., Piccione, F., Tonin, P., & Dam, M. (2005). Clinical correlation between motor evoked potentials and gait recovery in poststroke patients. *Archives of Physical Medicine and Rehabilitation, 86*(9), 1874–1878.

Pizzi, A., Carrai, R., Falsini, C., Martini, M., Verdesca, S., & Grippo, A. (2009). Prognostic value of motor evoked potentials in motor function recovery of upper limb after stroke. *Journal of Rehabilitative Medicine, 41*(8), 654–660.

Schaechter, J. D., Fricker, Z. P., Perdue, K. L., Helmer, K. G., Vangel, M. G., Greve, D. N., et al. (2009). Microstructural status of ipsilesional and contralesional corticospinal tract correlates with motor skill in chronic stroke patients. *Human Brain Mapping, 30*(11), 3461–3474.

Schwerin, S., Dewald, J. P., Haztl, M., Jovanovich, S., Nickeas, M., & MacKinnon, C. (2008). Ipsilateral versus contralateral cortical motor projections to a shoulder adductor in chronic hemiparetic stroke: implications for the expression of arm synergies. *Experimental Brain Research, 185*(3), 509–519.

Smania, N., Paolucci, S., Tinazzi, M., Borghero, A., Manganotti, P., Fiaschi, A., et al. (2007). Active finger extension: a simple movement predicting recovery of arm function in patients with acute stroke. *Stroke, 38*(3), 1088–1090.

Stinear, C. M. (2010). Prediction of recovery of motor function after stroke. *Lancet Neurology, 9*(12), 1228–1232.

Stinear, C. M., Barber, P. A., Smale, P. R., Coxon, J. P., Fleming, M. K., & Byblow, W. D. (2007). Functional potential in chronic stroke patients depends on corticospinal tract integrity. *Brain, 130*(Pt 1), 170–180.

Stinear, C. M., Barber, P. A., Coxon, J. P., Fleming, M. K. & Byblow, W. D. Priming the motor system enhances the effects of upper limb therapy in chronic stroke. *Brain, 131*, 1381–1390 (2008).

Stinear, J. W. & Byblow, W. D. Rhythmic bilateral movement training modulates corticomotor excitability and enhances upper limb motricity poststroke: a pilot study. *Journal of Clinical Neurophysiology, 21*, 124–131 (2004).

Swayne, O. B., Rothwell, J. C., Ward, N. S., & Greenwood, R. J. (2008). Stages of motor output reorganization after hemispheric stroke suggested by longitudinal studies of cortical physiology. *Cerebral Cortex, 18*(8), 1909–1922.

Talelli, P., Greenwood, R. J., & Rothwell, J. C. (2006). Arm function after stroke: Neurophysiological correlates and recovery mechanisms assessed by transcranial magnetic stimulation. *Clinical Neurophysiology, 117*(8), 1641–1659.

Traversa, R., Cicinelli, P., Pasqualetti, P., Filippi, M., & Rossini, P. M. (1998). Follow-up on interhemispheric differences of motor evoked potentials from the "affected" and "unaffected" hemispheres in human stroke. *Brain Research, 803*, 1–8.

Trompetto, C., Assini, A., Buccolieri, A., Marchese, R., & Abbruzzese, G. (2000). Motor recovery following stroke: a transcranial magnetic stimulation study. *Clinical Neurophysiology, 111*(10), 1860–1867.

Wandel, A., Jorgensen, H. S., Nakayama, H., Raaschou, H. O., & Olsen, T. S. (2000). Prediction of walking function in stroke patients with initial lower extremity paralysis: the Copenhagen Stroke Study. *Archives of Physical Medicine and Rehabilitation, 81*(6), 736–738.

Ward, N. S., Newton, J. M., Swayne, O. B., Lee, L., Frackowiak, R. S., Thompson, A. J., et al. (2007). The relationship between brain activity and peak grip force is modulated by corticospinal system integrity after subcortical stroke. *European Journal of Neuroscience, 25*(6), 1865–1873.

Ward, N. S., Newton, J. M., Swayne, O. B., Lee, L., Thompson, A. J., Greenwood, R. J., et al. (2006). Motor system activation after subcortical stroke depends on corticospinal system integrity. *Brain, 129*(Pt 3), 809–819.

Zarei, M., Johansen-Berg, H., Jenkinson, M., Ciccarelli, O., Thompson, A. J., & Matthews, P.M. (2007). Two-dimensional population map of cortical connections in the human internal capsule. *Journal of Magnetic Resonance Imaging, 25*(1), 48–54.

18 | DIRECTIONS FOR STROKE REHABILITATION CLINICAL PRACTICE AND RESEARCH

LEEANNE M. CAREY

18.1   INTRODUCTION

A paradigm shift is occurring in the way we think about stroke recovery and rehabilitation. The aim of this book has been to bring the evidence behind these new concepts and paradigms of recovery to practicing clinicians. This chapter highlights some of the key findings for the clinical practice of stroke rehabilitation explored in this book. Three concepts that have relevance across the field are then discussed. These are: (i) looking beyond the lesion to remote effects and impact on brain networks; (ii) the value and application of network-based models of recovery of specific functions to guide neuroscience-based rehabilitation; and (iii) tailoring interventions to the individual, based on viable brain networks with capacity for plasticity. Recommendations have been made to facilitate the translation of evidence to clinical practice. These are outlined. Future directions for stroke rehabilitation research are highlighted.

18.2   KEY FINDINGS FOR STROKE REHABILITATION CLINICAL PRACTICE

The potential for ongoing neural plastic changes in the mature human brain provides new hope for stroke survivors. These messages are relayed in the media regularly. Our clients are beginning to anticipate and seek this type of evidence-based contemporary treatment. As clinicians, our challenge is to set up the right conditions to facilitate this change for the particular individual. In this book we have reviewed current evidence to help inform clinicians of what might be the "right conditions." While we acknowledge that the paradigm shift is still emerging and there are many gaps in our knowledge, there are some key findings that can we can use in clinical practice now. Others will help guide us develop informed hypotheses for the future investigation of restorative approaches to rehabilitation.

We began by outlining a framework for stroke rehabilitation that highlighted the importance of active skill learning to achieve neural plastic change following brain injury (see Chapter 2). It includes the role of environment; active, learning-based approaches; and adjunct therapies in the context of how each may impact on neural plastic changes. The basis for these was further elaborated in the context of experience and learning-dependent plasticity (see Chapters 2 and 3). Each of these conditions may feed into a learning-based model of rehabilitation.

Motivation, goal-directed practice, intensive training, graded progression, and variation in task and practice conditions were identified as common core principles underlying learning and neural plastic changes in the model (Chapter 2). These principles were discussed further in the context of creating the right environment and conditions of training (Chapters 8 and 9) and have been incorporated in a number of training approaches. It is proposed that these principles may be used by clinicians in the context of active skill learning. They also complement components of enriched environments, as outlined below and in Chapter 3. Factors such as presence of depression and cognitive impairment will also influence these learning conditions and need to be taken into account, as discussed in Chapters 8, 14, and 15.

Skill-specific learning processes, such as targeted/facilitated feedback, calibration, goal identification and checking, and use of behavioral strategies were associated with learning-based rehabilitation of specific functions (Chapter 2). These were discussed and further elaborated in the context of rehabilitation of specific functions of movement, sensation, cognition, and language (Chapters

11 to 16). One of the primary benefits of these strategies is that they build on the abilities and capacities of the individual, rather than being reliant on externally imposed approaches. The individual can thus be more self-reliant and learn strategies that can be transferred to novel situations.

The environment was also identified as being important both in the context of skill-based learning (Chapter 2) and in the broader context of environmental enrichment (Chapter 3). Situated learning was identified as an important element in learning, together with the role of the clinician in enabling a positive learning environment (Chapter 2). The evidence behind environmental enrichment and multimodal stimulation is strong in animal studies but still requires systematic investigation in its translation to humans and stroke rehabilitation (Chapter 3). A number of conditions to achieve an "enriched" learning environment were discussed. It is suggested that these conditions may enhance the effect of other interventions (Johansson, 2011). The value of organized, multidisciplinary care (Chapter 7) was also highlighted and may be viewed as an important part of the environment.

Adjunctive therapies such as pharmacological agents and transcranial stimulation techniques have been developed and may be viewed as therapies to use in conjunction with behavioral interventions (Chapters 3 and 10). These neuromodulation approaches focus on influencing thresholds and activity levels in the brain so that it is more receptive to neural plasticity and learning. These methods may be important following brain damage. However, to produce lasting behavioral changes, the additional element of active skill-based learning is critical, as discussed in these chapters.

A number of interventions have been developed to treat specific functions such as movement, sensation, cognition, and language. Using evidence from neuroscience and neuroimaging, the authors of Chapters 11 to 16 explored the nature of the information processing deficit, evaluated current clinical interventions, provided experimental and clinical evidence of the potential value of these approaches, and suggested new interventions arising from neuroscience theory that may have potential. In the rehabilitation of movement (Chapter 11), the neural mechanisms underlying six interventions that have empirical evidence to support their use were discussed. These are repetitive task-specific training, constraint-induced movement therapy, mental practice, electrostimulation and electromyography (EMG) biofeedback, robot-assisted training, virtual reality, and visuomotor tracking training. The emerging picture is that techniques employing the principles of motor learning, such as repetition, progression, and variation (see also Chapter 9) can alter the neural control of movement of the paretic limbs, presumably via neural plasticity mechanisms (Chapter 11). In relation to touch and body sensations (Chapter 12), neuroscience evidence was presented for use

of goal-directed attention and deliberate anticipation, calibration across modality and within modality, and graded progression within and across sensory tasks. Examples of how these principles have been operationalized into training strategies are provided. A detailed knowledge of the visual system, its complexity and evidence of extraordinary plasticity within the system, supports the potential for restorative approaches to recovery of functions such as visual field deficits (Chapter 13).

The central role of attention and memory in rehabilitation and driving neural plastic change was discussed in Chapter 14. It was highlighted that attention is also guided by emotive and motivational evaluation of the stimuli to be attended to (Chapter 14). Executive dysfunction is common after stroke, yet there is no consensus about the exact cognitive and neural substrates supporting executive function as measured at the behavioral level (Chapter 15). It is recommended that a common language that covers neural, cognitive, and behavioral/performance levels be used. Interventions at the behavioral and performance levels were reviewed. The neuroscience evidence underpinning language and language rehabilitation was evaluated in Chapter 16. Clinical rehabilitation approaches for aphasia therapy, including constraint-induced aphasia therapy (CIAT), were outlined. Models of language and aphasia recovery were then reviewed, together with new insights from neuroimaging. The value of including cognitive principles of learning in rehabilitation was highlighted.

Together these findings highlight the potential value of a multimodal approach to rehabilitation based on neuroscience and neural plasticity. The components may be viewed as layers in creating the "right conditions" for neural plasticity and learning. New neural networks need to be formed or reorganized to take over the functions impaired by stroke. The individual has prior experience and abilities that he/she brings to the task. The brain has the demonstrated capacity to adapt and change in response to the environment and the goals of the individual. These neural plastic changes are synonymous with learning. The learning strategies used will influence which parts of the network are accessed, and the core learning principles will help to set up and reinforce the learning. Adjunct therapies may be helpful in modulating receptivity of the damaged brain, particularly when this is not able to be modulated internally or behaviorally by the individual himself/herself. On this basis it is argued that a combination of therapies is likely to maximize outcomes and plasticity (Figure 18.1).

This integrated multimodal approach may be likened to creating the right conditions when shaping the growth of a mature bonsai plant (Figure 18.2). The general growth of the plant will benefit from creating an enriched environment of light, water, fresh air, and sunshine—similar to the enriched environment with multimodal stimulation known to be associated with better recovery (Chapter 3). Plant cells have the organic ability to grow and form new branches

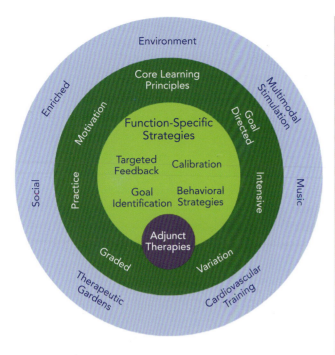

Figure 18.1 Stroke Rehabilitation: A multimodal approach to neural plasticity and skill learning.

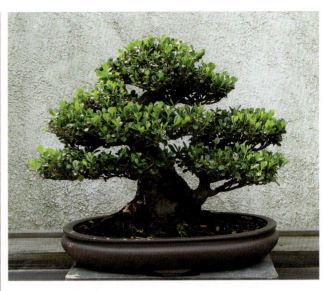

Figure 18.2 The science and art of bonsai: An analogy for a restorative approach to stroke rehabilitation.

and leaves. Similarly, there is compelling evidence for neural plastic changes in the mature human brain both in response to learning and injury. It is this capacity that may be nurtured and shaped to achieve the desired outcome. The untapped growth of the plant branches may be in the right direction or not, synonymous with adaptive and maladaptive plasticity. With the help of the bonsai master, these may be shaped in the right direction with training and careful pruning over a period of time. If the existing architecture of the plant does not achieve the desired outcome at a particular location then there is the potential to make new connections through grafting. In a similar way, the neurorehabilitation clinician can use knowledge from neuroscience to work with the client to craft the right conditions to achieve the desired outcome. They can draw on the core principles of learning as well as the function-specific learning strategies (Chapter 2). For example, they may use cross-modal calibration to reinforce connections with interconnected networks that usually do not have the lead role in a particular function. When necessary, there is also potential for external methods (adjunctive therapies) to reset the internal architecture for learning, as with grafting in a plant. This may be the case when the client–clinician team are not able to access necessary networks or connections through specific behavioral strategies. Critically, all the conditions that are designed to facilitate learning, including the behavioral training strategies, are still needed to achieve growth or adaptive plasticity in the right direction when these adjunctive therapies are used. An important distinction and potential value of the bonsai analogy is that it recognizes the innate and organic capacities of the plant (individual) as well as the skill of the bonsai master (clinician) to achieve the desired outcome. In this way it extends analogies that focus on a mechanical or externally driven rewiring of new networks.

18.3 BEYOND THE LESION: IMPACT OF FOCAL LESION ON BRAIN NETWORKS AND REHABILITATION

Stroke impacts beyond the lesion site. Focal lesions have important remote effects on the function of distant brain regions which contribute significantly to behavioral deficits observed (Carey & Seitz, 2007; Carter et al., 2010). Changes in remote locations and across hemispheres can be observed in animal models within the first hour after stroke (Mohajerani, Aminoltejari, & Murphy, 2011). Observations of transhemispheric diaschisis in humans (Seitz et al., 1999) support the concept that widespread interconnected regions can be functionally and structurally altered after a focal lesion. In addition, connected regions involved in information processing within a network may be affected. For example, in the field of neglect, attention deficits did not depend only on neuronal dysfunction at the site of injury, but were also mediated by impairment of connected neural systems that were structurally intact (Corbetta, Kincade, Lewis, Snyder, & Sapir, 2005). This dysfunction was reflected functionally by deactivation, hyperactivity or interhemispheric imbalance during task processing. A lesion may also critically disturb the complex balance of excitatory and inhibitory influences within a network (Grefkes & Fink, 2011; see Chapter 5). These findings highlight the importance of not only considering the focal lesion site but also the extent to which it may interrupt connections to distant brain regions and the contralesional hemisphere. This may be important for understanding the nature of the deficit, identifying remote changes that are susceptible to damage, and to identify viable brain networks with capacity for plasticity.

The brain operates as a functional unit with behaviors represented in distributed functional systems. The brain can be regarded as a system of elements (e.g., neuronal populations in distinct cortical areas) that interact with each other in a temporally and spatially specific fashion (Grefkes & Fink, 2011). For example, primary sensory area may be influenced by prefrontal areas that are themselves influenced by thalamic connections. Knowledge of how brain networks are interrupted is currently limited, but critical to better understand the clinical impairment and how neural plasticity can be manipulated by therapy. For example, recovery of spatial attention deficits was shown to correlate with the reactivation and rebalancing of normal activity within dorsal and ventral attention networks (He et al., 2007). The ventral network that was directly lesioned was diffusely disrupted but showed no recovery. In comparison, the dorsal network that was structurally intact showed early disruption but recovered. In recovery of motor deficits, extent of injury to specific motor tracts has been shown to predict behavioral gains from treatment in subjects with chronic stroke (Riley et al., 2011).

Within a network certain regions have more widespread connections. These regions are often defined based on whole brain analysis of resting networks and have been referred to as "hubs" (Sporns, Honey, & Kotter, 2007). Once network hubs have been identified, hubs may be classified on the basis of whether their connections are distributed mostly within or mostly between network modules. This may have implications relative to lesion location. For example, prefrontal and parietal regions have been identified as "connector hubs," and so interruption to these regions is likely to have more widespread impact (Honey & Sporns, 2008). Further, the structural network is vulnerable to deletion of highly central nodes, but more resilient to deletion of strong nodes, or randomly selected nodes (Alstott, Breakspear, Hagmann, Cammoun, & Sporns, 2009). It is suggested that while the effects of anatomical damage extend beyond the lesioned area, they typically remain within the borders of existing network connections (Nomura et al., 2010). Spatial distances between regions in a network may also impact the extent to which a network is interrupted or may experience interference (Grefkes & Fink, 2011).

Converging evidence from studies of functional connectivity also highlights the role of interhemispheric connectivity and its relationship to impairment and recovery (Grefkes, Eickhoff, Nowak, Dafotakis, & Fink, 2008; Carter et al., 2010; Grefkes & Fink, 2011). Interhemispheric functional connectivity, but not intrahemispheric functional connectivity, was correlated with motor impairment and

with neglect (Carter et al., 2010). The balance of activity between hemispheres may be particularly important in processing of information, for example in the somatosensory system (Blankenburg et al., 2008). Competition between hemispheres may also play a part (Nowak, Grefkes, Ameli, & Fink, 2009). Concepts of brain organization, such as the theory of interhemispheric rivalry and competitive feedback inhibition (Kinsbourne, 1977, 2006; Merzenich et al., 1983; Buonomano & Merzenich, 1998) will also have an impact.

Using this knowledge and advances in neuroimaging, we now have the opportunity to quantify the extent to which a lesion interrupts expected pathways and/or functional networks in individuals. For example, inferred interruption to trajectories of corticofugal fibers, characterized in healthy controls using probabilistic tractography, was associated with hand grip performance in individual stroke survivors (Newton et al., 2006). Similarly, we can investigate interruption to functional connections (Carter, et al., 2010) and regions of brain activation (Cramer et al., 2005). Knowledge of remote effects that impact functional activation and coherence across brain regions suggests that clinical practice and research studies should not be confined to conventional structural imaging techniques. It is recommended that acquisition of functional MRI data, such as resting-state MRI, be considered to inform rehabilitation. For example, the opportunity exists to observe functional connectivity across hemispheres using resting-state functional connectivity analysis. Use of a resting-state acquisition has particular advantages in that it has low demand on the patient and high yield, as different networks of interest may be investigated from the one dataset.

18.4 USE OF NETWORK-BASED MODELS OF RECOVERY IN STROKE REHABILITATION

Models provide a synthesized, evidence-based framework for the translation of science to practice. Models of recovery of motor function (Ward & Cohen, 2004; Carey & Seitz, 2007; Stinear et al., 2007;) and neglect (Corbetta et al., 2005) have been proposed based on neuroimaging and neurophysiological studies. Network-based models represent a paradigm shift from the standard lesion-deficit view, and can be used to guide and change clinical rehabilitation practices, as follows:

(i) *Characterize the deficit and recovery.* Network models can account for changes in the balance of activity across hemispheres and in functionally related remote locations, rather than focusing only on regional deficits at the lesion site. For example, in post-stroke neglect, Corbetta et al. (2005) describe a functional-anatomical model that identifies the cortical network and functional pathways involved in attention. The authors found that deficits of neglect depended not only on neuronal dysfunction at the site of injury, but also on connected neural systems structurally spared. This dysfunction presented functionally as deactivation, hyperactivity, or interhemispheric imbalance during task processing. Recovery correlated with reactivation and rebalancing of network activity (He, et al., 2007).

(ii) *Predict ability to benefit from therapy.* Models of recovery may provide guidance in predicting which patient will benefit most from which intervention. For example, Stinear et al.'s (2007) data-driven algorithm predicts motor improvements after therapy based on neurophysiological and structural integrity of the corticospinal tract (CST; see Chapter 17). Prediction based on interruption to brain networks has relevance in addition to clinical predictors. This approach helps to inform central mechanisms of recovery as well as identify capacities (viable networks) that may not be visible, but may be important to know about in therapy.

(iii) *Guide selection of individualized rehabilitation strategies.* Knowledge of viable brain networks may be used to tailor rehabilitation strategies for an individual. A network model can identify how different approaches to therapy may reestablish interhemispheric connections depending on part of the network disrupted, as depicted in a model of motor recovery (Carey & Seitz, 2007). For example, observation of functional integrity of corticospinal tract (CST) in an individual would recommend intense unilateral therapy, while a lack suggests an augmented or bilateral therapeutic approach for the individual based on Stinear et al.'s algorithm (Stinear, et al., 2007; Chapter 17).

The clinical value in developing such models is focused on identifying the strengths of an individual that may be used in therapy; specifically, the viability of distributed brain networks that have a known role in a particular function and recovery. Such an approach does not exclude individuals from treatment, rather it identifies brain networks that may be tapped into in therapy: individual strengths that are not necessarily visible via existing behaviors or known by clinical experience. There is currently a lack of evidence for rehabilitation interventions in stroke, let alone how they work. Studies of this type that provide clinicians with a model to predict outcomes based on brain mapping are overdue. By using modeling, patients may be selected for effective and cost-efficient stroke rehabilitation. These models may also be used to generate science-founded hypotheses for development of new interventions.

18.5 TARGETING STROKE REHABILITATION TO THE INDIVIDUAL

The value and need for individualized targeting of stroke interventions was identified by a number of authors in this book (e.g., Chapters 3 and 17). New therapies have been developed to help the brain recover after stroke. Yet, currently we do not have effective means of identifying individuals who have potential to benefit from these therapies nor do we have the means of selecting the most optimal therapy. In addition, determining whether a person with stroke has reached his or her full potential for recovery is difficult.

The individual brings a constellation of factors to the rehabilitation situation that will affect the potential to achieve neural plastic changes and recovery. These include personal, social and cultural, clinical, genetic, and environmental factors (Chapter 3). One factor that we could now add to this list is *neural networks*. Careful analysis of the impact of the lesion on brain networks, as well as knowledge of viable brain networks, has potential to guide rehabilitation clinicians in individualized stroke rehabilitation.

In order to tailor intervention to the individual, we need to ascertain what the individual's goals are and what motivates them. In the context of client-centered practice there are tools that can help in this regard. For example, the Canadian Occupational Performance Measure (COPM; Law et al., 2004) is designed to assist the individual in identifying tasks that he or she is experiencing problems with since the stroke, how important those tasks are, and what the individual's perceived performance and satisfaction ratings are for the tasks selected. There are also goal attainment scales that may be used in rehabilitation (Turner-Stokes, 2009). Individualized rehabilitation has an added benefit from being goal-directed, in that identification of client goals can guide selection of relevant tasks for relearning and help with motivation.

In addition, we now have the tools to assess the structural and functional changes in the brain and the capacity for plasticity. We can map how particular white matter tracts may be interrupted by the lesion, both directly and indirectly (Chapter 4). We can also map the residual architecture that may be accessed in therapy. Similarly, the lesion may be mapped relative to functional brain regions and networks that are known to be important for particular functions and tasks. Again, we may benefit not only from assessing the interruption to these functionally important regions, but also from identifying which connected regions and networks may be accessed in therapy. Given the complex interactions between networks, and widely distributed cognitive-emotional networks that may be impacted by the stroke (Chapter 14), it would also be beneficial to determine the extent to which these are directly or remotely affected by the stroke in an individual.

Changes in these networks may be evident even in mild stroke and may have an ongoing impact on the individual and his/her ability to benefit from rehabilitation.

In the context of rehabilitation, we may benefit from being able to identify and target viable brain networks that may be accessed through therapy. At one level, we can use knowledge of functional and structural integrity of connections to predict who is likely to benefit from therapy and guide selection of a particular rehabilitation approach. For example, in motor recovery, functional integrity of the corticospinal tract was found to be important in the prediction of outcome and in selection of unilateral compared to bilateral approaches to training (Stinear, et al., 2007; Chapter 17). An algorithm for predicting upper limb motor outcomes has been developed and may be used to help guide selection for an individual based on this data (Chapter 17).

At another level, knowledge of links between related functional networks and knowledge of goal-driven or task-driven pathways *within* a functional network may be used to guide and shape therapy. For example, we may use knowledge of the links between somatosensory and visual networks to target therapy and recalibrate the altered or poorly discriminated somatosensory information perceived after stroke (Chapter 12). An individual who has difficulty accessing the region responsible for this function (e.g., discriminating how rough or widely spaced a texture is) via the somatosensory network may be able to access the same or a similar region that is known to process and integrate touch and visual spatial (roughness) information via the linked visual network. It is known that pathways within a network may be specialized relative to particular goals or tasks. After damage to one of these, the potential exists to achieve a similar outcome via the related pathway. For example, if the "sensation for perception" pathway is interrupted, knowledge of the "sensation for action" pathway may be beneficial in therapy by focusing the goal of the task and guiding the therapist to link the touch sensation with the most optimal exploratory movement used to perceive that information. This may assist the client to better access the spatial touch information in relation to the goal of actively exploring the roughness of the object. This important link between sensation and action could also be accessed in the context of motor recovery.

Evidence suggests that the rules governing plasticity are distinctly different in different cerebral regions (Kolb, Teskey, & Gibb, 2010). Further, neural plasticity is experience-dependent, time-sensitive, and strongly influenced by features of environment (Cramer et al., 2011). No single pattern of neuroplastic change is observed during recovery; rather, they seem to depend on the training intervention and deficits caused by the initial lesion (Kreisel, Hennerici, & Bazner, 2007), as well as its impact on remote locations and networks (Grefkes & Fink, 2011). On this basis, individuals or subgroups "may require different rehabilitation strategies to target specific brain regions" (Kolb, et al., 2010, p.4). Recently the different impact of two training approaches (unilateral and bilateral motor arm training) on task-related brain activation was demonstrated after stroke (Whitall et al., 2011). Both groups had nonresponders. Based on evidence from Stinear et al. (2007) it is possible that nonresponders in each group were not matched with the most optimal intervention for the individual.

We also need to be mindful of interactions between mind, brain, and body. A stroke likely impacts an individual at the level of mind, brain, and body. The person's perception and consciousness of themselves may be altered, although this may not be obvious to those around (Lyons, 2010). Further, the individual will have an internally driven perspective on their recovery and rehabilitation. As stated in the words of a stroke survivor: "I am aware it is my responsibility alone to take control of my healing and it has to be a holistic approach. Not only do I have to consider my physical condition, but also be aware of my state of mind—how I think and how I feel—for all of these are intrinsically linked." Clearly the link between mind, brain, and body is important for the individual and potentially impacts the ability to benefit from rehabilitation. Further, as this stroke survivor with thalamic pain says, "Suffering is only one possible reaction to pain. One can experience pain without suffering from it." (Lyons, 2010). An active approach to neurorehabilitation can help link mind, brain, and body for the individual. The motivating context of the recovery and learning environment can help facilitate a positive state of mind. The potential of the brain to dynamically "change itself" may be facilitated through learning-dependent plasticity and knowledge of brain networks. Finally, at the body level the aim is often to improve bodily functions. This may be further supported by knowledge of the daily functions the brain has to solve.

18.6 GUIDELINES TO FACILITATE THE TRANSLATION OF EVIDENCE TO CLINICAL PRACTICE

Growing evidence from the literatures of basic science through to cognitive neuroscience and rehabilitation are helping to elucidate the neural substrates of recovery after stroke and the potential to influence these via rehabilitation. The challenge now is to facilitate the translation from neuroscience to clinical practice.

Despite advances in restorative approaches to rehabilitation, translation to clinical practice had been slow (Cheeran et al., 2009). Barriers to the "translational research pipeline" have been identified in relation to biological and process issues. These include: poor translation from animal studies to functional improvement in patients; small-scale studies; difficulty in recruitment to large-scale studies; ill-defined outcomes; and poor integration and

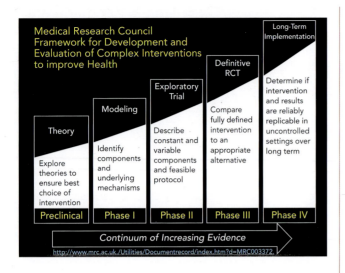

Figure 18.3 Framework for development and evaluation of complex interventions. Adapted from Medical Research Council, 2000.

partnership across researchers, hospitals, community, and patient stakeholders. A bidirectional approach to translation is advocated that includes proof-of-principle studies designed to look at efficacy (how well the intervention works under controlled circumstances) and clinical studies of effectiveness (how well an intervention performs under more typical circumstances) (Cheeran, et al., 2009). Other solutions recommended include improving the research culture, training clinicians in health services research, encouraging "patient pull," choice of outcome measures, and reference to biological and organizational catalysts.

The Medical Research Council of the United Kingdom has developed a "Framework for the Development and Evaluation of Complex Interventions to Improve Health" (Medical Research Council, 2000). It involves five steps that represent a continuum of increasing evidence: from theory to modeling, exploratory trials, definitive randomized control trial (RCT), and long-term implementation (see Figure 18.3). This framework may be useful to guide systematic development of novel approaches to therapy based on neuroscience. By way of example, the steps involved in development of a neuroscience-based approach to retraining body sensations, the SENSe (Study of the Effectiveness of Neurorehabilitation on Sensation) approach, are consistent with these guidelines (Carey, 2007, 2010; Carey, Macdonnell, & Matyas, 2011; also see Box 1).

BOX 1 DEVELOPMENT OF NEUROSCIENCE APPROACH TO SENSORY REHABILITATION.

Preclinical—Theory: The first step was to develop the training approach based on theories of perceptual learning, brain recovery, and neurophysiology of sensory processing, and operationalize these into a program of tactile and proprioceptive discrimination training (Carey, Matyas, & Oke, 1993). Each principle selected was based on complemen-

tary evidence from three bodies of literature (Carey, 2006; see Chapter 12). For example, use of calibration within and across modalities is associated with improved perceptual learning in healthy subjects, there is clear evidence of plasticity across modalities such as vision and touch, and there are preexisting connections within the system to support such change (see Chapter 12).

Phase I and II: Modeling & Exploratory Trials: Here, the components of the intervention are identified as well as the mechanisms that are thought to underlie outcomes. We used a series of controlled single case experiments to test clinical outcomes in relation to stimulus-specific training (Carey et al., 1993) with positive results. The approach was then modified to facilitate transfer of training effects to novel stimuli (Carey & Matyas, 2005) with positive outcomes. Repeated measurement of outcomes permitted quantification of a pattern of change, consistent with learning models. The intervention was systematically applied across subgroups of individuals with different characteristics, providing replication within the series of 30 single case experiments (Carey, 2006).

Phase III: Definitive RCT. The next step was to conduct a randomized control trial (RCT). The aim was to investigate the effectiveness of a clinical treatment package that uses the most optimal approach to training and applies it to training of texture discrimination, limb position sense, and recognition of everyday objects through the sense of touch. An RCT known as *SENSe: Study of the Effectiveness of Neurorehabilitation on Sensation* was conducted with positive outcomes (Carey et al., 2011). Significant improvement in the primary outcome, a composite index of functional sensory capacity, was found following SENSe training compared to exposure-only based training. Improvements were clinically significant, with maintenance of gains at 6-week and 6-month follow-ups.

Phase IV: Long-term Implementation: The final phase in development of the program is to establish the long-term and real-life effectiveness of the intervention when rolled out into wider practice (Medical Research Council, 2000). A planned and evidence-based approach to implementation (Graham et al., 2006) is critical to ensure that best evidence is successfully translated into clinical practice. In addition, it is important to work in partnership with key stakeholders (therapists, rehabilitation specialists, managers, and stroke survivors) to successfully address this knowledge–practice gap.

18.7 PERSPECTIVES AND DIRECTIONS FOR STROKE REHABILITATION RESEARCH

It is recommended that the agenda for stroke rehabilitation research be discussed by multidisciplinary groups ranging from basic scientists to clinicians. Such discussions have been initiated by groups such as the Cumberland Consensus Working Group (Cheeran et al., 2009) and the National Institutes of Health Blueprint for Neuroscience Research (Cramer et al., 2011). Potential research directions to support restorative approaches to stroke rehabilitation that are emerging from the literature are outlined below:

Investigation of combination of plasticity-enhancing interventions: A number of interventions have been developed for use in clinical settings that are supported by evidence of neural plastic change and better outcomes (see Chapters 3, 9, 11–16). The potential exists to examine use of a combination of these therapies that may enhance plasticity (see also Cramer et al., 2011). For example, it would be beneficial to examine the combined effects of enriched environment and task-specific motor training based on positive effects of both on neural plastic change following stroke. These investigations would also permit insight into the effects of nonspecific experience (enriched environment) and the additional effects of function-specific training on plasticity. Outcomes of brain networks associated with these interventions would help to elucidate the networks involved in recovery and skill-specific improvements.

Development of models for recovery of specific functions: It is proposed that models of recovery should be developed for each of the functions that are commonly addressed in stroke rehabilitation. Models also need to be developed to predict interactive effects of combined interventions. Models provide a synthesis of current research and direction for development of hypothesis-driven interventions (see section 18.4). The authors in this book have gone part way toward providing a foundation for the development of these models. They have reviewed the neuroscience in relation to the function, proposed guidelines and theoretical foundations for future practice, as well as critically reviewed current interventions. Future research would benefit from systematic development of data-driven network-based models, for example as have been developed by Stinear et al. (2007) and Corbetta et al. (2005). An ultimate aim is to predict which individuals will benefit from rehabilitation and target strategies accordingly.

Optimization of clinical interventions founded on neuroscience: Pre-post and proof-of-principle studies of the effects of different interventions on brain function and clinical outcomes are needed to better understand the adaptive changes that may occur in response to specific interventions in individuals, and in subgroups of patients. Understanding factors that differentiate responders from nonresponders will help define "treatment success" and improve prediction in individuals. These studies will benefit from stratifying patients, and from advances in neuroimaging and multimodal methods. For example, stratification may be according to the residual functional connectivity between key nodes in the relevant network,

such as between primary motor cortex and the spinal cord (Chapters 11 and 17). Findings will contribute to a better understanding of the neural mechanisms underlying the clinical benefits of learning-based rehabilitation techniques.

Longitudinal studies of recovery after stroke: Well-controlled longitudinal studies are needed to chart the changes in brain structure and function that occur after stroke. These would benefit from being linked with changes across a profile of outcomes, from changes in brain function and structure to behavioral performance and participation. Use of a profile of outcomes will help to further our understanding of the relationship between plasticity, activity limitations, societal participation, and quality of life (Chae, Duncan, Pugh, & Selzer, 2011). The potential interaction between time post-stroke and recovery has been discussed (Chapter 6). Longitudinal studies may provide valuable insight into critical therapeutic windows for interventions. Systematic investigation of the impact of time post-stroke on neural plastic changes is indicated.

Investigation of changes in brain structure and function using a combination of approaches: Different methodologies contribute different information in efforts to better understand changes that occur with specific training approaches. A convergence of multiple approaches, including structural and functional MRI as well as magnetoencephalography (MEG) and transcranial magnetic stimulation are advocated. Together, these will help to elucidate mechanisms related not only to the location of changes in the brain but also the timing of those changes. Links with computational modeling may be particularly valuable in investigations of perception and cognition. For example, dynamic system models can assess lawful relations between changes across multiple levels of analysis and may be useful in charting responses to treatment.

Use of common methods and paradigms across studies: Common use of valid acquisition protocols that may be readily applied, such as resting-state and diffusion tractography, are recommended to facilitate sharing and accumulation of data and knowledge across studies. Use of shared clinical measures is also advocated to facilitate comparison across studies. To facilitate this sharing, national and international research networks are encouraged (Cheeran, et al., 2009).

Implementation trials of plasticity-based clinical interventions: A few interventions that have strong foundations in neuroscience and have been tested in RCTs have potential to be implemented more broadly in clinical practice. These trials of clinical effectiveness will require large sample sizes. They will need to be optimized relative to the clinical setting and in relation to dose, intensity, and duration of treatment (Cheeran, et al., 2009). Focus on clinically relevant outcomes is recommended, including activity limitation, participation, and life satisfaction measures. Use of evidence-based approaches to guide implementation (Graham et al., 2006) is recommended.

Parallel studies in animals and humans: Translation from basic science to proof-of-principle studies in humans has been relatively limited (Cheeran et al., 2009; Cramer et al., 2011). Development of parallel studies that incorporate comparable measures across animals and humans may help to address this gap. For example, methods such as resting state BOLD and diffusion-weighted imaging are valid across species. Animal studies may also benefit from more sensitive measures of skill performance (Murphy & Corbett, 2009) comparable to those used in humans, and outcomes that reflect reengagement in activities (participation). Animal studies can then provide investigation of additional levels of analysis that are not possible in humans, for example the relationship between networks and cellular changes (Cheeran, et al., 2009).

18.8 CONCLUSION

Evidence of neural plastic changes after stroke provides an open window of opportunity for ongoing improvement, and thus new hope for stroke survivors. Stroke rehabilitation can create the right environment and learning conditions to facilitate positive adaptive changes in the brain. We still have a lot to learn, but through advances in neuroscience, neuroimaging, and related techniques, we can continue to gain new insights into how to maximize and shape these neural plastic changes. It is hoped that we will soon be able to use the knowledge of viable brain networks to tap into an individual's inherent capacities and select which intervention is most likely to benefit a particular individual. We encourage stroke rehabilitation clinicians to be involved in this era of discovery and translation. It is our responsibility to be informed and to deliver.

REFERENCES

Alstott, J., Breakspear, M., Hagmann, P., Cammoun, L., & Sporns, O. (2009). Modeling the impact of lesions in the human brain. *Public Library of Science Computational Biology, 5*(6). e1000408

Blankenburg, F., Ruff, C. C., Bestmann, S., Bjoertomt, O., Eshel, N., Josephs, O., et al. (2008). Interhemispheric effect of parietal TMS on somatosensory response confirmed directly with concurrent TMS-fMRI. *Journal of Neuroscience, 28*(49), 13202–13208.

Buonomano, D. V., & Merzenich, M. M. (1998). Cortical plasticity: from synapses to maps. *Annual Review of Neuroscience, 21*, 149–186.

Carey, L. M. (2006). Loss of somatic sensation. In M. E. Selzer, S. Clarke, L. G. Cohen, P. W. Duncan, & F. H. Gage (Eds.), *Textbook of Neural Repair and Rehabilitation. Vol II. Medical Neurorehabilitation* (Vol. II, pp. 231–247). Cambridge: Cambridge University Press.

Carey, L. M. (2007). Neuroplasticity and learning lead a new era in stroke rehabilitation. [editorial]. *International Journal of Therapy Rehabilitation, 14*(6), 200–201.

Carey, L. M. (2010). Neuroscience makes sense for occupational therapy. Viewpoint. [Special Issue on Stroke Rehabilitation]. *Australian Occupational Therapy Journal, 57*(3), 197–199.

Carey, L. M., Macdonnell, R., & Matyas, T. A. (2011). SENSe: Study of the effectiveness of neurorehabilitation on sensation: a randomized controlled trial. *Neurorehabilitation and Neural Repair, 25*(4), 304–313.

Carey, L. M., & Matyas, T. A. (2005). Training of somatosensory discrimination after stroke: facilitation of stimulus generalization. *American Journal of Physical Medicine and Rehabilitation, 84*(6), 428–442.

Carey, L. M., Matyas, T. A., & Oke, L. E. (1993). Sensory loss in stroke patients: effective training of tactile and proprioceptive discrimination. *Archives of Physical Medicine and Rehabilitation, 74*(6), 602–611.

Carey, L. M., & Seitz, R. (2007). Functional neuroimaging in stroke recovery and neurorehabilitation: conceptual issues and perspectives. *International Journal of Stroke, 2*(4), 245–264.

Carter, A. R., Astafiev, S. V., Lang, C. E., Connor, L. T., Rengachary, J., Strube, M. J., et al. (2010). Resting interhemispheric functional magnetic resonance imaging connectivity predicts performance after stroke. *Annals of Neurology, 67*(3), 365–375.

Chae, J., Duncan, P. W., Pugh, K., & Selzer, M. E. (2011). *Workshop White Paper.* Paper presented at the Eunice Kennedy Shriver National Institute of Child Health and Human Development: Scientific Vision Workshop on Plasticity.

Cheeran, B., Cohen, L., Dobkin, B., Ford, G., Greenwood, R., Howard, D., et al. (2009). The future of restorative neurosciences in stroke: driving the translational research pipeline from basic science to rehabilitation of people after stroke. *Neurorehabilitation and Neural Repair, 23*(2), 97–107.

Corbetta, M., Kincade, M., Lewis, C., Snyder, A., & Sapir, A. (2005). Neural basis and recovery of spatial attention deficits in spatial neglect. *Nature Neuroscience, 8*, 1603–1610.

Cramer, S. C., Benson, R. R., Himes, D. M., Burra, V. C., Janowsky, J. S., Weinand, M. E., et al. (2005). Use of functional MRI to guide decisions in a clinical stroke trial. *Stroke, 36*(5), e50–e52.

Cramer, S. C., Sur, M., Dobkin, B. H., O'Brien, C., Sanger, T. D., Trojanowski, J. Q., et al. (2011). Harnessing neuroplasticity for clinical applications. *Brain, 134*, 1591–1609.

Graham, I. D., Logan, J., Harrison, M. B., Straus, S. E., Tetroe, J., Caswell, W., et al. (2006). Lost in knowledge translation: time for a map? *Journal of Continuing Education in the Health Professions, 26*(1), 13–24.

Grefkes, C., Eickhoff, S. B., Nowak, D. A., Dafotakis, M., & Fink, G. R. (2008). Dynamic intra- and interhemispheric interactions during unilateral and bilateral hand movements assessed with fMRI and DCM. *NeuroImage, 41*(4), 1382–1394.

Grefkes, C., & Fink, G. R. (2011). Reorganization of cerebral networks after stroke: new insights from neuroimaging with connectivity approaches. *Brain, 134*(5), 1264–1276.

He, B. J., Snyder, A. Z., Vincent, J. L., Epstein, A., Shulman, G. L., & Corbetta, M. (2007). Breakdown of functional connectivity in frontoparietal networks underlies behavioral deficits in spatial neglect. *Neuron, 53*(6), 905–918.

Honey, C. J., & Sporns, O. (2008). Dynamical consequences of lesions in cortical networks. *Human Brain Mapping, 29*(7), 802–809.

Johansson, B. B. (2011). Current trends in stroke rehabilitation. A review with focus on brain plasticity. *Acta Neurologica Scandinavica, 123*(3), 147–159.

Kinsbourne, M. (1977). Hemi-neglect and hemisphere rivalry. *Advances in Neurology, 18*, 41–49.

Kinsbourne, M. (2006). From unilateral neglect to the brain basis of consciousness. *Cortex, 42*(6), 869–874.

Kolb, B., Teskey, G. C., & Gibb, R. (2010). Factors influencing cerebral plasticity in the normal and injured brain. *Frontiers in Human Neuroscience, 4*, Article 204.

Kreisel, S. H., Hennerici, M. G., & Bazner, H. (2007). Pathophysiology of stroke rehabilitation: The natural course of clinical recovery, use-dependent plasticity and rehabilitative outcome. *Cerebrovascular Diseases, 23*(4), 243–255.

Law, M., Baptise, S., Carswell, A., McColl, M. A., Polatajko, H. J., & Pollock, N. (2004). *Canadian occupational performance measure.* (4th ed ed.). Ottawa: CAOT Publications ACE.

Lyons, W. (2010). *Left of tomorrow.* Glen Waverley: Sid Harta Publishers.

Medical Research Council. (2000). *A framework for development and evaluation of RCTs for complex interventions to improve health.* (http://www.mrc.ac.uk accessed June 2006). UK: Medical Research Council. Update at: www.mrc.ac.uk/complexinterventionsguidance

Merzenich, M. M., Kaas, J. H., Wall, J., Nelson, R. J., Sur, M., & Felleman, D. (1983). Topographic reorganization of somatosensory cortical areas 3b and 1 in adult monkeys following restricted deafferentation. *Neuroscience, 8,* 33–55.

Mohajerani, M. H., Aminoltejari, K., & Murphy, T. H. (2011). Targeted mini-strokes produce changes in interhemispheric sensory signal processing that are indicative of disinhibition within minutes. *Proceedings of the National Academy of Sciences of the United States of America, 108*(22), E183–E191.

Murphy, T. H., & Corbett, D. (2009). Plasticity during stroke recovery: from synapse to behaviour. *Nature Reviews Neuroscience, 10*(12), 861–872.

Newton, J. M., Ward, N. S., Parker, G. J., Deichmann, R., Alesander, D. C., Friston, K. J., et al. (2006). Non-invasive mapping of corticofugal fibres from multiple motor areas—relevance to stroke recovery. *Brain, 129*(pt 7), 1844–1858.

Nomura, E. M., Gratton, C., Visser, R. M., Kayser, A., Perez, F., & D'Esposito, M. (2010). Double dissociation of two cognitive control networks in patients with focal brain lesions. *Proceedings of the National Academy of Sciences of the United States of America, 107*(26), 12017–12022.

Nowak, D. A., Grefkes, C., Ameli, M., & Fink, G. R. (2009). Interhemispheric competition after stroke: brain stimulation to enhance recovery of function of the affected hand. *Neurorehabilitation and Neural Repair 23*(7), 641–656.

Riley, J. D., Le, V., Dar-Yeghianian, L., See, J., Newton, J. M., Ward, N. S., et al. (2011). Anatomy of stroke injury predicts gains from therapy. *Stroke, 42,* 421–426.

Seitz, R. J., Azari, N. P., Knorr, U., Binkofski, F., Herzog, H., & Freund, H.-J. (1999). The role of diaschisis in stroke recovery. *Stroke, 30,* 1844–1850.

Sporns, O., Honey, C. J., & Kotter, R. (2007). Identification and classification of hubs in brain networks. *Public Library of Science One, 2*(10), e1049.

Stinear, C. M., Barber, P. A., Smale, P. R., Coxon, J. P., Fleming, M. K., & Byblow, W. D. (2007). Functional potential in chronic stroke patients depends on corticospinal tract integrity. *Brain, 130,* 170–180.

Turner-Stokes, L. (2009). Goal attainment scaling (GAS) in rehabilitation: a practical guide. *Clinical Rehabilitation, 23*(4), 362–370.

Ward, N. S., & Cohen, L. G. (2004). Mechanisms underlying recovery of motor function after stroke. *Archives of Neurology, 61*(12), 1844–1848.

Whitall, J., Waller, S.M., Sorkin, J. D., Forrester, L. W., Macko, R. F., Hanley, D. F., et al. (2011). Bilateral and unilateral arm training improve motor function through differing neuroplastic mechanisms: a single-blinded randomized controlled trial. *Neurorehabilitation and Neural Repair, 25*(2), 118–129.

INDEX

A

ACC. *See* anterior cingulate cortex
acetyl cholinesterase (AChE) inhibitors, 130
active motor threshold (AMT), 60
active-problem solving, with skills acquisition, 16
guided discovery, 16
strategies, 16
activities of daily living
skills acquisition for, 20
after somatosensory loss, with stroke, 158
timeline for recovery of, 84
activity-dependent plasticity, 13
acute stroke, rTMS for, 133–134
ADC. *See* apparent diffusion coefficient
adjunctive therapies, 8, 17. *See also* transcranial magnetic stimulation
animal models, 128–129
multiple session outcomes, 128–129
pharmacological studies, 129
with physical therapies, 129
direct cortical stimulation, 135–136
EMG feedback, 148–150
behavioural effects, 148–149
for finger tracking training tasks, 150
neural mechanisms, 149–150
neuroimaging for, 149–150
technical processes, 148
ES, 148–150
behavioural effects, 148–149
for finger tracking training tasks, 150
neural mechanisms, 149–150
neuroimaging for, 149
neuroprosthetic, 149
technical processes, 148
growth factors, 137
EPO, 137
G-CSF, 137
mental practices, 147–148
behavioural effects, 147–148
for motor learning, 120–121
neural mechanisms, 148
technical processes, 147
neuroprosthetics, 136
pharmacological, 129–130
amphetamines, 129
animal models, 129
cholinergic agents, 130
dopaminergic agents, 130
limitations of, 129
SSRIs, 130
rationale for, 128
Rehab-Learn model, 18
robot-assisted training, 150–151
advantages, 150
behavioural effects, 150–151
neural mechanisms, 151

technical processes, 150
robotic therapy, 136
MIT-MANUS robot, 136
rTMS, 27–28, 62–64, 133–134
for acute stroke, 133–134
for chronic stroke, 134
low frequency, 63–64
for post-stroke depression, 111
stem cell therapy, 136–137
hNT, 136–137
neuroplasticity after, 30
for stroke rehabilitation, 82–83
tDCS, 27–28, 133
anodal, 134–135
cathodal, 135
cost benefits of, 134
long-term effects of, 135
for post-stroke depression, 111–112
transcranial stimulation techniques, 131–135. *See also* transcranial magnetic stimulation
abnormal interhemispheric balance, 131–132
contraindications, 135
individual targeting for, 135
placebo trials, 133
rTMS, 62–64, 133–134
safety of, 135
seizure risks, 135
tDCS, 133
visuomotor tracking training, 151–153
VR therapy, 151–153
behavioural effects, 152
with finger tracking training tasks, 152–153
for motor learning, 152
neural mechanisms, 152–153
for neuroplasticity, 27
technical processes, 151–152
akinetopsia, 178
alexia without agraphia, 180
ALS. *See* amyotrophic lateral sclerosis
amnesia, 124
D-amphetamine, 28
amphetamines, in adjunctive therapies, 129
inconsistency of effects, 129
safety issues, 129
AMT. *See* active motor threshold
amyotrophic lateral sclerosis (ALS), 30
animal models
adjunctive therapies, 128–129
multiple session outcomes, 128–129
pharmacological studies, 129
with physical therapies, 129
for attention rehabilitation, post-stroke, 199
EE treatment therapy in, 111
infarct-induced disconnections, recovery potential for, 81

ipsilateral representation of vision, 176
stem cell therapy in, 30
anodal tDCS, 134–135
anterior cingulate cortex (ACC), 197
antidepressant therapy, 214
aphasia, 225, 226
Complexity Account of Treatment Efficacy principle, 228
diffuse tractography studies for, 227
functional connectivity studies for, 227
neuroscientifically-based rehabilitation model, 227–228
apparent diffusion coefficient (ADC), 37–38
DWI, 46
AROC. *See* Australasian Rehabilitation Outcomes Centre
astrocyte therapy, 30–31
ALS, 30
neuronal synapse function, 31
supernumerary synapse reduction, 31
VEGF, 30
attention
brain lesions and, 197–198
Balint's syndrome, 180, 198
unilateral spatial neglect, 198
cortical anatomy, 191–192
"what" pathway, 192
"where" pathway, 192
deficits
depression and, 190–191, 197
from stroke, 190
definition, 191
learning and, 195
MSI and, 194–195
at cortical level, 194–195
processing, 194
in TPJ, 195
neuroplasticity and, 195
non-spatial, rehabilitation training for, 200
rehabilitation post-stroke for, 198–200
animal models, 199
for non-spatial attention, 200
with TBI, 200
with training, 199–200
selective, 196–197
ACC and, 197
emotional evaluation of stimuli, 197
motivational evaluation of stimuli, 196–197
working memory and, 195–196
TEA for, 215
visual system and, 192–194
DAN in, 192–193
LIP cortex in, 193
for new learning, 193–194
supramodal function in, 194
VAN in, 193
working memory and, 195–196
selective attention, 195–196

attention deficits, from stroke, 190
depression and, 190–191
auditing, of health care services, 100
in Australia, 100
in Canada, 100
for quality of care, 99–100
in UK, 100
Australasian Rehabilitation Outcomes Centre (AROC), 99
Australia, health care services in, 96
auditing of, 100
characteristics of, 97
community-based, 97
Rural Stroke Project, 98
UK compared to, 100

B

backward chaining, 122–123
BADS. *See* Behavioural Assessment of the Dysexecutive Syndrome
Balint's syndrome, 180, 198
BDNF. *See* brain-derived growth factor
Behavioural Assessment of the Dysexecutive Syndrome (BADS), 215
behavioural experience, stroke rehabilitation and, 11
learning-dependent neuroplasticity, 13
bilateral practice training, 153
biomarkers, for stroke rehabilitation, 7
blindsight, 180
MRI studies, 183
retinotopic mapping for, 183
Riddoch syndrome, 183
blood oxygenation level dependent (BOLD) image contrast, 39–41, 54
amplitude and duration of, 40
for CBF, 41
for CBV, 41
with CIMT, 147
deoxyhaemoglobin concentration, 39–40
for executive functions, 213–214
neuronal activity, 40–41
neurovascular coupling, 41
for $rCMRO_2$, 41
RSFC studies, 43, 42–43
signaling, 42
spatial resolution, 40
time-course of signal changes, 40
in TMS multimodal studies, 64, 65
bombardment rehabilitation, 166
botulinum toxin, 84
brain activation maps, 7
brain-derived growth factor (BDNF), 31–32
brain function. *See also* executive function/dysfunction

brain function (Cont.)
    for attention, cortical anatomy, 191–192
        "what" pathway, 192
        "where" pathway, 192
    cortical networks
        after brain injury, 24–25
        executive functions, 208
        after spinal cord injury, 24–25
        stroke rehabilitation and, 8, 13–14
    focal lesions, 242–243
    frontal lobe, 209, 210–211
    learning-dependent neuroplasticity, by region, 13
    MRI for, 39–41
        BOLD image contrast, 39–41
    with post-stroke depression, changes in, 109–110
        cognition, 110
        cortical networks, 110
        functional, 109
        morphological, 110
        WMH, 110
        working model of, 109
    RSFC studies
        activation studies compared to, 43
        BOLD contrast imaging, 42–43
        episodic memory, 43
        ICA, 43
        language processing, 43
    task-specific training, regional activation, 116–117
        with active movements, 117
        MEPs during, 116
        with passive movements, 117
        SI activation, 117
    white matter
        DTI in, 45–46
        DWI in, 44–45
        tractography, 47–49
brain infarcts, after stroke
    in Type I strokes, 77, 78
    in Type II strokes, 77, 78
    in Type III strokes, 77, 78
    in Type IV strokes, 77, 78
    functional consequences of, 78–79
    interhemispheric connectivity alterations, 78–79
    intracortical excitability, 78
    lesions from, 78
        focal, 242–243
    after thrombolysis, 76, 77
brain injury, neuroplasticity after
    contralesional hemisphere, 25, 26
    cortical map rearrangements, 24–25
    corticospinal remodeling, 25–26
    SI, 24
    spontaneous recovery, 24
brain lesions
    attention and, 197–198
        Balint's syndrome, 180, 198
        unilateral spatial neglect, 198
    from infarcts, 78
        focal lesions, 242–243
    lateral geniculate nucleus, 179
    neuroimaging, 38–39
        limitations, 38–39
        mapping of, 39
        with MRI, 38
        VBM, 39
    recovery potential with, 81–82
brain perfusion, neuroimaging for, 35–37
    CT, 36, 37
    early development, 35–36
    MRI, 36–37
    rCBF, 35–36

brain stimulation. See noninvasive brain stimulation; repetitive transcranial magnetic stimulation; transcranial direct current stimulation
brain structure
    learning-dependent neuroplasticity and, 13
    stroke rehabilitation and
        cortical network changes, 8
        information processing recovery, 13–14
        neuroimaging for, 8
Broca's area, 224

C
Canada, health care services in, 96
    auditing guidelines, 100
    Telehealth, 97
    uptake of evidence in clinical practice, 101–102
Canadian Occupational Performance Measure (COPM), 244
CAP model. See computation-anatomy-psychology model
care. See health care, organization of
caregivers, role in rehabilitation, 96
cathodal tDCS, 135
CBF. See cerebral blood flow
CBV. See cerebral blood volume
central nervous system (CNS)
    neuroplasticity and, 24
    transfer of training phenomena, 123
cerebellum, 159
cerebral blood flow (CBF), 41
cerebral blood volume (CBV), 41
cerebral cortex, neuroplasticity and, 24
chaining technique, 15
cholinergic agents, in adjunctive therapies, 130
    AChE inhibitors, 130
chronic stroke, 134
CIAT. See constraint induced aphasia treatment
CIMT. See constraint induced movement therapy
cingulo-opercular network, 211–212
CIT. See constraint induced therapy
CNS. See central nervous system
cognitive capacity
    after NIBS, 28
    after stroke, 190–191
        post-stroke depression, 110
Cognitive Orientation to Daily Occupational Performance (CO-OP) therapy, 19
    for executive function, after stroke, 19
    task-specific skills acquisition in, 19
Cognitive Rehabilitation Research Group (CRRG), 209
colour perception, 178
community-based rehabilitation, 95
    in Australia, 97
    ESD, 95
    Telehealth, 95
    in UK, 97
compensation
    definition of, 5
    recovery compared to, 5
Complexity Account of Treatment Efficacy principle, 228
comprehensive stroke units, 94
computation-anatomy-psychology (CAP) model, 209
computed tomography (CT), 36, 37

constraint induced aphasia treatment (CIAT), 12, 20, 226–227
    shaping technique in, 20
constraint induced movement therapy (CIMT), 8, 12, 145–147
    behavioural effects, 145
    with fMRI, 146
    neural mechanisms, 145–147
    neuroimaging, 146–147
        with BOLD image contrast, 147
        with fMRI, 146
    neuroplasticity after, 6–7
    technical processes, 145
constraint induced therapy (CIT), 130
contralesional hemisphere, 25
    axonal remodeling, 26
    fMRI, 25
    transcranial stimulation techniques, 131–132
        abnormal interhemispheric balance, 131
CO-OP. See Cognitive Orientation to Daily Occupational Performance therapy
COPM. See Canadian Occupational Performance Measure
cortical networks, in brain
    after brain injury, 24–25
    executive functions, 208
    focal lesions, 242–243
    with post-stroke depression, 110
    after spinal cord injury, 24–25
    stroke rehabilitation and, 8
        information processing recovery, 13–14
corticospinal tract (CST), 234
crossed corticospinal tract (CST), 234
CRRG. See Cognitive Rehabilitation Research Group
CST. See corticospinal tract
CT. See computed tomography

D
DAN. See dorsal frontoparietal attention network
DEFUSE trial. See Diffusion and Perfusion Imaging Evaluation For Understanding Stroke Evolution trial
deliberate anticipation, in somatosensory recovery, 164
depression, post-stroke
    age factors for, 107
    assessment of, 107
    attention deficits and, 190–191, 197
    brain changes with, 109–110
        in cognition, 110
        in cortical networks, 110
        functional, 109
        morphological, 110
        WMH, 110
        working model of, 109
    clinical indications for, 106
    etiology of, 107–108
    frequency of, 106–107
    impact outcomes, 107
    MADRS for, 107
    overdiagnosis of, 108
    predictors of, 108–109
        inflammatory cytokines, 109
        serotonin polymorphism, 109
    as specific disorder, 108
    treatment therapies, 110–112
        EE, 111

non-pharmalogical, 111
    with physical activity, 112
    rTMS, 111
    SSRIs, 110–111
    tDCS, 111–112
    WHO ranking of, 106
Diffusion and Perfusion Imaging Evaluation For Understanding Stroke Evolution (DEFUSE) trial, 79
diffusion tensor imaging (DTI), 44, 45–46
    in white matter, 45–46
diffusion-weighted imaging (DWI), 37–38, 44–49
    ADC, 37–38
    biological parameter estimation, 46–49
        ADC, 46
        FA, 46
        fiber orientation, 47
    DTI and, 44, 45–46
        in white matter, 45–46
    higher order models, 46
        HARDI data, 46
    in stroke rehabilitation, 49
    structural connectivity, 44
    tractography, 47–49
        FACT algorithm, 48
        FOD, 48
    in white matter, 44–45
direct cortical stimulation, 135–136
direct teaching, 16
donepezil, 130
    in CIT, 130
dopamine augmentation, in executive function rehabilitation, 212–213
dopaminergic agents, in adjunctive therapies, 130
dorsal frontoparietal attention network (DAN), 192–193
DTI. See diffusion tensor imaging
DWI. See diffusion-weighted imaging

E
Early Supported Discharge (ESD), 95
Echoplanar Imaging Thrombolytic Evaluation Trial (EPITHET), 79
ECoG. See electrocorticography
EEG. See electroencephalography
EE therapy. See enriched environment therapy
EFPT. See Executive Function Performance Test
electrocorticography (ECoG), 66
electroencephalography (EEG), 55–60
    baseline physical fitness factors, 56–57
    conductivity values, 55–56
    development of, 55
    electrode localization, 56
    ERD, 57
    ERS, 57
    handedness and, 57
    head models, 55
    methodology, 55–58
        coherence measures, 57–58
        motor system reorganization, 56–57
        with MRI, 56
    mu rhythms, 57
    neurophysiological rhythms, 57–58
    single trial analysis, 57
    site recording, 55
    source modeling of data, 55–56
    TMS stimulation, 58

multimodal studies, sensorimotor cortex activity, 57, 58–60
  activation paradigms, 59
  contralateral limb monitoring, 59–60
  data analysis, 59
  fMRI compared to, 59
  stroke rehabilitation, 57–58
electromyogram (EMG) feedback, 148–150
  behavioural effects, 148–149
  for finger tracking training tasks, 150
  neural mechanisms, 149–150
  neuroimaging for, 149–150
  technical processes, 148
electrostimulation (ES), 148–150
  behavioural effects, 148–149
  for finger tracking training tasks, 150
  neural mechanisms, 149–150
  neuroimaging for, 149
  neuroprosthetic, 149
  technical processes, 148
EMG. *See* electromyogram feedback
enriched environment (EE) therapy
  definition of, 111
  for neuroplasticity improvement, 26–27
  for post-stroke depression, 111
  in animal models, 111
episodic memory, RSFC studies and, 43
EPITHET. *See* Echoplanar Imaging Thrombolytic Evaluation Trial
EPO. *See* erythropoietin
ERD. *See* event-related desynchronization
ERS. *See* event-related synchronization
erythropoietin (EPO), 137
ES. *See* electrostimulation
ESD. *See* Early Supported Discharge
event-related desynchronization (ERD), 57
event-related synchronization (ERS), 57
executive function/dysfunction
  CAP model, 209
  components of, 210
  cortical networks for, 208
  definition of, 208
  frontal lobe functions and, 209, 210–211
  measurement tests for, 214–217
    BADS, 215
    behaviour-related, 215–216
    brain-related, 215
    EFPT, 216–217
    Kettle Test, 217
    Multiple Errand Test, 217
    Patient Competency Rating Scale, 215–216
    performance-based, 216–217
    TEA, 215
    Trail Making Test, 215
    WAIS-IV, 215
    WCST, 215
  neural substrates of, 211–214
    antidepressant therapy, 214
    cingulo-opercular network, 211–212
    fronto-parietal network, 211
    rehabilitative interventions, 214
    top-down control from, 211–212
  neuroimaging for, 213–214
  MRI, 214
  performance-based approach to, 208
  purpose of, 208–209
  rehabilitation interventions, 217–218
    at behavioural level, 217–218

CO-OP therapy, 218
  dopamine augmentation, 212–213
  GMT, 217
  neurofunctional retraining approach, 217–218
  at performance level, 218
  strategy learning and awareness approach, 218
  research study on, 209
  future directions for, 218–219
Executive Function Performance Test (EFPT), 216–217
explicit learning, 123–124
  with amnesia, 124
  motor learning and, 124
explicit skills acquisition, after stroke, 15–16
extrageniculostriate pathway, 175–176
  components, 175–176
  efferents in, 176
extrastriate cortex pathway, 177
  akinetopsia, 178
  movement perception, 178
  visual object recognition, 177–178
  visual recovery rehabilitation, 181–182

F

FA. *See* fractional anisotropy
FACT algorithm. *See* fiber assignment continuous tracking algorithm
fading, in skills acquisition, 15
feedback, for skills acquisition, 18
feedback programs
  EMG, 148–150
    behavioural effects, 148–149
    for finger tracking training tasks, 150
    neural mechanisms, 149–150
    neuroimaging for, 149–150
    technical processes, 148
  graded exercises, for somatosensory system recovery, 166
  skills acquisition, after stroke, 16, 18
fiber assignment continuous tracking (FACT) algorithm, 48
fiber orientation distribution (FOD), 48
finger tracking training tasks, 150
  with VR therapy, 152–153
F-fluorodeoxyglucose, 38
fluoxetine, 28–29
fMRI. *See* functional magnetic resonance imaging
focal lesions, 242–243
FOD. *See* fiber orientation distribution
fovea-macular projection, 174
fractional anisotropy (FA), 46, 46
  for motor capacity rehabilitation, 235
frontal lobe, functions of, 209, 210–211
fronto-parietal network, 211
functional magnetic resonance imaging (fMRI), 41–44
  BOLD image contrast, 39–41, 54
    amplitude and duration of, 40
    for CBF, 41
    for CBV, 41
    with CIMT, 147
    deoxyhaemoglobin concentration, 39–40
    for executive functions, 213–214
    neuronal activity, 40–41
    neurovascular coupling, 41
    for rCMRO$_2$, 41
    RSFC studies, 42–43
    signaling, 42
    spatial resolution, 40
    time-course of signal changes, 40

in TMS multimodal studies, 64, 65, 65
  CIMT with, 146
  contralesional hemisphere, 25
  EEG compared to, in sensorimotor cortex studies, 59
  experimental design, 41–42
    block-design, 41
    event-related, 41–42
  language processes, 223, 224–225
  limitations of, 54, 58–59
  ME compared to, in sensorimotor cortex studies, 59
  for neuronal activity, 54
  perilesional tissue, 81
  RSFC studies
    activation studies compared to, 43
    BOLD contrast imaging, 42–43
    episodic memory, 43
    ICA, 43
    language processing, 43
    for stroke rehabilitation, 7, 43–44
      limitations, 43–44
      of motor learning, 54
  task-related activation studies, 41–42
    RSFC studies compared to, 43

G

G-CSF. *See* granulocyte-colony stimulating factor
generalized motor program (GMP), 123
geniculostriate pathway, 175
  arterial support, 175
  primary visual cortex, 175
  topographical structure, 175
genotypes, neurorehabilitation with, 238
GMP. *See* generalized motor program
GMT. *See* goal management training
goal directed action
  in stroke rehabilitation
    neuroplasticity and, 26
    somatosensory system processing, 163–164
  vision and, 191
goal-driven skills acquisition
  learning-dependent neuroplasticity, 13
  after stroke, 15–16
goal management training (GMT), 217
granulocyte-colony stimulating factor (G-CSF), 137
guided discovery, 16

H

HARDI data. *See* high angular resolution DW imaging data
health care, organization of
  access to, 97–99
  auditing of, 100
    in Australia, 100
    in Canada, 100
    for quality of care, 99–100
    in UK, 100
  in Australia, 96
    auditing practices, 100
    characteristics of, 97
    community-based, 97
    Rural Stroke Project, 98
    UK compared to, 100
  in Canada, 96
    auditing guidelines, 100
    Telehealth, 97
    uptake of evidence models in, for clinical practice, 101–102
  caregivers' role in, 96
  community-based, 95

ESD, 95
  Telehealth, 95
  in UK, 97
  innovations in, 102, 103
  inpatient care, 94. *See also* stroke units
    timing of rehabilitation, 94
  interdisciplinary approach, 98–99
  purpose of, 93
  quality of care, 99–103
    auditing practices, 99–100
    improvement programs, 103
    monitoring guidelines, 99–100
    in U.S., 99
  rehabilitation models, 94–97
    alternative, 95–96
    community-based, 95
    inpatient care, 94
    mixed methods in, 96
    stroke care pathways, 95–96
  services in, characteristics of, 96–97
    in Australia, 97
    in Canada, 96
  staffing resources, 98–99
  in UK
    auditing of services, 100
    Australian compared, 100
    community-based, 97
    uptake of evidence in clinical practice, 101–103
    in Canadian models, 101–102
    Knowledge to Action model for, 101
    pay-for-performance model, 101
Hebb, Donald, 13, 111
high angular resolution DW imaging (HARDI) data, 46
human teratocarcinoma (hNT), 136–137
hypoglycaemia, 191
hypoxia, 191

I

ICA. *See* independent component analysis
ICF. *See* intracortical facilitation
IHI. *See* interhemispheric inhibition
implicit learning, 123–124
  with amnesia, 124
  motor learning and, 124
independent component analysis (ICA), 43
individualized therapies
  neuroplasticity levels, 31–32, 245
    BDNF, 31–32
    genetic analysis, 31–32
  post-stroke rehabilitation, 244–245
    COPM, 244
    brain networks links in, 245
    neuroplasticity levels in, 31–32, 31–32, 245
    somatosensory system, 168
    mind, brain, body approach in, 245
  in transcranial stimulation techniques, 135
information processing, recovery of, 13–14
  neuroimaging for, 13–14
inosine therapy, 29
inpatient care models, 94
  with stroke units, 94
    comprehensive, 94
    mixed rehabilitation, 94
    rehabilitation, 94
  timing of rehabilitation, 94
insula, in somatosensory system, 159
interhemispheric inhibition (IHI), 62
  motor capacity rehabilitation, 235

intermittent theta burst stimulation (iTBS), 132–133
intracortical facilitation (ICF), 62
iTBS. *See* intermittent theta burst stimulation

J

James, William, 191

K

Kettle Test, 217
Knowledge to Action model, 101

L

language
  aphasia, 225, 226
    Complexity Account of Treatment Efficacy principle, 227–228
    diffuse tractography studies for, 227
    functional connectivity studies for, 227
    neuroscientifically-based rehabilitation model, 227–228
  Broca's area, 224
  CIAT, 12, 20
    in rehabilitation therapies, 226–227
    shaping technique in, 20
  lesion-symptom mapping of, 222
    with neuroimaging, 222
  neuroimaging of, 223–225
    fMRI, 223, 224–225
    lesion-symptom mapping with, 222
    MEG, 223
    with melodic intonation therapy, 223
    PET, 223
    white matter tractography, 223–224
  neuroscience of, 222
  perfusion-symptom mapping of, 222
  rehabilitation, after stroke, 225–226
    for aphasia, 225, 226, 227–228
    CIAT, 226–227
    cognitive neurolinguistic approach, 226
    cognitive neuropsychological approach, 225–226
    constraints in, 7
    practice intensity levels, 226–227
    remediation therapies, 225
    treatment principles, neuroscientifically-guided approach to, 226–227, 227–228
    TUF, 226
  RSFC studies, 43
  TMS for, 223
  Wernicke model for, 222
  Wernicke's area, 224
lateral geniculate nucleus (LGN), 174–175
  lesions, 179
lateral intraparietal (LIP) cortex, 193
learned non-use, 6, 12, 83
learning-based rehabilitation. *See also* task-specific training
  explicit learning in, 123–124
    with amnesia, 124
    motor learning and, 124
  goals of, 116
  implicit learning in, 123–124
    with amnesia, 124
    motor learning and, 124
  key clinical messages of, 124
  motor learning, 120–123
    backward chaining, 122–123

definition, 118
  GMP, 123
  mental practices for, 120–121
  neuroplasticity and, 118–119
  part-whole training strategies, 122–123
  repetitions in, 119, 121
  task-specific training, 118–119
  transfer of training effects, 121–123
learning-dependent neuroplasticity, 6, 13
  for attention, 195
  by brain region, 13
  experience effects, 13
  as goal-driven, 13
  Hebbian learning, 13
  motor learning and, 13
  in stroke rehabilitation, 6
  as task-oriented, 13
  task-specific rehabilitation training, 13
  as time-dependent, 13
lesions. *See* brain lesions; focal lesions
lesion-symptom mapping, of language, 222
  with neuroimaging, 222
levodopa, 130
LGN. *See* lateral geniculate nucleus
LIP cortex. *See* lateral intraparietal cortex
long-term depression (LTD), 13
long-term potentiation (LTP), 13
LTD. *See* long-term depression
LTP. *See* long-term potentiation

M

MADRS. *See* Montgomery-Asberg Depression Rating Scale
magnetic resonance imaging (MRI). *See also* functional magnetic resonance imaging
  for blindsight, 183
  BOLD image contrast, 39–41, 54
    amplitude and duration of, 40
    for CBF, 41
    for CBV, 41
    with CIMT, 147
    deoxyhaemoglobin concentration, 39–40
    for executive functions, 213–214
    neuronal activity, 40–41
    neurovascular coupling, 41
    for rCMRO$_2$, 41
    RSFC studies, 42–43
    signaling, 42
    spatial resolution, 40
    time-course of signal changes, 40
    in TMS multimodal studies, 64, 65
  brain function, 39–41
    BOLD image contrast, 39–41
  brain lesions, 38
  brain perfusion, 36–37
  DWI, 37–38
    ADC, 37–38
  EEG data, 56
  for executive functions, 214
  MEG data, 56
  for stroke rehabilitation, 7
  visual recovery studies, 183–184
    for blindsight, 183
    for visual field defects, 184
magnetoencephalography (MEG), 55–60
  baseline physical fitness factors, 56–57
  conductivity values, 55–56
  development of, 55
  handedness and, 57
  head models, 55

language processes, 223
  methodology, 55–58
    coherence measures, 57–58
    motor system reorganization, 56–57
    with MRI, 56
    mu rhythms, 57
    neurophysiological rhythms, 57–58
    single trial analysis, 57
    site recording, 55
    source modeling of data, 55–56
    TMS stimulation, 58
  multimodal studies, sensorimotor cortex activity, 57, 58–60
    activation paradigms, 59
    contralateral limb monitoring, 59–60
    data analysis, 59
    fMRI compared to, 59
    RF for, 56
  sensorimotor cortex and, 57
  stroke rehabilitation, 57–58
MCA stroke. *See* middle cerebral artery stroke
MEG. *See* magnetoencephalography
melodic intonation therapy, 223
memory
  episodic, RSFC studies and, 43
  working
    attention and, 195–196
    subtypes, 195
mental health. *See* depression, post-stroke
mental practices, 147–148
  behavioural effects, 147–148
  for motor learning, 120–121
    observational learning, 120
  neural mechanisms, 148
  technical processes, 147
mental training, as therapy, 27, 83–84
MEP. *See* motor evoked potential
metaplasticity, 13
middle cerebral artery (MCA) stroke, 179–180
mirror neurons, 120
mirror therapy, 27
MIT-MANUS robot, 136
mixed rehabilitation stroke units, 94
modeling, for skills acquisition, 15–16
Montgomery-Asberg Depression Rating Scale (MADRS), 107
motor capacity
  definition, 118
  learning-dependent neuroplasticity, 13
  after NIBS, 28
  rehabilitation for, 5
    connectivity measurement in, 233–237
    CST integrity, 234
    FA values, 235
    with fMRI, 54
    functional integrity of pathways, 234–235
    IHI, 235
    for lower limbs, algorithmic predictions, 236–237
    through motor learning principles, 8
    neuroimaging of, 235–236
    uncrossed corticospinal tract, 234–235
    for upper limbs, algorithmic predictions, 236
  restoration of, 5
  task-oriented motor training, 12
  TMS measurement, 60–62
    AMT, 60

cortical silent period, 62
  ICF, 62
  IHI, 62
  input-output curves, 62
  motor thresholds, 60
  SICI, 62
motor evoked potential (MEP), 60–62
  amplitude, 60–61
  central motor conduction time, 61–62
  latency, 61–62
  in multimodal studies, for stroke recovery, 64–65
  during task-specific training, 116
motor learning, 120–121
  backward chaining, 122–123
  definition, 118
  explicit learning and, 124
  GMP, 123
  implicit learning and, 124
  mental practices for, 120–121
    observational learning, 120
  neuroplasticity and, 118–119
  part-whole training strategies, 122–123
  repetitions in, 121
    in neurorehabilitation, 121
    in task-specific training, 119
  task-specific training, 118–119
    repetition intensity, 119
  transfer of training effects, 121–123
    for CNS, 123
    neuroimaging results, 123
    variability of practice, 122
  VR therapy for, 152
MRI. *See* magnetic resonance imaging
Multiple Errand Test, 217
multisensory integration (MSI), 194–195
  at cortical level, 194–195
  processing, 194
  in TPJ, 194
mu rhythms, 57
music therapy, 27

N

National Institute of Neurological Disorders and Health, 5
National Stroke Audit of Rehabilitation Services, 4
near-infrared spectroscopy (NIRS), 66–67
network-based models of recovery, for post-stroke rehabilitation, 243–244
neurofunctional retraining therapy, 217–218
neuroimaging. *See also* computed tomography; diffusion-weighted imaging; electroencephalography; functional magnetic resonance imaging; magnetic resonance imaging; magnetoencephalography; positron emission tomography; transcranial magnetic stimulation
  brain lesions, 38–39
    limitations, 38–39
    mapping of, 39
    VBM, 39
  brain perfusion, 35–37
    CT, 37
    early development, 35–36
    MRI, 37
    rCBF, 35–36
    with CIMT, 146–147
    development of, 35
    DWI, 44–49
    for EMG feedback, 149–150
    for ES, 149

for information processing recovery, 13–14
neuroimaging for, 13–14
of language processes, 223–225
fMRI, 223, 224–225
lesion-symptom mapping with, 222
with melodic intonation therapy, 223
white matter tractography, 223–224
motor capacity rehabilitation, 235, 235–236
rCMRO₂, 38
F-fluorodeoxyglucose, 38
for stroke rehabilitation, 7–8
of biomarkers, 7
brain activation maps, 7
for brain structure changes, 8
cortical networks, 8
functions of, 7
neuroplasticity changes, 7–8
for transfer of training, in motor learning, 123
neuroplasticity, 3
activity-dependent, 13
as adaptive, 6
astrocyte therapy, 30–31
ALS, 30
neuronal synapse function, 31
supernumerary synapse reduction, 31
VEGF, 30
attention and, with learning, 195
after brain and spinal cord injury, 24–26
contralesional hemisphere, 25, 26
cortical map rearrangements, 24–25
corticospinal remodeling, 25–26
SI, 24
spontaneous recovery, 24
cerebral cortex and, 24
CNS and, 24
definition, 5–6
future research study for, 247
individualized therapy strategies, 31–32, 245
BDNF, 31–32
genetic analysis, 31–32
learned non-use, 6
learning-dependent, 6, 13
by brain region, 13
experience effects, 13
as goal-driven, 13
Hebbian learning, 13
motor learning and, 13
in stroke rehabilitation, 6
as task-oriented, 13
task-specific rehabilitation training, 13
as time-dependent, 13
metaplasticity, 13
motor learning and, 118–119
NIBS for, 27–28
cognitive recovery, 28
motor recovery, 28
with rTMS, 27–28
with tDCS, 27–28
after RTT, 144–145
stem cell therapy, 30
in animal models, 30
neurogenesis, 30
stroke rehabilitation and, 5–7
animal studies, 6
behavioural experience, 11
CIMT, 6–7
constraint in language training, 7
fitness training, 26

goal-setting, 26
implications, 26
interventions for, 6–7
learning-dependent, 6
mitigating factors, 7
motivation engagement, 26
multidisciplinary teams for, 26
multimodal training and stimulation, 26
neuroimaging for, changes under, 7–8
post-hospital therapy, 26
spontaneous recovery, 24
task-specific approach, 26
timing of therapy, 26
therapy strategies, 26–31
D-amphetamine, 28
EE, 26–27
fluoxetine, 28–29
individualized, 31–32, 245
inosine, 29
mental training, 27
mirror therapy, 27
multimodal training and stimulation, 26–27
with music, 27
niacin, 29
Nogo-A inhibition, 29–30
pharmacological, 28–30
Sig-1R, 28
SSRIs, 28–29
stem cell, 30
tonic inhibition reduction, 30
with VR, 27
use-dependent, 6, 13
LTD, 13
LTP, 13
in stroke rehabilitation, 6
for visual recovery, after stroke, 180
cross-modal, 181–182
extrastriate pathway, 181–182
neuroprosthetics, 136
neurorehabilitation, 5
brain-computer interface interventions, 66–67
definition of, 11
future research study for, 238
motor learning repetitions, 121
priming approaches, 237–238
through genotypes, 238
Rehab-Learn model, 17–18
SENSe approach, 19–20
calibration in, 19
principles, 19–20
stroke rehabilitation and, 11
niacin therapy, 29
NIBS. See noninvasive brain stimulation
nicotinic acid. See niacin
NIRS. See near-infrared spectroscopy
Nogo-A receptors, inhibition of, 29–30
noninvasive brain stimulation (NIBS), 27–28
cognitive recovery, 28
motor recovery, 28
rTMS, 27–28
for post-stroke depression, 111
tDCS, 27–28
for post-stroke depression, 111–112
non-spatial attention, rehabilitation training for, 200

O

observational learning, 120
organization of care. See health care, organization of

P

parahippocampal place (PPA), 178
part-whole training strategies, 122–123
passive stimulation rehabilitation, 166
Patient Competency Rating Scale, 215–216
pay-for-performance model, 101
PCA stroke. See posterior cerebral artery stroke
penumbra, after stroke, 75–76, 79
recovery potential, 79
DEFUSE trial, 79
EPITHET for, 79
perceptual learning approach, to stroke rehabilitation, 8, 167
perilesional tissue, 79–81
fMRI for, 81
TMS for, 80
PET. See positron emission tomography
physical therapy, for stroke rehabilitation, 83
animal models, with adjunctive therapies, 129
learned non-use, 6, 12, 83
for post-stroke depression, 112
positron emission tomography (PET)
language processes, 223
rCMRO₂, 38
visual recovery studies, 182–183
posterior cerebral artery (PCA) stroke, 179–180
posterior parietal cortex (PPC), 159
PPA. See parahippocampal place
PPC. See posterior parietal cortex
primary somatosensory cortex (SI), 24, 158–159
during task-specific training, 117
prompting, in skills acquisition, 15
prosopagnosia, 180

Q

quality of life, after stroke, 4

R

radio frequency (RF), 56
rCBF. See regional cerebral blood flow
rCMRO₂. See regional cerebral metabolism of oxygen
recovery
compensation compared to, 5
definitions, 5
measurement guidelines, 5
regional cerebral blood flow (rCBF), 35–36
regional cerebral metabolism of oxygen (rCMRO₂), 38
BOLD image contrast, 41
F-fluorodeoxyglucose, 38
PET, 38
rehabilitation. See also health care, organization of
caregivers' role in, 96
community-based, 95
in Australia, 97
ESD, 95
Telehealth, 95
in UK, 97
Stroke Rehab Definitions Conceptual Framework guidelines, 5
WHO definition, 5
rehabilitation, post-stroke. See also adjunctive therapies; health care, organization of; inpatient care models; skills acquisition, after stroke
adaptive learning, 11–12

adjunctive approaches, 17
for attention, 198–200
animal models, 199
non-spatial, 200
with TBI, 200
with training, 199–200
biomarkers for, 7
brain structure, 8
cortical network changes, 8
neuroimaging for, 8
CIAT, 12, 20
for language processes, 226–227
shaping technique, 20
CIMT, 8, 12, 145–147
behavioural effects, 145
with fMRI, 146
neural mechanisms, 145–147
for neuroplasticity, 6–7
neuroplasticity after, 6–7
technical processes, 145
clinical practice guidelines, 4, 240–242
evidence translation, 245–246
community-based, 95
in Australia, 97
ESD, 95
Telehealth, 95
in UK, 97
compensatory approaches, 12
learned non-use, 6, 12
contextual application of, 17
CO-OP, 19
task-specific skills acquisition in, 19
definition, 5, 11
DWI in, 49
EEG in, 57–58
for executive functions, 217–218
at behavioural level, 217–218
CO-OP therapy, 218
dopamine augmentation, 212–213
GMT, 217
neurofunctional retraining approach, 217–218
at performance level, 218
strategy learning and awareness approach, 218
fMRI, 7, 43–44
limitations, 43–44
for motor learning, 54
focal lesions and, 242–243
functional outcomes, 11
funding models of, 95
future research study for, 246–248
with common methodology, 247
with longitudinal studies, 247
on multimodal approaches, 247
for neuroscientific-based interventions, 247
parallel animal/human model studies, 248
for plasticity-enhancing interventions, 247
for specific recovery functions, 247
goal directed action in
neuroplasticity and, 26
somatosensory system processing, 163–164
impacting factors for, 190–191
as impairment category, 4
individualized, 244–245
COPM, 244
brain networks links in, 245
neuroplasticity levels in, 31–32, 245
mind, brain, body approach in, 245
information processing recovery, 13–14

rehabilitation (Cont.)
  of language processes, 225–226
    for aphasia, 225, 226, 227–228
      CIAT, 226–227
      cognitive neurolinguistic approach, 226
      cognitive neuropsychological approach, 225–226
      constraints in, 7
      practice intensity levels, 226–227
      remediation therapies, 225
      treatment principles, neuroscientifically-guided approach to, 226–227, 227–228
      TUF, 226
  learning-dependent neuroplasticity in, 6
  MEG in, 57–58
  mental training therapy, 27, 83–84
  motor capacity, 5
    connectivity measurement in, 233–237
    CST integrity, 234
    FA values, 235
    functional integrity of pathways, 234–235
    IHI, 235
    for lower limbs, algorithmic predictions, 236–237
    through motor learning principles, 8
    neuroimaging of, 235–236
    restoration of, 5
    uncrossed corticospinal tract, 234–235
    for upper limbs, algorithmic predictions, 236
  National Institute of Neurological Disorders and Health guidelines, 5
  network-based models of recovery, 243–244
  neuroimaging, 7–8
    of biomarkers, 7
    brain activation maps, 7
    for brain structure changes, 8
    cortical networks, 8
    functions of, 7
    information processing recovery, 13–14
    neuroplasticity changes, 7–8
  neuroplasticity and, 5–7
    animal studies, 6
    behavioural experience, 11
    CIMT, 6–7
    constraint in language training, 7
    fitness training, 26
    goal-setting, 26
    implications, 26
    interventions for, 6–7
    learning-dependent, 6
    mitigating factors, 7
    motivation engagement, 26
    multidisciplinary teams for, 26
    multimodal training and stimulation, 26
    neuroimaging for, changes under, 7–8
    post-hospital therapy, 26
    spontaneous recovery, 24
    task-specific approach, 26
    timing of therapy, 26
    use-dependent, 6
  neurorehabilitation and, 11
  physical therapy in, 83
    learned non-use, 6, 12, 83
  recovery potential, 79–84
    from animal models, 81

from brain lesions, 81–82
  infarct-induced disconnections, 81–82
  for interhemispheric interactions, 82
  with mental training, 27, 83–84
  for motor cortical connectivity, 81
  penumbra, 79
  perilesional plasticity, 79–81
  with physical therapy, 6, 12, 83, 83
  with stem cell therapy, 82–83
Rehab-Learn model, 12, 17–18, 21
  adjunct therapies, 18
  environmental context, 18
  learning gaps, 17
  learning principles, 17–18
  skill specific strategies, 18
  environment/context, 18
  outcomes, 18
  skills acquisition, 18
SENSe approach, 19–20
  calibration in, 19
  principles, 19–20
somatosensory system, 5
  attended stimulation of specific sites, 166
  bombardment rehabilitation, 166
  core sensory network identification in, 168
  cortical network manipulation, 168
  deliberate anticipation in, 164
  goal-directed attentive processing, 163–164
  graded exercises with feedback, 166
  graded progression in, 165
  individual targeting in, 168
  lesion impact and, 168
  neuroscience-based models, 168, 246
  passive stimulation, 166
  processing-related networks, 168
  sensorimotor exercises, 166
  sensory discrimination approach, 166–167
  stimulus specific training, 165, 167
  task discrimination in, 164
  with transfer enhanced programs, 165, 167
  treatment principles, 162–165
spasticity in, botulinum toxin for, 84
stem cell therapy in, 82–83
task-oriented motor training, 12
therapy strategies
  mental training, 27, 83–84
  physical, 6, 12, 83
  stem cell therapy, 82–83
thrombolysis, 76
  brain infarcts after, 76, 77
timelines for, 84
  activities of daily living, 84
time windows for, 5
TMS studies, 64–66
  with BOLD fMRI, 64, 65
  MEP, 64–65
visual recovery, 180–182. See also blindsight
  acute phase, 180
  chronic phase, 180
  extrastriate pathway, 181–182
  hypotheses for, 182–184
  kinetic stimuli in, 184–185
  mechanisms, 180–181
  MRI studies, 183–184
  neuroplasticity, 180, 181–182
  oedema resolution, 180
  PET studies, 182–183
  prevalence rates, 180–181

restorative therapies, 184–185
  spared islands of tissue concept, 182
  VRT, 185
rehabilitation science, 12–13
  language for, 12
rehabilitation stroke units, 94
Rehab-Learn model, 12, 17–18, 21
  adjunct therapies, 18
  environmental context, 18
  learning gaps, 17
  learning principles, 17–18
  skill specific strategies, 18
  environment/context, 18
  outcomes, 18
  skills acquisition, 18
reinforcement, for skills acquisition, 16
repetitive task-specific training (RTT), 143–145
  behavioural effects, 143
  for lower limb function, 144
  neural mechanisms, 143–145
  neuroplasticity after, 144–145
  technical processes, 143
  for upper limb function, 144
repetitive transcranial magnetic stimulation (rTMS), 27–28, 62–64, 133–134
  for acute stroke, 133–134
  for chronic stroke, 134
  low frequency, 63–64
  for post-stroke depression, 111
resting-state functional connectivity (RSFC) studies
  activation studies compared to, 43
  BOLD contrast imaging, 42–43
  episodic memory, 43
  ICA, 43
  language processing, 43
  for somatosensory system recovery, 161–162
restitution, 5. See also restoration
restoration
  of motor capacity, 5
  of somatosensory capacity, 5
retinogeniculate pathway, 173–175
  LGN, 174–175
  lesions, 179
retinotopic mapping, 183
RF. See radio frequency
Riddoch syndrome, 183
robot-assisted training, 150–151
  advantages, 150
  behavioural effects, 150–151
  neural mechanisms, 151
  technical processes, 150
robotic therapy, 136, 150
  MIT-MANUS robot, 136
RSFC. See resting-state functional connectivity studies
rTMS. See repetitive transcranial magnetic stimulation
RTT. See repetitive task-specific training
Rural Stroke Project, 98

S
Schuell, Hildred, 225
secondary somatosensory cortex (SII), 159
seizure risk, with transcranial stimulation techniques, 135
selective attention, 196–197
  ACC and, 197
  emotional evaluation of stimuli, 197
  motivational evaluation of stimuli, 196–197
  working memory and, 195–196

selective serotonin reuptake inhibitors (SSRIs), 28–29
  in adjunctive therapies, 130
  for post-stroke depression, 110–111
sensations. See somatosensations; somatosensory system
SENSe approach. See Study of the Effectiveness of Neurorehabilitation on Sensation approach
sensorimotor cortex
  EEG/MEG multimodal studies, 57, 58–60
    activation paradigms, 59
    contralateral limb monitoring, 59–60
    data analysis, 59
    fMRI compared to, 59
  exercises, in somatosensory recovery, 166
  task-specific training as influence on, 117–118
    object size, 118
    task intention, 118
    timing adjustments, 118
sensory maps, 160
sensory perception, 157
Sentinel Stroke Audit Program, 99–100
serotonin
  post-stroke depression and, 109
  SSRIs, 28–29
    for post-stroke depression, 110–111
shaping technique, 15
  in CIAT, 20
short interval cortical inhibition (SICI), 62
SI. See primary somatosensory cortex
SICI. See short interval cortical inhibition
sigma-1 receptor (Sig-1R), 28
SII. See secondary somatosensory cortex
skills acquisition, after stroke, 14–17
  active-problem solving, 16
    guided discovery, 16
    strategies, 16
  chaining technique, 15
  direct teaching, 16
  explicit, 15–16
  fading, 15
  feedback for, 16, 18
  goal-driven, 15–16
  goals of, 14–15
  modeling, 15–16
  practice opportunities for, 16–17
  prompting, 15
  Rehab-Learn model, 18
  reinforcement for, 16
  response measurement for, 20
    for daily life functions, 20
    performance outcomes, 20
  shaping technique, 15
    in CIAT, 20
  task-specific, 15–16
  verbal guidance, 16
somatosensations, 157
somatosensory system, 157–161
  central processing, 158–161
    bottom-up influences, 160–161
    cerebellum, 159
    complexity of, 159
    graded progression in, 165
    insula, 159
    interhemispheric connections, 160, 161
    key features, 160–161

model of, 159–160
parallel, 160
PPC, 159
processing-related networks, 168
sensory maps, 160
serial, 160
SI, 24, 117, 158–159
SII, 159
thalamus, 159
top-down influences, 160–161
cross-modal neuroplasticity, 164
function, 157
interhemispheric connections, 160
after stroke, disruption of, 161
loss, after stroke, 157–158
activities of daily living and, 158
brain activation impairment, 161
deliberate anticipation in, 164
environmental impact of, 158
hypersensitivity, 158
impairment of discriminative
sensibility, 158
interhemispheric connection disruption, 161
network structural changes, 162
neural correlates for recovery,
161–162
neuropathic pain with, 158
prevalence, 157
resting-state functional connectivity
studies for, 161–162
symptoms, 158
purpose of, 157
rehabilitation for, 5
attended stimulation of specific
sites, 166
bombardment rehabilitation, 166
core sensory network identification
in, 168
cortical network manipulation, 168
deliberate anticipation in, 164
goal-directed attentive processing,
163–164
graded exercises with feedback, 166
graded progression in, 165
individual targeting in, 168
lesion impact and, 168
modality calibrations, 164–165
neuroscience-based models, 168,
246
passive stimulation, 166
processing-related networks, 168
sensorimotor exercises, 166
sensory discrimination approach,
166–167
stimulus specific training, 165, 167
task discrimination in, 164
with transfer enhanced programs,
165, 167
treatment principles, 162–165
sensory perception, 157
SI, 24, 158–159
during task-specific training, 117
SII, 159
somatosensations, 157
spared islands of tissue concept, for visual
recovery, 182
spinal cord injury, neuroplasticity after
contralesional hemisphere, 25, 26
cortical map rearrangements, 24–25
corticospinal remodeling, 25–26
SI, 24
spontaneous recovery, 24
SSRIs. See selective serotonin reuptake
inhibitors
stem cell therapy, 136–137

hNT, 136–137
neuroplasticity after, 30
in animal models, 30
neurogenesis, 30
for stroke rehabilitation, 82–83
stimulus specific training, 167
strategy learning and awareness approach,
for executive function rehabilitation, 218
striate cortex pathway, 177
stroke. See also depression, post-stroke;
rehabilitation, post-stroke; skills
acquisition, after stroke
attention deficits from, 190
depression and, 190–191, 197
brain infarcts
in Type I strokes, 77, 78
in Type II strokes, 77, 78
in Type III strokes, 77, 78
in Type IV strokes, 77, 78
animal models for, 81
functional consequences of, 78–79
interhemispheric connectivity alterations, 78–79
intracortical excitability, 78
lesions from, 78
after thrombolysis, 76, 77
cognitive impairments, 190–191
collateral occlusions, 76
general considerations after, 75
goal-driven skills after, 15–16
hypoglycaemia and, 191
hypoxia and, 191
incidence rates for, 4
with disability, 4
ischemic causes, 75–76
MCA, 179–180
pathophysiology, 75–79
of Type I strokes, 77, 78
of Type II strokes, 77, 78
of Type III strokes, 77, 78
of Type IV strokes, 77, 78
penumbra in, 75–76
primary effects, 76
secondary effects, 76
PCA, 179–180
prevalence rates, 190, 208–209
quality of life after, 4
somatosensory system loss after,
157–158
activities of daily living and, 158
brain activation impairment, 161
environmental impact of, 158
hypersensitivity, 158
impairment of discriminative
sensibility, 158
interhemispheric connection disruption, 161
network structural changes, 162
neural correlates for recovery,
161–162
neuropathic pain with, 158
prevalence, 157
resting-state functional connectivity
studies for, 161–162
symptoms, 158
symptoms, 75
thrombolysis, 76
brain infarcts after, 76, 77
visual syndromes after, 178–180
disorders of higher cognition, 180
hemianopic field defects, 179–180
homonymous visual deficits,
179–180
lateral geniculate nucleus lesions, 179
from MCA strokes, 179–180

monocular deficits, 179
from PCA strokes, 179–180
quandrantanopic field defects, 179
visual field deficits, 179
stroke care pathways model, 95–96
Stroke Quality Assessment Tool, 99
Stroke Rehab Definitions Conceptual
Framework, 5
stroke rehabilitation. See rehabilitation,
post-stroke
stroke units
comprehensive, 94
mixed rehabilitation, 94
rehabilitation, 94
Study of the Effectiveness of
Neurorehabilitation on Sensation
(SENSe) approach, 19–20
calibration in, 19
principles, 19–20
in transfer enhanced training, 167
substitution, 5
supernumerary synapses, 31

T
task-oriented motor training, 12
task-specific skills acquisition, after
stroke, 15–16
CO-OP, 19
neuroplasticity and, 26
task-specific training, 13
behavioural evidence, 119–120
stroke guidelines, 119
studies for, 119–120
biomechanics of, 120
brain region activation through,
116–117
with active movements, 117
MEPs during, 116
with passive movements, 117
SI activation, 117
definition of, 116
implementation of, 120
motor learning, 118–119
repetition intensity, 119
RTT, 143–145
behavioural effects, 143
for lower limb function, 144
neural mechanisms, 143–145
neuroplasticity after, 144–145
technical processes, 143
for upper limb function, 144
sensorimotor performance, 117–118
object size, 118
task intention, 118
timing adjustments, 118
task complexity, 119
TBI. See traumatic brain injury
TBS. See theta burst stimulation
tDCS. See transcranial direct current
stimulation
TEA. See Test of Everyday Attention
Telehealth, 95
in Canada, 97
temporoparietal junction (TPJ),
194–195
TES. See transcranial electrical
stimulation
Test of Everyday Attention (TEA), 215
thalamus, in somatosensory system, 159
theta burst stimulation (TBS), 132–133
iTBS, 132–133
thrombolysis, 76
brain infarcts after, 76, 77
TMS. See transcranial magnetic
stimulation

tonic inhibition reduction, as therapy
strategy, 30
TPJ. See temporoparietal junction
tractography, 47–49
FACT algorithm, 48
FOD, 48
Trail Making Test, 215
transcranial direct current stimulation
(tDCS), 27–28, 133, 134–135
anodal, 135–135
cathodal, 135
cost benefits of, 134
long-term effects of, 135
for post-stroke depression, 111–112
transcranial electrical stimulation
(TES), 60
transcranial magnetic stimulation
(TMS), 60–66, 132–133
EEG/MEG methodology, 58
language processes, 223
MEP, 60–62
amplitude, 60–61
central motor conduction time,
61–62
latency, 61–62
multimodal studies, for stroke
recovery, 64, 64–65
during task-specific training, 116
methodology, 60
current values, 60
motor cortex measurement, 60–62
AMT, 60
cortical silent period, 62
ICF, 62
IHI, 62
input-output curves, 62
motor thresholds, 60
SICI, 62
multimodal studies, for stroke recovery, 64–66
with BOLD fMRI, 64, 65
MEP, 64–65
for perilesional tissue, 80
pulse application, 132
resolution, 54
rTMS, 62–64
low frequency, 63–64
for post-stroke depression, 111
TBS, 132–133
iTBS, 132–133
TES compared to, 60
transfer enhanced training, 165, 167
SENSe approach in, 167
transfer of training phenomena, in motor
learning, 121–123
for CNS, 123
GMP, 123
neuroimaging results, 123
variability of practice, 122
traumatic brain injury (TBI), 200
Treatment of Underlying Forms (TUF),
226
Type I strokes, 77, 78
Type II strokes, 77, 78
Type III strokes, 77, 78
Type IV strokes, 77, 78

U
UK. See United Kingdom
unilateral spatial neglect, 198,
243–244
United Kingdom (UK), health care
services in
auditing, 97
Australia compared to, 100
community-based, 97

United States (U.S.), quality of health care in, 99
use-dependent neuroplasticity, 6, 13
  LTD, 13
  LTP, 13
  in stroke rehabilitation, 6

V

VAN. *See* ventral attention network
vascular endothelial growth factor (VEGF), 30
VBM. *See* voxel-based morphometry
VEGF. *See* vascular endothelial growth factor
ventral attention network (VAN), 193
ventral extrastriate cortex, 177–178
  PPA evidence, 178
verbal guidance, 16
virtual reality (VR) therapy, 151–153
  behavioural effects, 152
  with finger tracking training tasks, 152–153
  for motor learning, 152
  neural mechanisms, 152–153
  for neuroplasticity, 27
  technical processes, 151–152
vision
  anatomy of, for visual pathways, 173–176
    geniculostriate pathway, 175
  attention and, 192–194
    DAN in, 192–193
    LIP cortex in, 193
    for new learning, 193–194

supramodal function in, 194
  VAN in, 193
blindsight, 180
  MRI studies, 183–184
  retinotopic mapping for, 183
  Riddoch syndrome, 183
colour perception, 178
extrageniculostriate pathway, 175–176
  components, 175–176
  efferents, 176
extrastriate cortex pathway, 177
  akinetopsia, 178
  movement perception, 178
  visual object recognition, 177–178
  visual recovery rehabilitation, 181–182
fovea-macular projection, 174
geniculostriate pathway, 175
  arterial support, 175
  primary visual cortex, 175
  topographical structure, 175
goal direction action and, 191
information processing, 173–174
ipsilateral representation for, 176–177
  in animal models, 176
  in humans, 176–177
motion perception, 178
rehabilitation, after stroke, 180–182
  acute phase of, 180
  chronic phase of, 180
  extrastriate pathway, 181–182
  hypotheses for, 182–184
  kinetic stimuli in, 184–185

mechanisms, 180–181
MRI studies, 183–184
neuroplasticity, 180, 181–182
oedema resolution, 180
PET studies, 182–183
prevalence rates, 180–181
restorative therapies, 184–185
spared islands of tissue concept, 182
VRT, 185
retinogeniculate pathway, 173–175
  LGN, 174–175, 179
striate cortex pathway, 177
stroke-induced syndromes, 178–180
  disorders of higher cognition, 180
  hemianopic field defects, 179–180
  homonymous visual deficits, 179–180
  lateral geniculate nucleus lesions, 179
  from MCA strokes, 179–180
  monocular deficits, 179
  from PCA strokes, 179–180
  quandrantanopic field defects, 179
  visual field deficits, 179
ventral extrastriate cortex, 177–178
  PPA evidence, 178
vision restoration therapy (VRT), 185
visuomotor tracking training, 151–153
voxel-based morphometry (VBM), 39
VRT. *See* vision restoration therapy
VR therapy. *See* virtual reality therapy

W

WAIS-IV. *See* Weschler Adult Intelligence Scale-IV
WCST. *See* Wisconsin Card Sorting Test
Wernicke, Carl, 222
Wernicke's area, 224
Weschler Adult Intelligence Scale-IV (WAIS-IV), 215
"what" pathway, for attention, 192
"where" pathway, for attention, 192
white matter, in brain
  DTI in, 45–46
  DWI in, 44–45
  neuroimaging of, 223–224
  tractography, 47–49
  WMH, with post-stroke depression, 110
white matter hyperintensity (WMH), 110
WHO. *See* World Health Organisation
whole body approach, 245
Wisconsin Card Sorting Test (WCST), 215
WM. *See* white matter
WMH. *See* white matter hyperintensity
working memory
  attention and, 195–196
    selective, 195–196
  subtypes, 195
World Health Organisation (WHO)
  depression ranking for, as cause of burden, 106
  rehabilitation definition under, 5